OXFORD MEDICAL PUBLICATIONS

Oxford Handbook of Primary Care and Community Nursing

T0177471

Published and forthcoming Oxford Handbooks in Nursing

Oxford Handbook of Adult Nursing, 2e

Oxford Handbook of Cancer Nursing, 2e

Oxford Handbook of Cardiac Nursing, 2e

Oxford Handbook of Children's and Young People's Nursing, 2e

Oxford Handbook of Clinical Skills for Children's and Young People's Nursing

Oxford Handbook of Clinical Skills in Adult Nursing

Oxford Handbook of Critical Care Nursing, 2e

Oxford Handbook of Dental Nursing

Oxford Handbook of Diabetes Nursing

Oxford Handbook of Gastrointestinal Nursing

Oxford Handbook of Learning and Intellectual Disability Nursing, 2e

Oxford Handbook of Mental Health Nursing, 2e

Oxford Handbook of Midwifery, 3e

Oxford Handbook of Musculoskeletal Nursing, 2e

Oxford Handbook of Neuroscience Nursing

Oxford Handbook of Nursing Older People, 2e

Oxford Handbook of Orthopaedic and Trauma Nursing

Oxford Handbook of Perioperative Practice

Oxford Handbook of Prescribing for Nurses and Allied Health Professionals, 2e

Oxford Handbook of Primary Care and Community Nursing, 3e

Oxford Handbook of Renal Nursing

Oxford Handbook of Respiratory Nursing, 2e

Oxford Handbook of Surgical Nursing

Oxford Handbook of Women's Health Nursing, 2e

OXFORD HANDBOOK OF

Primary Care and Community Nursing

THIRD EDITION

EDITED BY

Judy Brook
Senior Lecturer, School of Health Sciences, City, University of London, UK

Caroline McGraw
Lecturer, Division of Health Services Research and Management, School of Health Sciences, City, University of London, UK

Val Thurtle
Educator, King's Centre for Global Health and Health Partnerships, King's College London, UK

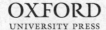

OXFORD
UNIVERSITY PRESS

OXFORD

UNIVERSITY PRESS

Great Clarendon Street, Oxford, OX2 6DP,
United Kingdom

Oxford University Press is a department of the University of Oxford.
It furthers the University's objective of excellence in research, scholarship,
and education by publishing worldwide. Oxford is a registered trade mark of
Oxford University Press in the UK and certain other countries.

© Oxford University Press 2021

The moral rights of the authors have been asserted

First edition published 2007
Second edition published 2014
Third edition published 2021

Impression: 2

Published in the United States of America by Oxford University Press
198 Madison Avenue, New York, NY 10016, United States of America

British Library Cataloguing in Publication Data
Data available

Library of Congress Control Number: 2013945066

ISBN 978–0–19–883182–2

Printed and bound by
Ashford Colour Press Ltd.

Preface

Primary care and community nurses carry out vital work to support the health of individuals and communities. Unlike nurses working in secondary care settings, primary care and community nurses may work alone or in small teams, in a variety of settings such as people's homes, community buildings, GP surgeries, or community hospitals. These nurses include practice nurses, health visitors, school nurses, district nurses, community children's nurses, occupational health nurses, community sexual health nurses, and specialist and advanced nurse practitioners. In their different roles, they address a wide variety of health issues ranging from the public health needs of specific community groups to the individual needs of patients with long-term conditions requiring them to take both preventative and reactive approaches to health and illness across the life course.

This handbook offers a valuable resource for nurses that cuts across traditional community roles and settings. In a landscape of changing health policy, funding, and service configuration, the comprehensive content of the handbook offers primary care and community nurses access to evidence-based information to support them in everyday clinical decision making. The fourteen chapters cover a broad range of conditions, including preventative care and treatment techniques, and offer information about the organizational structures that nurses are required to navigate when working in the community. It is written by primary care and community nurses who are specialists in their area of current practice, education, and policy development. One of the strengths of the handbook are the numerous references to sources of further information, ensuring that the content is embedded in a contemporary context and that accurate broader information can easily be accessed.

The handbook is particularly useful to nurses new to community working, but this revised and updated third edition will be a trusted reference source for any nurse working in a community role or setting.

Judy Brook, Caroline McGraw, and Val Thurtle

Acknowledgements

This third edition of the handbook builds on two previous editions. Our thanks go to the editors of the previous editions, Professor Vari Drennan MBE from the Centre for Health and Social Care Research at Kingston University London, St George's, and Professor Claire Goodman from the Centre for Research in Public Health and Community Care at the University of Hertfordshire. We would also like to thank all current and previous contributors to the handbook.

Acknowledgements

Contents

Contributors *xi*

Symbols and abbreviations *xiii*

1	The context of healthcare	1
2	Nursing in primary care	35
3	Quality and safety	67
4	Approaches to individual health needs assessment	109
5	Medicines management and nurse prescribing	127
6	Child health promotion	151
7	Child and adolescent health	257
8	Adult health promotion	333
9	Service users with extra needs	443
10	Adult care provision	503
11	Care of adults with long-term conditions	597
12	Adult health problems	677
13	First aid and emergencies	791
14	Useful information	831

Index *845*

Contents

Contributors
Symbols and abbreviations xiv

1 The context of healthcare
2 Nursing in primary care
3 Clarks and ethics
4 Approaches to individual health needs assessments
5 Medicine management and nurse prescribing
6 Child health promotion
7 Child and adolescent health
8 Adult health promotion
9 Service users with extra needs
10 Acute care provision
11 Care of adults with long-term conditions
12 Acute health problems
13 First aid and emergencies
14 Communication

Index 845

Contributors

Helen Bedford
Professor of Children's Health,
Great Ormond Street Institute of
Child Health, University College
London, UK

Louise Boole
Senior Lecturer, Department of
Health Care Practice, University of
Derby, UK

Sarah Bradley
Higher Trainee, Central and North
West London NHS Foundation
Trust, Mortimer Market Centre,
London, UK

Emily Chung
Locum Consultant, Central
and North West London NHS
Foundation Trust, Mortimer Market
Centre, London, UK

David Elliman
Consultant, Great Ormond Street
Hospital, London, UK and Hon.
Consultant in Community Child
Health, Whittington Health, and
Central and North West London
NHS Foundation Trust, London, UK

Francesca Entwistle
Professional Officer, Policy
and Advocacy, UNICEF UK,
London, UK

Lynda Filer
Lecturer, School of Health Sciences,
City, University of London, UK

Helen Hamilton
Midwife, Royal Surrey County
Hospital, Guildford, UK

Mary Harris
Macmillan Centre Manager,
Queen Alexandra Hospital,
Portsmouth, UK

Siobhan Hicks
Lecturer, School of Health Sciences,
City, University of London, UK

Pam Hodge
Lecturer, School of Health and
Education, Middlesex University,
London, UK

Ria Hunt
Advanced Nurse Practitioner,
Ravenswood Medical Practice,
Ipswich, UK

Nyree Kendall
Community Specialist Practice
District Nurse Lead, School of
Nursing and Midwifery, University
of Bolton, UK

Ashley Luchmun
Senior Teaching Fellow, Florence
Nightingale Faculty of Nursing,
King's College London, UK

Shereen Miller
Health Visitor, Tower Hamlets Care
Group, London, UK

Kat Millward
Lecturer, School of Health Sciences,
City, University of London, UK

Sophie Molloy
Lecturer, School of Health and
Education, Middlesex University,
London, UK

Phil Richardson
Independent Occupational Health Advisor, Ruislip, UK

Angela Robinson
Consultant in Sexual Health, Central and North West London NHS Foundation Trust, Mortimer Market Centre, London, UK

Melanie Rogers
Course Leader, School of Human and Health Sciences, University of Huddersfield, UK

Lorna Saunder
Senior Lecturer, School of Health Sciences, City, University of London, UK

Alison Schofield
Tissue Viability Service Lead and Clinical Nurse Specialist, North Lincolnshire and Goole NHS Foundation Trust, Scunthorpe, UK

Ellie Taylor
Deputy Designated Nurse Safeguarding Children, Cambridge and Peterborough Clinical Commissioning Group, Cambridge, UK

Jeremy Woods
Learning Disabilities Co-ordinator, Central and North West London NHS Foundation Trust, Archway Centre, London, UK

Jane Wright
Independent Nurse Consultant Specialist Public Health Nursing (School Nursing) High Wycombe, Buckinghamshire, UK

Symbols and abbreviations

↑	increased	BCG	Bacillus–Calmette–Guerin
↓	decreased	BG(L)	blood glucose (level)
→	leading to	BLF	British Lung Foundation
>	greater than	BLS	basic life support
<	less than	BMA	British Medical Association
≥	equal to or greater than	BMI	body mass index
≤	equal to or less than	BNF	British National Formulary
♂	male	BP	blood pressure
♀	female	BPE	benign prostate enlargement
°	degrees	BPH	benign prostatic hyperplasia
°C	degrees centigrade	BS	British Standards
°F	degrees Fahrenheit	BSA	Business Services Authority
1°	primary	BSL	British Sign Language
2°	secondary	CAMHS	Child and Adolescent Mental Health Service
⚠	warning		
➽	topic cross reference	CBT	cognitive behavioural therapy
℘	website	CCG	clinical commissioning group
A&E	accident and emergency	CD	controlled drug
AAA	abdominal aortic aneurysm	CDD	conduct disorder
ABPI	ankle-brachial pressure index	CE	Conformité Européenne
ABPM	ambulatory blood pressure monitoring	CF	cystic fibrosis
		CH	care home
ACE	angiotensin-converting enzyme	CHC	combined hormonal contraceptive
AD	autonomic dysreflexia		
ADHD	attention-deficit hyperactivity disorder	CHD	coronary heart disease
		CIN	cervical intraepithelial neoplasia
ADL	activities of daily living		
AED	automated external defibrillation	CKD	chronic kidney disease
		CMP	clinical management plan
AED	antiepileptic drug	CMSA	Case Management Society of America
AF	atrial fibrillation		
AHP	allied healthcare professional	CMV	cytomegalovirus
AM	antimicrobial	CNS	central nervous system
ANP	advanced nurse practitioner	CO	cardiac output
AO	accountable officer	COC	combined oral contraceptive
AR	anaphylactic reaction	COPD	chronic obstructive pulmonary disease
ART	antiretroviral therapy		
ASD	autistic spectrum disorder	COSHH	control of substances hazardous to health
AT	assistive technology		
AUDIT	Alcohol Use Disorders Identification Test	CP	cerebral palsy
		CPD	continuing professional development
AV	atrioventricular		
BCC	basal cell carcinoma	CPT	cardiopulmonary resuscitation
		CQC	Care Quality Commission

CrD	Crohn's disease
CT	computerized tomography
CVA	cardiovascular accident
CVD	cardiovascular disease
CYP	children and young people
D2A	discharge to access
DbHL	decibel hearing loss
DBS	Disclosure and Barring Service
DDH	development dysplasia of the hips
DHSC	Department of Health and Social Care
DI	donor insemination
DKA	diabetic ketoacidosis
DM	diabetes mellitus
DMARD	disease-modifying anti-rheumatic drug
DN	district nurse
DU	duodenal ulceration
DV	domestic violence
DVLA	Driver and Vehicle Licensing Agency
DVT	deep vein thrombosis
EC	emergency contraception
ECG	electrocardiogram
EDD	expected delivery date
EEA	European Economic Area
EEG	electroencephalogram
EHC	education and health care
EHO	environmental health officer
EIS	early intervention service
ENT	ear, nose, and throat
ESR	erythrocyte sedimentation rate
FBC	full blood count
FFT	Friends and Family Test
FGM	female genital mutilation
FH	family history
FIS	Family Information Service
FIT	faecal immunochemical test
FSH	follicle-stimulating hormone
FT	foundation trust
FTE	full-time equivalent
g	gram
GANTT	Generalized Activity Normalization Time Table
GDPR	General Data Protection Regulations
GI	gastrointestinal
GMC	General Medical Council
GMS	General Medical Service
GORD	gastro-oesophageal reflux disease
GP	general practitioner
GSF	gold standard framework
HAART	highly active antiretroviral therapy
Hb	haemoglobin
HbA1c	glycated haemoglobin
HBPM	home blood pressure monitoring
HCA	healthcare assistant
HCP	Healthy Child Programme
HF	heart failure
HIV	human immunodeficiency virus
HNA	health needs assessment
HPA	Health Protection Agency
HPV	human papilloma virus
HR	heart rate
hr	hour
HRT	hormone replacement therapy
HSC	health and social care
HSCB	Health and Social Care Board (NI)
HSE	Health and Safety Executive
HV	health visitor/visiting
IBD	inflammatory bowel disease
IBS	irritable bowel syndrome
ICSI	intracytoplasmic sperm injection
ID	identity
IM	intramuscular
INR	international normalized ratio
IRAS	Integrated Research Application System
IUD	intrauterine device
IUS	intrauterine system
IV	intravenous
IVF	*in vitro* fertilization
JHWS	Joint Health and Wellbeing Strategy
JIA	juvenile idiopathic arthritis
JSNA	joint strategic needs assessment
kcal	kilocalorie
kg	kilogram
khz	kilohertz
L	litre
LA	local authority
LBC	liquid-based cytology

LD	learning disability		NTSP	National Tracheostomy Safety Project
LFT	liver function test		O_2	oxygen
LH	luteinizing hormone		OA	osteoarthritis
LPA	lasting power of attorney		ODD	oppositional defiant disorder
LSCB	local safeguarding children board		OFSTED	Office for Standards in Education
LTC	long-term condition		ONS	Office for National Statistics
LTOT	long-term oxygen therapy		OTC	over the counter
MCA	Mental Capacity Act		PCP	personalized care plan
mcg	microgram		PD	Parkinson's disease
MDA	Misuse of Drugs Act		PDP	personal development plan
MDR	Misuse of Drugs Regulations		PE	pulmonary embolism
MDT	multidisciplinary team		PEFR	peak exploratory flow rate
mg	milligram		PEG	percutaneous endoscopic gastrostomy
MHRA	Medical and Healthcare Products Regulatory Agency		PEP	post-exposure prophylaxis
MI	myocardial infarction		PET	positron emission tomography
min	minute		PGD	patient group direction
MJ	megajoule		PHE	Public Health England
ml	millilitre		PID	pelvic inflammatory disease
MLD	manual lymphatic drainage		PKU	phenylketonuria
MM	malignant melanoma		PMS	Personal Medical Service
MMR	measles, mumps, and rubella		PMS	premenstrual syndrome
MND	motor neurone disease		PPE	personal protective equipment
MRI	magnetic resonance imaging		PRN	as needed (pro re nata)
MRSA	methicillin-resistant staphylococcus aureus		PSA	prostate-specific antigen
MS	multiple sclerosis		PSD	patient-specific direction
MSCC	metastatic spinal cord compression		PSHE	Personal, Social, and Health Education
MSK	musculoskeletal		PTSD	post-traumatic stress disorder
mth	month		PU	pressure ulcer
MUST	Malnutrition Universal Screening Tool		QNI	Queen's Nursing Institute
NCMP	National Child Measurement Programme		QoF	Quality and Outcomes Framework
NHS	National Health Service		RA	rheumatoid arthritis
NI	Northern Ireland		RCGP	Royal College of General Practice
NICE	National Institute for Health and Care Excellence		RCN	Royal College of Nursing
			RCT	randomized controlled trial
NIHR	National Institute for Health Research		RIG	radiologically inserted gastrostomy
NMC	Nursing and Midwifery Council		RPS	Royal Pharmaceutical Society
NMSC	non-melanoma skin cancer		RTA	road traffic accident
NPFS	National Pandemic Flu Service		SALT	speech and language therapy
NRT	nicotine replacement therapy		SARC	sexual assault referral centre
NSAID	non-steroidal anti-inflammatory drug		SC	subcutaneous
			SCC	squamous cell carcinoma
NSPCC	National Society for the Prevention of Cruelty to Children		SCD	sickle cell disease
			SCI	spinal cord injury

SCJ	squamocolumnar junction	TIA	transient ischaemic attack
sec	second	TM	trade mark
SEN	special educational needs	TOP	termination of pregnancy
SENDCO	Special Educational Needs and Disability Co-ordinator	TSE	testicular self-examination
		TSH	thyroid-stimulating hormone
SH	sexual health	tsp	teaspoon
SIDS	sudden infant death syndrome	UC	ulcerative colitis
SIGN	Scottish Intercollegiate Guidelines Network	UK	United Kingdom
		UN	United Nations
SL	sublingually	UPSI	unprotected sexual intercourse
SMP	statutory maternity pay	URTI	upper respiratory tract infection
SN	school nurse		
SOB	shortness of breath	USS	ultrasound scan
SOP	standard operating procedure	UTI	urinary tract infection
SPQ	Specialist Practice Qualification	UV	ultraviolet
SRE	Sex and Relationship Education	VAT	value added tax
STI	sexually transmitted infection	WHO	World Health Organization
SVC	superior vena cava	wk	week
TB	tuberculosis	yr	year
TFT	thyroid function test		

The context of healthcare

UK health profile 2
Key definitions of primary care and public health 4
Generic long-term conditions model 6
The National Health Service (NHS) 8
NHS entitlements 10
Commissioning of services 12
Public health in the NHS and beyond 14
Health needs assessment 15
Overview of services in primary care 16
General practice 18
Other primary healthcare services 20
Services to prevent unplanned hospital admission 22
Services to promote hospital discharge 23
Services for children, young people, and families 24
Homes and housing 26
Environmental health services 27
Social support 28
Social services 30
Care homes 32

UK health profile

The UK population was 66.4 million in 2018.[1] There were 607,172 deaths registered in the UK in 2017.[2] The majority of deaths occur in those aged >65yrs. The leading causes are: coronary heart disease (CHD), stroke, dementia, cancers, and respiratory diseases.[1–3] Leading causes of death vary with age and sex. For example, in terms of age: congenital abnormalities in 1–4yrs; brain cancer, acute respiratory disease, leukaemia, and lymphomas in 0–20yrs; CHD, stroke, and respiratory disease >50yrs; CHD, stroke, respiratory disease, and dementia >80yrs.

Health inequalities

Health is determined by a complex interaction between individual characteristics, lifestyle, and the physical, social, and economic environment. People are likely to suffer worse health than the rest of the population if they experience material disadvantage, lower educational attainment, and/or insecure employment.[4] Life expectancy at birth in the UK did not improve between 2015 and 2017, and remained 79.2yrs for ♂ and 82.9yrs for ♀[5] Infant mortality was 3.9 per 1,000 live births in England and Wales in 2018.[2] However, there is considerable variation by area and socioeconomic status, with higher rates in babies with fathers in manual occupations or where only the mother registered the baby. Highest rates are found for teenage mothers and lowest where the mother is 30–34yrs.

References

1. ONS (2019) *United Kingdom population mid-year estimate.* Available at: ℘ https://www.ons.gov.uk/peoplepopulationandcommunity/populationandmigration/populationestimates/timeseries/ukpop/pop
2. ONS (2018) *Vital statistics in the UK: births, deaths and marriages (2018 update).* Available at:℘ https://www.ons.gov.uk/peoplepopulationandcommunity/populationandmigration/populationestimates/datasets/vitalstatisticspopulationandhealthreferencetables
3. PHE (2018) *Trends in morbidity.* Available at: ℘ https://www.gov.uk/government/publications/health-profile-for-england-2018/chapter-2-trends-in-mortality
4. Marmot, M., Goldblatt, P., Allen, J., et al. (2010) *Fair society, healthy lives.* Available at: ℘ http://www.instituteofhealthequity.org/resources-reports/fair-society-healthy-lives-the-marmot-review
5. ONS (2018) *National life tables, UK: 2015–2017.* Available at: ℘ https://www.ons.gov.uk/peoplepopulationandcommunity/birthsdeathsandmarriages/lifeexpectancies/bulletins/nationallifetablesunitedkingdom/2015to2017

Further information

Public health profiles (PHE). Available at: ℘ https://fingertips.phe.org.uk/

Key definitions of primary care and public health

Primary care

The Declaration of Alma-Ata[6] stated that 1° care is the first level of contact that individuals, families, and communities have with a national health system, bringing healthcare as close as possible to where people live and work. More recently, the World Health Organization (WHO) reaffirmed the importance of 1° care to achieve universal health coverage and the sustainable development goals.[7] The WHO vision is summarized in Box 1.1.

> ### Box 1.1 **WHO vision for primary care**
>
> - Governments and societies that prioritize, promote, and protect people's health and well-being, at both population and individual levels, through strong health systems.
> - 1° healthcare and health services that are high-quality, safe, comprehensive, integrated, accessible, available, and affordable for everyone and everywhere, provided with compassion, respect, and dignity by professionals who are well-trained, skilled, motivated, and committed.
> - Enabling and health-conducive environments in which individuals and communities are empowered and engaged in maintaining and enhancing their health and well-being.
> - Partners and stakeholders aligned in providing effective support to national health policies, strategies, and plans.

1° care is made up of three main areas: empowered people and communities; multisectoral policy and action; and essential public health functions as the core of integrated health services.[8] This includes a range of services from prevention (i.e. vaccinations) to management of long-term conditions (LTCs) and palliative care. With 1° care concerned with proactive care, prevention, and health promotion, as well as treatment at a community level, there is much overlap with public health.

Public health

The purpose of public health is to create conditions so that people can be healthy, looking at the wider determinants of health. It is the science and art of preventing disease, prolonging life, and promoting physical and mental health through the organized efforts of society. It has a collective rather than an individual view of the health needs and healthcare of a population. The aim of public health bodies is to achieve this purpose by the: promotion of a safe environment; control of community infections; health promotion; organization of medical and nursing services for early identification and treatment of ill health and disease; and health protection. The underpinning values of public health are: equity and social inclusion; participation, collaboration, and community empowerment; and social justice, where health is a basic human right.

Related topics

➜ Overview of services in primary care p. 16; ➜ Health needs assessment p. 15; ➜ Public health in the NHS and beyond p. 14; ➜ UK health profile p. 2; ➜ Community approaches to health p. 338; ➜ The National Health Service (NHS) p. 8

References

6. Declaration of Alma-Ata. *International Conference on Primary Health Care, Alma-Ata (1978)*. Available at: http://www.who.int/publications/almaata_declaration_en.pdf

7. WHO (2018) *Declaration of Astana. Global Conference on Primary Health Care (2018)*. Available at: https://www.who.int/docs/default-source/primary-health/declaration/gcphc-declaration. pdf

8. WHO (2018) *What is primary care?* Available at: https://www.who.int/primary-health/en/

Generic long-term conditions model

This model (derived from the Kaiser Permanente model in the USA) shows how a population with LTCs can be stratified according to need. Case management (◆ Case management p. 114) is indicated at Levels 1 and 2.

Level 1: Support for self-care

Collaboratively helping patients and their carers (◆ Carers p. 458) to develop the knowledge, skills, and confidence to care for themselves and their condition effectively.

Level 2: Disease-specific case management (high risk)

Involves providing patients who have complex single needs or multiple conditions with responsive, specialist services using multidisciplinary teams (◆ Teamwork p. 58) and disease-specific protocols and pathways, such as the National Service Frameworks and Quality and Outcomes Framework (QoF) (◆ Evidence-based healthcare p. 72; ◆ Quality and Outcomes Framework p. 74). At this level, the case manager is most likely to be a qualified nurse, a social worker, or allied healthcare professional (AHP).

Level 3: Case management (high complexity)

Requires identification of the ↑ intensity users of unplanned 2° care (◆ Services to prevent unplanned hospital admission p. 22). Care of these patients is to be managed by a community matron or other professional using a case management approach to anticipate, co-ordinate, and join up health and social care.

The National Health Service (NHS)

Established on 5 July 1948 to provide a comprehensive range of health services to all in need. It is free at the point of delivery and paid for through taxation. Some services also incur subsidized charges (e.g. NHS prescriptions in 1° care in England).

Decisions about health policy have been devolved to each of the four countries of the UK. Consequently, structures and policy priorities are different in each country. The Isle of Man and the Channel Islands have independent health service structures.

In each country, there is a senior government minister responsible for health and publicly funded health services. Within government agreed policies, the central NHS administration sets overall priorities and some specific targets. Local NHS bodies plan, commission (➲ Commissioning of services p. 12), and sometimes also manage and monitor services for the residents of a defined area (usually co-terminus with a local authority (LA)). Each country has its own arrangements for assessing the quality of healthcare (➲ Quality governance p. 68). The NHS is subject to periodic re-organization and the latest information is on the country-specific websites.

In all countries, general practice (➲ General practice p. 18) is part of the NHS, but provided through specific contracts, not directly managed by the administrative structures of the NHS.

England

The Department of Health and Social Care (DHSC) provides central direction to both commissioning bodies and service-providing organizations within the NHS. There is a published NHS Constitution stating principles, rights, and responsibilities.[9] NHS England provides the overall commissioning direction and, at the local area level, clinical commissioning groups (CCGs). Public Health Departments are part of LAs.

NHS services are provided by a range of different organizations: acute non-specializing trusts (including foundation trusts (FTs)); acute specializing trusts (including FTs); mental health trusts (including FTs); community providers (including NHS trusts, FTs, social enterprises, and limited companies); ambulance trusts; and independent-sector organizations (including for-profit and not-for profit organizations). The patient and public involvement voice is through Health Watch (➲ Patient and public experience p. 75).

Northern Ireland (NI)

The Department of Health has responsibilities for health and social care: hospitals; family practitioner services (➲ General practice p. 18); community health services; personal social services; and public health and public safety. The Health and Social Care Board (HSCB) is a statutory organization which arranges or commissions health and social care services for the population. It is supported by five local commissioning groups. Five Health and Social Care (HSC) Trusts provide integrated health and social care services across NI, managing and administering hospitals, health centres, residential homes (➲ Care homes p. 32), day centres, and other health and social care residential facilities. The sixth HSC Trust is the NI Ambulance Service. The Patient and Client Council provides the focus for the patient voice.

Scotland

NHS Scotland is the publicly funded healthcare system in Scotland. Provision is the responsibility of 14 geographically based local NHS boards and seven national special health boards (e.g. public health and health education, and NHS 24 which provides a 24-hr telephone advice line). Health boards and councils in Scotland are concerned with 1° care services, such as general practitioners (GPs) and pharmacies, as part of the working arrangements between the NHS boards and LAs which includes responsibility for social care. The Scottish Health Council provides the patient voice.

Wales

The Department for Health and Social Services advises the Welsh Government on policies and strategies for health and social care. This includes contributing to relevant legislation and providing funding for the NHS and other related bodies. The NHS delivers services through seven Health Boards and three NHS Trusts. The local Health Boards plan, secure, and deliver health services in their area. These are matched by seven Community Health Councils providing the patient and public voice.

Related topics

➔ Overview of services in primary care p. 16

Reference

9. NHS (2015) *NHS constitution for England*. Available at: ℘ https://www.gov.uk/government/publications/the-nhs-constitution for-england

Further information

Department of Health (NI). Available at: ℘ https://www.health-ni.gov.uk/
NHS Scotland. Available at: ℘ https://www.scot.nhs.uk/about-nhs-scotland/
NHS Wales. Available at: ℘ https://www.wales.nhs.uk/nhswalesaboutus

NHS entitlements

The NHS is paid for through taxation (→ The National Health Service p. 8). People living or working in the UK are entitled to free or subsidized treatment at the point of care.

People coming from overseas

Treatment is always free at the point of care for: accidents and emergency treatment; compulsory psychiatric treatment; certain communicable diseases (e.g. tuberculosis (TB) (→ Tuberculosis p. 728)); family planning; treatment of a physical or mental condition caused by torture, female genital mutilation (FGM) (→ Female genital mutilation p. 492), domestic violence (→ Domestic violence p. 450), or sexual violence; and services provided via NHS111.

Non-European Economic Area (EEA) nationals

Need to pay a health surcharge when applying for a visa to stay in the UK for >6mths, unless they are exempt. They can then use the NHS on a similar basis as an ordinarily resident person while their visa remains valid, although they still need to pay for some services including prescriptions and dental treatment. There are some exceptions including those seeking asylum or applying for humanitarian protection, those identified as victims of human trafficking, and others applying for indefinite leave to remain.

Hospital treatment

Free to people classed as ordinarily resident in the UK, which is those living in the UK on a lawful and properly settled basis for the time being. Non-EEA nationals who are subject to immigration control must have the immigration status of indefinite leave to remain at the time of treatment and be properly settled, to be considered 'ordinarily resident'.

Those from countries with reciprocal healthcare agreements and those from the EEA

Those visiting from a country which has a bilateral healthcare agreement with the UK are exempt from charges for some NHS hospital treatments. People from EEA member states and Switzerland are exempt from charges for all medically necessary treatment, including monitoring and treatment of LTCs. They must show a valid European Health Insurance Card to receive free care.

Further information

NHS Wales (*Overseas visitors*). Available at: ℘ http://www.wales.nhs.uk/nhswalesaboutus/budgetcharges/overseasvisitors

Scottish Government (*Overseas visitors*). Available at: ℘ https://www2.gov.scot/Topics/Health/Services/Overseas-visitors

Commissioning of services

Commissioning of services

The process of assessing needs, planning, and prioritizing, purchasing, and monitoring health services → the best health outcomes. Commissioning uses competition to improve services and gives patients ↑ choice in the care they receive. Commissioning works differently in the four countries of the UK (◆ The National Health Service (NHS) p. 8). In England, commissioning arrangements were formalized by the Health and Social Care Act 2012. Services are commissioned by CCGs and NHS England on a local, regional, and national basis. CCGs commission most hospital and community services with responsibility for ~60% of the NHS budget. Each CCG has an elected governing body including GPs, clinicians, general managers, and patient representatives. Healthwatch exists to ↑ the public and user voice (◆ Patient and public experience p. 75).

NHS England sets the overall commissioning strategy and clinical priorities for the NHS. It also directly commissions some specialized services (e.g. treatments for rare conditions and secure mental healthcare), military and veteran health services (◆ Armed forces veterans p. 502), and services for people in prison. Other bodies involved in commissioning include LAs, who are responsible for commissioning public health services (◆ Public health in the NHS and beyond p. 14) as well as social care (◆ Social services p. 30) and a range of services that contribute to health and well-being, such as leisure services.

In England, there is no set list of the treatments that are available through the NHS. The care available depends on a series of decisions made at different levels: government decides how much money to give the DHSC; the DHSC and NHS England decide the overarching priorities and allocate money to CCGs and/or LAs who make decisions in terms of planning and purchasing services from local providers; local providers decide how to allocate money within their organization; and clinicians decide what care is clinically appropriate for that patient.

Commissioning arrangements have evolved significantly over the last 5yrs and continue to do so. Going forward, there is a need for commissioners to work more closely together, aligning their objectives with providers and taking a more strategic, place-based approach to commissioning. This will involve sustainability and transformation partnerships, integrated care systems, devolution, and co-commissioning (Table 1.1).[10,11]

Table 1.1 Evolution of commissioning in England

Sustainability and transformation partnerships (STPs)	Where the NHS and LAs come together to run services in a more co-ordinated way, to agree system-wide priorities, and to plan collectively how to improve the health of residents
Integrated care systems	Evolved from STPs and involve NHS organizations, in partnership with LAs and others, taking collective responsibility for managing resources, delivering NHS standards, and improving the health of the local population
Devolution	CCGs, LAs, and other local bodies come together to take responsibility for the entire local health and care budget (e.g. Greater Manchester, Cornwall, and the Surrey Heartlands)
Primary care co-commissioning	Giving CCGs the opportunity to take on greater responsibility for general practice commissioning

Related topics

◒ General practice p. 18; ◒ Overview of services in primary care p. 16

References

10. NHS England (2019) *How commissioning is changing*. Available at: ℘ https://www.england.nhs.uk/commissioning/how-commissioning-is-changing/
11. The King's Fund (2017) *What is commissioning and how is it changing?* Available at: ℘ https://www.kingsfund.org.uk/publications/what-commissioning-and-how-it-changing

Public health in the NHS and beyond

Public health focuses on health, as well as disease, and populations not in-dividuals (➔ Key definitions of primary care and public health p. 4). There is a focus on three main domains: health protection, health improvement, and healthcare public health. Public health seeks to protect health and pre-vent illness by studying health patterns/trends, and planning to address health needs. It goes beyond the view of individual responsibility for health choices to considering the role of policy, regulatory, and commercial forces in shaping the environment that promotes and/or potentially harms health. Health impact assessment is a defining feature of this work. In the UK, many public health teams operate within the LA, while the NHS offers preventative services such as immunizations (➔ Childhood immunization schedule (UK) p. 166; ➔ Targeted adult immunization p. 392), screening for different forms of cancers or different forms of disease (➔ UK screening programmes p. 362), diabetes prevention (➔ Diabetes: overview p. 660), and work on prevention both through general practice (➔ General practice p. 18) and through hospitals and other services. There are national and local public health team responsibilities for public protection (e.g. investigation and management of communicable disease outbreaks (➔ Infectious disease notifications p. 104)). Each of the four countries has separate public health strategies that provide the overarching targets for health improvement.

Current public health practice

Uses complementary approaches alongside epidemiology and demography that emphasize: equity, fairness, and social justice; cross-cutting approaches (known as partnership intersectoral work); community participation in the development of services; and participation in health service commissioning decisions (➔ Health needs assessment p. 15; ➔ Community approaches to health p. 338).

Health impact assessment

Intended to help decision making by predicting the health consequences (good and bad) if a proposal is implemented, whether the consequences are the same or different for groups within the population (e.g. socioeconomic groups), recommending how to maximize or minimize the consequences. There are different types of impact assessments including equity impact as-sessment (➔ Anti-discriminatory healthcare p. 81) and environmental im-pact assessment.

Nurses, midwives, and health visitors

All nurses, midwives, and public health nurses (health visitors (➔ Health visiting p. 46), school nurses (➔ School nursing p. 42) and others) are ex-pected to contribute to public health. Nurses on the Nursing and Midwifery Council (NMC) public health register are required to contribute to and in-fluence policies affecting health.

Health needs assessment

A systematic method for reviewing the health issues facing a population, →
agreed priorities and resource allocation that will ↑ health and ↓ inequalities
(● UK health profile p. 2). Health needs assessment (HNA) is central to
public health (● Key definitions of primary care and public health p. 4; ●
Public health in the NHS and beyond p. 14) and to making decisions as to
where to apportion resources.

The starting point is a defined population; the HNA seeks to identify
the needs and priorities of the population or community (as well as the
health assets) and will usually be those that ↓ health inequalities. The out-
puts are recommendations and an action strategy from the evidence about
that population, and a choice of interventions.

In England, LAs and CCGs have equal and joint duties to prepare
Joint Strategic Needs Assessments (JSNAs) and Joint Health and Well-
being Strategies (JHWSs), through the Health and Well-being Boards
(● Commissioning of services p. 12). JSNAs are assessments of the current
and future health and social care needs of the local community. JHWSs are
strategies for meeting the needs identified in the JSNAs.

HNA techniques

Statistical data, such as mortality rates, use of services, age of population,
and incidence and prevalence of disease/accidents are collated and ana-
lysed. These are plotted using geographical health information systems,
which can inform needs assessment at a macro level. The usefulness of statistical information is enhanced when combined with qualitative data, which
provides patient and public perspectives on a situation (e.g. why people do
not attend a clinic, how services might be developed, and the impact of
services on health).

Further information

Department of Health (*Statutory guidance on joint strategic needs assessments and joint health and
wellbeing strategies*). Available at: ℘ https://assets.publishing.service.gov.uk/government/up-
loads/system/uploads/attachment_data/file/277012/Statutory-Guidance-on-Joint-Strategic-
Needs-Assessments-and-Joint-Health-and-Wellbeing-Strategies-March-20131.pdf

Health Development Agency (*Health needs assessment: a Practical Guide*). Available at: ℘ https://
assets.publishing.service.gov.uk/government/uploads/system/uploads/attachment_data/
file/277012/Statutory-Guidance-on-Joint-Strategic-Needs-Assessments-and-Joint-Health-and-
Wellbeing-Strategies-March-20131.pdf

Overview of services in primary care

There are a wide range of NHS services available to the public, with some local variation. Different types of services have different relationships to the NHS: directly managed in NHS structures (e.g. foundation trusts); outside NHS management structures, but mainly only provide services under a nationally agreed contract to the NHS (e.g. GPs (◆ General practice p. 18)); independent of the NHS, but have a nationally agreed contract for NHS payment for particular activities (e.g. community pharmacists); or locally contracted by the NHS, via CCGs or NHS England, from not-for-profit and for-profit organizations.

Services in England are commissioned by CCGs, NHS England, or LAs (◆ Commissioning of services p. 12). CCGs are GP-led and, individually or together, they commission most mental health and community services. NHS England provides strategic oversight of the NHS and directly commissions services for 1° care including pharmacists and dentists, some public health services (e.g. screening programmes), as well as services for rare and complex conditions. LAs are responsible for commissioning publicly funded social care services. Since 2013, LAs have been also responsible for commissioning some public health services including health visitors (◆ Health visiting p. 46), school nurses (◆ School nursing p. 42), and sexual health services (◆ Sexual health: general issues p. 760).

In Scotland, healthcare is the responsibility of geographically based local NHS Boards and National Special Health Boards. Within NHS Wales, Local Health Boards are responsible for delivering all NHS services in Wales. In Northern Ireland, Health and Social Care Trusts are responsible for the delivery of 1°, 2°, and community healthcare and for providing integrated health and social care services (◆ The National Health Service (NHS) p. 8).

Core primary care health service elements

Available to all are: 24-hr NHS helplines (e.g. NHS 111); general or personal medical services and their out-of-hours services; dentistry, pharmacy, optometry; and community health services based in community clinics, health centres, and GP surgeries. These usually include: nursing in the home; public health nursing (e.g. health visiting and school nursing); sexual health and contraceptive services (◆ Contraception: general p. 400); podiatry; speech and language therapy; and physiotherapy. In addition, many 1° care organizations have: walk-in centres (assessment and treatment of minor injuries and health problems); multidisciplinary specialist teams (e.g. rapid response (◆ Services to prevent unplanned hospital admission p. 22) and palliative care); specialist nurses (e.g. incontinence (◆ Urinary incontinence p. 504); and community hospitals where admission and clinical management is typically provided by local GPs and 1° care nurses, often with consultant support.

General practice

General practice

In recent years, the number of GPs in England has ↓ along with the number of practices. There are now ~34,000 full-time equivalent GPs working in ~7,000 practices. Most are independent contractors and are not directly employed by the NHS. They work in general practices, which have a General Medical Service (GMS) contract negotiated nationally or a Personal Medical Service (PMS) contract negotiated locally.

GP specialty training includes placements in specialties such as: general medicine; elderly care medicine; paediatrics; obstetrics and gynaecology; psychiatry and old age; ear, nose, and throat; accident and emergency (A&E); dermatology; ophthalmology; palliative care; and 1yr as a GP registrar supervised by a GP trainer. During the 3-yr programme, doctors complete work-based assessments and prepare for membership of the Royal College of General Practice (RCGP). GPs with extended roles undertake tasks that are beyond the scope of GP training and RCGP membership, and which require additional training (e.g. skin surgery).

The GP contract

This is a contract between an individual practice and the NHS, either nationally or locally. It includes: global sum for essential services, some additional services, and adjustments for workload and costs incurred by features of the population served; QoF (❺ Quality and Outcomes Framework p. 74); and directed enhanced services (special services negotiated nationally, which practices can choose to provide or not). In addition, practices can bid for locally enhanced services to meet local healthcare needs (e.g. homeless people (❺ Homeless people p. 446)).

Essential services

These must be provided to all registered patients: day-to-day medical care, which includes management of minor and self-limiting illness, and referral to 2° and other services; non-specialist care of people who are terminally ill; and chronic disease management.

Additional services

The practice can opt out of these and receive less payment: cervical screening (❺ Cervical cancer screening p. 380); contraceptive services (❺ Contraception: general p. 400); vaccinations and immunizations, both childhood basic course, those >6yrs, missing the basic course and reinforcing doses (❺ Childhood immunization schedule UK p. 166); child health surveillance (❺ Overview of the Healthy Child Programme p. 154), excluding neonatal check; maternity services, excluding intrapartum care; and minor surgery procedures (e.g. curettage, cautery, and cryocautery).

Directed enhanced services

These are services that GP practices or primary care networks have to sign up for and which attract additional payment. Examples include: childhood immunizations for children <2yrs and pre-school boosters <5yrs (70% coverage to reach lower payment and 90% coverage to reach higher payment); influenza immunization for >65yrs and at-risk groups (❺ Targeted adult immunization p. 392); more complex minor surgery; reviews of medicines for people on long-term medication (➲ Principles of medication reviews p. 142); anticipatory care for patients with complex comorbidities (➲ Services to prevent unplanned hospital admission p. 22); and extended hours access.

Out of hours

Defined as from 8.30pm to 8.00am on weekdays, the whole of weekends, Bank Holidays, and public holidays. Usually provided by GP organizations, community interest companies, or business organizations.

Dispensing

Some practices are also dispensing practices (i.e. contracted to provide dispensing of medicines), particularly in rural and remote areas.

Registration, list closures, and removal from practice list

GP practices with open lists are required to take on anyone who lives within a practice's boundary area, and they can also take on those who do not. Temporary registrations can be given if the patient has been resident >24hrs and <3mths. Practices can only close their lists after application to NHS England. Patients can be removed from practice lists because of violence, or deception to receive treatment, or distance from the surgery.

Changes in general practice

In England, changes are coming to incorporate the NHS long-term plan[12] into a 5-yr framework for the GP services contract. It is expected changes will address workforce issues, support digital technologies, provide funding clarity, improve and extend service provision (e.g. early cancer diagnosis and medical care in care homes), improve the QoF, and help join up urgent care services.[13]

References

12. NHS England (2019) *The long-term plan*. Available at: ℗ https://www.longtermplan.nhs.uk/publication/nhs-long-term-plan/
13. BMA/NHS England (2019) *Investment and evolution: a 5-year framework for GP contract reform to implement The Long-Term Plan*. Available at: ℗ https://www.england.nhs.uk/wp-content/uploads/2019/01/gp-contract-2019.pdf

Further information

BMA (*General practice funding*). Available at: ℗ https://www.bma.org.uk/advice/employment/contracts/general-practice-funding

Other primary healthcare services

A range of services and professionals are available in 1° care. The following summarizes some of the most commonly used.

Dentists

Take private and NHS patients. NHS dentists have agreements to provide NHS dental services. Patients eligible for free NHS dental treatment include: those <18yrs (➔ Development and care of teeth for young children p. 196; ➔ Dental health in older children p. 226); ♀ who is pregnant or had a baby in previous 12mths (➔ Pregnancy p. 432; ➔ Postnatal care p. 438); those receiving dental treatment in an NHS hospital; people receiving some low-income benefits; and young people <20yrs who are dependent on someone receiving low-income benefits. All others pay a proportion of treatment costs, up to a set maximum.

Community dental service

NHS-funded to provide treatment to those who have difficulty accessing dental care (e.g. those with additional needs and people who are housebound). This service is on a referral basis. School oral dental screening may take place in some priority areas.

Podiatrists

Trained in all aspects of care of the feet and lower limbs. Some are also podiatric surgeons undertaking foot surgery. Services available in consulting rooms, at home, and in care homes (➔ Care homes p. 32). Most podiatry services are provided privately.

Community podiatry services

CCGs decide what foot care services to commission for specified vulnerable groups (e.g. patients with diabetes (➔ Principles of diabetes management p. 664) (➔ Commissioning of services p. 12). Local referral criteria apply.

Opticians

Provide eye sight tests and examine eyes for abnormalities (e.g. glaucoma). Also fit and supply spectacles to prescription. Dispensing opticians only fit and supply glasses. Free eye tests are available to certain groups including children, those aged >60yrs, those diagnosed with glaucoma, people >40yrs with a close relative diagnosed with glaucoma, individuals diagnosed as diabetic, individuals registered blind or partially sighted (➔ Blindness and partial sight p. 748), and some people receiving benefits. There is a mechanism for a domiciliary service for housebound people.

Pharmacists

Prepare and dispense medicines on prescription to the general public. They may own their business or work for a bigger company. The contract between local pharmacies and commissioners specifies services including dispensing medicines, waste disposal of medicinal products, and public health activities (e.g. smoking cessation (➔ Smoking cessation p. 356) and emergency contraception (➔ Emergency contraception p. 420)).

Community pharmacists also provide other services such as repeat prescribing through electronic transmission of prescriptions, medicine reviews (⊃ Principles of medication reviews p. 142), independent prescribing (⊃ Prescribing p. 136), home delivery services, and out-of-hours services.

Primary care pharmacists and medicines management teams

Pharmacists advise general practices, community health service staff, and local community pharmacists on issues related to supply, storage, and legislation concerning medicines, formularies, and prescribing budgets. They are also known as prescribing advisors.

Physiotherapists

Concerned with human function and musculoskeletal (MSK) movement (⊃ Common musculoskeletal problems p. 734). Physiotherapists deal with a wide range of issues (e.g. sports injuries, incontinence (⊃ Urinary incontinence p. 504), and back pain (⊃ Low back pain p. 604)). They work in a range of settings including hospitals, health centres, sports clubs, and private practice.

Community physiotherapists

Physiotherapists usually work as part of specialist multidisciplinary teams (MDTs) in stroke rehabilitation, intermediate care teams (⊃ Services to promote hospital discharge p. 23; ⊃ Services to prevent unplanned hospital admission p. 22), and services for children with special needs (⊃ Children with complex health needs and disabilities p. 238), providing clinic-based and domiciliary services. Local variation in eligibility.

Occupational therapists

Provide practical support to empower people to facilitate recovery and overcome barriers preventing them from doing the activities (or occupations) that matter to them. Community occupational therapists are usually employed by LAs to work with specific vulnerable groups (e.g. disabled adults) utilizing community care processes for aids and adaptions (⊃ Assistive technology and home adaptations p. 834). Also in NHS-commissioned services (e.g. community mental health teams and children with special needs teams). Local variation in eligibility.

Speech and language therapists

Work with children and adults with difficulties communicating, or with eating, drinking, and swallowing. Work as part of specialist teams (e.g. children with special needs) or more broadly across a client group (e.g. children or adults). Local variation in eligibility.

Services to prevent unplanned hospital admission

Hospitals are experiencing ↑ levels of emergency activity. Preventable emergency admissions put pressure on hospitals. They are also unpleasant experiences for patients. Many admissions are related to LTCs and could be prevented, if timely and effective care is provided in the community.[14] Various schemes exist to ↓ unplanned admissions. Some are similar to those promoting hospital discharges (➲ Services to promote hospital discharge p. 23) whilst others are tailored to prevention.

Approaches in general practice

Steps to preventing unplanned hospital admission in general practice (➲ General practice p. 18) include:[15]
- ↑ practice availability by timely telephone access.
- Identifying patients who are at ↑ risk of avoidable unplanned admissions, establishing a minimum 2% case management register and proactively managing these patients (➲ Case management p. 114; ➲ Generic long-term conditions model p. 6)).
- Developing personalized care plans for all patients on the register and undertaking at least one care review every 12mths.
- Reviewing and improving the hospital discharge process for patients on the register and co-ordinating delivery of care.
- Undertaking internal practice reviews of A&E attendances (➲ Clinical audit p. 70).

Changes to the urgent and emergency care pathway

Providing and promoting alternatives to A&E attendance including urgent care centres, walk-in centres, and NHS 111 or NHS Direct Wales (➲ Overview of services in primary care p. 16).

Case managers/community matrons for people at risk

Health or social care professionals who manage a caseload of people at risk of unplanned admission. Local organizations have different criteria for admission but often include people with a history of unplanned admissions, falls, or multiple health and social care needs.

References

14. The Health Foundation (2018) *Briefing: emergency hospital admissions in England. Which may be avoidable and how?* Available at: ℜ https://www.health.org.uk/sites/health/files/Briefing_Emergency%20admissions_web_final.pdf
15. NHS England (2016) Enhanced service specification: avoiding unplanned admissions. Proactive case finding and patient review for vulnerable people 2016/17. Available at: ℜ https://www.england.nhs.uk/commissioning/wp-content/uploads/sites/12/2016/04/aua-serv-spec.pdf

Services to promote hospital discharge

Patients should be discharged from hospital when they are clinically ready and have the right support to meet their needs. Initially, this support may relate to their short-term needs. Discharge to assess (D2A) is an approach advocated to address long-term needs.[16] It recommends that, wherever possible, people should be supported to return to their home for assessment for long-term care and support. Various services support the D2A approach.

Reablement schemes

Time-limited services (normally <6wks) focusing on restoring independent functioning and maximizing independence. Involves a range of integrated services including occupational therapists, physiotherapists. and support workers (➲ Teamwork p. 58). Provided at home or in designated beds in nursing or care homes (➲ Care homes p. 32).

Step-down schemes

Specially contracted beds in nursing or care homes. Patients will be transferred to these facilities when they no longer need acute care. Moving into a step-down bed allows further time to make arrangements for future care. Reablement services may also be provided during this period.

Rapid-response/hospital-at-home schemes

Short-term intensive support (usually ≤10 days) including nursing, therapy, and social care assessments. Provided mainly at home. Interventions may include IV therapy, nutritional support, and reablement. At the end of the support period, patients are referred to other appropriate services.

Virtual wards

A time-limited and enhanced package of healthcare within the home, typically involving reablement practitioners and rapid-response/hospital-at-home nurses or district nurses. While care is provided at home by the multidisciplinary team, the patient remains under the clinical responsibility of the hospital consultant or GP (➲ General practice p. 18).

Related topics

➲ Services to prevent unplanned hospital admission p. 22; ➲ Assistive technology and home adaptations p. 834; ➲ Social services p. 30)

References

16. NHS England (2016) *Quick guide: discharge to assess.* Available at: ℘ https://www.nhs.uk/NHSEngland/keogh-review/Documents/quick-guides/Quick-Guide-discharge-to-access.pdf

Services for children, young people, and families

The United Nations (UN) Convention of the Rights of the Child (1989)[17] is the basis of government policies for children in the UK. These focus on priority outcomes of being healthy, staying safe, enjoying and achieving, making a positive contribution, and achieving economic well-being. The policies emphasize multi-agency planning (❸ Teamwork p. 58) and provision of publicly funded services for children and families. In any area, there is a wide range of state-funded, voluntary organizations and private services for children and families. Sources of information include: LA family information services (FIS); public libraries; children centres; and family centres.

Early years: social support and play

Provision ranges from groups to one-to-one support. For example, meetings in community centres organized by a paid worker (e.g. parent and toddler groups) or meetings in cafes organized by such as the National Childbirth Trust or Meet a Mum. Organizations such as Family Action and Home-Start UK offer one-to-one befriending and practical support schemes for new parents and parents under stress (❸ Support for parenting p. 172).

Early years: childcare, play, and education

Working parents have a range of options, depending on availability and what they can afford (e.g. childminders, au pairs, nannies, group care in nurseries). LA FIS provide local information on childcare. All childminders and group care settings for <8yr olds have to be registered and meet national standards. Children in need are usually prioritized for funded support in day-care facilities (❸ Safeguarding children p. 248). All 3yr olds and 4yr olds in England are entitled to 570hrs funded early education or childcare a year (with more for working parents). 2yr olds can get free early education and childcare in England if the family is in receipt of certain benefits or if the child is looked after by the council (❸ Looked-after children p. 254), has a current statement of special educational needs (❸ Children with special educational needs p. 242), or gets disability allowance. Similar provision is available in Wales, Scotland, and Northern Ireland.

Education

Every child has to receive education from 5yrs to 16yrs, either at a state school, private school, or home. Many schools have breakfast and after-school clubs. Pupil referral units or home tutoring is provided by each LA for children who need alternative provision (e.g. have been excluded from mainstream school). State schools are supported by LA-wide services, such as education psychology services. Young people must continue in education or work-based training until 18yrs. Education for 16–18yr olds is in schools, sixth form colleges, or further education colleges.

Young people's health services

Many areas provide open-access young people's drop-in health clinics, most providing sexual health (→ Sexual health: general issues p. 760) and contraceptive services (→ Contraception: general p. 400).

Leisure activities and sport

Schools, LA services (e.g. education, youth, and leisure), voluntary organizations (e.g. guides and scouts, Woodcraft Folk, faith groups), and the private sector provide a range of different sports and leisure activities.

Young offenders

The youth offending team is a multi-agency team co-ordinated by a LA and overseen by the Youth Justice Board. It deals with young offenders, sets up community services and reparation plans, and attempts to prevent youth reoffending and incarceration.

Reference

17. UN Convention of the Rights of the Child (1989). Available at: ℜ www.unicef.org/crc/index_30184.html

Further information

Children in Scotland (*Bringing voices together*). Available at: ℜ www.childreninscotland.org.uk

Family Action (*Early years*). Available at: ℜ https://www.family-action.org.uk/what-we-do/early-years/

Home-Start (*Things we can help with*). Available at: ℜ https://www.home-start.org.uk/Pages/Category/things-we-can-help-with

Northern Ireland (*Direct pre-school development and learning*). Available at: ℜ https://www.nidirect.gov.uk/information-and-services/parents/pre-school-development-and-learning

Welsh Government (*Childcare*). Available at: ℜ https://gweddill.gov.wales/topics/people-and-communities/people/children-and-young-people/childcare/?lang=en

Homes and housing

Grenfell Tower is a 24-storey residential tower block in North Kensington, London. On 14 June 2017, the tower was destroyed by fire, killing 72 residents. Homes, housing, and health are inextricably linked. In the UK, there is a mix of owner-occupied, socially rented (LA and housing association), and privately rented homes. The home should be a place of warmth, rest, security, and safety. Poor health is associated with: homes that are cold, damp, or otherwise hazardous (unhealthy homes); homes that do not meet the household's needs due to risks such as overcrowding or inaccessibility (unsuitable homes); and homes that do not provide a sense of safety and security, including precarious living circumstances and/or homelessness (➔ Homeless people p. 446) (unstable homes). Housing can play a part in preventing people from being admitted to hospital (➔ Services to prevent unplanned hospital admission p. 22), in helping people to be discharged from hospital (➔ Services to promote hospital discharge p. 23), and in supporting people to remain independent in the community (➔ Healthy ageing p. 366).

Rented accommodation

In most areas, there is a central waiting list for socially rented properties. Each provider has different systems for accepting applicants and prioritizing people on their waiting lists, including people who are homeless, people living in poor conditions, people with medical conditions, people who have served in the armed forces (➔ Armed forces veterans p. 502), people with urgent housing needs (e.g. domestic violence (➔ Domestic violence p. 450)), and people needing to live in a particular area (e.g. care leavers (➔ Looked-after children p. 254)). Privately rented accommodation offers renters choice. It is also possible to find somewhere to live quickly. Disadvantages include short-term contracts and cost. Some private landlords will not let people on housing benefit rent their property.

Landlord responsibilities

Legal obligations vary depending on tenancy type. However, landlords must always ensure their rental properties are safe and free from health hazards (particularly those related to gas, electric, and fire (see ✆ https://www.gov.uk/renting-out-a-property)). Concerns about health and safety hazards should be brought to the attention of the environmental health team in the LA (➔ Environmental health services p. 27).

Supported housing

Combines housing with support for older people or people with physical or mental health problems. Often referred to as sheltered housing. Provided by LAs, housing associations, and voluntary organizations. Also available to purchase on a lease. There may be eligibility criteria and waiting lists. Some supported housing is staffed 24hrs/day, while support in others is only provided intermittently.

Environmental health services

Practitioners frequently come across environmental health issues that impact on their patients and users. Each LA has an environmental health department (sometimes called consumer protection department) employing environmental health officers (EHOs). Their role is to prevent, detect, and control environmental hazards that affect human health. The department's core functions are usually: private sector housing (➲ Homes and housing p. 26); food hygiene and safety (➲ Food-borne disease p. 730); noise and pollution control; pest control; occupational health and safety (➲ Health and safety at work p. 92); and notifiable and reportable diseases control (with public health departments) (➲ Infectious disease notifications p. 104) (Box 1.2). It may also include other functions such as waste disposal and cleansing services, and animal wardens for stray dogs. EHOs are also involved in public health and health promotion campaigns.

Box 1.2 Environmental health department functions
Private sector housing
- EHOs can inspect rented properties and enforce basic living standards.
- Noise and pollution control
- EHOs have powers to deal with noise problems from industry, continual neighbourhood noise (e.g. barking dogs, music). They can seize noisy equipment or serve notices to stop. Failure to comply can result in prosecution.
- Occupational health and safety
- EHOs inspect non-manufacturing premises under the Health and Safety at Work Act (1974) and can stop work activities immediately, require improvements to be made, and/or prosecute businesses. EHOs also investigate workplace accidents.

Food hygiene and safety
- Food premises are inspected according to the food safety risk they pose to the public. Premises found to contravene basic food hygiene standards can be closed down and prosecuted.
- Pest control
- Advice and action to remove ants, bees, mice, rats, wasps, and other pests from homes and businesses. Fees are usually charged, reduced for those on low-income benefits or pension.
- Notifiable and reportable diseases
- LAs appoint a 'proper officer' to be notified of legally reportable infectious diseases (usually the medical consultant for environmental health or consultant in communicable disease control). EHOs investigate the causes of notifiable and reportable diseases and food poisoning in conjunction with NHS public health leads for communicable diseases (forming a team for infectious disease outbreak control), as well as other 'reportable diseases'.

Social support

Social support is the existence or availability of networks of people on whom you can rely, who let you know that you are cared about, valued, and loved. The main source of social support comes from family, friends, and involvement in local organizations (e.g. schools and faith groups). In contrast, social isolation is an objective measure of the number of contacts that people have and loneliness is a subjective feeling about their social connections. Social isolation and loneliness are associated with ↑ morbidity and mortality.

Assessing whether someone is socially isolated or lonely

Questions to assess levels of social support include:

- Is someone available to talk with, who will listen?
- Is someone available to help with activities of daily living?
- Is there someone who can provide emotional support?
- What is the frequency of contact with those you feel close to and who you trust and confide in?

Statements used by the Campaign to End Loneliness to measure loneliness include:[18]

- I am content with my friendships and relationships.
- I have enough people I feel comfortable asking for help at any time.
- My relationships are as satisfying as I would want them to be.

Sources of social support

- Local community-based organizations (e.g. faith organizations, political parties, schools, community centres, tenants associations, youth clubs)
- Local support groups for people in the same situation (e.g. carers support groups (→ Carers p. 458) and self-management support groups (→ Expert patients and self-management programmes p. 340))
- Local branches of national charities and voluntary organizations (e.g. Alzheimer's Society, Gingerbread (→ Support for parenting p. 172), Family Welfare Association)
- Local volunteer organizations and good neighbour schemes
- Online and telephone support (e.g. ChildLine, ParentLine, SilverLine)

Related topics

→ Community approaches to health p. 338

References

18. Campaign to End Loneliness (no date) *Measuring your impact on loneliness in later life*. Available at: ℘ https://campaigntoendloneliness-rspmbr9ezvmofjn.netdna-ssl.com/wp-content/up-loads/Loneliness-Measurement-Guidance1-1.pdf

Social services

Social care departments (England and Wales), social work departments (Scotland), or health and social services boards (NI) have wide-ranging legal responsibilities to use public funds to provide a range of care, support, and protection services for: children, young people, and their families; vulnerable adults who, by reason of age or disability, need assistance to live an independent life; and carers of vulnerable adults (➲ Carers p. 458). These departments form part of the LA (except in NI). They work in partnership with health, education, housing, the police, and voluntary sector to meet the needs of vulnerable children, young people, and adults (➲ Teamwork p. 58).

Contacting social services

Social services take direct enquiries from the public, as well as take referrals by professionals. People are assessed by a social worker to determine needs. Social workers can provide: information about the care and support services that are available; an assessment of need; practical help and support for some people according to local eligibility criteria; and information about other organizations that may help.

Many services are charged for, following an individual assessment of ability to pay (varies in each country of the UK).

Support for children, young people, and their families

- Protection for children and young people from abuse and neglect (➲ Child protection processes p. 252)
- Support for vulnerable families to prevent family breakdown
- Looking after children who cannot live at home (➲ Looked-after children p. 254)
- Support for families with a child who has a permanent and substantial disability (➲ Children with complex health needs and disabilities p. 238)
- Work to reduce likelihood of young people committing offences

Services likely to be available include: safeguarding children (➲ Safeguarding children p. 248); family support; short-term breaks; equipment and adaptations to the home (➲ Assistive technology and home adaptations p. 834); residential care and support for young people leaving care; and youth justice teams.

Support for vulnerable adults

- Older people with physical disabilities
- Older people with dementia (➲ People with dementia p. 498)
- People with sensory disabilities (➲ Deafness p. 696; ➲ Blindness and partial sight p. 748)
- People with learning disabilities (➲ People with learning disabilities p. 456)
- People with mental health needs
- People with problems of substance misuse (➲ Alcohol p. 360; ➲ Substance use p. 476)

Services likely to be available include: home care; day centres; short-term breaks; equipment and home adaptations; and registration for disabled people. Adult social care services may directly provide services or commission other providers (→ Commissioning of services p. 12). Some people may have direct payments to purchase their own care with public funds. There are increasing and ongoing concerns that people who need social care miss out because councils have insufficient funds.[19]

Social work teams

Teams will be comprised of social workers and support workers. The former are registered professionals; the latter are not registered. Social work teams can be organized in different ways (e.g. covering a geographical area) and work generically or be part of a joint service with health (e.g. community mental health teams). Some teams specialize in children in families, adult services, or specific groups (e.g. people with sensory disabilities). Most social services have a duty system, where designated social workers/ teams take new enquiries or referrals.

Every nurse in 1° care needs to identify local referral processes to social services for children, young people, their families, and adults.

Reference

19. The Nuffield Trust (2017) *Focus on: social care for older people*. Available at: ℘ https://www.nuffieldtrust.org.uk/research/focus-on-social-care-for-older-people

Care homes

UK government policy promotes support to enable people to live in their own homes (➲ Healthy ageing p. 366); however, some people require extra support that is only available in an institutional setting (e.g. a care home (CH)). This might be long-term care, respite care, intermediate care, or palliative care. There is a mixed economy of care home providers including private, not for profit, and public (NHS and LA). The term 'care homes' describes two formerly distinct types of facility: those that provide onsite nursing and personal care (formerly called nursing homes); and those offering personal care only and dependent on 1° care nursing services to meet nursing needs (formerly called residential care homes).

Regulation and inspection

Each of the four countries have their own regulator. In England, both residential CHs and nursing homes for adults are registered with the Care Quality Commission (CQC). Children's homes are registered with Ofsted, and those providing healthcare will need to be registered with the CQC (➲ Looked-after children p. 254).[20] In Scotland, there is the Care Inspectorate; in Wales, the Care Inspectorate Wales; and in NI, the Regulation and Quality Improvement Authority.

General and enhanced medical services

People in CHs have complex healthcare needs. All residents are entitled to a GP (➲ General practice p. 18). The relationship between resident and GP is critical to health and well-being. In some areas, GPs can seek additional funding to provide a range of enhanced medical services (e.g. weekly visits). Whilst district nurses (➲ District nursing p. 50) will not usually visit nursing homes (due to the presence of onsite nurses), residents should have access to specialist nursing services (e.g. stoma nurses).

Paying for a care home

Systems of funding vary across the UK. Legislation and guidance is changing rapidly, so always check for updated information. The starting point in all four countries for public assistance is an assessment of needs. In Scotland, the local council will pay a flat rate contribution towards CH fees for people with assessed personal care needs. In England, personal care needs are means tested. In Scotland and England, a flat rate contribution will be paid for those with nursing needs. The accommodation costs in both countries are means tested. Local councils will have a set ceiling for fees. These may be topped up by a third party (e.g. family members).

NHS continuing healthcare

Some people with long-term complex health needs qualify for free social care arranged and funded solely by the NHS. NHS continuing care is for adults.[21] Children and young people may receive a continuing care package if they have needs arising from disability, accident, or illness that cannot be met by existing universal or specialist services alone (➲ Children with complex health needs and disabilities p. 238).[22]

References

20. CQC/Ofsted (2011) *Registration of healthcare at children's homes: joint guidance for CQC and Ofsted staff, and providers.* Available at: ℜ https://www.cqc.org.uk/sites/default/files/documents/rp_poc1a2a4a_100840_20110320_v1_00_cqc_and_ofsted_joint_guidance_for_publication.pdf
21. Department of Health and Social Care (2018) *National framework for NHS continuing healthcare and NHS-funded nursing care.* Available at: ℜ https://assets.publishing.service.gov.uk/government/uploads/system/uploads/attachment_data/file/746063/20181001_National_Framework_for_CHC_and_FNC_-_October_2018_Revised.pdf
22. Department of Health (2016) *National framework for children and young people's continuing care.* Available at: ℜ https://assets.publishing.service.gov.uk/government/uploads/system/uploads/attachment_data/file/499611/children_s_continuing_care_Fe_16.pdf

Further information

Age Scotland Factsheets (*Care home guide: funding*). Available at: ℜ https://www.ageuk.org.uk/globalassets/age-scotland/documents/ia---factsheets/care-5-care-home-guide-funding.pdf
Age Cymru Factsheets (*Paying for a permanent care home placement in Wales*). Available at: ℜ https://www.ageuk.org.uk/global/Age-Cymru/Factsheets%20and%20information%20guides/FS10w.pdf?dtrk=true

Chapter 2

Nursing in primary care

Work roles 36
Learning to work in primary care 38
General practice nursing 40
School nursing 42
Working in schools 44
Health visiting 46
District nursing 50
Clinical supervision and appraisal 52
Continuing professional development 53
Facilitating learning in practice 54
Research in primary care and community nursing 56
Teamwork 58
Leadership 60
Innovation and project planning 62
Using information for practice 64

Work roles

1° care services are those services that can be accessed directly by the public without referral from another professional. Nurses and health visitors (HVs) (**Ⓔ** Health visiting p. 46) work in a variety of 1° care settings, delivering a range of interventions including:

- Public health interventions (**Ⓔ** Key definitions of primary care and public health p. 4; **Ⓔ** Public health in the NHS and beyond p. 14)
- Preventative interventions
- Curative interventions
- Treatment interventions
- Self-management interventions
- End-of-life care (**Ⓔ** Palliative care in the home p. 550; **Ⓔ** Services for the dying patient p. 552)

The main work roles are categorized as providing first-contact services, providing chronic disease-management services, and providing public health services. Some groups of nurses focus more on one category (e.g. HVs on public health) while others may combine all three categories (e.g. practice nurses (**Ⓔ** General practice nursing p. 40)). The service provided can be reactive (in response to people seeking them out or referring to them) or proactive (actively seeking out people or particular populations). Nurses in 1° care can be:

- Generalists (e.g. practice nurses)
- Specialists working with only one type of condition (e.g. people with sickle cell disorders (**Ⓔ** Sickle cell disorders p. 308))
- Specialists working with only one part of the population (e.g. Gypsy Travellers (**Ⓔ** Gypsies and travellers p. 448))
- Specialists only providing one type of service (e.g. sexual health (**Ⓔ** Sexual health: general issues p. 760) or contraceptive services (**Ⓔ** Contraception; general p. 400))

In the UK, over 35,000 full-time equivalent (FTE) nurses and 8,000 (FTE) HVs[1] are employed by organizations providing 1° care. The organizations could be NHS Foundation Trusts, Social Enterprises, private providers, or LAs in England, Local Health Boards in Wales, NHS Boards in Scotland, and Health and Social Care Trusts in Northern Ireland. Other NHS organizations employ nurses who reach out into the community, and over 22,976 nurses[2] are employed directly by general practice organizations. The numbers are changing as more healthcare is delivered in 1° healthcare settings. The largest groups of nurses are within:

- District nursing (**Ⓔ** District nursing p. 50)
- Health visiting
- Practice nursing
- School nursing (**Ⓔ** School nursing p. 42)

However, there are also significant numbers in specialist services such as family planning, sexual health services, community children's nursing, walk-in centres, out-of-hours centres, and occupational health services. Some specialist nurses also work in 1° care as outreach from the hospital-based services (e.g. diabetes specialist nurses).

1° care offers a very dynamic environment for career development
(➔ Continuing professional development p. 53). Local as well as national
advice should always be sought on educational pathways and competencies required of different roles (➔ Learning to work in primary care p. 38).

References

1. NHS Digital (2018) *General and personal medical services, England: final 31 March and
provisional 30 June 2018, Experimental Statistics.* Available at: https://digital.nhs.uk/
data-and-information/publications/statistical/general-and-personal-medical-services/
final-31-march-and-provisional-30-june-2018-experimental-statistics
2. NHS Digital (2018) *NHS workforce statistics, December 2017.* Available at: https://
digital.nhs.uk/data-and-information/publications/statistical/nhs-workforce-statistics/
nhs-workforce-statistics-december-2017#summary

Further information

NHS Careers (*Working in health*). Available at: ✆ www.nhscareers.nhs.uk

Learning to work in primary care

Working in 1° care and domiciliary settings is very different to working in the hospital environment. ⚠ Nurses new to 1° care, irrespective of prior clinical experience and seniority, become novice practitioners again (➔ Professional accountability p. 83). This is because:

- The patient is in control of the interaction; the nurse is a guest in the home (➔ Homes and housing p. 26).
- Patients and their carers (➔ Carers p. 458) undertake most of their own care; the overall nursing contribution is small.
- Many systems and infrastructures support the delivery of health and social care (➔ Social services p. 30; ➔ Overview of services in primary care p. 16) and are locally specific and variable; it takes time to familiarize oneself with the full range of available services.
- Clinical decision making, care delivery, and management of the daily workload are often done independently and at a physical distance from other colleagues.
- Nurses work with uncertainty, changing situations, and services; this requires flexibility and assertiveness to work on the patient's behalf.

Orientation to primary care

Nobody knows how long it will take individual nurses to become orientated to working in 1° care. Some adapt rapidly, others take much longer. In addition, the different responsibilities of the range of posts mean that nurses need different preparation. However, all nurses new to working in 1° care should ensure that they have:

- An orientation and induction process from their employer
- A mentor or preceptor to review and discuss work with
- Opportunities to work with and shadow other professionals
- Access to information (e.g. organizational intranet) about the local service environment: the range of local services, referral mechanisms, key contacts, eligibility criteria, and funding mechanisms
- Knowledge of risk assessment processes for both patient and personal safety (➔ Clinical risk management p. 78; ➔ Lone working p. 94; ➔ Health and safety at work p. 92)
- Information on how to get about within the area

Related topics

➔ Clinical supervision and appraisal p. 52; ➔ Facilitating learning in practice p. 54

Further information

Queen's Nursing Institute (*Transition to working in the community and primary care*). Available at: ℬ https://www.qni.org.uk/nursing-in-the-community/transition-community-nursing/

General practice nursing

The majority of practice nurses are directly employed by general practices (➲ General practice p. 18). They mainly work as self-directing practitioners within the practice organization, often in small nursing teams that may include advanced nurse practitioners and/or HCAs.

Focus of practice nurses' work

- Provide appropriate care/treatment in conjunction with the GP or independently where care has been transferred to the nurse by the GP
- Assess nursing needs of patients registered with GP practice
- Document the process of assessment of need and delivery of care
- Evaluate the outcome of care and make changes to care plan
- Liaise with other members of 1° healthcare team
- Provide counselling (➲ Talking therapies p. 472) and health education (➲ Models and approaches to health promotion p. 334)
- Contribute to clinical governance (➲ Quality governance p. 68), QOF (➲ Quality and outcomes framework p. 74), and risk management of practice (➲ Clinical risk management p. 78).

In addition, those working as Advanced Nurse Practitioners (ANPs) may:
- Provide telephone triage
- Receive patients with undifferentiated and undiagnosed problems and assess their healthcare needs using advanced-level nursing skills and knowledge, including physical examination
- Make differential diagnoses using decision-making and problem-solving skills
- Initiate treatment plans/investigations/referrals
- Provide counselling and health education
- Work collaboratively with other healthcare professionals
- Provide leadership (➲ Leadership p. 60), management, and consultancy functions as required.

The practice nurse role and the focus of their work will be directed by the GP. In contrast, the ANP role is largely autonomous, depending on level of education/experience.

Main areas of responsibility and skills

Each practice nurse agrees their responsibilities with their employer. They require a range of clinical skills and knowledge for general patient care, developed through experience and training. Depending on their work role, these skills may include:
- Chronic disease management
- Cervical cytology (➲ Cervical cancer screening p. 380; ➲ Cervical sample taking p. 384)
- Travel health (➲ Travel healthcare p. 394; ➲ Travel health promotion p. 396; ➲ Travel vaccinations p. 399)
- Child and adult immunization (➲ Childhood immunization p. 164; ➲ Childhood immunization schedule (UK) p. 166; ➲ Targeted adult immunization p. 392)

- Wound care (➲ Wound assessment p. 522; ➲ Wound dressing p. 532)
- Ear care (➲ Ear care p. 590)
- ♀ health, i.e. HRT (➲ Menopause p. 364) and contraception (➲ Contraception: general p. 400)
- Health education and promotion
- Triage assessment
- Management and care of patients with acute and/or chronic illness
- Audit (➲ Clinical audit p. 70) and record keeping (➲ Record keeping p. 86), particularly for QOF indicators

Those working as ANPs will have additional skills including: physical examination; screening patients for disease risk factors and early signs of illness (➲ UK Screening programmes p. 362); ordering necessary investigations; and admitting and discharging patients from the caseload.

Education, training, and responsibilities

Practice nurses

Registered nurses, usually with some post-registration experience (➲ Learning to work in primary care p. 38; ➲ Continuing professional development p. 53). Can access degree- and postgraduate-level education in practice nursing (including NMC recordable Specialist Practice Qualification (General Practice Nursing)) or disease-specific topics (e.g. diabetes management (➲ Diabetes: overview p. 660; ➲ Principles of diabetes management p. 664) and asthma management (➲ Asthma in children p. 306; ➲ Asthma in adults p. 608)).

Advanced nurse practitioners

Royal College of Nursing (RCN) defines advanced practice as a level of practice rather than a type of practice. ANPs are educated at masters level in clinical practice and have been assessed as competent in practice using their expert clinical knowledge and skills. They have the freedom and authority to act, making autonomous decisions on the assessment, diagnosis, and treatment of patients. Debates continue in the UK as to possible future regulation by the NMC. In the meantime, ANPs can get formal recognition of their expertise through credentialiing managed by the RCN.

Further information

NHS Careers (*Practice nursing*). Available at: ℘ www.nhscareers.nhs.uk
RCN (*Credentialing*). Available at: ℘ https://www.rcn.org.uk/professional-development/professional-services/credentialing

School nursing

The main focus of school nurse (SN) work (➔ Working in schools p. 44) is
to contribute to giving children and young people the best start in life. This
includes enabling children and young people to achieve their full potential
by building resilience in order to stay physically and emotionally healthy according to individual circumstances. The Healthy Child Programme 0–19yrs
emphasizes the importance of education: being ready to learn at 2yrs and
being school-ready at 5yrs[3] (➔ Overview of the Healthy Child Programme
p. 154). SNs are key professionals in working towards these priority outcomes and this requires working with a range of individuals and services
including children, young people, and their families; multidisciplinary teams
such as education, health, safeguarding services (➔ Safeguarding children
p. 248); and the voluntary sector (➔ Teamwork p. 58).

Main areas of responsibility

The work of SNs varies across the UK but, fundamentally, they work with
school-aged children and young people and their families to:

* Assess health and social care needs, monitor, and refer as necessary
  (➔ Assessment of children, young people, and families p. 156)
* Promote healthy lifestyles through health-promoting activities either in
  groups or 1:1 (➔ Health promotion in schools p. 230; ➔ Group health
  promotion p. 336)
* Identify those in need of protection (➔ Identifying the child in need
  of protection p. 250), monitor, refer, and contribute to safeguarding
  children in accordance with local/national policies (➔ Child protection
  processes p. 252)
* Provide support for those with special/complex needs (➔ Children with
  complex health needs and disabilities p. 238)
* Provide advice, support, and teaching for school staff, parents, carers,
  children, and young people

Team and work organization

Statutory duties for public health, including child health services, were conferred on LAs in the Health and Social Care Act 2012. LAs are responsible
for providing services that improve the health of their local population. The
commissioning of these services has varied across the UK and, in some
areas, social enterprises have been commissioned to provide child health
services (➔ Commissioning of services p. 12). Therefore, SNs are organized in a variety of ways according to local organizations and population
needs. For example:

* SNs may be named nurses with responsibility for a number of schools
  (either 1° or 2° or both)
* SNs may be based in a secondary school, with the same responsibilities
  as a community school nurse for promoting health and well-being
* SNs may work in teams with nursery nurses and HCAs, led by a
  senior SN.

The work of SNs is organized to follow recommendations from national child health programmes.[3] It may involve specific clinical or health promotion sessions in schools, as well as offering open access drop-in sessions for school children. This will be dependent on local commissioning requirements.

Employment and education

SNs are qualified nurses either employed by NHS Foundation Trusts, social enterprises, LAs, or private providers. Independent schools may also employ their own nurses or receive a limited school nursing service from their local provider. Qualified school nurses are level 1 nurses on part 1 and part 3 of the NMC Register[4] (➲ Learning to work in primary care p. 38).

References

3. PHE (2018) Best start in life and beyond: improving public health outcomes for children, young people and families. Guidance to support the commissioning of the Healthy Child Programme 0–19: health visiting and school nursing services. Available at https://assets.publishing.service.gov.uk/government/uploads/system/uploads/attachment_data/file/686928/best_start_in_life_and_beyond_commissioning_guidance_1.pdf

4. NMC (2004) Standards of proficiency for specialist community public health nurses. Available at https://www.nmc.org.uk/globalassets/sitedocuments/standards/nmc standards-of-proficiency-for-specialist-community-public-health-nurses.pdf

Further information

NHS Careers (School nursing). Available at ✍: https://www.healthcareers.nhs.uk/search/school%20nursing

NHS Wales (The new school nursing framework). Available at ✍: http://www.wales.nhs.uk/news/45033

Queen's Nursing Institute (Transition to school nursing). Available at ✍: https://www.qni.org.uk/resources/transition-school-nursing/

RCN (Toolkit for school nurses). Available at ✍: https://www.rcn.org.uk/professional-development/publications/pub-006316

School and Public Health Nurses Association (Contact). Available at ✍: http://www.saphna.co/contact.html

Working in schools

Health provision for school-aged children is delivered in different ways, within a variety of sites, in order to meet the needs of young people, their parents, and carers. School nurses (SNs) (➔ School nursing p. 42) work flexible hours, e.g. prior to and after normal school hours. Services are predominantly provided in the school setting, but additionally at other sites, e.g. health centres/clinics, children's centres, youth centres.

The SN needs to develop effective communication processes with key school members including:

- Head teacher/deputy head teacher/teachers
- Special educational needs and disability coordinator (SENDCO) (➔ Children with special educational needs p. 242)
- Child protection/safeguarding children co-ordinator (➔ Safeguarding children p. 248; ➔ Identifying the child in need of protection p. 250; ➔ Child protection processes p. 252)
- Personal, social, and health education co-ordinator

SNs identify health needs through profiling (➔ Using information for practice p. 64) and plan key health promotion activities with school staff according to local needs and priorities (➔ Health promotion in schools p. 230). Policy changes in health and education may influence the ways in which services are commissioned, and this will impact on school health services around the UK (➔ Commissioning of services p. 12). The head teacher and school governors are responsible for developing school health-related policies, e.g. sex and relationship education (➔ Sex and relationship education p. 236), health, and safety. SNs contribute by providing evidence-based information (➔ Evidence-based healthcare p. 72).

Year and term planning

The academic year dates and most school activities are planned a year in advance. SNs and other professionals liaise with relevant school staff, to contribute towards health promotion and curriculum planning, during the summer term for the next school year. Some activities/sessions can be organized on a termly basis, but it would be wise to do this a term in advance. The school terms, in most areas, run as follows:

- Autumn: September–December
- Spring: January–April
- Summer: May–July

Medicines in schools

There are national and local policies to help education staff and health professionals in meeting the needs of children/young people requiring medicines in schools. Responsibility for giving or supervising medicines is usually undertaken by teachers or classroom helpers who are often trained by school health advisers, children's community nurses, or specialist nurses. The process involves careful planning within the multidisciplinary team (➔ Teamwork p. 58), including:

- Training for parents (➔ Working with parents p. 170), carers, and school staff regarding storage, administration, and disposal (➔ Storage, transportation and disposal of medicines p. 148)

- Proper discharge planning from hospital (→ Services to promote hospital discharge p. 23) and suitable drug regimens to facilitate smooth administration (→ Medicines optimization p. 128)
- GP for medication review (→ Principles of medication reviews p. 142)

Children with statements of special educational needs

SNs may be involved with drawing up education and health care (EHC) plans for children and young people up to 25yrs who need extra support if there is a health need. EHC plans identify specific educational, health, and social needs and set out any additional support that children and young people may require.

Working in special schools/units

Special schools cater for children and young people with complex needs (→ Children with complex health needs and disabilities p. 238) requiring a multi-disciplinary approach involving: speech and language therapists (→ Adults and children with additional communication needs p. 122), occupational therapists, physiotherapists, education staff, parents, and social services (→ Social services p. 30). Arrangements for nursing cover vary; some areas have nurses on site, while others visit on a regular basis. Generally, nurses working in special schools will perform a wider range of hands-on nursing care compared to those in mainstream schools. Some members of the school staff may also be trained to undertake some tasks such as feeding (→ Enteral tube feeding p. 594), administration of emergency medicines (→ Anaphylaxis p. 810), and catheter care (→ Indwelling urinary catheter care p. 508).

Some children/young people who are excluded from school will attend pupil referral units. Some schools also provide for children with hearing/vision impairment or language difficulties in special units. SNs and the medical team support the families and school in meeting their needs.

Further information

Department of Education (*Special educational needs and disability: code of practice, 0 to 25 years*). Available at: ℘ https://assets.publishing.service.gov.uk/government/uploads/system/uploads/attachment_data/file/398815/SEND_Code_of_Practice_January_2015.pdf

Department of Education (*Supporting pupils at school with medical conditions*). Available at: ℘ https://www.gov.uk/government/publications/supporting-pupils-at-school-with-medical-conditions--3

Health visiting

Health visiting (HV) is a public health nursing specialism (➔ Key definitions of primary care and public health p. 4; ➔ Public health in the NHS and beyond p. 14). Its focus is the promotion of health and the prevention of ill health. The main principles of HV activity are:

- The search for health needs (➔ Health needs assessment p. 15)
- The stimulation of an awareness of health needs
- The facilitation of health-enhancing activities
- The influence on policies affecting health

This public health focus can be directed to any individual, family, or group in the population (➔ Group health promotion p. 336), or to the community (➔ Community approaches to health p. 338). The search for health needs can be through formalized health needs assessment of a community, a caseload, or an individual (➔ Using information for practice p. 64). The locus of the activity may be in the client's home, health centre, GP surgery, children's centre, or community setting. Each country has its own programme and plans for HV services.

Main area of responsibility

The majority of HVs are employed to work with families with young children (➔ Working with parents p. 170; ➔ Promoting the health of children p. 152). Evidence from neuroscience and social sciences shows that the early years are crucial to a child's future development and adult health. HVs lead and deliver on nationally agreed, evidence-based public health programmes for a healthy child, starting in pregnancy (➔ Pregnancy p. 424) through early childhood (e.g. the Healthy Child Programme (HCP) (➔ Overview of the Healthy Child Programme p. 154) in England), and different types of services.

Community approach

The community-centred approach is adopted by HVs to develop community resources for health. It involves mobilizing assets within communities, promoting equity, and increasing people's control over their health and lives.

Health promotion and support

HVs offer health promotion and support to all families with young children, to access the HCP and local services at key points: antenatally (➔ Antenatal education and preparation for parenthood p. 425; ➔ Antenatal care and screening p. 426); soon after the birth of the baby (➔ New birth visits p. 174); postnatal contacts at 6–8wks; and, health reviews at 1 and 2yrs. Health promotion includes:

- Advice on adult health, including maternal mental well-being (➔ Postnatal depression p. 440) to enable strong early attachment and infant emotional well-being (➔ Emotional development in babies and children p. 210)
- Advice and support on parenting (➔ Support for parenting p. 172) and child development <5yrs (➔ Child development 0–1 years p. 192; ➔ Child development 1–5 years p. 204) to support emotional well-being and to develop improved school readiness

- Advice and support on nutrition including breastfeeding
  (➔ Breastfeeding p. 182) and infant nutrition for individual good health
  and to address rising obesity rates (➔ Bottle feeding p. 186; ➔ Weaning
  p. 188; ➔ Food and the under-fives p. 212)
- Advice and information on child immunization for the individual and
  to achieve population immunity (➔ Childhood immunization p. 164;
  Childhood immunization schedule (UK) p. 166)
- Early identification of health (physical, social, emotional, and mental)
  needs of babies, children, and adults, and negotiating and agreeing an
  action plan with clients which may involve more contact with HV team,
  e.g. for listening visits or referral to other services
- Expert help from the HV team, with more frequent contact (known
  as Universal Plus in England) in response to an identified need, e.g.
  breastfeeding problems or postnatal depression. Ongoing support from
  the HV team, and a range of other services, to address more complex
  issues over a period of time. Examples are children with disabilities
  (➔ Children with complex health needs and disabilities p. 238) and child
  protection needs (➔ Safeguarding children p. 248; ➔ Child protection
  processes p. 252).

There are times when the more vulnerable families and children require
co-ordinated support from a number of different professionals and organizations. HVs work closely with these professionals and the families to de-
vise plans of support, based upon the child and family's needs (known as
Universal Partnership Plus in England).

Team and work organization

HVs work collegiately with other HVs. Some share their caseloads (known
as 'corporate caseloads') in order to ensure equity in workloads and improve access and services to clients. Caseloads (of clients) are created from
either those living in a geographical area or a GP patient population. HVs
proactively make contact, offering services, as well as receiving referrals
from other services. They work closely with others, e.g. early years practitioners, midwives, GPs (➔ General practice p. 18), and social workers
(➔ Social services p. 30), and other agencies both statutory and voluntary.
Some HVs have specialist roles to work with specific vulnerable groups (e.g.
homeless families (➔ Homeless people p. 446) or specific health promotion
programmes (e.g. specialize in community development).

Many HVs lead teams of other staff, e.g. nursery nurses, staff nurses, and
HCAs, to deliver the public health agenda and HCP. HVs may also be part
of wider initiatives in multi-agency settings, e.g. public health departments.
HVs are active in programmes such as the Family Nurse Partnership and
Maternal Early Childhood Sustained Home Visiting.

Education and training for health visiting

All HVs are registered with the NMC as nurses or midwives before com-
mencing specialist practitioner training, a 1-yr full-time or 2-yr part-time
course at degree or postgraduate level (➔ Learning to work in primary
care p. 38). Apprenticeship schemes as a means of preparing HVs are being
developed in England. Newly qualified HVs are recorded on the specialist
community public health register of the NMC, with an annotation to show
they are HVs.

Further information

Institute of Health Visiting (*Health visitors*). Available at: www.ihv.org.uk/

NHS Careers (*Health visiting*). Available at: https://www.healthcareers.nhs.uk/explore-roles/public-health/roles-public-health/health-visitor

Scottish Government (*Universal health visiting pathway in Scotland: pre-birth to pre-school*). Available at: https://beta.gov.scot/publications/universal-health-visiting-pathway-scotland-pre-birth-pre-school/pages/1/

District nursing

District nurses (DNs) are commissioned to deliver a wide range of nursing interventions to people aged ≥18yrs in their own homes and care homes (◆ Care homes p. 32) (but not nursing homes). Patients are usually only eligible if housebound due to physical or psychological illness. Referrals received from hospitals, health and social care professionals, patients, and carers (◆ Carers p. 458). DN teams work geographically and/or by GP attachment. As well as a core daytime offer, many provide evening and overnight nursing care. DN teams are skill-mixed, including district nurses, community staff nurses, and support workers (◆ Teamwork p. 58).

District nurses and community staff nurses

A DN is a registered nurse with a specialist practitioner qualification (SPQ) in DN, recordable with the NMC (◆ Learning to work in primary care p. 38). These nurses often hold senior or management positions within the team. A community staff nurse is a registered nurse without a specialist practitioner qualification. Work at varying levels of seniority depending on their experience and pay banding. Possible for nurses without DN qualification to hold management positions.

Nursing support staff and healthcare support workers

Staff working in clinical roles who are not registered nurses, e.g. HCAs and assistant practitioners.

Key colleagues

Colleagues in the 1° and community care team include (◆ Overview of services in primary care p. 16): GPs, occupational therapists, physiotherapists, community matrons (◆ Services to prevent unplanned hospital admission p. 22), nurse specialists (e.g. palliative care nurse specialists (◆ Services for the dying patient p. 552), speech and language therapists, pharmacists, social workers (◆ Social services p. 30), home carers (◆ Social support p. 28), and carers.

Care provided

DN services play a key role in supporting independence, managing LTCs, and preventing and treating acute illnesses. Regarded as a key service to ↓ unplanned hospital admissions and promote hospital discharge (◆ Services to promote hospital discharge p. 23). Key activities include:

- Bowel care and continence management (◆ Urinary incontinence p. 504; ◆ Faecal incontinence p. 514)
- End-of-life care (◆ Palliative care in the home p. 550)
- IV therapy (◆ Care of central venous catheters p. 582), injections (◆ Injection techniques p. 576), and medication administration
- PEG feeding (◆ Enteral tube feeding p. 594)
- Wound care (◆ Wound assessment p. 522; ◆ Wound dressing p. 532), and pressure ulcer prevention and management (◆ Pressure ulcer prevention p. 520)
- Urinary catheterization and ongoing catheter management (◆ Indwelling urinary catheter care p. 508)

- Support for self-management
- Carer support
- Case management/co-ordination (➔ Case management p. 114)
- Non-medical prescribing (➔ Prescribing p. 136)

Contemporary challenges

Pressures include issues relating to: ↑ in the number of people needing DN care; ↑ complexity of care delivered in the community; staff shortages and a significant capacity gap; variable provision of other community-based services; and, resourcing and commissioning of DN services (➔ Commissioning of services p. 12).

Preparation for specialist practitioner qualification

To be recorded as a SPQ DN, nurses have to complete a post-registration training programme. All programmes, which lead to a recordable SPQ DN, must meet standards for specialist education and practice[5] (➔ Learning to work in primary care p. 38). Programme providers are also encouraged to meet new Queen's Nursing Institute (QNI) voluntary standards for DN education and practice,[6] which focus on four competency domains: clinical care; leadership (➔ Leadership p. 60) and operational management; facilitation of learning (➔ Facilitating learning in practice p. 54); and evidence (➔ Evidence-based healthcare p. 72), research (➔ Research in primary care and community nursing p. 56), and development (➔ Continuing professional development p. 53).

References

5. NMC (2001) *Standards for specialist education and practice*. Available at: https://www.nmc.org.uk/globalassets/sitedocuments/standards/nmc-standards-for-specialist-education-and-practice.pdf
6. QNI (2015) *Voluntary standards for DN education and practice*. Available at: https://www.qni.org.uk/wp-content/uploads/2017/02/District_Nurse_Standards_WEB.pdf

Further information

Department of Health (*Care in local communities: a new vision and model for district nursing*). Available at: ℜ https://www.qni.org.uk/wp-content/uploads/2016/09/vision-district-nursing.pdf
King's Fund (*Understanding quality in district nursing services: learning from patients, carers and staff*). Available at: ℜ https://www.kingsfund.org.uk/publications/quality-district-nursing
Queen's Nursing Institute (QNI) (*Transition to district nursing service*). Available at: ℜ https://www.qni.org.uk/wp-content/uploads/2017/01/Transition-to-District-Nursing.pdf

Clinical supervision and appraisal

Clinical supervision

Clinical supervision is a practice-focused professional relationship that enables staff to reflect on practice with the support of a skilled supervisor. It supports practitioners to modify and develop their practice and identify continuing professional development (CPD) needs (➜ Continuing professional development p. 53). The principles are aligned to the NMC revalidation process and, as such, it is an element of clinical governance (➜ Quality governance p. 68) as it helps to support quality improvement, managing risks (➜ Clinical risk management p. 78) and increasing accountability (➜ Professional accountability p. 83).

Clinical supervision has some or all of these purposes: normative (i.e. maintaining professionalism); educative (i.e. developing competence); and, supportive (i.e. helping staff to manage professional demands).

Approaches to clinical supervision vary according to the needs of staff and the services they provide. The frequency of supervision can also vary and will depend on the type of work the practitioner undertakes and the requirements of the relevant professional body. It is important to ensure a supervision contract is shared so that all parties are aware of the aims of the supervision, responsibilities, roles, and boundaries.

Appraisal

Appraisal is a formal opportunity for practitioners to review and develop their performance in the context of their organization's goals, their own job description, and the linked NHS Knowledge and Skills Framework. It is a formal system to: review past performance, set new objectives, and identify training and development needs in a personal development plan; highlight individual potential and discuss short-, medium-, and long-term career development; acknowledge and record employee achievements, as well as performance concerns.

In the independent sector, it may link to performance-related pay and bonus systems. In the NHS, it links to the Agenda for Change gateways in pay bands.

Further information

NMC (*Guidance on revalidation*). Available at: ✒ http://revalidation.nmc.org.uk/welcome-to-revalidation

Continuing professional development

Healthcare and professional practice are continuously changing. All professionals have to maintain and develop competence through a lifelong learning process known as continuing professional development (CPD). CPD needs should be identified through everyday reflection on practice, clinical supervision, and a personal development plan (PDP) developed during induction and appraisal processes (➲ Clinical supervision and appraisal p. 52).

NMC requirements

Revalidation is the process that all nurses and midwives in the UK and nursing associates in England need to follow to maintain their registration with the NMC. As part of revalidation, nurses must undertake 35hrs of CPD relevant to their scope of practice in the 3-yr period since registration was last renewed. The 35hrs of CPD must include ≥20hrs of participatory learning. The learning must be recorded and linked with part of the NMC Code.[7] An instance of CPD may lead to one of the five written reflective accounts in the 3-yr period which is also part of revalidation.

Sources of support

- Electronic access to NHS Evidence
- Professional organizations' (e.g. Queen's Nursing Institute) provision of study days and conferences, as well as financial support opportunities
- Access to Open Athens for various databases (℅ https://openathens.org/about-us/)
- E-Learning for Healthcare
- Healthcare libraries in universities and employing organizations
- General practice (➲ General practice p. 18) and 1° care multidisciplinary learning events
- In-house training and development programmes
- Employing organizations' learning and development plans that commission places for nurses on formal education courses at universities (➲ Learning to work in primary care p. 38)

Reference

7. NMC (2018) The code: professional standards of practice and behaviour for nurses, midwives and nursing associates. Available at: https://www.nmc.org.uk/globalassets/sitedocuments/nmc-publications/nmc-code.pdf

Further information

E-Learning for Health (Programmes). Available at: ℅ https://www.e-lfh.org.uk/programmes/
NICE (Evidence search). Available at: ℅ https://www.evidence.nhs.uk/
NMC (Revalidation). Available at: ℅ http://revalidation.nmc.org.uk/

Facilitating learning in practice

The NMC have set standards for student supervision and assessment that 1° care and community nurses should follow when working with student health visitors and pre- or post-registration nurses[8]. The standards set out expectations for the learning, support, supervision, and assessment of students in the practice environment. Students are generally supernumerary, although the apprenticeship model of education is becoming more common and apprentices will be working for some of their time in their substantive role.

Students should be able to learn in a safe and effective environment from a range of different practitioners in 1° care or the community. There should be a nominated person in each practice setting to support students and, depending on the extent of the role, these positons may attract additional salary or designated time for teaching.

Supervision and assessment of students is allocated to different practitioners as an assessor cannot simultaneously be supervisor for the same student. All nurses or midwives can be practice supervisors following appropriate preparation. Practice supervisors should:

- Act as role models in accordance with The Code[9]
- Have relevant and current knowledge and expertise
- Provide feedback on student progress, including raising concerns on conduct or proficiency
- Contribute to student assessments
- Receive ongoing support to supervise students

Students are allocated a practice assessor from the same field of practice (nurse, midwife, or specialist community public health nurse), who will be able to objectively assess the proficiency of the student and raise any concerns. Assessors rely on the feedback from supervisors as well as their own observations to form their decisions about assessment and will liaise with the higher education institute that runs the education programme. Practice assessors must undertake preparation to carry out the role.

Effective practice learning

Principles to consider when working with adult learners in practice include:

- Students should be empowered to be proactive and take responsibility for their learning.
- Students will benefit from learning from a range of different people, including service users, non-registered practitioners, and practitioners from other disciplines (❺ Teamwork p. 58).
- Student needs will be diverse as they will bring a wide range of prior experience with them.
- The level of supervision required will vary according to their needs and stage of learning.
- A successful supervisory relationship is based on trust, respect, and clear objectives.
- Learning should be two-way; supervisors should also learn from the student.

Consent of patients to teaching

The teacher practitioner should gain the full consent (➜ Consent p. 82) of patients/clients before students 'sit in' on consultations or provide clinical/professional services. It is good practice to have public information about the teaching in the practice/service and the right of patients/clients to decline to participate.

References

8. NMC (2018) *Realising professionalism: standards for education and training*. Available at: https://www.nmc.org.uk/standards-for-education-and-training/standards-for-student-supervision-and-assessment/

9. NMC (2018) *The code: professional standards of practice and behaviour for nurses, midwives and nursing associates*. Available at: https://www.nmc.org.uk/standards/code/

Research in primary care and community nursing

Research is the systematic inquiry to develop or contribute to the development of new knowledge that can be generalizable. It is essential for provision of high-quality healthcare (➲ Evidence-based healthcare p. 72). Methodologies may be quantitative, qualitative, or mixed, as appropriate to the question to be answered. Data collection methods range from clinical drug trials through to surveys, questionnaires, ethnographies, and in-depth case studies. All research follows a systematic process (see Fig. 2.1).

All countries' central health departments have research policies and funding for research and research careers. In England and Wales, this is the National Institute for Health Research (NIHR). The UK Clinical Research Network supports the infrastructure for clinical research UK wide.

Ethics

Ethical review of research, where research participants are patients (and sometimes staff) or users of social care services, is undertaken by one of a network of NHS Research Ethics Committees. An electronic application

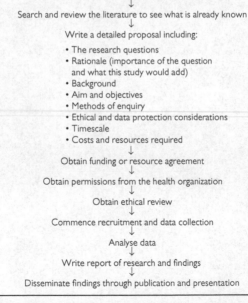

Turn the issue or idea into a specific question
↓
Search and review the literature to see what is already known
↓
Write a detailed proposal including:

• The research questions
• Rationale (importance of the question
  and what this study would add)
• Background
• Aim and objectives
• Methods of enquiry
• Ethical and data protection considerations
• Timescale
• Costs and resources required

↓
Obtain funding or resource agreement
↓
Obtain permissions from the health organization
↓
Obtain ethical review
↓
Commence recruitment and data collection
↓
Analyse data
↓
Write report of research and findings
↓
Disseminate findings through publication and presentation

Fig. 2.1 The research process.

goes through the Integrated Research Application System (IRAS). Research outside the remit of this body and undertaken as a student, or in collaboration with a university, follows university research ethics procedures. Research should be undertaken in partnership with patients and service users. For consent (→ Consent p. 82) to be considered both legal and ethical it must be given voluntarily by a person with capacity (→ Mental capacity p. 470) and who has been adequately informed, hence the importance of participant information sheets and consent forms.

Research governance and permissions

Research governance is concerned with setting standards to improve the quality of research and safeguard patients and the public. All research projects have to gain written permission from the organization in which they will take place (usually via clinical governance (→ Quality governance p. 68) or a research and development office).

Further information

International Collaborations for Community Health Nursing Research (ICCHNR) (*About ICCHNR*). Available at: ℳ http://icchnr.org/about-icchnr/

NIHR (*Primary care*). Available at: ℳ https://www.nihr.ac.uk/nihr-in-your-area/primary-care/

NIHR (*Public health*). Available at: ℳ https://www.nihr.ac.uk/nihr-in-your-area/public-health/

NIHR (*Involve: public involvement in research*). Available at: ℳ www.invo.org.uk

NHS Health Research Authority (*Research ethics service and research ethics committees*). Available at: ℳ https://www.hra.nhs.uk/about-us/committees-and-services/res-and-recs/

RCN (*Research society*). Available at: ℳ https://www.rcn.org.uk/get-involved/forums/research-society

UK Clinical Research Network (*Research infrastructure*). Available at: ℳ https://www.ukcrc.org/research-infrastructure/clinical-research-networks/uk-clinical-research-network-ukcrn/

Teamwork

Modern healthcare is delivered by teams rather than individuals (➋ Overview of services in primary care p. 16). The nature of teams is varied, including: teams that draw from a single professional group; multi-disciplinary teams; teams that are co-located; teams that are geographically distributed; teams with constant membership; and teams with constantly changing membership. Teamwork is the way people work together co-operatively and effectively.

Team characteristics

Effective teams have been shown to improve patient outcomes, ↑ productivity, and enhance job satisfaction in a range of settings. Such teams are characterized by common purpose, measurable goals, effective leadership, effective communication, good cohesion, and mutual respect.[10] In contrast, dysfunctional teams are characterized by absence of trust, fear of conflict, lack of accountability, and inattention to results.[11]

Teamwork competencies

Competencies for effective teamwork include:
- Leadership (➋ Leadership p. 60)
- Ability to influence
- Decision making
- Listening
- Planning
- Communication
- Negotiation
- Motivating others
- Self-management
- Peer counselling
- Conflict management

Tuckman's team formulation theory

According to Tuckman,[12] there are five stages that all newly formed teams go through.

Forming

Group members come together and start getting to know each other. At this stage, you should engage in ice-breaking activities, work out strategies for staying in touch, and agree ways of working.

Storming

Conflict can arise as people try to sort out confusion relating to allocated tasks and disagree about rules of behaviour. People seek to assert their authority and get challenged. Whilst this stage is uncomfortable, it is one that will pass. Refer back to agreed ways of working.

Norming

The group begins to settle down, co-operation begins, and people communicate their feelings more positively. Remember to keep up the goodwill and do what you say you will do.

Performing
Group starts delivering task effectively. Keep in contact and encourage one another.

Adjourning
The break-up of the group when the task is completed and everyone moves on to new things. Given there can be a sense of loss, stay in contact and look for opportunities to work together in the future.

Belbin's team roles theory

According to Belbin,[13] there are nine team roles that people assume:
- Resource investigator: uses inquisitive nature to find ideas to bring to the team
- Team worker: helps the team to gel, using their versatility to identify the work required and complete it on behalf of the team
- Co-ordinator: needed to focus on the team's objectives, draw out team members, and delegate work appropriately
- Plant: tends to be creative and good at solving problems in unconventional ways
- Monitor/evaluator: provides a logical eye, making impartial judgements where required, and weighs up the team's options in a dispassionate way
- Specialist: brings in-depth knowledge of a key area to the team
- Shaper: provides the necessary drive to ensure that the team keeps moving and does not lose focus or momentum
- Implementer: needed to plan a workable strategy and carry it out as efficiently as possible
- Completer/finisher: most effectively used at the end of tasks to polish and scrutinize the work for errors, subjecting it to the highest standards of quality control.

Each role has strengths and weaknesses. The strongest teams have members for each role type.

References

10. WHO (2012) *Being an effective team player*. Available at: http://www.who.int/patientsafety/education/curriculum/who_mc_topic-4.pdf
11. Thistlewaite, J. (2012) *Values-based interprofessional collaborative practice*. Cambridge University Press: Cambridge
12. Tuckman, B. (1965) Developmental sequence in small groups. *Psychological Bulletin*, 65(2), 384–99
13. Belbin Associates (2018) *The nine Belbin team roles*. Available at: https://www.belbin.com/about/belbin-team-roles/

Leadership

To lead is to influence and guide in a direction, course of action, or opinion. Acts of leadership can come from anyone, not just someone in a position of authority. The success of an organization is not dependent on one heroic leader but the efforts of the whole team.[14] Leadership is a set of skills, qualities, and behaviours which all nurses are expected to demonstrate. Leadership qualities are key to developing compassionate and high-quality services that improve patient experiences (➲ Patient and public experience p. 75) and health outcomes, and meet population needs.

Principles of leadership

The Healthcare Leadership Model identifies nine dimensions of leadership behaviour.[15]

Inspiring a shared purpose
- Valuing a service ethos
- Curious about how to improve services and patient care
- Behaving in a way that reflects the principles and values of the NHS

Leading with care
- Having the essential personal qualities for leaders in health and social care
- Understanding the unique qualities and needs of the team (➲ Teamwork p. 58)
- Providing a caring, safe environment (➲ Health and safety at work p. 92) to enable everyone to do their jobs effectively

Evaluating information
- Seeking out varied information (➲ Using information for practice p. 64)
- Using information to generate new ideas and make effective plans for improvement or change (➲ Innovation and project planning p. 62)
- Making evidence-based decisions (➲ Evidence-based healthcare p. 72) that respect different perspectives and meet the needs of all service users (➲ Anti-discriminatory healthcare p. 81)

Connecting our service
- Understanding how health and social care services fit together and how different people, teams, or organizations interconnect and interact (➲ Learning to work in primary care p. 38; ➲ Overview of services in primary care p. 16)

Sharing the vision
- Communicating a compelling and credible vision of the future in a way that makes it feel achievable and exciting

Engaging the team
- Involving individuals and demonstrating that their contributions and ideas are valued and important for delivering outcomes and continuous improvements to the service

Holding to account
- Agreeing clear performance goals and quality indicators
- Supporting individuals and teams to take responsibility for results
- Providing balanced feedback (◑ Facilitating learning in practice p. 54)

Developing capability
- Building capability to enable people to meet future challenges
- Using a range of experiences as a vehicle for individual and organizational learning
- Acting as a role model for personal development

Influencing for results
- Deciding how to have a positive impact on other people
- Building relationships to recognize other people's passions and concerns
- Using interpersonal and organizational understanding to persuade and build collaboration

Leadership development

Leadership development (training, coaching, and mentoring) should be addressed within the context of continuing professional development (◑ Continuing professional development p. 53), appraisal processes, and clinical supervision (◑ Clinical supervision and appraisal p. 52).

Reference

14. King's Fund (2011) *The future of leadership and management in the NHS: no more heroes.* Available at: https://www.kingsfund.org.uk/publications/future-leadership-and-management-nhs
15. NHS Leadership Academy (2013) *Healthcare Leadership Model: the nine dimensions of leadership behaviour.* Available at: https://www.leadershipacademy.nhs.uk/wp-content/uploads/2013/10/NHSLeadership-LeadershipModel-10-Print.pdf

Innovation and project planning

Innovation is the introduction and application of ideas, processes, products, or procedures that are new, relevant, and beneficial. In 1° and community care, innovations include new:

- Services (e.g. new clinical sessions and specialist teams)
- Clinical roles (e.g. physician assistant)
- Ways of working (e.g. remote consultations (➔ Assessment by remote consultation p. 124))

Critical to the success is stakeholder management and detailed project planning.

Stakeholder management

Stakeholders are those people who the innovation will impact upon (e.g. colleagues, managers, and patients). These people could be strong supporters or opponents of the innovation. Need to win them over.

Stakeholder analysis
- Identify stakeholders
- Assess their power, influence, and interest
- Understand the most important stakeholders

Stakeholder planning
Work out how to communicate with each stakeholder:
- For patients, refer to patient and public involvement protocols (➔ Patient and public experience p. 75)
- For staff, refer to human resources policies and procedures

Project plans
Aim and objectives
The aim is a broad statement of what is to be achieved. Objectives are derived from the broader aim and will focus on the benefits that the innovation is expected to produce (e.g. ↓ avoidable hospital admissions, ↓ morbidity and mortality). Expressed in a SMART format:
- Specific: clear about what will be achieved
- Measurable: quantify results
- Achievable: agreed, attainable
- Relevant: related to the project
- Timed: attainable within a specified timescale

Risk management
All projects involve an element of risk (➔ Clinical risk management p. 78). A risk analysis addresses the following questions:
- What could possibly go wrong?
- What is the likelihood of it going wrong?
- How will it affect the project?
- What can be done about it?

Costing
- Staff salary costs for the time involved in the project (including employer's contributions to pensions and national insurance)

- Organizational overheads: usually expressed as a % of the salary costs and covers central services that keep the organization functioning (e.g. running and maintenance of premises)
- All materials, equipment, non-staff resources to be used
- Additional expenses (e.g. hire of rooms, payment for speakers)

Planning tools
- Computer software can be bought to aid project planning
- Tools such as Generalized Activity Normalization Time Table (GANTT) charts outline detailed steps and time frames in a diagrammatic way and monitor progress (see Fig. 2.2)
- Other tools include critical pathway analysis which diagrammatically shows when activities can happen in parallel or are dependent on each other

Evaluation
- Formative evaluation of the process of implementation
- Summative evaluation of whether objectives have been achieved

Task	Person Responsible	Week 1	Week 2	Week 3	Week 4
Collect information	Nurse A	×			
Write draft report	Nurse B		×		
Revise report	Nurse A and B			×	
Present report to general practice meeting	Nurse A to speak. Nurse B to answer questions				×

Fig. 2.2 GANTT chart.

Related topics

➔ Leadership p. 60; ➔ Teamwork p. 58; ➔ Quality governance p. 68.

Further information

NHS Improvement (*Project management: an Overview*). Available at: ℛ https://improvement.nhs.uk/resources/project-management-overview/

Using information for practice

A key 1° care and community nursing activity is to use data to inform and change practice. This is often called profiling. Three types of profiling activities are used: community profiling; caseload profiling; and workload profiling and resource management. Nurses working in or closely with general practice may also be using practice patient profiles or QOF returns (➋ Quality and Outcomes Framework p. 74).

Community profiling

This means using local public health data to understand the health needs of the community/population that practitioners work with, combined with LA and community data on resources to help address identified needs (➋ Community approaches to health p. 338). This informs the nurse of what the key local needs are, and where their attention should be directed. This links to health needs assessment activities (➋ Health needs assessment p. 15).

Caseload profiling

Caseload profiling is a technique for understanding the collated health and social care needs of those within the 'caseload' held by the nurse or team of nurses. The purpose is to assist with planning, prioritizing, and identifying particular issues/groups/trends that need addressing either by the team or by alerting others to, or making a business case for, more or different resources. It is usually undertaken on an annual basis as a snapshot.

Demographic information
- Age and sex
- Ethnicity and first language

Presence of morbidity and key health and social issues
- LTCs
- Substance misuse (➋ Substance use p. 476)
- Carers, including child carers (➋ Carers p. 458)
- Violence or neglect to children (➋ Safeguarding children p. 248), older adults (➋ Adults at risk from harm and abuse p. 454), and ♀ (➋ Domestic violence p. 450)
- Children with special needs (➋ Children with complex health needs and disabilities p. 238; ➋ Children with special educational needs p. 242)
- Adults requiring care and support as per the Care Act 2014
- People in short-term or temporary accommodation (➋ Homeless people p. 446)
- Asylum seekers and refugees (➋ Asylum seekers and refugees p. 444)

Key public health indicators
- Breastfeeding rates (➋ Breastfeeding p. 182)
- Influenza vaccination rates (➋ Targeted adult immunization p. 392)
- Smoking cessation rates (➋ Smoking cessation p. 356)
- Obesity rates (➋ Overweight and obesity p. 348)

Dependency scores
Many district nursing services (➲ District nursing p. 50) have a dependency scale or care objective scale that assigns patients to different categories that indicates both the objectives of care and how much nurse time their pursuit involves. Health visiting services (➲ Health visiting p. 46) may also assign clients/families to a grouping that indicates whether or not a family receives more support than those receiving the locally determined core service (in England, Universal Plus services). Likely to include families with children who are or have had a child protection plan (➲ Child protection processes p. 252) and families receiving additional supportive/listening visits (e.g. after detection of postnatal depression (➲ Postnatal depression p. 440)).

Performance data
Any service outcome/performance data in addition to public health indicators: e.g. venous leg ulcer (➲ Venous leg ulcer p. 540) healing rates; from electronic record systems such as Rio, SystmOne, EMIS; early identification of speech and language problems in children (➲ Adults and children with additional communicaiton needs p. 122); audit data (➲ Clinical audit p. 70).

Referral and discharge data
The total volume of patients/clients that have been admitted to the caseload in a given period, e.g. annual/6mths, and the total volume of patients/clients that have been discharged/left the caseload through moving or death. Caseload profile information only becomes meaningful when it is compared to wider information, e.g. national or regional rates, or compared year on year or against a benchmark. Some areas provide proformas, with local public health data inserted, for instant comparison.

Workload profiling and resources

Nationally, there is no recommended ratio of population to number of nurses. This is because the number of staff required is dependent on what types of nursing work, for different populations, are commissioned. Caseload and workload profiling assist practitioners and managers in determining: equitable distribution of staffing to work; and ↑ or ↓ demand on the nursing staff resource. Beyond the aggregate caseload data, workload includes all the other activities that are part of the nursing team's responsibilities, e.g. nurse education (➲ Facilitating learning in practice p. 54), attending GP link/clinical meetings, liaison sessions with other services (➲ Teamwork p. 58).

All patients/clients/work activities do not make equal demands on nursing time. In order to determine the impact on the nursing resource, weighted scoring systems are applied to the caseload and the extra work activities. In district nursing teams, the weighted scoring system is linked to patient dependency on the nursing team (rather than self-care/informal carers or home carers). In health visiting, the score is linked to issues such as child protection, although the receipt of income support can act as an accurate proxy for high demands on health visiting team time. In school nursing teams (➲ School nursing p. 42), the weighted score is linked to numbers of children in schools with special needs and child protection needs (➔ Working in schools p. 44). Weighted scores are also given to issues such as travel distances or number of GP practices or schools linking with the service.

The weighted scoring results are triangulated with the regular monitoring data of nursing activity levels, outcomes, and quality indicators. Experienced staff and managers then also use their expert knowledge in determining manageable workloads and decisions are made including: shifting or changing team staffing or team activity focus, and discussing increasing demand with commissioners.

Further information

National Quality Board (*Safe, sustainable and productive staffing: an improvement resource for the district nursing service*). Available at: ℜ https://improvement.nhs.uk/documents/816/Safe_staffing_District_Nursing_final.pdf

PHE (*LA health profiles*). Available at: ℜ https://fingertips.phe.org.uk/profile/health-profiles

PHE (Supporting the public health nursing workforce: health visitors and school nurses delivering public health for children and young people 0–19). Available at: ℜ https://assets.publishing.service.gov.uk/government/uploads/system/uploads/attachment_data/file/686922/PH_nursing_workforce_guidance_for_employers_and_employees.pdf

PHE (*Child health profiles*). Available at: ℜ https://fingertips.phe.org.uk/profile/child-health-profiles/data#page/1/gid/1938133228/pat/46/par/E39000030/ati/154/are/E38000010

Queen's Nursing Institute (*Developing a national district nursing workforce planning framework*). Available at: ℜ https://www.qni.org.uk/wp-content/uploads/2016/09/district_nursing_workforce_planning_report.pdf

Quality and safety

Quality governance 68
Clinical audit 70
Evidence-based healthcare 72
Quality and Outcomes Framework 74
Patient and public experience 75
Complaints procedures 76
Clinical risk management 78
Professional conduct 80
Anti-discriminatory healthcare 81
Consent 82
Professional accountability 83
Chaperones 84
Whistleblowing 85
Record keeping 86
Access to records 88
Confidentiality 89
Client and patient-held records 90
Health and safety at work 92
Lone working 94
Patient moving and handling 96
Hand hygiene 98
Personal protective equipment 100
Occupational exposure to blood-borne viruses 102
Infectious disease notifications 104
Managing healthcare waste 106
Sharps injuries 108

Quality governance

Provides a framework for organizations and individuals to improve standards of care and create a culture of improvement. There are country-specific mechanisms. In England, NHS Improvement is responsible for overseeing NHS foundation trusts, NHS trusts, and independent providers, helping them give patients consistently safe and financially sustainable care of increasing quality. In Scotland, Healthcare Improvement Scotland is responsible for inspecting and regulating care. Healthcare Inspectorate Wales is the independent inspectorate and regulator of healthcare in Wales.

NHS Improvement works closely with the Care Quality Commission (CQC), NHS England, and the Department of Health and Social Care to support and hold healthcare organizations to account around five key areas: safe, effective, caring, and responsive care; finance and use of resources; operational performance; strategic change; and leadership and improvement capability (➜ Leadership p. 60).

Those responsible for commissioning (➜ Commissioning of services p. 12) or planning health services will also use these domains in their service specifications. The expectation is that each organization will use nationally available, evidence-based clinical guidelines (➜ Evidence-based healthcare p. 72) and nationally set quality indicators (e.g. NHS Outcomes Framework and QOF (➜ Quality and Outcomes Framework p. 74)) as criteria against which to measure themselves (➜ Clinical audit p. 70) and plan for improvement, through both service change and staff development (➜ Continuing professional development p. 53). In addition, organizations will have named clinicians and managers responsible for quality, safety (➜ Clinical risk management p. 78), and patient experience (➜ Patient and public experience p. 75).

Further information

NHS Improvement (*About us*). Available at: ℳ https://improvement.nhs.uk/about-us/who-we-are/

CQC (*About us*). Available at: ℳ https://www.cqc.org.uk/about-us

Healthcare Improvement Scotland (*About us*). Available at: ℳ http://www.healthcareimprovementscotland.org/about_us.aspx

Healthcare Inspectorate Wales (*About us*). Available at: ℳ http://hiw.org.uk/about/?lang=en

NHS Outcomes Framework (*NHS outcomes framework indicators—November 2018*). Available at: ℳ https://digital.nhs.uk/data-and-information/publications/clinical-indicators/nhs-outcomes-framework/current

Clinical audit

Fig 3.1 Clinical audit cycle

Clinical audit

A quality improvement process to improve patient care and outcomes. The audit cycle (Fig. 3.1) systematically reviews current care (what is happening) against explicit criteria (what should be happening), to identify deficiencies or problems (what changes are needed), so that practice can be modified where necessary. Further monitoring is then used to make sure improvement continues.

Audits may arise from significant events, complaints (◑ Complaints procedures p. 76), guidelines, or protocols (◑ Evidence-based healthcare p. 72). National clinical audit programmes are also in place. In England, the National Clinical Audit and Patient Outcomes Programme[1] comprises over 30 national audits related to common conditions, which healthcare organizations are obliged to complete. These allow local organizations to benchmark against national performance.

Every healthcare organization has an annual programme of priority areas for audits based on quality standards in service specifications, contracts, QOF (◑ Quality and Outcomes Framework p. 74), and national guidance. The audit process should incorporate the views of service users (◑ Patient and public experience p. 75). Audit should be undertaken in a culture of supportive development.

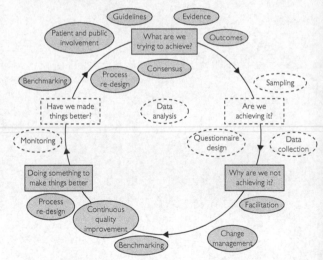

Fig. 3.1 Clinical audit cycle

© NICE (2002) *Principles of best practice in clinical audit.* Available from https://www.nice.org.uk/media/default/About/what-we-do/Into-practice/principles-for-best-practice-in-clinical-audit.pdf. All rights reserved. Subject to Notice of rights. NICE guidance is prepared for the National Health Service in England. All NICE guidance is subject to regular review and may be updated or withdrawn. NICE accepts no responsibility for the use of its content in this product/publication.

How to conduct an audit

Preparing to undertake an audit

Ensure the team and organization support the audit, with resources, skills, and commitment to act on findings. Clarify whether the audit will be conducted at individual practitioner level, service level, or organizational level, and how findings will be reported back.

Choosing a topic for audit

The topic should be important, manageable, clearly defined, and preferably have data easily available.

Choosing audit criteria

Audit criteria should be explicit and evidence-based (e.g. statements in national or local clinical guidance). Statements should also be agreed about the expected standard (i.e. % of cases in which the criteria should be fulfilled).

Measuring current performance against the criteria

Methods of gathering data depend on the criteria being measured and available resources. They can include computer and medical records, data collection sheets, or surveys. Results should be compared with recognized standards and any other available audit data (e.g. published audits from other practices or teams).

Planning for improvement

Identifying areas for modification and continued monitoring of change implementation requires a team and organizational approach. Change may also involve addressing individual practice in professional development plans (◑ Continuing professional development p. 53). Following implementation, the cycle leads back into re-auditing.

Reference

1. Healthcare Quality Improvement Partnership (*National clinical audit programme*). Available at: ℜ https://www.hqip.org.uk/a-z-of-nca/#.XA4qd9v7TRZ

Further information

Burgess, R. (2011) *New principles of best practice in clinical audit* (2nd edn). Oxford: Radcliffe Medical Press.

NICE (*Audit and service improvement*). Available at: ℜ https://www.nice.org.uk/about/what-we-do/into-practice/audit-and-service-improvement

Evidence-based healthcare

One of the central pillars of modern care delivery (⊖ Quality governance p. 68). Making decisions that affect the care of patients, provision of health services, and public health by drawing on all valid, relevant information is especially important due to ↑ healthcare costs and variations in practice. Evidence-based clinical practice is when professionals consider current best research evidence, clinical expertise, and patient values to decide on the best course of action.

Critical appraisal

The process of assessing and interpreting evidence by systematically considering its validity, relevance, and usefulness. Evidence is classified into a hierarchy dictated by the source (Box 3.1). Results from type 1 studies are considered strongest and type 4 weakest.

Guidelines

Statements written to inform decision making and recommend how professionals should care for patients with specific conditions. They are compiled from critically appraised research evidence and clinical data. Usually produced at national or international level and aim to increase standards of care, reduce risk, and achieve cost effectiveness. NICE is a UK government-funded body producing evidence-based guidelines.

Protocols

These usually refer to specific guidelines on evidence-based professional activities and treatments required for particular conditions and situations, and are more directive than guidelines.

Box 3.1 Hierarchy of evidence

Type 1
- Meta-analyses
- Systematic reviews of randomized controlled trials (RCTs)
- RCTs (including cluster RCTs)

Type 2
- Systematic reviews of, or individual, non-RCTs
- Case-control studies
- Cohort studies
- Controlled before-and-after studies
- Interrupted time-series studies
- Correlation studies

Type 3
- Expert opinion
- Formal consensus

Type 4
- Non-analytical studies (e.g. case reports, case series)

Integrated care pathways

These are structured multidisciplinary care plans that outline steps in the care journey of a patient with a specific condition (● Teamwork p. 58). They are evidence-based documents designed to help translate national guidance into local protocols. Care pathways are useful to support communication with patients and other professionals so they know what to expect at each point in their care (● Continuity of care p. 598).

Further information

Cochrane Collaboration (*About*). Available at: ✍ https://www.cochrane.org/about-us
European Pathway Association (*About EPA*) Available at: ✍ http://e-p-a.org/about-epa/
NICE (*Evidence search*). Available at: ✍ https://www.evidence.nhs.uk/
SIGN (*Who we are*). Available at: ✍ http://www.sign.ac.uk/who-we-are.html

Quality and Outcomes Framework

The QOF is part of the General Medical Services contract for general practices (◆ General practice p. 18) introduced in April 2004. QOF is a voluntary reward and incentive programme that rewards GP practices for the quality of care they provide (◆ Quality governance p. 68). QOF helps standardize improvements in the delivery of 1° care and fund further improvements. The results are published every year in all four UK countries but by different organizations (e.g. NHS England works with NHS Digital and the Department of Health and Social Care to provide general practices with individual GP-level data on the care provision for their patients).

QOF domains

- Clinical care
- Public health (◆ Public health in the NHS and beyond p. 14)
- Quality and productivity
- Patient experience (◆ Patient and public experience p. 75)

General Practice Extraction Service reports on many QOF indicators from patient record read codes. QOF and point-system indicators are reviewed annually and new indicators are added and others removed.

Further information

Department of Health Northern Ireland (*QOF—Northern Ireland*). Available at: ℘ https://www.health-ni.gov.uk/topics/doh-statistics-and-research/quality-outcomes-framework-qof

Information Services Division (ISD) Scotland (*QOF—Scotland*). Available at: ℘ http://www.isdscotland.org/Health-Topics/General-Practice/Quality-And-Outcomes-Framework/

NHS Digital (*QOF—England*). Available at: ℘ https://digital.nhs.uk/data-and-information/data-tools-and-services/data-services/general-practice-data-hub/quality-outcomes-framework-qof

NHS Employers (*QOF*). Available at: ℘ https://www.nhsemployers.org/your-workforce/primary-care-contacts/general-medical-services/quality-and-outcomes-framework

NHS Wales (*QOF—Wales*). Available at: ℘ http://www.wales.nhs.uk/sites3/page.cfm?orgid=480&pid=6063

Patient and public experience

Feedback by patients on their experience of services is integral to health service governance (➲ Quality governance p. 68). Patient views on the care they receive in the NHS are collected via the Overall Patient Experience Survey programme, which produces statistics about specific areas of care such as community mental health or cancer care. The NHS Friends and Family Test (FFT) is another example, created to help service providers and commissioners understand patient satisfaction and where improvements are needed. The FFT is used in most NHS services, including community care and GP practices (➲ General practice p. 18). The CQC in England, Healthcare Inspectorate Wales, and Healthcare Improvement Scotland draw on patient feedback to monitor the quality of care delivered.

Patients should be able to comment on areas of service delivery such as clinical care and health-promoting activities, administrative processes, and healthcare environment. Professionals and healthcare organizations can capture information about that experience in different ways and feed it into their quality governance systems. Examples of ways to receive feedback (positive and negative) include: suggestion boxes in reception areas; on-line comments and feedback systems; waiting-room kiosks for electronic feedback; patient surveys, through national programmes and local initiatives; complaints processes (➲ Complaints procedures p. 76); patient representative groups; and as part of clinical audit (➲ Clinical audit p. 70) and QOF activities (➲ Quality and Outcomes Framework p. 74).

In addition, patient-reported outcome measures are structured evaluation tools to measure health gain in patients undergoing certain procedures such as hip replacement or knee replacement surgery in England, based on responses to questionnaires before and after surgery.

Further information

NHS Digital (*Patient reported outcome measures*). Available at: ℘ https://digital.nhs.uk/data-and-information/data-tools-and-services/data-services/patient-reported-outcome-measures-proms

NHS England (*Overall patient experience scores*). Available at: ℘ https://www.england.nhs.uk/statistics/statistical-work-areas/pat-exp/

NHS England (*Friends and Family Test data*). Available at: ℘ https://www.england.nhs.uk/fft/friends-and-family-test-data/

Complaints procedures

Anyone using healthcare services who is unhappy with the treatment or service is entitled to make a complaint, have it considered, and receive a response from the healthcare organization. Every NHS organization and general practice (➔ General practice p. 18) has to publicize its complaints procedures. People generally want: their complaint to be heard and investigated promptly; to be dealt with courteously and sympathetically; to receive an apology if mistakes have occurred; to have the problem rectified promptly if possible; and to be assured that steps will be taken to prevent a recurrence. Complaints procedures are a key part of quality governance (➔ Quality governance p. 68).

Timescale and form of complaint

The complaint can be made by the affected individual or someone acting on their behalf with their consent (➔ Consent p. 82). It should be made within 6mths of the event(s) or from the time they became aware that they had cause for complaint. Can be to any member of staff. Can be to the NHS service provider directly (e.g. hospital) or to the commissioner of the services (➔ Commissioning of service p. 12). Can be by letter, email, phone, or in person. There are several organizations that provide advice and support: Citizens Advice; Local Healthwatch (England); NHS Inform (Scotland); NHS Complaints Advisory Service; Patient Advice and Liaison Service; Health in Wales; and Independent Sector Complaints Adjudication Service. Initial response from the NHS organization should be within 3 days.

Complaint handling at the local level

Every organization should have a named complaints manager who receives all complaints, responds in a timely way, and signposts to local advice or advocacy services. Complaints manager contacts all involved, investigating facts and actions to be taken, and reports progress and outcome back to the complainant. Complaints manager has to summarize findings, assess need for apology, and consider actions taken to both rectify situation and prevent recurrence. Response to complainant may be by letter or face-to-face meeting. Reconciliation should also be offered. All attempts should be made to resolve complaint at local level.

Failure to resolve complaint at the local level

Complainants have right to take their complaint to independent review (e.g. Health Service Ombudsmen (England)).

Further information

Citizens Advice (*NHS and social care complaints*). Available at: ♒ https://www.citizensadvice.org.uk/health/nhs-and-social-care-complaints/

Clinical risk management

Risk is defined as any situation involving exposure to danger. Patient safety is everyone's responsibility. Risk management refers to the process of preventing and controlling the risk of errors and harmful events. Organizations and nurses have a duty to manage risks. Risk management programmes consist of proactive and reactive components. These programmes are a key part of quality governance (◆ Quality governance p. 68).

Risk management in the proactive mode

Efforts are directed at identifying the circumstances and opportunities that put patients, staff, and visitors at risk, and then acting to prevent or control those risks. Involves three-step risk assessment process (Box 3.2).

Risk management in the reactive mode

An adverse incident is any event that could have or did lead to unintended or unexpected harm, loss, or damage. It includes accidents and near misses. On discovering any adverse incident, the person discovering the incident must: ensure the immediate safety of those directly affected by the incident; inform the appropriate senior member of staff or line manager; complete an adverse incident form (usually online); instigate professional duty of candour requirement, being open and honest with the patient and those close to them; and document in patient records (◆ Record keeping p. 86).

All organizations must have systems for centrally reporting incidents. The NHS aims to encourage a 'blame-free' culture that acknowledges most adverse incidents are part of system failure, rather than individual failure. However, a blame-free culture does not override the need for disciplinary or criminal processes in the event of negligent or criminal acts (◆ Professional accountability p. 83). Some adverse incidents must also be

---

Box 3.2 Risk assessment process

Step 1: Identification of possible risks
- Gathering information about how a process works
- Mapping the process
- Identifying all potential risks that might occur during the process

Step 2: Assessment of their potential likelihood and impact
- Assessing the likelihood of the risk occurring (score 1 (rare), 2 (unlikely), 3 (possible), 4 (likely), and 5 (almost certain))
- Assessing the impact if the risk occurs (score 1 (negligible), 2 (minor), 3 (moderate), 4 (major), and 5 (catastrophic))
- Calculating a total risk score by multiplying the likelihood score by the impact score

Step 3: Developing plans to eliminate risk/minimize negative effects
- Ensuring that a strategy is put in place
- Review risk assessment strategy

reported to external bodies such as: MHRA; CQC; health and safety executive; professional regulatory bodies; LA child protection teams (→ Child protection processes p. 252); and LA safeguarding adults referral points (→ Adults at risk from harm and abuse p. 454).

The National Reporting and Learning System receive anonymised data from all patient safety incidents reported by NHS provider organizations. This information is used to identify national patient safety issues.

When an adverse incident happens, it is important to ensure lessons are learnt. Specific root-cause analysis models may be used to help trace errors back to their root. The findings from such investigations will inform the development of precautionary measures to reduce the risk of a similar event happening to another patient, staff member, or visitor in the future.

Multi-agency investigations (e.g. after a child death associated with abuse or neglect) have agreed processes.

Related topics

→ Health and safety at work p. 92

Further information

Healthcare Improvement Scotland (*Scottish patient safety programme*). Available at: ℗ http://www.scottishpatientsafetyprogramme.scot.nhs.uk/

NHS Improvement (*Patient safety improvement hub*). Available at: ℗ https://improvement.nhs.uk/improvement-hub/patient-safety/

Patient Safety Wales (*Supporting NHS organizations to improve patient safety*). Available at: ℗ http://www.patientsafety.wales.nhs.uk/home

Professional conduct

Respect for human rights is the basis for all healthcare practice. Human rights rest on three key principles: every human has certain rights, which are not conferred on him or her, but which arise in him or her by virtue of their humanity alone; a person cannot be deprived of those rights by another or by their own acts; and just laws must be applied consistently, independently, impartially (without fear or favour), and with fair procedures.

UK Human Rights Act 1998

Incorporates into domestic law certain rights from the European Convention and has three main effects: an allegation of a breach of rights can be brought in the UK courts; it is unlawful for a public body (including the NHS) to breach rights; and in situations where courts find that legislation is incompatible with rights set out in the Act, judges can make a 'declaration of incompatibility' where legislation will be referred back to Parliament for reconsideration. Examples of rights set out in the Human Rights Act that relate to healthcare include:

- Article 2: Right to life
- Article 3: Prohibition of torture
- Article 8: Right to respect for private and family life
- Article 14: Prohibition of discrimination
- Article 17: Prohibition of abuse of rights

Professional codes of conduct

Beyond practicing in ways that respect human rights, the NMC Code specifies that registered nurses, health visitors (➲ Health visiting p. 46), and midwives must: act in the best interests of people at all times; treat people as individuals and uphold their dignity; respect people's right to privacy and confidentiality (➲ Confidentiality p. 89); uphold the reputation of the profession at all times; and share their skills, knowledge, and experience for the benefit of people receiving care and of their colleagues.[2] A registered nurse, midwife, or health visitor is personally accountable for their practice, must act lawfully, and be able to justify decisions. Failure to act within The Code can bring fitness to practice into question and, with it, registration.

Reference

2. NMC (2018) *The Code: professional standards of practice and behaviour for nurses and midwives.* Available at: ✍ https://www.nmc.org.uk/standards/code/

Further information

Council of Europe (*Convention for the Protection of Human Rights and Fundamental Freedoms*). Available at: ✍ http://conventions.coe.int/Treaty/en/Treaties/Html/005.htm

Anti-discriminatory healthcare

The Equality Act 2010, underpinned by the Human Rights Act (➔ Professional conduct p. 80), prohibits discrimination, victimization, or harassment of a person. The Act makes it illegal to discriminate on a wide range of grounds including: age; disability; marriage and civil partnership; pregnancy and maternity; race; religion or belief; sex; gender reassignment; and sexual orientation.

Anti-discriminatory practice is required in all aspects of healthcare, from individual practitioners to entire organizations who may (often unintentionally) discriminate against certain groups of people (e.g. by printing leaflets in only one language or not making provision for breastfeeding mothers). The Equality Act 2010 is the legal framework that is used to protect people from discrimination from healthcare providers and employers. Public sector organizations in particular need to comply with the public sector Equality Duty in order to: eliminate discrimination, advance equality of opportunity, and foster good relations with people.

Equality impact assessments are a tool used by NHS organizations to understand whether their policies or activities may affect people differently. Their purpose is to identify and address existing or potential inequalities resulting from policy and practice development, so that they can be addressed.

Further information

Equality and Human Rights Commission (*Our work*). Available at: ℘ https://www.equalityhumanrights.com/en/our-work

Government Equalities Office (*Equality Act 2010: guidance*). Available at: ℘ https://www.gov.uk/guidance/equality-act-2010-guidance

Government Equalities Office (*Public sector: quick start guide to the public sector Equality Duty*). Available at: ℘ https://www.gov.uk/government/publications/public-sector-quick-start-guide-to-the-public-sector-equality-duty

NHS Education for Scotland (*Equality and diversity*). Available at: ℘ https://www.nes.scot.nhs.uk/about-us/equality-and-diversity.aspx

NHS Employers (*Equality analysis and equality impact assessments*). Available at: ℘ https://www.nhsemployers.org/your-workforce/plan/diversity-and-inclusion/tools-and-resources/external-resources/equality-analysis-and-equality-impact-assessments

NHS Wales (*NHS Centre for Equality and Human Rights*). Available at: ℘ http://www.equalityhumanrights.wales.nhs.uk/home

Consent

It is important that a person receiving healthcare agrees to receive it by providing their consent. For consent to be valid, it must be: voluntary (i.e. made by the person themselves, and given without undue pressure or coercion); informed (i.e. the person must understand what the treatment involves, including the benefits and risks and alternatives, and what will happen if treatment does not go ahead); and made by a competent person with capacity (i.e. the person must understand the information given to them and be able to use it to make an informed decision) (➔ Mental capacity p. 470).

Competency is 'function-specific'. This means someone may have capacity to make some healthcare decisions, but may lack capacity to decide more complex matters. All adults (≥18yrs in England and Wales, and ≥16yrs in Scotland) are presumed to be competent, but that presumption can be questioned and refuted. If an adult has the capacity to consent to or refuse a particular treatment, their decision must be respected, even if refusing treatment would result in their death, or the death of their unborn child. If a person does not have the capacity to make a decision about their treatment, and they have not appointed a lasting power of attorney, the healthcare professionals treating them can go ahead and give treatment if they believe it is in the person's best interests. They must however take reasonable steps to seek advice from people who know the person before making these decisions.

Parents can give consent for their child to have treatment if they have parental responsibility and the child is ≤16yrs. The child should consent for themselves if they are believed to have enough intelligence, competence, and understanding to fully appreciate what is involved in their treatment.

The professional providing the care, treatment, or investigation should seek consent. It can be: implied (e.g. holding out arm for blood pressure measurement); verbal (for minor procedures such as venepuncture); or written (for procedures with risk such as surgery). Consent forms act as a record in case of future disputes. In an emergency, treatment can be provided without consent as long as it is limited to saving life or preventing serious injury, and known not to be contrary to previous wishes of a competent patient.

Further information

NHS Wales (*Governance e-manual: patient consent*). Available at: ℬ http://www.wales.nhs.uk/governance-emanual/patient-consent

Royal College of Nursing (*Principles of consent*). Available at: ℬ https://www.rcn.org.uk/professional-development/publications/pub-006047

Professional accountability

Accountability means being responsible for someone or something. All nurses are accountable for their professional practice; individually, they are answerable for their actions and omissions. Nurses can be called to account via: professional regulation (i.e. NMC); criminal law (e.g. law of assault); civil law (e.g. tort of negligence); and employment law (e.g. through enforcement of contract).

Duty of care and negligence

Nurses have a legal and professional duty of care for patients and clients. This means taking reasonable care to avoid acts or omissions that can be reasonably foreseen as likely to be injurious. Patients and clients can make complaints to the organization and NMC about negligent care (€ Complaints procedures p. 76). They can also sue through the civil court. Any court considering a claim of negligence would apply the Bolam test (i.e. that the nurse had acted competently as an ordinary nurse in the view of expert opinion). The Bolam case amended this to state that the expert opinion had to demonstrate a logical basis. Both the employer and the nurse have a responsibility to ensure the latter is competent.

New roles, students, and junior staff

Nurses performing roles usually undertaken by other professionally qualified staff would be judged against the ordinary competent other professional performing that role. Students and junior staff actions are also judged against the ordinary competent professional, and not that of a student or junior. Nurses have a duty to ensure that the care that they delegate to juniors or students is carried out at a reasonably competent standard. This means they remain accountable for the delegation of the work and ensuring that the person who does the work is able to do it.

Vicarious liability

Employers are vicariously liable for the actions and omissions of their staff, which means that if a patient successfully sues for negligence, the employer will usually pay the compensation, not the nurse. However, this only includes those activities within the job description and contract. It does not cover 'Samaritan' acts or acts not specified in the job description. Some employers may seek reimbursement of compensation paid out from the staff member who committed the negligent act. Most nurses pay for professional indemnity through a professional or indemnity organization.

Further information

NHS Resolution (*What we do*). Available at: ℰ https://resolution.nhs.uk/about/our-work/
NMC (*The Code*). Available at: ℰ https://www.nmc.org.uk/standards/code/

Chaperones

All consultations, examinations, and investigations are potentially distressing. Patients can find intimate examinations, investigations, or photography particularly intrusive. Consultations involving dimmed lights, the need for patients to undress, or intensive periods of being touched may also make a patient feel vulnerable. A chaperone is an independent person, appropriately trained, whose role it is to independently observe the examination or procedure undertaken by the health professional and to assist with the appropriate professional–patient relationship. A chaperone is a safeguard for all parties (patient and practitioners) and is a witness to continuing consent to the procedure (➔ Consent p. 82). Every healthcare organization is expected to have a chaperone policy.

Good practice principles

The General Medical Council (GMC) has produced good practice guidance about intimate examinations and recommends[3]:
- Use of a chaperone should be routinely offered.
- Use of a chaperone must be the patient's decision.
- Chaperones should be Disclosure and Barring System checked.
- Patient's family and friends should not be expected to chaperone.
- Children and young people should always be offered a chaperone.

In addition:
- Patients should be made aware of the availability of chaperones through notices and practice leaflets.
- The same principles for offering and use of chaperones should apply in all settings, including home visits and out-of-hours centres.
- Any discussion about chaperones should be recorded in the patient's medical record, including the outcome, the identity of the chaperone, or the reason for declining (➔ Record keeping p. 86).
- If, for justifiable practical reasons, a chaperone cannot be offered, this should be explained to patient and, if possible, the examination delayed until one is available; however, the patient's clinical needs should take precedence.

Reference

3. GMC (2013) *Guidance on intimate examinations and chaperones*. Available at: https://www.gmc-uk.org/ethical-guidance/ethical-guidance-for-doctors/intimate-examinations-and-chaperones

Whistleblowing

Following the Francis Report,[4] NHS organizations have recognized the need to develop a more open and supportive culture that encourages staff to raise any issues of patient care quality or safety (◆ Quality governance p. 68; ◆ Clinical risk management p. 78). Someone is a whistleblower if they are a member of staff and report concerns and certain types of wrongdoing (e.g. poor clinical practice or other malpractice which may harm patients, failure to safeguard patients, maladministration of medicines, and untrained or poorly trained staff).

Protecting practitioners

Practitioners may be too afraid to report something because of fear of victimization, being shunned by their peers, or losing their job. The Public Interest Disclosure Act 1998 sets out the mechanisms for promoting whistleblowing and provides legal protection to people who do this. The practitioner will be 'protected' if they make the disclosure in good faith and reasonably believe that the information disclosed is true.

Action to take

If you have a concern, you should: make an immediate note of your concerns (e.g. what was said, date, time, and names of people involved); convey your suspicions to someone with the appropriate authority and experience (all health organizations should have policies for whistleblowing); and deal with the matter promptly, as delay may cause your organization or patients to suffer or ↑ the risk of harm. Key points:

- Do not ignore poor practice.
- Recognize there may be an innocent or good explanation.
- Do not be afraid of making your concerns known.
- Do not approach or accuse any individuals directly.
- Do not try to investigate the matter yourself.
- Only convey your suspicions to those with the proper authority.

Reference

4. Francis, R. (2013) The Mid Staffordshire NHS Foundation Trust public inquiry. Available at: http://webarchive.nationalarchives.gov.uk/20150407084003/http://www.midstaffspublicinquiry.com/

Further information

NHS England (Whistleblowing) Available at: ℰ https://www.england.nhs.uk/ourwork/whistleblowing/

Record keeping

Good record keeping promotes continuity of care (➔ Continuity of care p. 598; ➔ Teamwork p. 58), acts as a means to demonstrate the quality of care, and provides a resource if nurses are called to account at a later date (➔ Professional accountability p. 83). It may be difficult to convince a court something happened if it was not recorded.

Personal data

The General Data Protection Regulations (GDPR) 2018 define personal data concerning health as 'personal data related to the physical or mental health of a natural person, including the provision of healthcare services, which reveal information about his or her health status'.[5] This could be in the form of audio tapes, emails, photographs, text messages, messages on social media, websites that provide information to patients and staff, or computerized records. Processing of personal health data is only allowed if the patient has given explicit consent (➔ Consent p. 82), it is necessary for reasons of public interest in the area of public health, or it is necessary for preventative or occupational medicine.

General principles for good record keeping

Employees are responsible for any records that they create or use in the course of their duties. Any records created or received by an employee of the NHS are public records and may be subject to both legal and professional (e.g. NMC) obligations. Records should:

- Be contemporaneous
- Include date and time information
- If a paper version, be legible, using black permanent ink, and be signed and name printed
- Be clear, comprehensive, and focused on provision of accurate, objective, factual, and relevant information relating to client's diagnosis/ needs and care/treatment
- Be written in collaboration with patients.

Records should not, in general, include anything you are not prepared to say or reveal to the client. They should not be altered, except to correct inaccurate information. Any alterations should be clearly marked as such and signed/dated.

Details to include when making entries to patient records

- Information on which decisions have been based
- Impressions of the current situation
- Action plan
- Information shared and advice given
- Other essential information (e.g. correspondence with others)

Storage of records

When not in use, records should be stored (including laptops and tablets) under lock and key (Box 3.3). If records are held by the patient or parent/ child, then reinforce the need to keep information secure (➔ Client and patient-held records p. 90).

Box 3.3 Securing patient records

Electronic records
- Do not leave a terminal/laptop unattended and signed-in
- Never share passwords, and change passwords regularly
- Use password-protected screen-savers

Manual records
- Store files closed and in a logical order
- Use a tracking system to monitor whereabouts of files
- Return files as soon as they are no longer needed

Retention of records

The Information Governance Alliance suggests the following as minimum retention periods:[6]
- Children and young people: until their 25th birthday or 26th if young person was 17yrs at time of conclusion of treatment, or 8yrs after patient's death if death occurred before 18th birthday
- Maternity (including midwifery and obstetric): 25yrs
- Patients with mental health problems: 20yrs after no further treatment or 8yrs after patient's death
- Oncology: 30yrs or 8yrs after patient has died
- General: 8yrs after conclusion of treatment
- GP records: 10yrs after death

Destruction of records should be through a secure process organized by the healthcare organization.

Related topics

➔ Access to records p. 88

References

5. Information Commissioner's Office (2018) *GDPR*. Available at: https://ico.org.uk/for-organisations/guide-to-the-general-data-protection-regulation-gdpr/
6. Information Governance Alliance (2016) *Records management code of practice for health and social care 2016*. Available at: https://digital.nhs.uk/data-and-information/looking-after-information/data-security-and-information-governance/codes-of-practice-for-handling-information-in-health-and-care/records-management-code-of-practice-for-health-and-social-care-2016

Further information

Information Commissioners Office (*General data protection regulation: FAQs*). Available at: M https://ico.org.uk/for-organisations/health/health-gdpr-faqs/

Access to records

Patients have legal rights to privacy in the processing of personal data and rights of access to those data.

General Data Protection Regulations

Gives patients (known as 'data subjects') formal rights of access. The right of access (referred to as 'subject access') gives individuals the right to obtain a copy of their personal data and other supplementary information.

Requesting access

An individual can make a subject access request verbally or in writing (including by social media) to any part of an organization. The request does not have to be to a specific person or contact point. You have a maximum of 1mth to comply with the request.

Circumstances when access may be restricted

Access may be restricted when it would be likely to cause serious harm to the physical or mental health of the data subject; also when access would reveal identity of a third person. Does not apply if third person is a health professional involved in care of the data subject, unless giving access is likely to cause serious harm to that health professional.

People who can seek access

- Any competent person (including a competent child/young person)
- Person with parental responsibility for a child (<18yrs old in England and Wales, <16yrs old in Scotland). ⚠ A competent child/young person has a right to confidentiality (➔ Confidentiality p. 89)
- Person appointed by a court on behalf of a person who is incapacitated
- Third party when authorized by data subject
- Executor or administrator of deceased person's estate

Freedom of Information Act 2000

This gives right to access recorded information held by public sector organizations. There are no restrictions on who can request information. Requests are handled under the Data Protection Act 2018, which is the UK's implementation of the General Data Protection Regulations. An organization can refuse a request if the information is too sensitive or the costs of providing it are unreasonable.

Further information

Data Protection Act 2018 (*Your rights and the law*). Available at: ℵ https://www.gov.uk/data-protection

Information Commissioner's Office (*Right of access*). Available at: ℵ https://ico.org.uk/for-organisations/guide-to-the-general-data-protection-regulation-gdpr/individual-rights/right-of-access/

Confidentiality

Confidentiality is when you ensure that information shared by patients is not disclosed to a third party without permission. Preserving confidentiality is: important for maintaining trust between patient and professional; recognized in statue and UK case law; stated by the NMC in The Code; and stated or implied in your employment contract. Although nurses often routinely share information, this should be with patient consent (→ Consent p. 82).

Refusal of consent to share information

The patient should be made aware of the implications of refusal. Their choice should be documented and respected. However, circumstances exist when patient confidentiality can be breached. These include:

- When the patient consents
- In the best interests of the patient (e.g. in emergency)
- To protect a child (e.g. from actual or threatened abuse or under a court order) (→ Child protection processes p. 252)
- To protect an adult at risk of harm (e.g. from abuse of others or self-harm such as threats of suicide) (→ Adults at risk from harm or abuse p. 454; → Suicidal intent and deliberate self-harm p. 494)
- Where disclosure is required by law (e.g. notification of infectious diseases or prevention of terrorism) (→ Infectious disease notifications p. 104)
- In the public interest (e.g. to prevent, detect, or prosecute crime). ⚠ Risk should be serious and substantially reduced by disclosure.

Information disclosed should be limited to that necessary to protect the patient/client/public.

Issues around disclosure and confidentiality may not be clear-cut. It is good practice to discuss the issues with senior colleagues/managers if a situation of potential disclosure arises.

Caldicott guardians and principles

Caldicott guardians are appointed to ensure Caldicott principles of disclosure of patient-identifiable information are applied. These principles state that: disclosure should justify the purpose; patient-identifiable information should not be used unless absolutely necessary, and then only the minimum necessary amount; access to patient-identifiable information should be on a strict 'need-to-know' basis; everyone with access to patient-identifiable information should be aware of their responsibilities and understand and comply with relevant legislation.

Further information

National Data Guardian (*Information: to share or not to share*). Available at: ℘ https://www.gov.uk/government/publications/the-information-governance-review

Client and patient-held records

Patients are increasingly holding their own health and social care records in the UK, although they remain the property of the issuing organization. Local policies will exist as to whether duplicates or summaries are held by the organization or if the patient-held record is the sole record.

Benefits

- Facilitates partnership
- Empowers patients/clients to be involved in their care
- Encourages all contact to be recorded in one place
- Ensures key information is available to the next professional

Limitations

Research studies indicate that while client-/patient-held records are generally of practical benefit, they may place unwanted responsibility on patients or informal carers, and are not always completed by professionals.[7]

Commonly encountered client and patient-held records

- Personal maternity records or co-operation card (◆ Antenatal care and screening p. 426)
- District nursing home records (◆ District nursing p. 50)
- Parent-held child health records
- School child health records (◆ School nursing p. 42)
- Personal health records of asylum applicants and refugees (◆ Asylum seekers and refugees p. 444)
- Local disease-specific patient-held records (e.g. diabetes care (◆ Diabetes: overview p. 660))

Related topics

◆ Access to records p. 86; ◆ Record keeping p. 86

Reference

7. Sartain, S., Stressing, S., & Preito, J. (2016) Patients' views on the effectiveness of patient-held records: a systematic review and thematic synthesis of qualitative studies. *Health Expectations*, 18(6), 2666–77.

Further information

Royal College of Paediatrics and Child Health (*Personal child health record*). Available at: ℜ https://www.rcpch.ac.uk/resources/personal-child-health-record-pchr

Health and safety at work

Poor staff health and well-being has a significant impact on the performance of organizations, so investing in health and well-being has clear benefits for healthcare organizations, staff, and ultimately patients. To comply with the Health and Safety at Work Act 1974, employers also have a legal duty to ensure staff health, safety, and welfare at work.

Employers

Employers must consult staff or their safety representatives on matters relating to health and safety at work (often through safety committees, set up to monitor systems). Employers must:

- Assess and address risks to staff health and safety
- If there are >five staff, record risk assessment and plans, and draw up a health and safety policy available to all
- Appoint a competent person responsible for health and safety
- Set up emergency procedures and provide first-aid facilities
- Ensure the workplace satisfies health, safety, and welfare requirements (e.g. temperature, lighting, and sanitary and rest facilities)
- Ensure work equipment is suitable, maintained, and used properly
- Prevent or control exposure to damaging substances (Control of Substances Hazardous to Health (COSHH) legislation) and protect against danger from flammable, electrical, or explosive hazards, noise, and radiation
- Ensure no hazardous manual handling operations and reduce likelihood of injury (◆ Patient moving and handling p. 96)
- Provide health surveillance as appropriate
- Provide free personal protective equipment (PPE) when risks are not controlled in other ways (◆ Personal protective equipment p. 100)
- Ensure there are safety signs
- Report certain occupational diseases, injuries, and dangerous events to authorities (Reporting of Injuries, Diseases, and Dangerous Occurrences Regulations (RIDDOR)) (◆ Clinical risk management p. 78; ◆ Occupational lung disease p. 752)

Employees

Employees also have legal duties, including:

- Taking reasonable care for their own and others health and safety
- Co-operating with employer on health and safety issues
- Correctly using work items provided by employers (including PPE)
- Not interfering with or misusing anything provided for health and safety

Safety representatives

Safety representatives are appointed by trade unions to represent their members on health and safety issues, and may represent entire workforces. They are entitled to paid time off to carry out their role. Unions offer full training and information backup.

Health, safety, and welfare in healthcare organizations

Key areas of attention in the NHS are: ↓ accidents and MSK injuries (❍ Common musculoskeletal problems p. 734); reducing stress and violence to staff (❍ Managing stress p. 358; ❍ Lone working p. 94); providing smoke-free workplaces; tackling bullying and harassment; reducing risk of blood-borne viruses (❍ Occupational exposure to blood-borne viruses p. 102) and latex allergies (❍ Hand hygiene p. 98; ❍ Allergies p. 694); ensuring occupational health services are offered to all staff; and ensuring sickness absence and opportunities for rehabilitation and redeployment are managed well.

Health and safety at work concerns

Concerns should be raised with the employer or manager, or through the safety representative. If they fail to act or respond satisfactorily, the employee or safety representative can contact health and safety inspectors of the enforcing authority. Anyone can get health and safety information confidentially from the Health and Safety Executive's (HSE) information line (☎ 0300 003 1647).

Related topics

❍ Targeted adult immunization p. 392; ❍ Whistleblowing p. 85

Further information

HSE (*Health and Safety at Work Act 1974*). Available at: ℅ http://www.hse.gov.uk/legislation/hswa. htm

HSE (*COSHH*). Available at: ℅ http://www.hse.gov.uk/coshh/

HSE (*RIDDOR 2013*). Available at: ℅ http://www.hse.gov.uk/riddor/

NHS Employers (*NHS health and well-being framework*) Available at: ℅ http://www.nhsemployers. org/case-studies-and-resources/2018/05/nhs-health-and-wellbeing-framework

NHS Employers (*Health and safety*). Available at: ℅ https://www.nhsemployers.org/ staffwelfareissues

Lone working

Lone workers are those who work by themselves without close or direct supervision, out of sight or earshot of another colleague. Employers have a duty to assess risks to lone workers and take steps to avoid or control risks where necessary, as lone workers should not be put at ↑ risk compared to other employees (➔ Clinical risk management p. 78; ➔ Health and safety at work p. 92). Working in the health and social care sector may mean dealing with unpredictable client behaviour and situations arising from impatience, frustration, anxiety, resentment, drink or drugs, and inherent aggression or poor mental health. Employers should conduct risk assessments to help decide the right level of supervision or other measures that are required. Wherever possible and legally permissible, health and other public sector providers should share information on individuals and addresses known to be a risk. All services should have a system for keeping staff details required in an emergency (e.g. mobile and home numbers, next of kin, car registration and model, staff photographs).

Good practice guidance for lone working and home visiting

There is a wide range of technology that can support lone workers. Some devices are integrated into mobile phones and some are stand-alone units, such as SIM cards within ID badge holders. Staff should make sure a lone worker device is well maintained, charged, and is carried in line with local procedures.

Scheduling appointments and reporting movements

Ensure colleagues are aware of one another's movements including full addresses, details of home visiting, journey details, telephone numbers, and anticipated arrival and departure times. Some areas use texting to let a colleague know when a staff member has safely left after each home visit. All staff need to know procedures if colleagues do not return when expected.

If the patient, relative, or carer has a history of violence or the location is considered unsafe

Do not visit alone. If possible, contact should take place at a neutral location or within a secure environment.

Key safety equipment to be carried

Safety equipment includes ID badge, map of the local area, personal attack alarm, torch, and mobile phone. The phone should be kept fully charged and close at hand, with emergency contacts on speed dial. It is important to check the mobile signal before entering lone worker situations. Do not use phones overtly in open spaces, to avoid theft.

Arriving at and conducting the appointment

- When the front door is opened, carry out a 10-sec risk assessment
- Have an excuse ready should it be deemed necessary not to enter
- Request that animals be secured prior to entry
- Shut the front door and be familiar with the door lock
- Maintain awareness of entrances and exists
- If uncomfortable, do not sit down and do not spread belongings out
- If feeling unsafe, make an excuse and leave immediately

If something happens

Incidents and 'near misses' provide details about violent individuals, unsafe environments, and other important information on the risks faced, so they should always be reported to the manager.

Good practice principles for travelling

Lone working and vehicles

Ensure enough petrol and join a recovery breakdown service. Do not leave valuables visible. Avoid nurse-on-call badges, as they may encourage thieves looking for controlled drugs (⊃ Controlled drugs p. 144). Hold keys when leaving premises to avoid looking for them outside. Lock doors/shut windows at slow speed and traffic lights. Park in well-lit locations, facing the direction you wish to leave.

Lone working and public transport

Use a busy bus stop or train station that is well-lit. Keep a transport timetable. Sit near the driver, in an aisle seat and near emergency alarm. Avoid upper decks, empty carriages, or carriages occupied by only one other person.

Lone working and travelling by foot

Walk briskly and do not stop in unfamiliar areas. If carrying equipment, use bags that do not advertise what is carried. In the event of attempted theft, relinquish property at once. Keep house keys and mobile phone separate from handbag. Remain aware of location and surrounding people. Avoid waste ground, isolated pathways, and subways.

Further information

Health and Safety Executive (*Lone working*). Available at: ℵ www.hse.gov.uk/treework/site-management/lone-working.htm

NHS Employers (*Improving safety for lone workers: a guide for staff*). Available at: ℵ http://www.nhsemployers.org/case-studies-and-resources/2018/03/improving-safety-for-lone-workers-a-guide-for-staff-who-work-alone

Suzie Lamplugh Trust (*About us*). Available at: ℵ www.suzylamplugh.org

Patient moving and handling

Manual handling is defined by the Manual Handling Operations Regulations 1992 as any transporting or supporting of a load (including lifting, putting down, pushing, pulling, carrying, or moving) by hand or bodily force. Patient moving and handling is a part of the everyday role of the nurse. However, poor moving and handling can cause: back pain and MSK disorders (➔ Common musculoskeletal problems p. 734); moving and handling accidents, injuring the patient and nurse; and lack of dignity for the patient.

Legislation

The following legislation is relevant to moving and handling:
- Health and Safety at Work Act 1974
- Manual Handling Operations Regulations 1992 (as amended 2002)
- Provision and Use of Work Equipment Regulations 1998
- Lifting Operations and Lifting Equipment Regulations 1998

⚠: Employees have a duty to obey reasonable instructions and cooperate with employers in manual handling procedures (➔ Health and safety at work p. 92).

Risk assessment

Action must be taken to prevent or ↓ the risk of injury (➔ Clinical risk management p. 78). Manual handling should be avoided where reasonable and practicable. If not reasonable and practical, legislation requires that a moving and handling risk assessment is undertaken. The LITE mnemonic is helpful (Box 3.4). Control measures (including the provision of equipment) should be introduced in response to the risk assessment. The risk assessment and associated control measures should be documented (➔ Record keeping p. 86). Reassess if there is a change to the load, the individual, the task, or the environment, as per local policy.

Moving and handling equipment

Patient handling aids should be used whenever they can ↓ the risk of injury (➔ Assistive technology and home adaptations p. 834). Their selection should be based on individual patient assessment and consideration of handler safety. Equipment may include:
- Hoists (including ceiling hoists and mobile hoists) and slings
- Bath lifts and adjustable height baths
- Slide sheets
- Turning tables
- Electric profiling beds
- Wheelchairs
- Handling belts
- Lifting cushions
- Bed levers, support rails and poles
- Emergency evacuation equipment
- Suitable walking aids, hand rails, etc.
- Raised toilet seats
- Transfer boards and swivel seats

Box 3.4 LITE mnemonic

Load (the patient)

- Expectations, co-operation, and level of understanding
- Rehabilitation potential
- Ability to weight bear, history of falls
- Pain or arthritis
- Problems with sight or spatial awareness
- Body weight and distribution (including amputation)
- Medication that might affect mobility
- Ataxia or balance disorders

Individual capacity (the handler)

- Physical capabilities, health, and fitness
- Up-to-date moving and handling training
- ⚠: All employers have a duty to provide training and regular updates for staff involved in the moving and handling of patients
- Suitability of clothing and footwear
- Heights of people working together
- Familiarity with chosen equipment

Task

- The task to be performed (e.g. move from bed to chair)

Environment

- Location of the task (e.g. clinic room or patient bedroom)
- Space available
- Presence of hazards (e.g. obstacles or slippery surfaces)
- Gradients or distances involved

Some items may be ordered by nurses from the local loans service. Others may be classified as specialist equipment and will need to be ordered by a physiotherapist or occupational therapist. If the patient refuses equipment, negotiation skills are important. Staff need to report such refusal to the line manager as the risk of injury to staff has to be considered alongside the risk to the patient if a particular procedure is not carried out.

⚠: Moving and handling equipment may be classified as medical devices and regulated by the MHRA. Devices should be used as per manufacturer instructions. See local policies on both medical devices and decontamination of medical devices.

Further information

Health and Safety Executive (*Moving and handling in health and social care*). Available at: ℘ http://www.hse.gov.uk/healthservices/moving-handling.htm

Hand hygiene

⚠ Hand decontamination is the single, most important practice to prevent healthcare-associated infection. Nurses should ensure they have access to liquid soap, disposable paper towels, hand moisturizer, and alcohol hand rub. Nurses visiting patients in their own homes should consider the benefits of carrying their own hand decontamination kit. Occasions when hands must be decontaminated include:

- Before starting and when finishing work
- Whenever hands become soiled
- Before and after every patient contact
- Before different care activities for the same patient
- After handling equipment used by patients
- After handling specimens, wasted and used linen
- After removing gloves (⊃ Personal protective equipment p. 100)
- Before preparing, handling, and eating food (⊃ Home food safety and hygiene p. 352)
- After going to the toilet
- After coughing and blowing nose

Preparation for hand decontamination

Nurses should ensure that their hands can be decontaminated throughout the duration of clinical work by:

- Being bare below the elbow when delivering direct patient care
- Removing wrist and hand jewellery
- Making sure fingernails are short, clean, and free of nail polish
- Covering cuts and abrasions with waterproof dressings

Decontamination by alcohol hand rub

Decontamination of hands can be carried out either by handwashing with liquid soap or by the use of alcohol hand rub. The current recommendation is that alcohol hand rub should be the main way of decontaminating hands, except in situations where hands are visibly soiled, and in cases of diarrhoea where there is the potential for organisms resistant to alcohol to spread (e.g. Clostridium difficile). Using alcohol hand rub should take 20–30secs (Box 3.5).

Box 3.5 Seven steps to using alcohol hand rub

- Apply a palmful of the product in a cupped hand
- Rub hands palm to palm
- Right palm over left dorsum with interlaced fingers, and vice versa
- Palm to palm with fingers interlaced
- Backs of fingers to opposing palms with fingers interlocked
- Rotational rubbing of left thumb clasped in right palm, and vice versa
- To clean fingertips, rotational rubbing backwards and forwards with clasped fingers of right hand in left palm and vice versa

Decontamination by hand washing

Hand washing should take 40–60secs. To wash hands effectively:
- Wet hands with water and apply enough liquid soap to cover all hand surfaces
- Rub hands palm to palm
- Right palm over left dorsum with interlaced fingers, and vice versa
- Palm to palm with fingers interlaced
- Backs of fingers to opposing palms with fingers interlocked
- Rotational rubbing of left thumb clasped in right palm, and vice versa
- To clean fingertips, rotational rubbing backwards and forwards with clasped fingers of right hand in left palm, and vice versa
- Rinse hands with water
- Dry hands thoroughly with a single use towel
- Use towel to turn off tap

Related topics

➲ Managing healthcare waste p. 106; ➲ Principles of working with someone with an infectious disease p. 467

Further information

NICE (*Healthcare-associated infections: prevention and control in primary and community care* [CG139]). Available at: ℗ https://www.nice.org.uk/Guidance/CG139

WHO (*Hand hygiene: why, how and when?*) Available at: ℗ http://www.who.int/gpsc/5may/Hand_Hygiene_Why_How_and_When_Brochure.pdf

Personal protective equipment

Personal protective equipment (PPE) protects the user against health and safety risks at work (✪ Health and safety at work p. 92). Selection is based on an assessment of the risk of transmission of micro-organisms to the patient or healthcare practitioner, and the risk of contamination of the healthcare practitioner's clothing and skin by patients' blood, body fluids, secretions, or excretions (✪ Occupational exposure to blood-borne viruses p. 102). In community settings, common types of equipment include gloves and aprons, and sometimes goggles and masks. These items are for single use only. Employers have legal duties relating to the provision and use of PPE at work. Practitioners should be trained in using the PPE they need in their role.

Gloves

Should be used for invasive procedures including contact with sterile sites, non-intact skin, or mucous membranes, and for all activities that have been assessed as carrying a risk of exposure to blood, body fluid, or infectious respired aerosols or droplets. They must be applied immediately before an episode of patient contact and removed as soon as the episode of care is completed. They should be changed when soiled. Instructions for application: select either sterile or non-sterile gloves as appropriate; select appropriate hand size glove; decontaminate hands; and extend to cover wrist. Outside of the glove is contaminated. Instructions for removal: hold the outside of the glove with the opposite gloved hand; peel off; hold the removed glove in the gloved hand; slide the fingers of the ungloved hand under the remaining glove at the wrist; peel the second glove off over the first; discard as per local policy (✪ Managing healthcare waste p. 106); and decontaminate hands.

Materials include plastic, latex, nitrile, or neoprene. Different materials provide different levels of protection. For example, plastic gloves are not recommended in clinical practice other than when preparing or serving food. All materials can potentially cause contact dermatitis (✪ Eczema/dermatitis p. 684). ⚠ Latex is hazardous to human health. Latex allergy is hypersensitivity to latex proteins in individuals with latex-specific antibodies from previous exposure and sensitization (✪ Allergies p. 694). Signs and symptoms include contact urticarial, itching of the skin and eyes, sneezing, bronchospasm, asthma (✪ Asthma in adults p. 608), and anaphylaxis (✪ Anaphylaxis p. 810). These symptoms can occur in people previously not known to be sensitized. Evidence suggests that powdered gloves have ↑ latex allergen content than powder-free gloves. Employers should consider the risks and benefits when selecting gloves for use by healthcare practitioners (✪ Clinical risk management p. 78); making a judgement on whether to use latex-free or powder-free latex gloves.[8] Practitioners with latex allergy, latex sensitivity, or latex-induced asthma should use non-latex gloves.

Gloves are not a substitute for effective hand washing (✪ Hand hygiene p. 98); nor are they required where there is a ↓ risk of cross infection between patients and healthcare practitioners and no blood/body fluid exposure (e.g. measuring blood pressure, temperature, and pulse).

Plastic aprons

Plastic aprons must be worn when in close contact with patients, materials, or equipment that pose a risk of contamination with blood or body fluids. Practitioners should ensure aprons/gowns are changed when visibly soiled and are worn for one procedure or episode of patient care only. Instructions for application: pull apron over the head and fasten at the back of the waist. Apron front is contaminated. Instructions for removal: unfasten or break ties at the back; pull apron away from the neck and shoulders, lifting over the head, touching inside only; fold or roll into a bundle; discard as per local policy; and decontaminate hands.

Face masks and eye protection

Fluid-repellent masks and eye protection should be worn when there is a risk of blood or body fluid splashing onto the eyes and face of the healthcare practitioner, and to protect against respired infectious aerosols/droplets (e.g. pulmonary TB (◆ Tuberculosis p. 728) and avian influenza (◆ Pandemic influenza p. 726)). Selection of the appropriate mask will be guided by the infection control team and take into account the infective micro-organism, anticipated activity, and duration of exposure. Respiratory masks rely on a good seal with the wearer's face and should be face fit tested. Face masks should be removed at the end of the clinical procedure and changed if reliability is compromised (e.g. if wet). They should be removed by pulling strings (or other securing devices) away from the side of the face. Always refer to manufacturer's instructions for use.

PPE must be removed in the following order to minimize the risk of cross/self-contamination: gloves, then apron, and lastly eye protection and face mask.

Related topics

◆ Principles of working with someone with compromised immunity p. 466;
◆ Principles of working with someone with infectious disease p. 467

Reference

8. Royal College of Physicians and NHS Plus (2008) *Latex allergy: occupational aspects of management*. Available at: https://www.nhshealthatwork.co.uk/images/library/files/Clinical%20excellence/Latex_allergy_hc_professionals_leaflet.pdf

Further information

NHS Education for Scotland (*Cleanliness champions: personal protective equipment*). Available at: ♫ https://www.nes.scot.nhs.uk/media/4011312/ccp_unit_4.pdf

Occupational exposure to blood-borne viruses

Occupational exposure to blood-borne viruses is unnecessarily common and most frequently associated with Hepatitis B and C (➔ Viral hepatitis p. 724), and HIV (➔ Human immunodeficiency virus p. 462). Many exposures result from a lack of training or a failure to follow recommended procedures, including safe handling and disposal of needles and syringes (➔ Sharps injuries p. 108), or wearing personal protective eyewear where indicated (➔ Personal protective equipment p. 100). All healthcare workers, including temporary staff, should be vaccinated against Hepatitis B (➔ Targeted adult immunization p. 392). It is important to remember that healthcare workers providing care to people in the community and care homes (➔ Care homes p. 32) should also be protected. Other high-risk workers are prison staff. Wherever possible, the use of 'safer sharps' is recommended (➔ Health and safety at work p. 92; ➔ Sharps injuries p. 108).

Accidental exposure to blood and body fluids can occur through:

- Percutaneous injury (e.g. used needles, bone fragments, significant bites that break the skin)
- Exposure of broken skin (e.g. abrasions, cuts, eczema (➔ Eczema/dermatitis p. 684))
- Exposure of mucous membranes (including the eyes and mouth)

Increased risk of exposure is associated with:

- Deep injury
- Visible blood on the device which caused the injury
- Injury with a needle, which had been placed in the source patient's artery or vein
- Terminal HIV-related illness in the source patient

Not associated with saliva, urine, vomit, or faeces, unless blood is present. There is no risk of HIV transmission where intact skin is exposed to HIV-infected blood. Every employer should have a policy on the management of occupational exposures to blood-borne viruses. All nurses must have immediate 24-hr access to advice, through either an occupational health service or out-of-hours cover provided by A&E departments.

Post-exposure response

Following accidental exposure to blood and body fluids, regardless of whether or not the source is known to pose an infection risk, you should:

- Immediately stop what you are doing and attend the injury
- Encourage bleeding of the wound by applying gentle pressure. ⚠ Do not suck
- Wash wound well under running water
- Dry and apply a waterproof dressing as necessary
- If blood and body fluids splash into eyes, irrigate with cold water
- If blood and body fluids splash into your mouth, do not swallow, and rinse out several times with cold water

Report the incident in line with local policy and complete an accident/incident form (➔ Clinical risk management p. 78). If the injury is from a used needle or instrument, risk assessment should be carried out by an occupational health adviser, virologist, or other suitable professional. The assessment will include the type and depth of the wound, whether gloves were worn, and the health worker's Hepatitis B antibody levels. Should the staff member have low immunity to Hepatitis B, a booster is normally given straight away. Consent is required if blood needs to be taken from the source, if known (**➲** Consent p. 82).

Post-exposure prophylaxis (PEP) following exposure to HIV consists of a combination of antiretroviral drugs that, ideally, should be started within 1hr. PEP may still be considered up to 2wks following exposure. Exposed nurses should be encouraged to:

Post-exposure prophylaxis

- Provide a baseline blood sample for storage for up to 2yrs and a follow-up sample for testing
- Seek psychological support (**➲** Talking therapies p. 472)
- Report any sickness absence associated with adverse effects of PEP drugs following an occupational exposure; such absence does not contribute to an individual's sickness absence record

Further information

PHE (*Blood-borne viruses in healthcare workers: report exposures and reduce risks*). Available at: ↪ https://www.gov.uk/guidance/bloodborne-viruses-in-healthcare-workers-report-exposures-and-reduce-risks

RCN (*Essential practice for infection prevention and control*). Available at: ↪ https://www.rcn.org.uk/professional-development/publications/pub-005940

Infectious disease notifications

Since the beginning of the 19th century, certain infectious diseases have been notifiable (Box 3.6). The statutory process aims to ensure speed in identifying possible outbreaks and epidemics, and prevention of spread of infectious disease. The specific diseases are selected for notification because they are potentially life-threatening, spread rapidly, and cannot be easily treated. Occasionally, notification is used to monitor success of immunization programmes (❸ Childhood immunization schedule (UK) p. 166) and the development of localized outbreaks.

If a GP (❸ General practice p. 18) becomes aware/suspects that a patient has a notifiable disease or is suffering from food poisoning, there is

---

Box 3.6 Notifiable diseases

- Acute encephalitis
- Acute poliomyelitis
- Anthrax
- Cholera
- Coronavirus (COVID19)
- Diphtheria
- Dysentery*
- Food poisoning
- Leptospirosis
- Malaria
- Measles
- Meningitis (including meningococcal, pneumococcal, haemophilus influenzae, viral, other specified, and unspecified)
- Meningococcal septicaemia (without meningitis)
- Mumps
- Ophthalmia neonatorum
- Paratyphoid fever
- Plague
- Rabies
- Relapsing fever
- Rubella
- Scarlet fever
- Smallpox
- Tetanus
- Tuberculosis
- Typhoid fever
- Viral haemorrhagic fever
- Viral hepatitis (including Hepatitis A, B, and C)
- Whooping cough
- Yellow fever

NB. Leprosy is also notifiable, but directly to the HPA.

* Causes of dysentery or bloody diarrhoea include amoebiasis, caused by a single-cell parasite entamoeba histolytica frequently picked up abroad, and bacillary dysentery (shigellosis), caused by shigella bacteria, and the most common type of dysentery in the UK. Both types of dysentery can also be transmitted sexually.

a statutory duty in England and Wales to notify the 'proper officer' (usually the medical consultant for environmental health or consultant in communicable disease control) (◆ Food-borne disease p. 730). For local contact details see the Health Protection Agency (HPA).

The notification form to be completed is available online ℘ (https://www.gov.uk/government/publications/notifiable-diseases-form-for-registered-medical-practitioners). If urgent action is required, information should be phoned/communicated electronically. Information must include: name, age and sex of patient; current address and location of the patient; details of disease or poisoning, and date of onset; and other relevant information (e.g. if individual has been abroad).

In Scotland, healthcare providers and other agencies should report to NHS organizations who are required to notify the Common Services Agency, who inform Health Protection Scotland.

Schools

OFSTED (England) (◆ Working in schools p. 44) should be notified of:
- Any food poisoning affecting two or more children
- Any child having meningitis or the outbreak on the premises of any notifiable disease identified as such in the Public Health (Control of Disease) Act 1984 or because the notification requirement has been applied to them by relevant regulations (Public Health (Infectious Diseases) Regulations 1988)

Further information

Health Protection Scotland (*Notifiable disease data*). Available at: ℘ https://www.hps.scot.nhs.uk/publichealthact/NotifiableInfectiousDiseaseData.aspx

NHS Wales (*About the notification of infectious disease in Wales*). Available at: ℘ https://www.wales.nhs.uk/sites3/page.cfm?orgid=457&pid=48544

PHE (*Notifiable diseases and causative organisms: how to report*). Available at: ℘ https://www.gov.uk/guidance/notifiable-diseases-and-causative-organisms-how-to-report

Managing healthcare waste

Disposal of clinical waste

An essential part of an employer's overall health and safety management system and staff training (➲ Working in schools p. 44). The organization should have access to a dedicated, qualified waste manager. Hypodermic needles and other hazardous healthcare wastes should never be disposed of in the domestic waste stream (➲ Sharps injuries p. 108). Nurses have a responsibility to protect the health of their patients and the natural environment. Categories of waste are summarized in Table 3.1. Clinical waste is classified as 'hazardous waste' and should be transported as an infectious substance. An 'offensive' waste stream describes non-infectious wastes. Local policies and guidance should be followed.

Identification of infectious waste

Only waste generated from healthcare practice undertaken by a suitably qualified health professional will be considered infectious waste. Bodily fluids that may be infectious include blood, semen, and vaginal secretions.

Non-infectious bodily fluids include faeces, nasal secretions, sputum, tears, urine, and vomit. However, these may be considered infectious if they contain visible blood or the source patient has been assessed as having an infection that might be transmitted via the waste (i.e. an infection pathway exists, e.g. faeces known/suspected of contamination with enteric pathogens such as Salmonella spp. or Shigella spp., or vomit from patient with acute vomiting virus).

Collection of waste

- Infectious waste should be collected weekly
- Sharps bins should be collected at least every 3mths
- Waste transfer note to be completed to keep track of the waste
- All sites producing hazardous waste must notify the Environment Agency

Table 3.1 Categories of waste and receptacles

Waste category	Receptacle/colour coding	Examples of contents
Domestic waste	Black bag	General refuse (e.g. newspapers)
Infectious waste	Orange bag	Infectious and potentially infectious waste (e.g. soiled dressings)
Offensive waste	Yellow bag with black stripes	Incontinence pads, nappies, sanitary pads, plaster casts, etc.
Sharps	Yellow bin	Not contaminated with cytotoxic products; sharps from phlebotomy
Sharps	Yellow bin with blue top	Contaminated with cytotoxic and/or cytostatic medicinal products

- Vehicles used by community nurses are exempt from regulation procedures regarding registered waste carriers
- If patients are treated in their home by a community nurse, any waste produced as a result is considered to be the nurse's waste

Aims of waste management

- Waste reduction and prevention
- Reusable/recyclable products
- Reduction of disposal of waste to landfills
- The use of cleaner technologies
- Energy recovery
- An integrated network of waste management facilities

Further information

Department of Health and Social Care (*Management and disposal of healthcare waste*). Available at 🖰 https://www.gov.uk/government/publications/guidance-on-the-safe-management-of-healthcare-waste

Health and Safety Executive (*Management of healthcare waste*). Available at: 🖰 http://www.hse.gov.uk/healthservices/healthcare-waste.htm

Royal College of Nursing (*Essential practice for infection prevention and control*). Available at: 🖰 https://www.rcn.org.uk/professional-development/publications/pub-005940

Sharps injuries

Employers are required to assess the risk of sharps injuries and, where possible, eliminate the use of sharps (➋ Health and safety at work p. 92; ➋ Clinical risk management p. 78). Sharps include needles, blades, suture cutters, broken glass. Sharps injuries are a major cause of transmission of blood-borne viruses (➋ Occupational exposure to blood-borne viruses p. 102) and should be treated as a serious event.

⚠ All staff at risk of sharps injuries should have up-to-date Hepatitis B vaccination (➋ Viral hepatitis p. 724; ➋ Targeted adult immunization p. 392).

Prevention of sharps injuries

- Ensure workforce has received training.
- Always assume there is a risk following a sharps injury.
- Keep sharps handling to a minimum.
- Use needle safety devices if available.
- Sharps containers should be as close as possible to the point of use.
- Sharps must not be passed directly from hand to hand.
- Needles must not be recapped, bent/broken, or disassembled after use.
- Containers in public areas must be located in a safe position.
- Used sharps must be disposed of at the point of use by the user.
- Containers must not be filled above the indicator marking they are full.

Where a patient uses sharps as part of their self-treatment, they are responsible for safe disposal. They can arrange for the local authority to collect sharps bins for disposal.

There is no specific guidance available on the carriage of sharps containers in cars but the employer should agree practice with the infection control committee. The car should be securely locked when unoccupied and the sharps container kept out of sight. Containers must always be disposed of by the licensed route (➋ Managing healthcare waste p. 106).

If someone sustains a sharps injury, follow the steps set out in ➋ Occupational exposure to blood-borne viruses p. 102.

Related topics

➋ Injection techniques p. 576; ➋ Immunization administration p. 390

Further information

Royal College of Nursing (*Essential practice for infection prevention and control*). Available at: ⟡ https://www.rcn.org.uk/professional-development/publications/pub-005940

Chapter 4

Approaches to individual health needs assessment

Principles, theories, and models *110*
Integrated assessment for adults *112*
Case management *114*
Consultation models and frameworks *116*
Standardized assessment tools *118*
Principles of good communication in patient assessment *120*
Adults and children with additional communication needs *122*
Assessment by remote consultation *124*
Motivational interviewing in consultations *126*

Principles, theories, and models

The purpose of assessment at an individual level is to establish a baseline of the health and well-being of the person and create a mutually agreed plan of care. Comprehensive assessment of ↑ quality is the means by which people access care and services that are tailored to their needs. Assessment strategies are influenced by: the problem-solving framework of the nursing process (i.e. assessment, planning, implementation, and evaluation); nursing models, theories, and values (e.g. focus on ADL, self-care, and health promotion); specialism (e.g. health visiting (🢂 Health visiting p. 46), district nursing (🢂 District nursing p. 50), or general practice nursing (🢂 General practice nursing p. 40)); patient group (e.g. children, young people, older people); national and local policy (e.g. integrated assessments for children, young people, and families (🢂 Assessment of children, young people, and families p. 156)); and electronic patient record systems that dictate how assessment data is collected, recorded, and shared.

Principles

- Assessment is one aspect of case management (🢂 Case management p. 114).
- Assessment should incorporate a sense of the person's own ratings of health status.
- Assessment should focus on the health needs of people and their carers (🢂 Carers p. 458); what is available from the service should not limit the assessment.
- Objective and quantifiable data, plus subjective and person-focused data, is important for a rounded assessment.
- Assessment includes the extent to which and the ways in which identified needs and problems are currently being addressed, plus factors that ameliorate or reduce the impact of the needs and problems (i.e. a strengths-based approach); it is important that assessments do not focus exclusively on what the person cannot do.
- Assessment should lead to the identification of agreed problems and needs for which a plan of care can be devised in collaboration with the person.
- Assessment and the identification of agreed problems and needs provides the basis for selection of nursing interventions and referrals to other professionals and organizations.
- After implementation of the plan of care, further assessment serves to evaluate outcomes and effect, as well as identify new problems and needs.

Most individual health needs assessments will include a biographical profile; physiological, psychological, and sociocultural development; and spiritual domains.

Theories influencing assessment

Maslow's 'Hierarchy of Needs'

Comprises a five-tier model of human needs, often depicted as hierarchical levels in a pyramid. Needs lower down in the hierarchy must be satisfied before people can attend to needs higher up. From the bottom of the hierarchy upwards, the needs are: physiological, safety, love and belonging, esteem, and self-actualization.

Bradshaw's 'Taxonomy of Needs'

Developed to help services understand the different ways in which needs are perceived, expressed, and measured. Four types of needs are identified: normative (those accepted in society or by professionals as the norm); felt (as perceived by the individual); expressed (as felt and acted upon in some way by the individual); and comparative (compared with others).

Models directing assessments by nurses

Activities of daily living model

Draws on Roper, Logan, and Tierney's 'Model of Nursing'. Uses the 12 ADL as units of assessment to encourage a focus on health rather than ill health: breathing; maintaining a safe environment; communication; eating and drinking; elimination; washing and dressing; controlling temperature; mobilizing; working and playing; expressing sexuality; sleeping; and death and dying.

Self-care model

Draws on Orem's 'Self-Care Deficit Theory of Nursing'. Widely used in disease prevention and health promotion. Assessment based on self-care requisites and self-care deficits.

Biomedical or diagnostic model

Comprises history taking, physical examination, and clinical investigations to arrive at a working diagnosis. A model often used by advanced nurse practitioners.

Related topics

➔ Consultation models and frameworks p. 116; ➔ Integrated assessment for adults p. 112; ➔ Standardized assessment tools p. 118

Integrated assessment for adults

Five Year Forward View sets out to deliver models of care that break the artificial boundaries between hospitals and 1° care, between health and social care, and between generalists and specialists, to deliver care that is co-ordinated around what patients need and want[1] (➔ Teamwork p. 58). Assessment is central to identifying needs. As the health and social care of older people and people with multiple co-morbidities becomes more complex, there is ↑ requirement for co-ordinated, effective, and efficient assessment.[2]

Single or integrated assessments are seen as a way to ↓ bureaucracy, duplication, and administration for frontline staff; conserve resources; and improve the patient experience, given they will only have to tell their story once.[3,4] Assessments must be holistic and patient-centred, and consider areas that might previously have been the preserve of one professional group:[4]

- Physical and mental health and emotional well-being
- Protection from abuse and neglect
- Education, training, and recreation
- Domestic, family, and personal relationships
- Contribution made to society
- Securing rights and entitlements
- Social and economic well-being

Single or integrated assessments require a different type of professional; someone who is not tied by traditional boundaries and has a broader range of skills. Development activities (➔ Continuing professional development p. 53) include: talking to a colleague from another discipline about how they approach assessment; undertaking some joint visits with a colleague from another discipline and reflecting together on the differences in approach ; and sharing or teaching skills.[2]

References

1. NHS England (2014) *Five Year Forward View*. Available at: https://www.england.nhs.uk/wp-content/uploads/2014/10/5yfv-web.pdf
2. Health Education England (undated) *Introducing integrated care and assessment*. Available at: https://www.hee.nhs.uk/our-work/integrated-care
3. NHS England (2012) *A narrative for person-centred, coordinated (integrated) care*. Available at: https://www.england.nhs.uk/wp-content/uploads/2013/05/nv-narrative-cc.pdf
4. Welsh Government (2013) *Integrated assessment, planning and review arrangements for older people*. Available at: https://www.rcpsych.ac.uk/pdf/131217reporten.pdf

Case management

Case management is a generic term, with various definitions. The Case Management Society of America (CMSA) describe it as a collaborative process of assessment, planning, facilitation, care co-ordination, evaluation, and advocacy for options and services to meet a patient's and family's comprehensive health needs through communication and available resources, to promote quality and cost-effective outcomes.[5] It is an approach characterized by one person (e.g. nurse, social worker, AHP) having designated responsibility to co-ordinate and oversee care to ensure it is integrated and actively managed (⊃ Continuity of care p. 598). Case management is indicated at Levels 1 and 2 of the generic long-term conditions model (⊃ Generic long-term conditions model p. 6).

Core components of a case management programme

Case finding

Systematic method to identify patients at ↑ risk of hospital admission or other adverse events (⊃ Services to prevent unplanned hospital admission p. 22). There are a number of statistical tools and techniques that can be used alongside clinical judgement to predict a patient's risk of future admission.

Assessment

Patient assessment will include: clinical background and current health status; current level of mobility; current ability and needs in terms of ADL; current level of cognitive functioning; current formal care arrangements; current informal care arrangements; social history; physical care needs; medication review (⊃ Principles of medication reviews p. 142); social care needs; and wider needs (e.g. housing, welfare, employment, education). Assessment of carer needs should also be considered (⊃ Carers p. 458).

Care planning

Personal care planning is at the heart of case management. The care plan should be co-produced with the patient and, where appropriate, involve carers and other members of the health and social care team (⊃ Teamwork p. 58). The care plan supports the care manager to: make referrals to other services; co-ordinate all the different services they need to liaise with to ensure that referrals have been received and acted upon; and monitor whether the patient has made any progress.

Care co-ordination

Care co-ordination is the essence of care management, requiring continual communication with the patient, carers, and members of the health and social care team. Key elements of care will include: medication management (⊃ Medicines optimization p. 128); self-care support (⊃ Expert patients and self-management programmes p. 340); advocacy and negotiation; psychosocial support; and monitoring and review.

Case closure

The duration of case management intervention will be dependent on local policies and programme guidelines. Possible discharge criteria include: death, self-discharge, decision by the case manager/multidisciplinary team that care has been optimized, and ↓ in the patient's risk of hospital admission.

Case management competencies

The Case Management Competences Framework,[6] sets out the competencies associated with case management (◆ Continuing professional development p. 53). Domains include: leading complex care co-ordination; proactively managing complex LTCs; managing cognitive impairment and mental well-being; supporting self-care, self-management, and enabling independence; professional practice and leadership (◆ Leadership p. 60); identifying ↑ risk patients, promoting health, and preventing ill health; managing care at the end of life; and interagency and partnership working. In addition, community matrons will need to demonstrate competency in advanced clinical nursing practice.

References

5. CMSA (2017) *What is a case manager?* Available online: http://www.cmsa.org/who-we-are/ what-is-a-case-manager/
6. NHS Modernization Agency and Skills for Health (2005) *Case management competences framework for the care of people with long-term conditions.* Available at: https://webarchive.nationalarchives. gov.uk/20130105053725/http://www.dh.gov.uk/prod_consum_dh/groups/dh_digitalassets/ @dh/@en/documents/digitalasset/dh_4118102.pdf

Consultation models and frameworks

Developed to provide a potential structure for the complex interactions that occur between patients and GPs.[7] With 1° care nurses increasingly consulting independently, these models are relevant to nursing practice.[8] They are not fixed rules but learning aids (➔ Continuing professional development p. 53) to help practitioners develop their own consultation style.

Calgary-Cambridge consultation guide

- Initiating the session: preparing for the consultation, establishing rapport with the patient, and discovering the reason(s) for the consultation
- Gathering information: exploring the patient's perspective, exploring the biomedical perspective, and exploring background information
- Physical examination
- Explanation and planning: planning decision making together, providing appropriate information, and using strategies that aid accurate recall and understanding
- Closing the session: planning, final checking, and safety netting.

There are two additional key threads: building the relationship, and providing structure. These are used continuously throughout the consultation.

Pendleton model of consultation

- Define the reasons for the patient's attendance including: the nature and history of the problem(s); their aetiology; the patient's ideas, concerns, and expectations; and the effects of the problem(s).
- Consider other problems including: continuing problems, and at-risk factors.
- With the patient, choose an appropriate action for each problem.
- Achieve a shared understanding of the problem with the patient.
- Involve the patient in the management of the problem, and encourage and enable them to accept appropriate responsibility. Agree targets, monitoring, and follow-up.
- Use time and resources appropriately (both in the consultation and in the longer term).
- Establish or maintain a relationship with the patient which helps to achieve other tasks and to consider other problems not yet presented, ongoing problems, and risk factors.

Neighbour: the inner consultation

- Connecting: establishing rapport
- Summarizing: understanding the reason the patient has presented
- Handing over: formulating a management plan with the patient
- Safety netting: developing a contingency plan to manage risks, and organizing appropriate follow-up
- Housekeeping: prompting healthcare practitioner to be mindful of any emotions that have arisen as a consequence of the consultation. Ensure receptive to the next patient.

Related topics
➔ Principles of good communication in patient assessment p. 120

References
7. Denness, C. (2013) What are consultations models for? *InnovAiT*, 6(9), 592–9
8. Lakasing, E. (2007) 50 years of consultation models: tips for nurses. *Primary Health Care*, 17(7), 22–4

Further information
Neighbour, R. (1987) *The Inner Consultation*. Radcliffe Medical Press: Oxford

Pendleton, D., Schofield, T., Tate, P., & Havelock, P. (1984) *The consultation: an approach to learning and teaching*. Oxford University Press: Oxford

Pendleton, D., Schofield, T., Tate, P., & Havelock, P. (2003) *The new consultation*. Oxford University Press: Oxford

Silverman, J., Kurtz, S., & Draper, J. (2004) *Skills for communicating with patients* (2nd edn). Radcliffe Publishing: Abingdon

Standardized assessment tools

Effective patient assessment is key to the safety, continuity, and quality of patient care, and to the equitable allocation of resources. The appropriate use of standardized assessment tools can enhance patient assessment by facilitating greater patient engagement, and encouraging decisions based on objective data rather than solely subjective measures.

Types of standardized assessment

Mini-assessment tools

Give a snapshot based on a quick visual and physical assessment (e.g. the Airway, Breathing, Circulation, Disability, and Exposure (ABCDE) approach to assessing and treating deteriorating or critically ill patients).

Comprehensive assessment tools

Provide an in-depth and holistic assessment (e.g. assessment frameworks used by health visitors (◆ Health visiting p. 46) to assess whether a child is in need (◆ Assessment of children, young people, and families p. 156), and first-contact assessment tools used by district nurses (◆ District nursing p. 50)).

Focused assessment tools

These explore specific issues, problems, or risks; for example, the Whooley Questions for Depression screening (◆ Postnatal depression p. 440), the Ages and Stages Questionnaire for childhood development screening, the Mini-Mental State Examination to test cognitive function (◆ People with dementia p. 498), the Waterlow Score Card to assess the risk of pressure ulceration (◆ Pressure ulcer prevention p. 520), and the Caregiver Strain Index to identify families with potential caregiving concerns (◆ Carers p. 458).

Acceptability

To be useful in clinical practice, an assessment tool must be simple, culturally sensitive, have a clear and interpretable scoring system, and demonstrate reliability and validity (◆ Evidence-based healthcare p. 72). Shorter versions are preferable where available. ⚠ Clinical judgement is essential and should support the use of standardized assessment tools. Some tools are subject to copyright. In some cases, the copyright owner has entered into an agreement with the NHS to make their tool available. Where this is not the case, you may be charged for using the tool. For further information, visit NHS Digital, National Clinical Content Repository (Copyright Licensing Service) at ℘ https://digital.nhs.uk/services/national-clinical-content-repository-copyright-licensing-service

Principles of good communication in patient assessment

Effective patient assessment is not only dependent on clinical skills and knowledge, but interviewing skills and the relationship between the nurse and the patient. Good communication helps patients feel at ease and in control, and makes them feel valued.[9]

Prior to scheduled appointment

Anticipate potential barriers to effective communication such as sensory problems (◆ Deafness p. 696; ◆ Blindness and partial sight p. 748), confusion (◆ People with dementia p. 498), or language barriers. Plan appropriate interventions (e.g. minimize ambient noise, and arrange the use of translation and interpreting services).

Opening the consultation

Greet the patient using their preferred form of address. Dr Kate Granger MBE made the stark observation that many people looking after her when she was in hospital did not introduce themselves. She subsequently launched a campaign called '#hello my name is . . .' In a clinic setting, invite the person to be seated. If visiting the patient in their own home, ask permission to be seated. Ascertain whether the person wants a family member or friend to be present (◆ Carers p. 458). Seek consent to note taking.

Key principles during the consultation

Listening

Avoid interrupting as long as the patient remains on track and providing useful information. Demonstrate active listening:

- Sit squarely facing the person
- Open posture
- Lean forward towards the other person
- Eye contact with the other person
- Relax and avoid fidgeting

⚠: The above should be used judiciously (e.g. be aware that direct eye contact is not acceptable in all cultures).

Non-verbal communication

Position yourself at the same level as the other person. Maintain awareness and control of facial expressions. ⚠: Touch has been used in nursing to demonstrate care and compassion. However, there are potential harms associated with touch. It is important that patients give their consent (◆ Consent p. 82) to be touched.

Verbal communication

Ensure verbal communication is clear, accurate, honest, and appropriate (e.g. avoid medical jargon and speaking too quickly). Tone of voice can convey different feelings. Use a combination of open questions, that encourage the patient to speak in depth, and closed questions for clarification.

Allow the patient adequate time to respond to questions. Use empathetic phrases:

- Reflection phrases: summarizing/paraphrasing what the patient has said
- Affirmation phrases: confirming what the patient is experiencing
- Partnership phrases: expressing a desire to help the patient
- Respect phrases: conveying admiration for the patient's efforts

Closure

When closing the consultation, it is important to:

- Summarize the session
- Confirm the established plan of care
- Clarify the next steps
- Provide safety netting
- Final check the patient agrees and is comfortable with the plan

Written information

Provide written information to reinforce that given in the consultation and to be kept for future reference. Ensure information is up to date and presented in an appropriate format.

Related topics

➔ Consultation models and frameworks p. 116

Reference

9. Silverman, J., Kurtz, S., & Suchman, A. (2013) *Skills for communicating with patients* (3rd edn). CRC Press: London

Adults and children with additional communication needs

Information is a crucial part of any patient journey and central to their experience of care (➔ Patient and public experience p. 75). The form and medium of communication can vary according to patient needs and preferences: verbal, written, signed, Braille, audio, pictorial, drama, translated, etc. It is good practice to reinforce verbal communication with another form (e.g. leaflet).

Identify with the individual what, if any, communication support is needed (➔ Deafness p. 696; ➔ Deafness in children p. 268; ➔ Blindness and partial sight p. 748; ➔ People with learning disabilities p. 456; ➔ Communication and learning problems p. 224).

Many of those with English as a second language are fluent. However, there will be others: without any knowledge of English; who speak it well, but may understand comparatively little; or who understand a great deal, but may be unable to speak any. Try to ascertain how much English the person understands.

Once identified, organize the appropriate support: induction loops for people with a hearing impairment; palantypists (speech to text reporting); Makaton (which uses speech, signs, and symbols to help people communicate); signers for the hearing impaired; touch signers for people with visual and hearing impairments; and interpreters for people who do not speak English. Language and communication support needs should be recorded in the patient's records (➔ Record keeping p. 86).

Good practice points

- Find a suitable place to talk, with good lighting and away from noise and distractions.
- Speak at a moderate pace, directly to the patient, even when using communication support.
- Do not shout.
- Use natural facial expressions and gestures.
- Use clear, simple language, avoiding jargon, ambiguity, and medical terminology.
- Check throughout the consultation that you are understood.
- Use illustrations and pictures where suitable.
- If the patient is required to do something, make this obvious.
- If talking to a child, try to adjust language to their age.

Interpreters and translators

Official interpreters translate without adding, changing, or omitting anything. They will ask for clarification when needed, will not enter into a discussion or give advice or express opinions, and are bound by rules of confidentiality (➔ Confidentiality p. 89). Different types of interpreting are available including face-to-face, telephone, video remote, and video relay. The patient may prefer a gender-specific interpreter. Some people may prefer to use their children as an interpreter, desiring family privacy. However, this should be discouraged as the burden of responsibility may be too great for the child. When an interpreter is required, additional time will be needed for the consultation.

Advocates

Advocates provide advice and support, facilitate cultural and linguistic communication, voice patient concerns and expectations, advise on how to access healthcare, and help patients to become more informed and to make choices (→ Mental capacity p. 470). Various organizations provide advocacy support:

- PohWER ☎ 0300 456 2370 Available at: ✆ https://www.pohwer.net/Pages/Category/in-your-area
- SeAp Advocacy ☎ 0330 440 9000 Available at: ✆ https://www.seap.org.uk/im-looking-for-help-or-support/
- VoiceAbility ☎ 01223 555800 Available at: ✆ https://www.voiceability.org/
- Age UK ☎ 0800 055 6112 Available at: ✆ https://www.ageuk.org.uk/

Further information

NHS England (*Guidance for commissioners: interpreting and translation services in primary care*). Available at: ✆ https://www.england.nhs.uk/wp-content/uploads/2018/09/guidance-for-commissioners-interpreting-and-translation-services-in-primary-care.pdf

NHS England (*Accessible information and communication policy*). Available at: ✆ https://www.england.nhs.uk/wp-content/uploads/2016/11/nhse-access-info-comms-policy.pdf

Assessment by remote consultation

The use of telephone triage has been commonplace for many years. ↑ numbers of healthcare providers are now going beyond telephone triage and using remote systems (including over the telephone, via video link, or online) to conduct full consultations. Remote consultations can save time, benefit patients, and help meet the demand for faster access to healthcare.

⚠ There are limitations, as visual information cannot be ascertained from the patient's general appearance and behaviour, and from more formal physical examination and non-verbal cues. These limitations pose a potential threat to patient safety. Remote consultations with third parties introduce additional risks relating to consent and confidentiality.[10] Risks need to be identified and managed. Familiarity with information governance issues is important. Some practical risk-reduction methods include: dedicated and protected remote consultation times; enhanced documentation (➔ Record keeping p. 86); standardized protocols for managing common conditions (➔ Evidence-based healthcare p. 72); and ensuring all staff have received appropriate training (➔ Continuing professional development p. 53).[11]

Should a face-to-face consultation be arranged?

Remote consultations are not always the right choice.[12] As a starting point, consider:

• What do I know about the patient's needs and wishes?
• What are the limitations and risks of communicating remotely?
• Will I need to carry out a physical examination or other assessment?
• Do I have access to the patient's medical records and do I need them?
• Will the patient need follow-up or ongoing management?

⚠: A second contact from a patient about the same problem, within a short period of time, may best be dealt with face to face, either because the problem is unresolved or because it is escalating.

Tips for effective remote consultations

Introductions

• Introduce yourself with your full name, title, and service/practice.
• Identify the caller (should be the patient whenever possible).
• Sound friendly, interested, and empathetic.

Gathering information

• Listen to speech (e.g. content, rate, tone, and emotion) and non-speech sounds (e.g. cough, wheeze, background noises).
• Use good questioning techniques.
• Speak clearly, distinctly, and vary voice timbre.
• Avoid jargon and emotive words.
• Address both the clinical history and the patient's perspective.

Next steps and goodbye
- Summarize the call and give your interpretation of the patient's problem.
- Negotiate and agree actions.
- State what you are going to do next.
- Check that the patient has understood and agreed.
- Make follow-up arrangements and provide safety netting advice.

Writing up
Make a through, contemporaneous record, including the means of remote consultation used (including the patient telephone number, etc.).

Related topics
→ Consultation models and frameworks p. 116

References
10. Medical Protection Society (2015) *Risks of telephone consultations.* Available at: http://www.medicalprotection.org/uk/practice-matters-june-2015/risks-of-telephone-consultations
11. Frame, A. (2015) *Telephone consultations: advice for GPs.* Available at: https://www.gponline.com/telephone-consultations-advice-gps/article/1376349
12. General Medical Council (2018) *Remote consultations.* Available at: https://www.gmc-uk.org/ethical-guidance/ethical-hub/remote-consultations

Motivational interviewing in consultations

Originally designed to help people with addiction (➲ Alcohol p. 360; ➲ Substance use p. 476), motivational interviewing research has broadened to include behaviour change associated with medication adherence (➲ Medicine concordance and adherence p. 132), dietary change (➲ Nutrition and healthy eating p. 342), smoking cessation (➲ Smoking cessation p. 356), and physical activity (➲ Exercise p. 354). Includes four essential elements:

- Collaboration between practitioner and client
- Evoking or drawing out the client's ideas about change
- Emphasizing the autonomy of the client
- Practicing compassion in the process

General principles

- Express empathy: client should experience the practitioner as seeing the issue from their perspective
- Support self-efficacy: highlighting previous successes, skills, and strengths
- Roll with resistance: avoid engaging with resistance; accepting ambivalence is part of the process
- Highlight discrepancies: helping client to become aware of the gap between their current behaviours and their goals

Communication style

- Open-ended questions
- Affirmations
- Reflections
- Summaries

Talk of change

The more someone talks of change, the more they are likely to change. The practitioner seeks to guide the client to expressions of change as a pathway to behaviour change.

Further information

Royal College of Nursing (Supporting behaviour change: online learning resource). Available on-line: ℜ https://www.rcn.org.uk/clinical-topics/supporting-behaviour-change

Medicines management and nurse prescribing

Medicines optimization *128*
Medicine concordance and adherence *132*
Help with costs of medicines *134*
Prescribing *136*
Prescribing for special groups *138*
Principles of medication reviews *142*
Controlled drugs *144*
Antimicrobial stewardship *146*
Storage, transportation, and disposal of medicines *148*

Medicines optimization

The legislation for the prescription (➔ Prescribing p. 136), dispensing, safe custody (➔ Storage, transportation, and safe disposal of medicines p. 148), and administration of medicines applies across the UK, but each country's department of health determines some aspects (e.g. non-medical prescribing).

Non-medical prescribing

A range of healthcare professionals other than doctors can prescribe medicines for patients, as either independent or supplementary prescribers. They must have a registered first-level qualification and a recordable prescribing qualification with their regulatory body (➔ Professional accountability p. 83).

Independent prescribers

Are responsible and accountable for the assessment of patients with either undiagnosed or diagnosed conditions, and for the decisions about the clinical management required, including prescribing. They can prescribe any licensed drug which lies within their field of competency, from anywhere in the BNF, including some controlled drugs (CDs) (➔ Controlled drugs p. 144). Independent nurse prescribers can also prescribe unlicensed drugs if they are competent, have considered the risks and benefits, have the support of their employing organization, and can justify their actions in the light of the patient's best interests.[1]

Community practitioner nurse prescribers

Nurses, with or without a community specialist practice qualification, but with a NMC-recorded prescribing qualification, can prescribe from a limited formulary.

Supplementary prescribing

A partnership between an independent prescriber and a supplementary prescriber to implement an agreed clinical management plan (CMP). Nurses, pharmacists, and designated allied health professionals with recordable qualifications can undertake supplementary prescribing. This includes prescribing of CDs and unlicensed medicines where the doctor agrees with a patient's CMP.

Prescriptions

NHS prescriptions are made on FP10 (GP10 in Scotland, HS21 in Northern Ireland, WP10 in Wales) forms or computer generated on FP10(C). The NHS Business Services Authority (NHS BSA) provides prescriptions to NHS organizations and they are then distributed free of charge to medical and non-medical prescribers, dentists, and other organizations as required. Prescription pads can be personalized with the NMC number (for nurses) and can be ordered up to 42 days before the nurse joins an organization. The patient's GP code will need to be added if the prescriber is not employed by a GP. The NHS BSA records the costs from each prescription by practice and prescriber, and provides reports for monitoring and auditing prescribing (➔ Clinical audit p. 70).

Dispensing medication

Medicines are usually dispensed (supplied) as a response to a prescription by local pharmacists (or a dispensing GP) and are the property of the patient. Some nurses working in specialist services may also supply medicines provided by the organization (e.g. family planning clinics (● Contraception: general p. 400) and sexual health clinics (● Sexual health: general issues p. 760)). All dispensed or supplied medicines must be labelled with the patient's name and accompanied by a patient information leaflet. Local policies apply.

Administration of medicines

- In 1° care, many people administer their own medicines.
- Vulnerable and frail adults (● Frailty p. 678) at home may be assisted in taking medicines by both nursing and home care services. Local guidance applies on division of responsibilities, accountabilities, and mechanisms for shared record keeping (● Record keeping p. 86).
- In schools, staff must not give prescription medicines without appropriate training and updates (● Working in schools p. 44).
- Nursing staff are directed to administer medication by either:
  - A written patient-specific direction (PSD) for a named patient, either as directed on the patient's pharmacy supplied medicine label or through a written direction by an independent prescriber (e.g. GP request).
  - A patient group direction (PGD) that provides a legal mechanism for medicines to be supplied and/or administered by named registered health professionals to groups of patients without prescriptions having to be written. There is specific guidance on the authorization process by a senior doctor and pharmacist. For example, immunizations (● Childhood immunizations p. 164; ● Childhood immunization schedule UK p. 166); ● Targeted adult immunization p. 392), travel vaccines (● Travel vaccinations p. 399), contraceptives.

Prescribed and supplied/administered medicines and appliances should be recorded in any clinical and personally held records (● Client- and patient-held records p. 90).

Errors in medication dispensing or administration

- Report to the prescriber and consult doctor with responsibility for clinical care (e.g. GP).
- Take an appropriate action, advised with regard to the patient.
- Report incident to line manager; complete incident and accident form in line with local policies (● Quality governance p. 68; ● Clinical risk management p. 78).

Monitoring adverse drug reactions

Any prescriber or patient can report suspected adverse drug reactions to any drug (including those self-medicated by the patient, reactions to blood products, vaccines, radiographic contrast media, and herbal products (→ Complementary and alternative therapies p. 838) to the MHRA online (see ℰ https://yellowcard.mhra.gov.uk/) or by using the yellow card in the BNF.

Reference

1. NMC (2009) *Nurse and midwife independent prescribing of unlicensed medicines.* Available at: www.nmc-uk.org/Documents/Circulars/2010circulars/NMCcircular04_2010.pdf

Further information

Beckwith, S. & Franklin, P. (2011) *The oxford handbook of prescribing for nurses and allied health professionals* (2nd edn). Oxford: Oxford University Press.

BNF (*Access to the BNF online*). Available at: ℰ https://www.bnf.org/products/bnf-online/

Department for Education (*Supporting pupils with Medical Conditions at School*). Available at: ℰ https://www.gov.uk/government/publications/supporting-pupils-at-school-with-medical-conditions--3

NHS BSA (*NHS prescription services*). Available at: ℰ https://www.nhsbsa.nhs.uk/nhs-prescription-services

NICE (*Medicines information resources*). Available at: ℰ https://bnf.nice.org.uk/about/medicines-information-services.html

NICE (*Information on the nurse prescribers' formulary*). Available at: ℰ https://bnf.nice.org.uk/nurse-prescribers-formulary/

Medicine concordance and adherence

The cost of NHS prescriptions dispensed in the community in England was >£9 billion in 2017.[2] 30–50% of people do not take medicines as directed to reach therapeutic effect.[3] Reasons include:
- Lack of information about their condition and the importance of treatment
- Beliefs about medicines (e.g. unnatural or should be able to manage without)
- Unwilling to tolerate side effects
- Practical difficulties, such as getting the prescription dispensed, remembering to take medicines, opening containers
- Prescription costs (➔ Help with costs of medicines p. 134)

Medicine concordance

Concordance is defined as a partnership process between professional and patient that addresses the beliefs, experiences, and wishes of the patient as well as other factors that contribute to successful prescribing and medicine taking.

Patient involvement in decisions about medicines

Good communication between healthcare professional and patient is essential (➔ Principles of good communication in patient assessment p. 120). It is also important to involve patients in decisions about medicines. Also:
- Consider physical or learning disabilities (➔ People with learning disabilities p. 456), language, and hearing (➔ Deafness p. 696) or sight difficulties (➔ Blindness and partial sight p. 748).
- Use pictures, an interpreter, or patient advocate (➔ Adults and children with additional communication needs p. 122).
- Acknowledge patient views about their condition and treatment, and ensure they have a role in making decisions.
- Clarify what the patient would like the outcome to be.
- Focus on benefits and risks rather than misconceptions.
- Accept the patient has the right to decide not to take the medicine.
- Assess patient's mental capacity (➔ Mental capacity p. 470) to make decisions as per the Mental Capacity Act 2005.

Understand the patient's knowledge, beliefs, and concerns about medicines, and provide information about their condition and possible treatments and answer any questions.

Medicine adherence

The purpose of assessing adherence is not to monitor patients but to find out whether they need more information and support. Patients are more likely to take medicines as prescribed when they:
- Recognize consequences of not treating their condition
- Agree with course of action and the proposed treatment
- Understand or are able to minimize side effects
- Have the simplest regimen that can fit with their routine
- Use aids such as a multi-compartment medicines system

- Have clear verbal instructions, reinforced with written instructions they can read (e.g. appropriate font size and language)
- Have an opportunity for a follow-up discussion with a professional in 2–3wks if a long-term regimen or difficult technique (e.g. inhalers)
- Have an opportunity for medication review if long-term use (➋ Principles of medication reviews p. 142)

Related topics

➋ Motivational interviewing in consultations p. 126; ➋ Consultation models and frameworks p. 116; ➋ Consent p. 82

References

2. NHS Digital (2018) *Prescription cost analysis*. Available at: ✎ https://digital.nhs.uk/data-and-information/publications/statistical/prescription-cost-analysis/prescription-cost-analysis-england-2017
3. NICE (2009) *Medicines adherence: involving patients in decisions about prescribed medicines and supporting adherence [CG76]*. Available at: ✎ https://www.nice.org.uk/guidance/cg76/chapter/1-Guidance#supporting-adherence

Help with costs of medicines

NHS prescriptions are free in Scotland, Wales, and Northern Ireland, but not England (➲ NHS entitlements p. 10). Some medicines are cheaper bought OTC. There is also help with the cost of prescription items for people on low incomes, with particular conditions, or with multiple medication costs.

Free prescription entitlement

See information on NHS leaflet HC11 (England). Also see tick box on reverse of prescription. Free for: contraception; >60yrs, <16yrs, or 16–18yrs if in full-time education; and patient or family receiving Income Support or Income-Based Job Seeker Allowance, Income-Related Employment and Support Allowance, Pension Credit or Guarantee Credit, or Universal Credit.

Maternity Exemption (MatEx) Certificate

For pregnant women (➲ Pregnancy p. 424), for 12mths after the expected delivery date, or women who gave birth <12mths ago (➲ Postnatal care p. 438).

War Pension Exemption Certificate

Prescriptions related to the war pensioner's accepted disability (AFCS/WPS001 form (see ☞ https://www.gov.uk/government/publications/war-pension-scheme/war-pension-scheme-what-you-need-to-know))

Medical Exemption (MedEx) Certificate

For certain conditions, using form FP92A signed by doctor (or authorized member of practice staff). The conditions are:

* Diabetes insipidus or other forms of hypopituitarism (➲ Diabetes: overview p. 660; ➲ Principles of diabetes management p. 664)
* Forms of hypoadrenalism (e.g. Addison's disease) for which specific substitution therapy is essential (➲ Adrenal disorders p. 700)
* A permanent fistula (e.g. colostomy (➲ Stoma care p. 516) or laryngostomy (➲ Tracheostomy care p. 586) requiring continuous surgical dressing (➲ Wound dressing p. 532) or an appliance
* Diabetes mellitus, except where treatment is by diet alone
* Hypoparathyroidism (➲ Thyroid p. 702)
* Myasthenia gravis
* Myxoedema
* Epilepsy requiring continuous anticonvulsants (➲ Seizures and epilepsy p. 740)
* A continuing (not temporary) physical disability so person cannot go out without the help of another person
* Treatment for cancer or the effects of treatment for cancer

Pre-payment certificate

May be cheaper for patients who have to pay for >three items in 3mths or 14 items in 12mths to buy pre-payment certificate (PPC). Can only be used by applicant for own prescriptions. Cost of PPC (as at 2019): £29.10 for 3mths; £104 for 12mths. Apply to NHS Business Services Authority (NHS BSA) online (see 🕮 https://apps.nhsbsa.nhs.uk/ppc-online/patient.do) or by phone 📞 0300 330 1341 or use form FP95 available in surgeries and pharmacies. Apply for refunds to issuer. Claims for payments made while awaiting certificates can be made with form FP57, with official receipts from pharmacist sent to NHS BSA.

Further information

Beckwith, S. & Franklin, P. (2011) *The oxford handbook of prescribing for nurses and allied health professionals* (2nd edn). Oxford: Oxford University Press.

Prescribing

Competency framework for all prescribers

The Royal Pharmaceutical Society (RPS) has developed a competency framework for all prescribers and this has been adopted by the NMC. Keeping the patient at the centre of prescribing, the framework outlines ten steps.

The consultation

- **Step 1:** Assess the patient—including a social and medication history, allergies, and a clinical assessment in order to reach diagnosis (→ Consultation models and frameworks p. 116; → Standardized assessment tools p. 118; → Principles of good communication in patient assessment p. 120).
- **Step 2:** Consider the options—including pharmacological and non-pharmacological options, risks, and benefits (→ Clinical risk management p. 78).
- **Step 3:** Reach a shared decision—working in partnership with the patient to make an informed choice (→ Medicine concordance and adherence p. 132).
- **Step 4:** Prescribe—generic medicines where practical and safe, and with awareness of contraindications, interactions, cautions, and unwanted effects.
- **Step 5:** Provide clear and accessible information—through leaflets or reliable online sources.
- **Step 6:** Monitor and review—including effectiveness of treatment and reporting of any adverse drug reactions (→ Principles of medication reviews p. 142).

Prescribing governance

- **Step 7:** Prescribe safely—within own scope of practice (→ Professional accountability p. 83).
- **Step 8:** Prescribe professionally—maintaining own competency and acknowledging and dealing with influences on prescribing.
- **Step 9:** Improve prescribing practice—using reflection, patient feedback, and prescribing analysis and cost (ePACT) data and Scottish prescribing analysis (→ Clinical audit p. 70; → Continuing professional development p. 53; → Patient and public experience p. 75).
- **Step 10:** Prescribe as part of a team—including developing relationships with other prescribers and seeking support and supervision (→ Teamwork p. 58; → Clinical supervision and appraisal p. 52).

Prescription writing

Prescriptions should be completed as per specimen given on the inside cover of this book, ensuring either the words 'no more items on this prescription' are written immediately after last item or unused space is deleted with 'Z'. Each prescription requires nurse's NMC PIN number and patient's GP code (for costing to NHS prescribing budget).

Handwritten prescriptions

Write legibly; sign in ink. State patient's full name and address, preferably include their age and date of birth (date of birth is a legal requirement for a child <12yrs), and date of issue.

BNF recommendations

Avoidance of unnecessary decimal point (e.g. 3mg not 3.0mg); put zero in front of unavoidable decimal point (e.g. 0.5mL). Use units that give whole numbers where possible (e.g. paracetamol 500mg rather than paracetamol 0.5g). Units, micrograms, and nanograms should not be abbreviated. Use the term millilitre (mL)—not cubic centimetre, cc, or cm^3.

Computer-generated prescriptions

Must print the date of issue, the patient's surname, one forename, any other forenames as initials, address, age of those <12yrs or >60yrs. The prescriber's name, surgery address, telephone contact number, and reference number should be printed. Must be signed in ink. Controlled drugs have specific criteria when prescribing (❷ Controlled drugs p. 144).

Security of NHS prescriptions

Must be kept in locked drawer; not left in cars or unattended. Record serial numbers of prescriptions held so that these can be circulated if a pad is stolen (❷ Record keeping p. 86). Blank prescriptions should not be signed in advance. Any loss or suspected theft must be reported immediately to line manager and police.

Related topics

❷ Quality governance p. 68; ❷ Evidence-based healthcare p. 72; ❷ Medicines optimization p. 128.

Further information

BNF (*Access to the BNF Online*). Available at: ✆ https://www.bnf.org/products/bnf-online/
MHRA (*Yellow Card Scheme*). Available at: ✆ https://yellowcard.mhra.gov.uk/
NICE (*Medicines information resources*). Available at: ✆ https://bnf.nice.org.uk/about/medicines-information-services.html
NICE (*Information on the nurse prescribers' formulary*). Available at: ✆ https://bnf.nice.org.uk/nurse-prescribers-formulary/
RPS (*Competency framework for all prescribers, with NMC endorsement*). Available at: ✆ https://www.nmc.org.uk/standards/standards-for-post-registration/standards-for-prescribers/royal-pharmaceutical-societys-competency-framework-for-all-prescribers/

Prescribing for special groups

Particular consideration needs to be given to the altered pharmacokinetics and pharmacodynamics of the old (➲ Frailty p. 678), very young, pregnant (➲ Pregnancy p. 424) and breastfeeding ♀ (➲ Breastfeeding p. 182), people with reduced renal function, and people with liver disease (➲ Problems of the liver, gallbladder, and pancreas p. 718). The BNF gives prescribing guidance for all groups (➲ Prescribing p. 136).

Older people

Important to recognize the diversity and individuality of older people. Essential to assess not only the presenting problem but also: altered pharmacodynamics and kinetics due to natural ageing process rather than disease; any underlying pathologies and polypharmacy (four or more medicines); use of alternative therapies (➲ Complementary and alternative therapies p. 838), herbal remedies, and OTC medicine; and possible drug interactions and food–drug interactions. Common to initially prescribe at the lower end of a range of adult doses. Consider mental capacity (➲ Mental capacity p. 470), physical dexterity required to undo medication containers, the need for large-print labels on containers (➲ Blindness and partial sight p. 748), and ability to swallow solid-dosage forms (➲ Medicine concordance and adherence p. 132). Explain clearly and write full instructions on each prescription. Review repeat prescriptions regularly. Stop drugs or reduce doses if renal function declines (➲ Principles of medication reviews p. 142).

> ### Box 5.1 Altered pharmacokinetics in older people
> **Altered elimination**
> - Assume at least mild renal impairment when prescribing for older people. ↓ renal clearance results in slower drugs' excretion and ↑ susceptibility to nephrotoxic preparations.
> - ↓ renal clearance exacerbated by routine illnesses, such as urinary tract infection (➲ Urinary tract infection p. 756). Can result in adverse effects or overdose in a patient previously stabilized on a drug with a narrow therapeutic margin (e.g. digoxin) (➲ Poisoning and overdoses p. 822).
>
> **Altered absorption**
> - Total body water ↓ = ↑ plasma levels of water-soluble drugs
> - ↓ body mass, ↓ saliva production, atrophy of intestinal epithelium, slower gastric emptying
>
> **Altered distribution**
> - ↓ cardiac output, ↓ renal mass, ↓ renal blood flow
> - ↓ plasma proteins = ↑ in 'active' free protein-binding drugs
>
> **Altered metabolism**
> - ↓ hepatic blood flow, first pass metabolism ↓
> - Liver size ↓, blood flow ↓, enzyme production ↓, ↑ likelihood of toxicity with repeated doses

Altered pharmacokinetics in older people
That is, altered ways in which the body processes the drug (see Box 5.1).

Altered pharmacodynamics in older people
That is, altered number, specificity, and responsiveness of receptors to the drug.

- ↑ sensitivity to drugs due to changes in the responsiveness of target organs. Commonly, ↑ sensitivity to: opioid analgesics (➲ Pain assessment and management in palliative care p. 554), benzodiazepines (➲ People with anxiety and depression p. 478), antipsychotics (➲ People with psychosis p. 486), anti-hypertensives (➲ Hypertension p. 628), and non-steroidal anti-inflammatory drugs.
- Common adverse reactions affecting older people are gastrointestinal and haematological in nature.

Infants and children

Pharmacokinetics and pharmacodynamics are often different for children, especially in the very young.

- Always refer to the BNF/BNF Online for Children.
- Consult with senior clinician or specialist if in doubt.
- Many drugs are not licensed for children, so independent prescribers must be working within scope of practice (➲ Professional accountability p. 83), have an evidence-based rationale (➲ Evidence-based healthcare p. 72), and have support of employer.
- Doses are generally calculated using child's body weight in kilograms.
- Prescribe sugar-free solutions (➲ Development and care of teeth for young children p. 196).
- Legal requirement to write the child's age if <12yrs.
- State the strength of the tablets, capsules, or liquid. Involve the child or parent in choosing the formulation (➲ Medicine concordance and adherence p. 132).
- Advise parents not to add the drug to the child's feed (there may be an interaction or the child may not complete their feed).
- Avoid intramuscular injections as they are painful (➲ Injection technique p. 576).
- Report all adverse drug reactions using the yellow card scheme, as drugs are less extensively tested on children or not specifically licensed for children (➲ Clinical risk management p. 78).

Pregnant women

Drugs can have a harmful effect on the embryo or fetus at any time during the pregnancy. In the first trimester, they can produce congenital malformations; and in the second and third trimesters, drugs can affect the growth or functional development of the fetus.

Only prescribe for pregnant women when it is essential. Where possible, avoid prescribing for pregnant women during the first trimester. Prescribe drugs that have been tried and tested as safe in pregnancy, and only if benefit outweighs risk to the fetus. BNF/BNF Online identifies drugs known to be harmful and not harmful in pregnancy.

Breastfeeding women

There is little known about the effect of drugs taken by the mother on the baby through breastfeeding. The amount of drug transferred is rarely sufficient to produce a discernible effect on the infant, but this could happen.

Only absolutely necessary drugs should be taken when breastfeeding as may harm infant or inhibit sucking reflex or suppress lactation. BNF/BNF Online identifies drugs that should be used with caution or are contraindicated in breastfeeding, and drugs present in milk but not known to be harmful.

People with renal disease

Reduced renal function affects ability to excrete drugs, which increases the toxicity of the drug (➋ Renal problems p. 754). Problems can be avoided by reducing dose or using different drugs. Dose adjustment depends on grade of renal failure (mild, moderate, severe) measured by blood values. BNF/BNF Online provides prescribing guidance on drugs to be avoided or used with caution/dose reduction.

People with liver disease

Liver disease may impair drug metabolism and alter the body's response to drugs, e.g. ↑ toxicity and ↑ sensitivity (➋ Problems of the liver, gallbladder, and pancreas p. 718). Drug prescribing should be kept to a minimum in severe liver disease. See BNF/BNF Online.

Related topics

➋ Medicines optimization p. 128; ➋ Falls prevention p. 368

Further information

BNF (*Access to the BNF Online, including BNF for Children*). Available at: ℛ https://www.bnf.org/products/bnf-online/

NICE (*Medicines management: general and other*). Available at: ℛ https://www.nice.org.uk/guidance/service-delivery--organisation-and-staffing/medicines-management/medicines-management--general-and-other#panel-pathways

Principles of medication reviews

Prescribing medication is the most common medical intervention in the UK and 80% of drugs prescribed are repeat prescriptions (➲ Prescribing p. 136). QOF medicines management section (➲ Quality and Outcomes Framework p. 74) includes recorded medication reviews within last 15mths for all patients on repeat prescriptions and all patients on ≥ four medicines. A medication review is: 'a structured, critical examination of patient's medicines with the objective of reaching an agreement with the person about treatment, optimising the impact of medicines, minimising the number of medication-related problems and reducing waste'.[4] There are three levels of medication review.

Level 0: an ad hoc opportunist review

Done by anyone without access to patient's notes and without the patient. Perhaps to verify name or dose of medication or as a triage to indicate patients requiring prioritization for higher-level review.

Level 1: prescription review

This can be either a prescription intervention, where patient is not present and with no access to their notes, or medicines use review, with patient present but still no access to their notes. These are undertaken by a community pharmacist, pharmacy technician, or practice nurse (➲ General practice nursing p. 40).

Level 2: full medication review

Full access to the notes, but the patient is not present. Undertaken by a doctor, pharmacist in specific practice schemes, nurse prescriber, or specialist nurse.

Level 3: clinical medication review

Full access to patient's notes; patient present and consulted; all medications and all conditions reviewed. Undertaken by a doctor, nurse prescriber, or specialist nurse.

Only Levels 2 and 3 count in QOF for reviews of repeat medication.

Principles of medication review

Seeks to optimize the treatment for an individual patient (➲ Medicines optimization p. 128). Is undertaken in a systematic way, by a competent person (➲ Professional accountability p. 83). Any changes resulting from the review are agreed with the patient (➲ Medicine concordance and adherence p. 134). The clinical medication review gives patients an opportunity to ask questions and highlight problems regarding their medicines. Review is documented in the patient's notes (➲ Record keeping p. 86). Impact of any change is reviewed. Medication reviews should consider:

- The person's, family members', or carers' views (➲ Carers p. 458), understanding, questions, concerns, or problems with the medicines
- All prescribed or OTC medicines that are being taken
- Safety, appropriateness, effectiveness of the drugs (➲ Clinical risk management p. 78), and whether they are used in line with current national guidance (➲ Evidence-based healthcare p. 72)

- Risk factors for adverse drug reactions (check for interactions, duplications, or contraindications) (➔ Prescribing for special groups p. 138)
- Risk reduction and prevention (opportunistic screening (➔ UK Screening programmes p. 362), e.g. risk of falls (➔ Falls prevention p. 368), BP (➔ Hypertension p. 628))
- Whether the regimen can be simplified

Setting up a medication review system

Often, local guidance available from pharmacy advisors and medicine management teams. Guidance is also available on the NICE website (see ℘ https://www.nice.org.uk/sharedlearning/a-medicines-optimisation-service). Documentation important for auditing for: clinical outcomes, patient views, cost effectiveness indicators, and quantitative data (e.g. number reviewed) (➔ Clinical audit p. 70).

Reference

4. NICE (2016) *Medicines optimisation [CGS120]*. Available at: https://www.nice.org.uk/guidance/qs120/chapter/quality-statement-6-structured-medication-review

Further information

Beckwith, S. & Franklin, P. (2011) *Oxford handbook of prescribing for nurses and allied health professionals* (2nd edn). Oxford: Oxford University Press.

QOF Database (*Medicines management*). Available at: ℘ https://www.gpcontract.co.uk/browse/UK/Medicines%20Management/18

Controlled drugs

Relevant legislation includes the Misuse of Drugs Act (MDA) 1971, which classified different drugs according to the amount of harm they can cause when misused. There are three classes: A, B, and C. The Misuse of Drugs Regulations (MDR) 2001 (and subsequent amendments) divided drugs into five schedules—1, 2, 3, 4 (part 1 and 2), and 5—that govern production, supply, possession and storage, prescribing, administration, and record keeping. Different schedules have different requirements in relation to the aforementioned activities. Following expert advice, and in the public interest, the government may decide to amend the legal status of a drug. For example, in April 2019, Gabapentin was controlled under the MDA 1971 as a Class C substance and scheduled under the MDR 2001 as a Schedule 3 drug.

Governance

All aspects of the management of controlled drugs (CDs) are underpinned by the Health Act 2006 and Controlled Drugs (Supervision of Management and Use) Regulations 2013. Every healthcare organization or designated body has to appoint an accountable officer (AO) responsible for the safe management, supply, disposal, and administration of CDs, plus right of entry and inspection of CD records (➔ Quality governance p. 68). All organizations must have standard operating procedures (SOPs) for responsibilities and procedures for total management of CDs. Local procedures apply for reporting to AO any concerns regarding a healthcare professional and their use of CDs (➔ Professional conduct p. 80). AOs should record and manage information arising from their duties and prevent inappropriate handling of that information.

Prescribing controlled drugs

Prescriptions (➔ Prescribing p. 136) must be written legibly, indelibly, and include:

- Name, address, and age or date of birth (if <12yrs of age); if patient is homeless (➔ Homeless people p. 446), 'no fixed abode' is an acceptable address
- NHS number or Community Health Index number (Scotland)
- Name and form of drug, even if only one form exists
- The strength, dose interval, and the dose to be taken
- The total quantity of the preparation ≤30 days, or the number of dose units, to be supplied in both words and figures
- The NMC PIN and UK address of the prescriber, plus date

Prescriptions for CDs are only valid for 28 days from the date they are signed and cannot be issued as repeat dispensing prescriptions. Prescriptions for Schedule 5 CDs are valid for 6mths, and Schedule 4 and 5 CDs can be dispensed by repeat prescription.

⚠ Nurse prescribers should be aware that under current legislation, except in very restricted circumstances, mixing more than one drug in a syringe driver (➔ Syringe drivers p. 570) creates an unlicensed medicine (see ⌖ https://www.gov.uk/drug-safety-update/medical-and-non-medical-prescribing-mixing-medicines-in-clinical-practice) (➔ Professional accountability p. 83).

Administration of controlled drugs

CDs are only administered under the specific written, not verbal, directions of an independent prescriber. Details of prescriptions must always be recorded in patients' records (➔ Record keeping p. 86). There is no legal requirement for administration to be witnessed by a second person.

Related topics

➔ Storage, transportation, and disposal of medicines p. 148

Further information

Department of Health (2013) (*Controlled drugs (supervision of management and use) Regulations 2013*). Available at: ℜ http://www.legislation.gov.uk/uksi/2013/373/contents/made

NHS Business Services Authority (*NHS drug tariff—England & Wales*). Available at: ℜ http://www.ppa.org.uk/ppa/edt_intro.htm

NICE (*Controlled drugs safe use and management*). Available at: ℜ https://www.nice.org.uk/guidance/ng46/chapter/recommendations

NICE (*Medicines and prescribing support*). Available at: ℜ https://www.nice.org.uk/about/nice-communities/medicines-and-prescribing

Antimicrobial stewardship

Antimicrobial (AM) stewardship refers to a set of co-ordinated strategies to improve the use of AM medications, with the goal of enhancing patient health outcomes, ↓ resistance to antibiotics, and ↓ unnecessary costs. All health and social care practitioners, healthcare organization managers, and patients and their families need to be aware of what they can do to help.

Antimicrobial stewardship programmes

NICE suggest the following should be included in AM stewardship programmes:
- Monitoring and evaluating of AM prescribing (➲ Prescribing p. 136)
- Regular feedback to prescribers about amount of prescribing and patient safety incidents linked to AM prescribing (➲ Clinical risk management p. 78)
- Education and training about AM stewardship (➲ Continuing professional development p. 53)
- Audit of programmes linked to AM stewardship (➲ Clinical audit p. 70)
- Establish AM stewardship teams (➲ Teamwork p. 58)

Recommendations for antimicrobial prescribers

- Prescribe the shortest effective course.
- Follow local or national guidelines on the most appropriate dose and route of administration (➲ Evidence-based healthcare p. 72).
- Take account of risk to the individual patient and population as a whole.
- Take microbiological samples, where possible, before prescribing.
- Discuss the benefits and harm with patients.
- Do not issue an immediate prescription to patients who are likely to have a self-limiting condition.
- Do not issue repeat prescriptions for AM unless needed for a specific condition.
- Do not issue for >6mths without review.

Further information

NHS England (*Guide to antimicrobial stewardship*) Available at: ℘ https://www.england.nhs.uk/ourwork/clinical-policy/sepsis/antimicrobial-stewardship/

NICE (*Guidance on antimicrobial stewardship*). Available at: ℘ https://www.nice.org.uk/guidance/NG15/chapter/1-Recommendations#all-antimicrobials

Storage, transportation, and disposal of medicines

In the course of using medicines for therapeutic benefit, it is important to comply with current legislation, follow guidance issued by government departments (e.g. Department of Health and Social Care, the Home Office), and manage the risks to patients and staff arising from the use of medicines (→ Quality governance p. 68; → Clinical risk management p. 78). Pharmacist advisors employed by 1° care organizations or medication management teams provide up-to-date local guidance.

Storage on community sites and general practice

- Each service should have SOPs (including designated responsible person) for the safety and security of medicines.
- Medicines that are not required for the treatment of anaphylaxis (→ Anaphylaxis p. 810) or resuscitation (→ Child basic life support p. 800; → Adult basic life support and automated external defibrillation p. 792) should always be kept locked in a cupboard or refrigerator (designated for the storage of medicines) as applicable.
- The cupboard or refrigerator must conform to British Standards (BS) 2881 (1989) NHS Estates and Building Note No. 29
- Maximum/minimum thermometers should be used to monitor the temperature of the refrigerator (usually 2–8°C). These temperatures should be recorded each working day and records kept for 6mths.
- Medicines held for clinical emergencies should be in packs labelled as such and available in those clinical sessions; otherwise securely stored.
- If controlled drugs (CDs) are held as stock (e.g. in the GP practice), it is a legal requirement to hold a CD register, and to hold CDs in a fixed, locked cupboard sited away from the public (→ Controlled drugs p. 144). The key should be secured, and never left in the cupboard door.

Storage in the patient's home

Patients' medicines are their property. Key messages to promote:
- Keep medicines in cool, dark places away from light and heat (including steam), or as directed on instructions (e.g. fridge) (→ Weather extremes p. 370).
- Always read medicine information leaflets for storage instructions.
- Keep in original container as it has instructions, expiry date, etc. If a medication reminder device is used (→ Medicine concordance and adherence p. 132), the contents must be labelled. Some drugs are unsuitable for these devices if they are affected by light, moisture, or temperature.
- Keep out of reach and sight of children (→ Accident prevention p. 168; → Poisoning and overdoses p. 822).

Administering home-stored medicines

- Nursing staff should be aware of individual medicine storage requirements. If drug potency is compromised by poor storage, new supplies need to be obtained.
- Local guidelines apply to involvement of nursing staff in filling and prompting from medicine reminder devices (➲ Professional accountability p. 83). Many types available, but widespread safety concerns relate to labelling and opportunities for mix-ups, particularly if person has cognitive impairment (➲ People with dementia p. 498) or there are multiple carers (➲ Carers p. 458) helping with medication. Many areas have schemes for pharmacist to dispense into sealed, monitored dosage systems (e.g. blister packs).

Key principles for transportation

- Wherever possible, the patient, their carer, or agent should collect any prescribed items from pharmacy. Some pharmacists have local delivery systems.
- Legally, nurses can transport prescribed CDs from pharmacy (requires ID and signature) to a named patient if latter unable to collect or return unwanted prescribed medicines. Only done if there is no alternative. If necessary to transport CDs, these should be in locked bag/box and kept out of sight.
- Do not leave medicines in the car overnight or for long periods.
- Ensure temperature-sensitive preparations are transported in conditions to maintain the appropriate temperature range (i.e. preserve the cold chain).
- Cool boxes and bags should be monitored and maintained at the correct temperature (e.g. for vaccines, this is between 2–8°C).
- Local guidelines should be followed on the transportation of medicines and vaccines.

Key principles for disposal

Disposal into the sewerage system is an environmental hazard. Patients/carers/agents should be encouraged to return unwanted and out-of-date medicines to supplying pharmacy for safe disposal. Patients/carers can return unused CDs to any pharmacy. A nurse can do this if no alternative. Local guidelines should be followed on the disposal of out-of-date or unwanted medicines or medicinal products from clinic/surgery held stocks. This includes records of disposal.

Further information

NMC (*Standards for medicines management*). Available at: ℅ https://www.nmc.org.uk/globalassets/sitedocuments/standards/nmc-standards-for-medicines-management.pdf

Royal Pharmaceutical Society (*Professional guidance on the safe and secure handling of medicines*). Available at: ℅ https://www.rpharms.com/recognition/setting-professional-standards/safe-and-secure-handling-of-medicines/professional-guidance-on-the-safe-and-secure-handling-of-medicines

Child health promotion

Promoting the health of
 children 152

Overview of the Healthy Child
 Programme 154

Assessment of children, young
 people, and families 156

Children and young people in
 need 158

Child screening tests 160

Eyes and vision screening 162

Hearing screening 163

Childhood immunization 164

Childhood immunization schedule
 (UK) 166

Accident prevention 168

Working with parents 170

Support for parenting 172

New birth visits 174

Pre-term infants 176

New babies 178

Twins and multiple births 180

Breastfeeding 182

Bottle feeding 186

Weaning 188

Growth 0–2 years 190

Child development 0–1 years 192

Baby hygiene and skin care 194

Development and care of teeth for
 young children 196

Crying babies 198

Babies, children, and sleeping 200

Promoting baby development
 safely 0–1 years 202

Child development 1–5 years 204

Growth 2–4 years 206

Promoting development in the
 under-fives 208

Emotional development in babies
 and children 210

Food and the under-fives 212

Toilet training 214

Understanding behaviour
 1–5 years 216

Speech and language
 acquisition 218

Child development
 5–11 years 220

Growth and nutrition
 5–11 years 222

Communication and learning
 problems 224

Dental health in older children 226

Puberty and adolescence 228

Health promotion in schools 230

Working with teenagers 232

Growth and nutrition
 12–18 years 234

Sex and relationship
 education 236

Children with complex health
 needs and disabilities 238

Children with special educational
 needs 242

Child and adolescent mental
 health 246

Safeguarding children 248

Identifying the child in need of
 protection 250

Child protection processes 252

Looked-after children 254

Promoting the health of children

The UK ratified the UN Convention on the Rights of the Child in 1989. The Children Act 2004 created children's commissioners to promote the views and rights of children. The Act also places a responsibility on practitioners to work together to help a child:

- Be healthy
- Stay safe
- Enjoy and achieve
- Make a positive contribution
- Achieve economic well-being

Children in the UK

- There are ~13.5 million children <16yrs.
- 4.5 million children live in households with income poverty.[1]
- Infant mortality is considerably higher in deprived areas.[2]
- ~240 babies die each year from sudden infant death syndrome (SIDS)[3] (→ Sudden infant death syndrome p. 278).
- International comparisons show the UK has some of the ↑ rates of children 2–15yrs diagnosed with asthma (→ Asthma in children p. 306), eczema (→ Eczema in childhood p. 284), and hay fever (→ Allergies p. 694).[4]
- In 2018, ~54,000 children had a child protection plan (→ Child protection processes p. 252).[5]
- 7% children <15yrs have a severe disability.[6] Disabilities are more frequent in children from lower-incomes families (→ Children with complex health needs and disabilities p. 238).
- Boys and young ♂ aged 11–20yrs are at ↑ risk of committing suicide[7] (→ UK health profile p. 2).

Health promotion activities

Should include:

- Supporting breastfeeding (→ Breastfeeding p. 182)
- Prevention of infectious diseases (→ Infectious diseases in childhood p. 290; → Childhood immunization p. 164; → Childhood immunization schedule (UK) p. 166)
- Encouraging good nutrition (→ Growth 0–2 years p. 190; → Growth 2–4 years p. 206; → Growth and nutrition 5–11 years p. 222; → Growth and nutrition 12–18 years p. 234) and prevention of obesity (→ Overweight and obesity p. 348)
- Encouraging dental care and caries prevention (→ Development and care of teeth for young children p. 196; → Dental health in older children p. 226)
- ↓ the risk of SIDS

The personal child health record should be used (→ Client- and patient-held records p. 90). There are clear care pathways for children with health or development problems (→ Child development 0–1 years p. 192; → Child development 1–5 years p. 204; → Child development 5–11 years p. 220).

Statutory responsibilities are fulfilled in respect of child protection, looked-after children (➋ Looked-after children p. 254), adoption procedures, and children with special educational needs (➋ Children with special educational needs p. 242).

Health professionals working with adult patients should recognize the impact of adult problems on children.

Healthcare for children and young people in school (➋ Working in schools p. 44) should include: support of children with problems and special needs; participation in public health programmes (➋ Health promotion in schools p. 230); provision of agreed screening and immunization programmes; and promotion of personal, social, and sexual health including emotional literacy (➋ Sex and relationship education p. 236).

References

1. Social Metrics Commission (2018) *A new measure of poverty for the UK*. Available at: http://socialmetricscommission.org.uk/MEASURING-POVERTY-SUMMARY-REPORT.pdf
2. ONS (2018) *Child mortality in England and Wales: 2016*. Available at: https://www.ons.gov.uk/peoplepopulationandcommunity/birthsdeathsandmarriages/deaths/bulletins/childhoodinfantandperinatalmortalityinenglandandwales/2016
3. Lullaby Trust (2018) *Statistics on SIDs*. Available at: https://www.lullabytrust.org.uk/professionals/statistics-on-sids/
4. Asthma UK (2018) *Asthma facts and statistics*. Available at: https://www.asthma.org.uk/about/media/facts-and-statistics/
5. ONS (2018) *Characteristics of children in need: 2017 to 2018 England*. Available at: https://assets.publishing.service.gov.uk/government/uploads/system/uploads/attachment_data/file/762527/Characteristics_of_children_in_need_2017-18.pdf
6. Department of Work and Pensions (2017) *Family Resources Survey 2016/17*. Available at: https://assets.publishing.service.gov.uk/government/uploads/system/uploads/attachment_data/file/600465/family-resources-survey-2015-16.pdf
7. ONS (2018) *Suicides in the UK: 2017 registrations*. Available at: https://www.ons.gov.uk/peoplepopulationandcommunity/birthsdeathsandmarriages/deaths/bulletins/suicidesintheunitedkingdom/2017registrations#suicide-patterns-by-age

Overview of the Healthy Child Programme

This is a universal programme that outlines how health professionals will work together to promote the health and well-being of children, young people, and their families[8]. Care begins in the antenatal period (➲ Antenatal care and screening p. 426, continuing until the child is aged 19yrs. The programme is delivered in two parts: 0-5yrs and 5-19 yrs. The focus of the programme is on: acknowledging social, as well as biological determinants of health; the importance of community-based approaches (➲ Community approaches to health p. 338) to improving health; partnerships with parents to help them make healthy choices for their children and families (➲ Working with parents p. 170); and public health nurses (e.g. health visitors (➲ Health visiting p. 46) and school nurses (➲ School nursing p. 42)) as key health service providers (➲ Teamwork p. 58).

Every child and parent should have access to a universal or core programme of preventative pre-school care based on: delivery of agreed screening procedures (➲ Child screening tests p. 160); delivery of health promotion and support for parenting (➲ Support for parenting p. 172) programmes; and the need to establish which families have more complex needs and to respond appropriately to those following full assessment (➲ Assessment of children, young people, and families p. 156).

Formal screening confined to those activities agreed by the National Screening Committee. In addition, professionals elicit and respond to all parental concerns with appropriate assessment and action.

Each UK country has produced its own version of the programme and these should be checked for updates.[8-11] Table 6.1 provides an overview of the current programme in England.

Table 6.1 Overview of the Healthy Child Programme

Age	Intervention
Soon after birth (<72hrs)	General physical examination including inspection of eyes and red reflex, semi-automated hearing screening, Ortolani and Barlow tests for developmental dysplasia of hips (DDH), examination of the heart and testes
5–6 days (ideally 5 days)	Newborn blood-spot screening
By 14 days	New baby review to assess child and family needs; information/ support to parents on key health issues
6–8wks	General physical examination including inspection of the eyes and red reflex, Ortolani and Barlow tests for DDH, examination of the heart and testes
	Review of general progress and delivery of key health promotion messages: usually at the same time as the 1st set of immunizations
	Review of parental mood/ transition to parenthood, assessment of baby's health and well-being

(Continued)

Table 6.1 (*Contd.*)

Age	Intervention
2mths (8wks)	1st set of immunizations
3mths (12wks)	2nd set of immunizations
4mths (16wks)	3rd set of immunizations
By the 1st birthday	Overall review of the child and family, and 8–12mth health review; assessing growth and development; age-appropriate health promotion
12–13mths	1st measles, mumps, and rubella (MMR) vaccine and boosters of Hib, Men C, Men B, and PCV vaccines
2–2.5yrs	Health review, face-to-face contact, assessing growth and development. Like the 3–4mth and 8–12mth health review, this review assesses the child's communication, gross motor, fine motor, personal/social, and problem-solving skills. Parental mood is assessed in view of the fact that postnatal depression may develop any time in the years postnatally.
3–4yrs	Preschool booster and 2nd MMR vaccine; review of child's progress and delivery of key health promotion messages Review of child's progress where there is vulnerability (safeguarding, medical)
4–5yrs	Assessment of visual acuity
School entry	General review; hearing screening; height and weight measurement
Throughout school years	Ongoing support by the school health service; no further routine screening procedures recommended
Girls 12–13yrs	HPV vaccine
13–14yrs	Teenage booster and Men C vaccines

References

8. Healthy Child Programme England (2009) *Healthy Child Programme: pregnancy and the first five years of life*. Available at: www.gov.uk/government/publications/healthy-child-programme-pregnancy-and-the-first-5-years-of-life

9. Scotland Child Health Programme (2017) *Child Health Programme*. Available at: https://www.isdscotland.org/Health-Topics/Child-Health/Child-Health-Programme/Child-Health-Systems-Programme-Pre-School.asp

10. Welsh Government (2016) *Healthy Child Wales Programme*. Available at: https://gweddill.gov.wales/topics/health/publications/health/reports/healthy-child/?lang=en

11. Department of Health, Social Services and Public Safety (2010) *Healthy child, healthy future: a framework for the Universal Child Health Promotion Programme in Northern Ireland*. Available at: https://www.health-ni.gov.uk/sites/default/files/publications/dhssps/healthychildhealthyfuture.pdf

Assessment of children, young people, and families

Promotion of children's and young people's health involves consideration of their developmental needs, the quality of parental care, and the circumstances and environment in which they grow up in. Each dimension has a number of elements (Fig. 6.1). These form the basis for structuring and recording in the parent-held child health record (➔ Client and patient-held records p. 90) assessments of children in routine practice as part of the Healthy Child Programme (➔ Overview of the Healthy Child Programme p. 154). The dimensions are also essential in determining whether a child or young person is in need or suffering significant harm (➔ Identifying the child in need of protection p. 250; ➔ Safeguarding children p. 248).

All assessments should be carried out in partnership with parents and young people to identify strengths, problems, and opportunities for health promotion (➔ Working with parents p. 170). The next step is to plan to provide information, advice, supporting resources, practical help, and referral to other services as appropriate. Like all individual health needs assessments, the plan and its outcome should be jointly reviewed with child, parents, and practitioners who are involved, and amended as the child develops (➔ Teamwork p. 58).

In England, the Common Assessment Framework has been used as a tool for assessing and co-ordinating multi-agency support to children with additional needs (and their families), below the threshold of all statutory

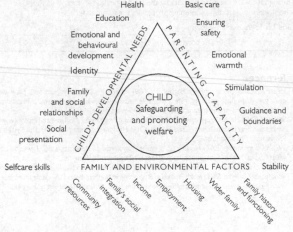

Fig. 6.1 The assessment framework.

Department of Health (2000) *Framework for the assessment of children in need and their families.* Reproduced under the Open Government License for public sector information (➔ https://www.nationalarchives.gov.uk/doc/open-government-licence/version/3/).

services for children who may be vulnerable or at risk in some way. It forms the basis of local assessment systems and provides for identification of a child's or young person's needs, early assessment, decision making, and co-ordinated service delivery in response and review.

Further information

HM Government (*Working together to safeguard children: a guide to inter-agency working to safeguard and promote the welfare of children*). Available at: ℅ https://assets.publishing.service.gov.uk/government/uploads/system/uploads/attachment_data/file/779401/Working_Together_to_Safeguard-Children.pdf

Children and young people in need

Under the Children Act 1989, a child or young person is considered in need if:

- They are unlikely to achieve or maintain, or to have the opportunity of achieving or maintaining, a reasonable standard of health or development without provision of services by the LA.
- Their health or development is likely to be significantly or further impaired without such provision.
- They are disabled.

This Act, together with the Children Act 2004, provides a comprehensive framework for the safeguarding and promotion of the welfare of children, i.e. protecting children from abuse and neglect, preventing impairment of their health or development, and ensuring they receive safe and effective care. LAs are required to provide services for children in need for the purposes of safeguarding and promoting their welfare (🔂 Identifying the child in need of protection p. 250; 🔂 Safeguarding children p. 248).

Integrated assessment frameworks

All UK countries are developing integrated or common assessment frameworks (and records) for use by staff of all agencies providing services to children (🔂 Assessment of children, young people, and families p. 156). The assessment, planning, and monitoring processes should be undertaken in partnership with parents, children, and young people. Parents and children should be kept fully informed and supported to participate in meetings and services (🔂 Working with parents p. 170; 🔂 Support for parenting p. 172). Assessment will look at whether the child or young person appears: healthy; safe from harm; to be learning and developing (🔂 Communication and learning problems p. 224); to have a positive impact on others; and free from the negative impact of poverty. Children identified as vulnerable and in need are referred to specialist and targeted services. Local child protection procedures are followed if there is risk of harm (🔂 Child protection processes p. 252).

Full common assessment frameworks cover:

- General health
- Physical development (🔂 Growth 0–2 years p. 190; 🔂 Growth 2–4 years p. 206; 🔂 Growth and nutrition 5–11 years p. 222; 🔂 Growth and nutrition 12–18 years p. 234)
- Speech, language, and communications development (🔂 Speech and language acquisition p. 218)
- Emotional and social development (🔂 Emotional development in babies and children p. 210)
- Behavioural development (🔂 Understanding behaviour 1–5 years p. 216)
- Self-esteem, self-image, and identity
- Family and social relationships
- Self-care skills and independence
- Understanding, reasoning, and problem solving
- Participation in learning, education, and employment

- Progress and achievement in learning
- Aspirations
- Basic care, ensuring safety, and protection (➲ Accident prevention p. 168)
- Emotional warmth and stability
- Guidance, boundaries, and stimulation
- Family history, functioning, and well-being
- Parents' health, ill health, or disability, and impact on child
- Wider family
- Housing, employment, and financial considerations (➲ Homes and housing p. 26)
- Social and community elements and resources, including education

Impact of adult health problems on children

Professionals should assess the impact and needs of children and young people when working with adults with health problems, particularly if they are: parents with mental health problems; parents with long-term conditions and disabilities; or parents with addictions (➲ Alcohol p. 360; ➲ Substance use p. 476).

Care planning, management, monitoring, and evaluation

A child in need plan operates under Section 17 of the Children Act 1989. Assessment should be part of a care management process with an identified lead professional, key worker, or care manager who will work closely with the family to help co-ordinate: a plan to address the identified and agreed needs; the delivery of services and support; and the monitoring and review of the plan.

Further information

Healthy Child Programme England (*Healthy Child Programme: pregnancy and the first five years of life*). Available at: ℬ www.gov.uk/government/publications/healthy-child-programme-pregnancy-and-the-first-5-years-of-life

HM Government (*Working together to safeguard children: a guide to inter-agency working to safeguard and promote the welfare of children*). Available at: ℬ https://assets.publishing.service.gov.uk/government/uploads/system/uploads/attachment_data/file/779401/Working_Together_to_Safeguard-Children.pdf

Child screening tests

Nationally agreed child screening tests are carried out on the whole population. Where there is professional or parental concern, additional interventions may be appropriate. Children who are at ↑ risk of a condition may need extra investigations, despite a normal screening test.

Consent (➔ Consent p. 82) should be sought from a person with parental responsibility before any screening test is undertaken.

Physical examination

The following form part of routine physical examination carried out at 72hrs old and again between 6–8wks old by a competent practitioner:

- Eyes (eye problems requiring treatment) (➔ Eyes and vision screening p. 162)
- Heart (congenital heart defect needing treatment) (➔ Congenital heart defects p. 260)
- Hips (development dysplasia of the hips (DDH))
- Testes (undescended testes)
- Hearing (➔ Hearing screening p. 163)

Early treatment can reduce disability:

- Early surgery for cataracts improves visual outcome.
- Surgery for congenital heart disease before symptoms develop is beneficial in more severe forms.
- Early treatment (splinting) of DDH ↓ need for surgical intervention.
- Early surgery (referral by 1yr of age) for undescended testes may improve fertility (➔ Problems with fertility p. 784) and facilitate early diagnosis of malignancy.

Whilst not part of the formal 'screening' programme, birthweight and head circumference at birth act as a baseline for future measurements (➔ New birth visits p. 174). At 6–8wks. weight can provide reassurance that a baby is growing appropriately during a period of rapid growth (➔ Growth 0–2 years p. 190; ➔ Growth disorders p. 298). Weight should be measured using appropriately calibrated scales, and head circumference using a tape measure around the occipito-frontal circumference.

Neonatal blood spot screening

- Phenylketonuria (PKU) (➔ Congenital impairments p. 262)
- Congenital hypothyroidism (CHT) (➔ Thyroid p. 702)
- Cystic fibrosis (➔ Cystic fibrosis p. 318)
- Sickle cell disease (➔ Sickle cell disorders p. 308)
- Medium-chain acyl-CoA dehydrogenase deficiency (MCADD)
- Glutaric aciduria type 1 (GA1)
- Homocystinuria (pyridoxine unresponsive) (HCU)
- Isovaleric acidaemia (IVA)
- Maple syrup urine disease (MSUD)

Preventative treatment ↓ the risk of disability and, in some, early death. Heel prick blood sample (usually by midwife) at 5–8 days (ideally 5 days). Standards for performance have been agreed nationally.[12] All results from laboratories are sent to child health record departments/child health information systems who are responsible for monitoring coverage and informing health visitor/GP. Health visitors are responsible for informing parents of negative results (➲ Health visiting p. 46). Positive results are reported to hospital paediatricians and GPs, by the laboratory, for follow-up, and copied to child health record departments/child health information systems.

Related topics

➲ UK screening programmes p. 362; ➲ Thalassaemia p. 312; ➲ Overview of the Healthy Child Programme p. 154

References

12. PHE (2017) *NHS newborn blood spot screening programme standards*. Available at: https://www.gov.uk/guidance/newborn-blood-spot-screening-programme-overview

Further information

Public Health Agency (Northern Ireland) (*Newborn screening*). Available at: ℘ http://www.publichealth.hscni.net/directorate-public-health/service-development-and-screening/newborn-screening

PHE (*Newborn and infant physical examination*). Available at: ℘ https://www.gov.uk/guidance/newborn-and-infant-physical-examination-screening-programme-overview

PHE (*Sickle cell and thalassaemia screening: programme overview*). Available at: ℘ https://www.gov.uk/guidance/sickle-cell-and-thalassaemia-screening-programme-overview

PHE (*NHS population screening explained*). Available at: ℘ https://www.gov.uk/guidance/nhs-population-screening-explained

NHS Scotland (*National screening programmes*). Available at: ℘ https://www.nsd.scot.nhs.uk/services/screening/

NHS Wales (*Newborn blood spot screening Wales*). Available at: ℘ http://www.newbornbloodspotscreening.wales.nhs.uk/home

Eyes and vision screening

Congenital ocular opacities

Looking for cataracts, retinoblastoma, and congenital glaucoma
(➔ Congenital impairments p. 262). Early treatment leads to improved
prognosis. Inspection is conducted within 72hrs of birth and again at 6–
8wks. It includes red reflex. Carried out by a healthcare professional trained
to do this.

Impaired visual acuity

Looking for amblyopia—suppression of vision in a healthy eye due to different images falling on the two retinae—and other causes of impaired
visual acuity. Early intervention with glasses and/or patching may lead to improved visual function. Visual acuity of both eyes assessed separately using
standard charts in an appropriately lit environment. Carried out by trained
personnel at 4–5yrs or on school entry, ideally by an orthoptist or as part
of an orthoptic-led service.

Related topics

➔ Overview of the Healthy Child Programme p. 154; ➔ Child screening
tests p. 160

Further information

PHE (*Child vision screening*). Available at: ℘ https://www.gov.uk/government/publications/
child-vision-screening

Hearing screening

Neonatal

To identify congenital sensorineural hearing impairment (◆ Congenital impairments p. 262). Conducted either in the first days in hospital or in the community in the first 5wks of life (◆ Child screening tests p. 160). Early detection allows implementation of optimal management (hearing aids and parental interaction) with improvement of language development. Semi-automated techniques employed. Oto-acoustic emissions and auditory brain responses are measured by specially trained personnel.

Targeted ongoing surveillance may be undertaken irrespective of the newborn screening outcome if: parental or professional concern; meningitis, measles (◆ Infectious diseases in childhood p. 290), chronic middle-ear effusion, or craniofacial abnormalities; ↑ levels of ototoxic drugs; and other risk factors for late-onset, progressive or acquired deafness (◆ Deafness in children p. 268).

Primary school entry

To identify acquired hearing impairment and late-onset/progressive impairments linked to prenatal or perinatal infection or to hereditary factors. Hearing loss may contribute to problems with learning (◆ Communication and learning problems p. 224). Appropriate management can minimize this. Pure-tone audiometry by trained personnel, usually audiometricians or school nurses (◆ School nursing p. 42), involves using a regularly tested and calibrated audiometer in a quietened room and presenting tones (usually at each octave between 125 and 8kHz) through headphones at amplitudes related to expected thresholds for a normal hearing person. The child indicates when they can hear the tones and this is charted. Local protocols specify referral pathways for identified hearing loss.

Related topics

◆ Overview of the Healthy Child Programme p. 154

Further information

NHS Scotland (*Universal newborn hearing screening programme*). Available at: ℛ https://www.nsd. scot.nhs.uk/services/screening/UNhearingscreening/index.html

NHS Wales (*Newborn hearing screening Wales*). Available at: ℛ http://www.wales.nhs.uk/sitesplus/ 980/home

Northern Ireland Direct Government Services (*Newborn screening*). Available at: ℛ https://www. nidirect.gov.uk/articles/newborn-screening#toc-0

PHE (*Newborn hearing screening: programme overview*). Available at: ℛ https://www.gov.uk/guidance/newborn-hearing-screening-programme-overview

Childhood immunization

Childhood immunization is important for both the individual and public health.[13] It is an essential part of the Healthy Child Programme (➔ Overview of the Healthy Child Programme p. 154). Information (including leaflets) about immunization programmes is usually given to parents at the new baby review (➔ New birth visits p. 174) and opportunities offered for parents to discuss any issues or concerns. Information on Bacillus–Calmette–Guerin (BCG) (➔ Tuberculosis p. 728) and Hepatitis B (➔ Viral hepatitis p. 724) for ↑ risk babies should be provided by the midwives prior to delivery. Consent (➔ Consent p. 82) should be sought from a person with parental responsibility before immunization (➔ Immunization administration p. 390).

Each 1° care organization should have a named person who has oversight of the programme. This person should act as a source of expert advice and, if they cannot answer clinical queries, be able to call on a local clinician. There are national targets for immunization uptake. Child health record departments or child health information systems act as a repository for immunization data, recording consent or refusal. In some areas, they also provide parent and professional reminder systems, although this is done independently by many GP practices (➔ General practice p. 18). The 1° course of immunization is part of the general medical services contract (global sum), but may also form enhanced services or personal medical services contracts for areas or populations with particular challenges in reaching coverage targets.

Immunization should be offered as in the UK immunization schedule (➔ Childhood immunization schedule (UK) p. 166). On every occasion a child is seen by a healthcare professional, their immunization status should be checked and appropriate immunizations made available.

Vaccines

Routine childhood vaccines are purchased nationally and are free to patients. Information on suppliers of vaccines is available on the 'Green Book' website.[14] Vaccines must be stored at 2–8°C and must not be frozen. The cold chain must be preserved if transported to other sites (➔ Storage, transportation, and disposal of medicines p. 148).

Safety and side effects

All vaccines are carefully tested, both for their efficacy and safety, before being introduced. Each batch of vaccine is tested before release and close post-marketing surveillance is in place. Part of this is the 'Yellow Card' system.[15]

Measles, mumps, and rubella (MMR) vaccine

Much research has been conducted on the vaccine and it has been shown to have a good safety profile with no link to autism or chronic bowel disease.

Thiomersal

Some vaccines used to contain thiomersal, a mercury-containing preservative. No research has shown it to be toxic in doses contained in vaccines but, based on the 'precautionary principle', it is being phased out and none of the routine childhood vaccines contain any.

Homeopathy

↑ numbers of people are turning to alternative forms of healthcare (➲ Complementary and alternative therapies p. 838). There is no evidence that any of these are effective in preventing the diseases against which vaccines are used.

Vulnerable children

Some children (e.g. looked-after children (➲ Looked-after children p. 254)) are at risk of not receiving all the routine immunizations. Others with chronic disorders (e.g. cardiac and neurological) may need extra immunizations. Both groups should be closely monitored.

References

13. PHE (2016) *Vaccines work.* Available at: https://upload.wikimedia.org/wikipedia/commons/1/16/Infographic_Vaccines_Public_Health_England.pdf
14. PHE (2013) *Immunisation against infectious diseases (The Green Book).* Available at: https://www.gov.uk/government/collections/immunisation-against-infectious-disease-the5green-book
15. MHRA (2015) *The Yellow Card Scheme: guidance for healthcare professionals.* Available at: https://www.gov.uk/guidance/the-yellow-card-scheme-guidance-for-healthcare-professionals

Childhood immunization schedule (UK)

The immunization schedule (as at 2018) is given in Table 6.2. Other vaccines or extra doses may be indicated for ↑ risk individuals. These include: pneumococcal polysaccharide vaccine, influenza vaccine, Hepatitis B

Table 6.2 UK childhood immunization schedule: 2018

Age	Vaccine	Mode of delivery	Site
8wks	Diphtheria, tetanus, acellular pertussis, inactivated polio vaccine, Haemophilus influenzae type b, and Hepatitis B (DTaP/IPV/Hib/Hep B)	One injection One injection One injection Oral	IM thigh Same time, different limb or different site (2.5cm apart)
	Pneumococcal conjugate vaccine (PCV)		
	Meningococcal B (Men B)		
	Rotavirus vaccine (Rota)		
12wks	DTaP/Hib/IPV/Hep B	One injection	IM thigh
	Rota	Oral	Injections guidance as 8wks
16wks	DTaP/Hib/IPV/Hep B	One injection	IM thigh
	PCV	One injection	Injections
	Men B	One injection	guidance as 8wks
12–13mths	Hib/Men C	One injection	IM upper arm or thigh
	MMR	One injection	
	PCV	One injection	Injections
	Men B	One injection	guidance as 8wks
2yrs (just before the flu season)	Influenza	Nasal spray	Intranasal in each nostril
3yrs (just before the flu season)	Influenza	Nasal spray	Intranasal in each nostril
Preschool (3yrs 4mths)	DTaP/IPV or DTaP/IPV (Preschool booster)	One injection	IM upper arm
	MMR (2nd dose)	One injection	Injections guidance as 8wks
Primary school Yrs R and 1–6 (just before the flu season)	Influenza	Nasal spray	Intranasal in each nostril
12–13yrs, girls only	HPV	Three injections over 6mths	IM upper arm
13–14yrs	Tetanus, low-dose diphtheria, IPV (Td/IPV; teenage booster)	One injection	IM upper arm
	Men ACWY	One injection	Injections guidance as 8wks

(➔ Viral hepatitis p. 724) vaccine, and BCG (➔ Tuberculosis p. 728). BCG is only offered to ↑ risk groups:

- Infants in areas where tuberculosis (TB) ≥40/100,000
- Infants and children <16yrs old whose parents or grandparents were born in a country with a TB incidence ≥40/100,000
- Previously unvaccinated new immigrants <16yrs old from ↑ TB prevalence countries
- Children and young people who are going to stay or have stayed in close contact with the indigenous population in ↑ TB prevalence countries for at least a month

Infants (i.e. those <6yrs) do not need Mantoux test prior to BCG. For older groups, consult the 'Green Book'.[16]

Where and by whom

Routine vaccines for young children are usually given in 1° care and for older children by the school health service (➔ School nursing p. 42). Given by someone trained in the administration of vaccines and ↑ level of knowledge about vaccines and immunization (➔ Immunization administration p. 390). Nurses and health visitors (➔ Health visiting p. 46) often administer vaccines under patient group directives (➔ Medicines optimization p. 128). Anyone administering vaccines should be competent in cardiopulmonary resuscitation (➔ Child basic life support p. 800) and dealing with anaphylaxis (➔ Anaphylaxis p. 810).

Contraindications

Anaphylaxis to a previous dose of vaccine or a component of vaccine is a contraindication to vaccination. In addition, particular live vaccines, such as MMR vaccine, may be contraindicated in some immunosuppressed individuals (➔ Principles of working with someone with compromised immunity p. 466). Before withholding a vaccine from such patients, consult patient's specialist. In children who are moderately or severely systemically unwell with a fever, vaccination should be delayed.

References

16. PHE (2013) *Immunisation against infectious diseases (The Green Book)*. Available at: https://www.gov.uk/government/collections/immunisation-against-infectious-disease-the-green-book

Further information

E-Learning for Healthcare (*Immunisation*). Available at: ✌ https://www.e-lfh.org.uk/programmes/immunisation/

Health Protection Scotland (*Immunisation and vaccine preventable diseases*). Available at: ✌ www.hps.scot.nhs.uk/immvax/index.aspx#

NHS Wales (*Vaccines for children*). Available at: ✌ http://www.wales.nhs.uk/sitesplus/888/page/59487

Oxford Vaccine Group (*Vaccine Knowledge Project*). Available at: ✌ http://vk.ovg.ox.ac.uk/

PHE (*Vaccine uptake guidance and the latest coverage data*). Available at: ✌ www.hpa.org.uk/Topics/InfectiousDiseases/InfectionsAZ/VaccinationImmunisation/

Public Health Agency (Northern Ireland) (*Immunisation/vaccine preventable diseases*). Available at: ✌ http://www.publichealth.hscni.net/directorate-public-health/health-protection/immunisationvaccine-preventable-diseases

Accident prevention

Accidental injury to children is a major public health and inequalities issue. Accidental injury is one of the biggest killers of children. The patterns and types of injury are closely linked with child development stages. The group most at risk are children <4yrs (➲ Child development 0–1 years p. 192; ➲ Promoting baby development safely 0–1 years; Promoting baby development; ➲ Child development 1–5 years p. 204). Many accidents are preventable.

UK statistics

~55 children aged <5yrs die each year due to an unintentional injury. Annually, 370,000 children attend A&E and 40,000 are admitted to hospital as an emergency.[18] Unintentional injuries are a major health inequality; e.g. emergency hospital admission rate for unintentional injuries among the under-fives was 38% higher for children from the most deprived areas compared with the least deprived[17](➲ UK health profile p. 2).

Types of unintentional injuries amongst the under-fives

- Choking, suffocation, and strangulation: including inhalation of food and vomit, and suffocation and strangulation from, for example, entrapment in cot bumpers (➲ Child choking p. 806; ➲ Food and the under-fives p. 212)
- Falls: including falls from furniture, on and off the stairs, and buildings (including windows and balconies)
- Poisoning: including medicines, button batteries, and household chemicals (such as liquid detergent capsules) (➲ Poisoning and overdoses p. 822)
- Burns and scalds: including scalds from hot drinks, contact with hot household appliances (including hair straighteners), and bath water scalds (➲ Burns and scalds p. 816)
- Drowning: including in the bath, fish ponds, and open water
- Road traffic accidents (RTAs): the single biggest cause of accidental death in children aged 12–16yrs, including as a pedestrian, as a passenger in a vehicle (particularly if unrestrained or inappropriately restrained), and bicycle accidents
- Dog bites

Emotional, family, and relationship consequences

These can be far-reaching, leading to parents/carers experiencing acute stress disorder or significant traumatic stress symptoms >6mths after the initial injury (➲ People with anxiety and depression p. 478; ➲ Post-traumatic stress disorder p. 490). Caring for a child who has been seriously injured can stop a parent from returning to education or work, or plunge an already disadvantaged family further into poverty.

Action for prevention

Accident prevention is most successful at a public health and legislative level, e.g. traffic-calming measures, child-resistant medication containers, compulsory use of seat belts in all parts of a car. Parents also need to be aware of:
- Risks at different child developmental stages, and preventative action

- Use of home safety equipment and schemes that loan equipment or provide for free (e.g. stair gates and smoke detectors)
- Risks associated with different leisure and sport activities, and preventative action (e.g. cycling and the use of helmets)
- Correct use of in-car safety equipment for the age group

There are also opportunities for education of children and young people on safety issues including crossing roads, learning to swim, and cycling proficiency. These types of learning opportunities may be provided by parents, local leisure organizations, early years education, and/or through Personal, Social, Health, and Economic (PSHE) curriculum in schools (➲ Working in schools p. 44).

References

17. PHE (2018) *Reducing unintentional injuries in and around the home among children under five years.* Available at: https://assets.publishing.service.gov.uk/government/uploads/system/uploads/attachment_data/file/696646/Unintentional_injuries_under_fives_in_home.pdf

Further information

Child Accident Prevention Trust (*Safety advice*). Available at: ℜ https://www.capt.org.uk/Pages/Category/safety-advice-injury-types

Dogs Trust (*Be safe around dogs*). Available at: ℜ https://www.dogstrust.org.uk/help-advice/factsheets-downloads/bds%20parents%20leaflet.pdf

Royal Society for the Prevention of Accidents (*Accidents to children*). Available at: ℜ www.rospa.com/home-safety/advice/accidents-to-children/

UNICEF (*Caring for your baby at night*). Available at: ℜ www.unicef.uk/caringatnight

Working with parents

This might involve parents expecting a first child or those living with adolescents. Work might be preventative or in response to significant problems defined by parents, teachers, health practitioners, social care, or wider society. A supportive role may be adopted in order to protect the health and well-being of the child/adolescent and support parents to achieve health outcomes (➔ Child protection processes p. 252). Problems affecting the child's health and well-being may include sleep problems (➔ Babies, children, and sleeping p. 200) and aggression towards other children (➔ Understanding behaviour 1–5 years p. 216; ➔ Behavioural disorders in children p. 326).

The aim is to work with parents to attune their parenting in order to protect the child and promote physical, intellectual, emotional, and social development (➔ Emotional development in babies and children p. 210; ➔ Emotional problems in children p. 330). Parents should be supported with the relevant skills from before the birth of the child until early adulthood. Different approaches exist, which may have various theoretical underpinnings:

• Behavioural modification: concentrates on the behaviour to be changed, e.g. attention seeking or bed wetting (➔ Nocturnal enuresis p. 296), by rewarding acceptable behaviour.
• Parent advisory models: seek to understand individual context in which child and parent live. Helper–parent relationship is seen as central, with helper an active listener, followed by negotiated plan to meet individual family's needs.
• Brief interventions: short-term interactions focused on a particular issue.
• Child development programme: sees developmental achievements of child as central. Considering what a child can do, the parents develop ideas for care and stimulation, including health factors such as diet.

Many approaches draw from different perspectives—humanistic, counselling, social learning, and active listening. Integrating these views can lead to an approach specific for the family. Widely used models include: Solihull Approach (see ℘ https://solihullapproachparenting.com/), Mellow Parenting (see ℘ http://www.mellowparenting.org/), and Triple-P (see ℘ http://www.triplep.net/glo-en/home) (➔ Support for parenting p. 172).

Relationship-building approaches

Health practitioners build effective and lasting relationships by demonstrating empathy, enthusiasm, confidence, and expertise whilst seeking to empower the parent. Regular contact, sharing records, transparency, and adopting a non-judgemental approach are crucial to building successful relationships. Partnership working is key, with parents and practitioners agreeing on what they can contribute to the relationship.

Two-way sharing of knowledge, experience, and responsibility

The health worker draws on their expertise in child development, health promotion, or adolescent health (➔ Child and adolescent mental health p. 246). The parents know the child, family circumstances, and the socio-cultural context in which the family lives. Both contributions are valued, as neither party can 'solve' the problem alone. Interactions will lead to the development of skills of both parent and professional. Reflection on the situation clarifies the issues and establishes the priorities for action.

Getting parent (and child or young person) to set own goals

The family need to 'own' the issue, to define what they want to achieve and what is manageable. This may be different from the professional or parents' views. Practitioners will advocate for the child and help parents to provide the best opportunities for their children.

Recognizing and celebrating success

Small, positive developments need to be noted and celebrated. This builds up the confidence of all involved, empowers parents, and ↑ expectations of success.

Accessing other parenting support if necessary

This may include early years' provision, attending children's centres, assessing health assets, engaging with local services, and attending activities in the community (**⊃** Support for parenting p. 172).

Impact of other issues

Parents may have problems or issues that impact on parenting. Interventions in terms of domestic violence (**⊃** Domestic violence p. 450), family breakdown, mental illness (**⊃** People with psychosis p. 486; **⊃** People with bipolar affective disorder p. 482), alcohol (**⊃** Alcohol p. 360), and substance use (**⊃** Substance use p. 476) may be appropriate.

Parenting and child mental health

Parenting may be linked with child mental health work. School nurses, health visitors, GPs, nursery nurses, teachers, and youth workers should be involved at the first level, promoting sound parenting and child mental health (**⊃** Teamwork p. 58). Entrenched difficulties may need the involvement of mental health and multidisciplinary teams. Building good parenting skills needs to begin early in life, and so can feature in personal, social, and health promotion, and citizenship in schools, together with youth organizations, pre-conceptual care (**⊃** Preconceptual care p. 422), and early antenatal interventions (**⊃** Antenatal education and preparation for parenthood p. 425).

Further information

Department of Health and Social Care (*Healthy Child Programme: pregnancy and the first five years of life*). Available at: ℒ https://www.gov.uk/government/publications/healthy-child-programme-pregnancy-and-the-first-5-years-of-life

Institute of Health Visiting (*Developing your practice*). Available at: ℒ https://ihv.org.uk/for-health-visitors/developing-you-in-practice/

Support for parenting

All national policies on children have support for parenting as a key standard. 'Good enough parenting' providing love, care, and commitment, acts as a buffer against adversity, e.g. poverty. It contributes to emotional well-being (➲ Emotional development in babies and children p. 210) and ↓ the need for later reactive intervention. Good parenting will include: provision of resources to facilitate growth and development (➲ Child development 0–1 years p. 192; ➲ Child development 1–5 years p. 204; ➲ Promoting development in the under-fives p. 208; ➲ Child development 5–11 years p. 220); meeting the child's needs for love and security; realistic expectations of the child linked to their development and maturity; and provision of appropriate stimulation and opportunities for social development. A quality environment, providing appropriate accommodation (➲ Homes and housing p. 26) and nutrition, good nursery provision, play spaces, maternity/paternity leave, family friendly working patterns, and financial support also support parenting.

Family and networks

Traditionally, extended families have provided practical and emotional encouragement. This still exists for some groups. However, when families are spread throughout the country/world, support may come from community links and faith/cultural groups. Those without support may not be obvious and may include lone parents and those whose previous focus was on career development.

Home visits

Visits by health workers or volunteers are effective in developing parenting skills (➲ Working with parents p. 170), promoting the child's development, improving breastfeeding rates (➲ Breastfeeding p. 182), and reducing unintentional injury (➲ Accident prevention p. 168). Healthcare organizations promote the use of specific techniques and programmes such as the Solihull Approach (see ♫ https://solihullapproachparenting.com/), Mellow Parenting (see ♫ http://www.mellowparenting.org/), and Triple-P (see ♫ http://www.triplep.net/glo-en/home).

Peer support

Support is available in groups facilitated by health visitors (➲ Health visiting p. 46) and school nurses (➲ School nursing p. 42), such as postnatal support groups (➲ Postnatal care p. 438), parent drop-ins, and parenting groups. These seek to build parental confidence and local networks. Mother and toddler groups, and local branches of the National Childbirth Trust and Meet a Mum, may have similar aims.

Programmes, groups, and communities

A variety of programmes, groups, and communities seek to support parenting. Some are local, some nationally based. They generally aim to: take a partnership approach; raise parents' self-esteem; build up parent support networks; take a positive approach to discipline, setting clear boundaries; understand how families see issues; and recognize there are different parenting styles. Examples of programmes, communities, and groups include:

- First parenting programmes (for new mothers and fathers as they make the transition to parenthood)
- Home-Start (voluntary organization providing informal support for families with young children in their own home)
- Children's centres (bringing together early education, childcare, health, and family support)

Setting up such programmes should involve partnership with parents in the planning, development, and monitoring of services (⊃ Patient and public experience p. 75). Parents might be involved in writing the mission statement, recruitment and appraisal of staff, design and evaluation of the service, and contributing to new ways of working for both staff and users.

Further information

Home Start (About us). Available at: ♒ https://www.home-start.org.uk/about-us

National Childbirth Trust (Local branches). Available at: ♒ http://www.nct.org.uk/branches

Parenting UK (Parenting professionals). Available at: ♒ http://www.parentinguk.org/

University of Kent (TOPSE: a tool to measure parenting self-efficacy). Available at: ♒ https://www.topse.org.uk/site/

Welsh Government (Parenting support). Available at: ♒ https://gov.wales/topics/people-and-communities/people/children-and-young-people/parenting-support-guidance/?lang=en

New birth visits

A new birth visit is the first contact (usually at home) with a family with a new baby. These visits are completed by a health visitor (HV) (➔ Health visiting p. 46) at 10–14 days after birth. It is a core component of the Healthy Child Programme (HCP) (➔ Overview of the Healthy Child Programme p. 154). The HV may have met the mother (and partner) previously at an antenatal visit (➔ Antenatal education and preparation for parenthood p. 425) or from contacts with previous children.

Information about a new birth

Every maternity unit provides the details of all births to the local child health department. The child health department informs the HV service, which is either assigned to provide services in the area where the mother resides or to the GP surgery (➔ General practice p. 18) that she is registered to.

Key principles of the new birth visit

- To introduce themselves, HVs discuss the services and care delivered in line with the HCP to the mother and partner (➔ Working with parents p. 170; ➔ Support for parenting p. 172)
- To begin to establish relationship of trust with mother and family so they feel safe to raise issues
- To encourage and support all aspects of learning to nurture the baby and being a parent, often through using techniques such as the Brazelton approach (see ℰ http://www.brazelton.co.uk/) to sensitize parents to newborn abilities
- To encourage and support all aspects of ensuring good physical and emotional health in mother and baby (➔ Postnatal depression p. 440; ➔ Emotional development in babies and children p. 210)
- To support mother and infant to bond and develop a secure attachment
- To assess and identify any maternal, baby, family health (physical, mental, and emotional), or social problems, and offer advice and agree steps to addressing the problems
- To identify children in need (➔ Identifying the child in need of protection p. 250) and plan appropriate action with parent
- To provide information on the HCP (particularly childhood immunizations (➔ Childhood immunization p. 164)) and information about local services, including children's centres, information about health assets, health services, and birth registration (➔ Registration of births, marriages, and deaths p. 842)
- To agree a pattern of future contact and provide information about how to contact the HV service

Key topics

Local healthcare organizations have guidelines, which are informed by national guidance and the HCP. Content will include: establishing infant feeding, especially breastfeeding (➔ Breastfeeding p. 182); promoting positive parenting and parent–baby relationship; prevention of sudden infant death syndrome (➔ Sudden infant death syndrome p. 278); maternal mental health; parents' relationship; sex and contraception (➔ Sexual health: general issues p. 760); and keeping the baby safe (➔ Accident prevention p. 168), including passive smoking (➔ Smoking cessation p. 356).

Style of contact

Visits are holistic. HVs should adopt motivational interviewing techniques (➔ Motivational interviewing in consultations p. 126), with open-ended questions, paraphrasing, and self-awareness. HVs often start by asking what the birth was like, as a way into understanding the experience so far (➔ Complicated labour p. 436). Some organizations provide standard operating procedures that must be adhered to when assessing the baby and the family setting, but most HVs use these as an aide memoire, rather than as a yes/no checklist.

Records

All organizations have record-keeping guidance (➔ Record keeping p. 86). Records should be contemporaneous, accurate, and written following local guidelines. All contacts and communications should be recorded on local electronic healthcare records. When contact is made in person, it should also be recorded in the personal child health record (Redbook) (➔ Client-and patient-held records p. 90). Electronic personal child health records are being trialled across the UK.

Further information

Department of Health and Social Care (*Healthy Child Programme: pregnancy and the first five years of life*). Available at: ℰ https://www.gov.uk/government/publications/healthy-child-programme-pregnancy-and-the-first-5-years-of-life

Institute of Health Visiting (*New birth visit: the second of the child development reviews of the Healthy Child Programme (England)*). Available at: ℰ https://ihv.org.uk/wp-content/uploads/2015/06/IHV_Why_a_health_visitor_NEW_BIRTH_2.pdf

NICE (*Postnatal care up to 8 weeks after birth [CG37]*). Available at: ℰ https://www.nice.org.uk/guidance/cg37/ifp/chapter/Every-postnatal-contact

Pre-term infants

Pre-term describes infants born <37wks. Approximately 60,000 babies are born prematurely in the UK/yr (1 in every 13 babies)[18] (➔ UK health profile p. 2). Infants born at 23–26wks' gestation have 30–80% chance of survival. They often have problems including respiratory distress, hypotension, and metabolic problems, and require many weeks in intensive and special care. Very ↓ birthweight babies (<1500g) have ↑ risk of neurodevelopmental problems, including visual impairment, hearing loss (➔ Deafness in children p. 268), cerebral palsy (➔ Cerebral palsy p. 320), and learning difficulties (➔ People with learning disabilities p. 456). Multiple pregnancies, where a mother is carrying twins and triplets, often result in premature labour (➔ Twins and multiple births p. 180). The average delivery date for such pregnancies (➔ Pregnancy p. 424) is 33–37wks, often resulting in a planned premature labour. Planned premature labour may also occur where there is a risk to mother or baby, e.g. where there is ↓ fetal heart rate or mother has pre-eclampsia (➔ Common problems in pregnancy p. 432). Those born >32wks have good prognosis with few problems.

On returning home from hospital

Parents may need extra reassurance and support. Very premature and ↓ birthweight babies have ↑ risk of hospital readmission in first year. Key areas of support and advice from 1° care professionals are described below.

Bonding

May have been difficult while in hospital and added to by fear of baby dying.

Feeding

Pre-term babies are 'suck and swallow' poor, and so require frequent feeding. Breast milk (sometimes with calorie supplements) or special low birthweight formula is used (➔ Breastfeeding p. 182; ➔ Bottle feeding p. 186). Vitamin and iron supplements are routine. Weaning advice for each baby will be different, so parents should ask for advice from paediatric team (➔ Weaning p. 188).

Temperature control

May be poor at first. Controlled environment temperature of 18°C/65°F needed, and adequate insulation with clothes and blankets.

Respiratory problems

Sometimes sent home on oxygen via nasal cannulae. ↑ risk from respiratory infections. Possibly advise use of apnoea monitor at home.

Vision problems

As a result of ↑ partial pressures of oxygen in special care. May need follow-up in 1° care (➔ Eyes and vision screening p. 162).

Hearing

↑ risk of hearing problems. Should have neonatal screening and follow-up (➔ Hearing screening p. 163).

Sudden infant death

Pre-term babies have ↑ risk. Lullaby Trust has material on safe sleeping (➲ Babies, children, and sleeping p. 200) to contribute to prevention (➲ Sudden infant death syndrome p. 278; ➲ Child basic life support p. 800).

References

18. BLISS (for babies born premature or sick) (2017) *Prematurity statistics in the UK*. Available at: https://www.bliss.org.uk/research-campaigns/research/neonatal-care-statistics/prematurity-statistics-in-the-uk

Further information

BLISS (for babies born premature or sick) (*Our prematurity message*). Available at: ℘ https://www.bliss.org.uk/support-bliss/world-prematurity-day/prematurityis

Lullaby Trust (*The best sleeping position for your baby*). Available at: ℘ https://www.lullabytrust.org.uk/safer-sleep-advice/sleeping-position/

New babies

Many parents, particularly first-time ones, need reassurance and advice about the changes and minor problems that arise with their new baby.

Head

May appear elongated or misshapen as a result of the bones moving during the birth process. Resolves spontaneously during the first weeks.

Umbilicus

After birth, the umbilicus dries, becomes black, and separates at about 1wk of age. Potential problems include: infected stump—symptoms include offensive odour, exudate, and malaise (refer to GP for treatment (➋ General practice p. 18)); sometimes a granuloma forms (refer to GP for treatment); and hernia, due to weak abdominal wall allowing intestines to bulge out (this is common and usually resolves by 1yr).

Skin

The vernix protects against minor skin problems, such as peeling and flaking. Peeling (common in those born after due date) is best dealt with by a non-irritant moisturizer such as coconut oil, sunflower oil, or almond oil (⚠ do not use nut oils when there are nut allergies in the immediate family (➋ Allergies p. 694; ➋ Baby hygiene and skin care p. 194). Olive oil should not be used as this often makes dry skin worse. Skin may be blotchy as blood vessels are unstable. Babies of black parents are often light-skinned at birth, then produce melanin and reach permanent skin colour by 6mths.

Birth marks

- Strawberry (stork) marks: pink areas; may grow, but fade. Sometimes raised bumps that shrivel and go by second year
- Spider naevi: network of dilated vessels, usually go by second year
- Port wine stains: found anywhere; can be treated with lasers or camouflaged, or embraced as something that makes the baby different (but should be protected from the sun (➋ Skin cancer prevention p. 374))
- Blue spots: dark-skinned children often have harmless bluish black areas on back or base of spine known as congenital dermal melanocytosis; fade by 2yrs

Common skin problems

- Milia: tiny, pearly white papules on the nose and face (caused by blocked sebaceous ducts), which disappear spontaneously
- Neonatal urticaria: red blotches with a central, white vesicle, which are common in first week but disappear spontaneously
- Heat rash: small, red spots on face, which can be relieved by not overwrapping or overheating rooms
- Harlequin colour change: a harmless vasomotor effect where one side of body flushes red, while the other stays pale

Hair

The baby may be bald or have full head of hair. Hair colour may change. Lanugo (downy hair on body) will fall off soon after birth.

Eyes

May have broken blood vessels following birth; this is harmless and resolves within a couple of weeks. Sticky eyes are common and are usually due to blocked tear duct. They can be treated by swabbing with cooled boiled water at each nappy change. Infective causes of neonatal conjunctivitis include Chlamydia trachomatis and Neisseria gonorrhoea (➔ Sexually transmitted infections p. 764). Chlamydia presents 5–14 days after birth. Gonococcal conjunctivitis presents within the first 24 hours of delivery until 5 days post birth. Suspicion of either will require GP review and opthalmology follow-up.

Nose

Sneezing and snuffling are very common to clear amniotic fluid. Reassure parents.

Genitals

Many babies, ♂ and ♀, may appear to have enlarged genitals and swollen 'breasts' shortly after birth, due to maternal hormones in their bloodstream. This will subside spontaneously.

First nappies

Meconium (blackish-green) is the first bowel movement passed within 24hrs. Stools then change to greenish-brown, then yellow semi-solid. Stools of bottle-fed babies often resemble scrambled eggs. Most babies have bowel movements soon after feeding. A red-stained nappy is common and is usually due to urinary urates, but may be due to blood from vagina through oestrogen withdrawal. Reassure parents.

Further information

NHS (*Start for life*). Available at: ℜ https://www.nhs.uk/start4life/baby
NICE (*Postnatal care up to 8 weeks after birth*). Available at: ℜ https://www.nice.org.uk/guidance/CG37

Twins and multiple births

Occur in 1 in 64 pregnancies (➲ Pregnancy p. 424) in the UK. More common in ♀ treated for problems with fertility (➲ Problems with fertility p. 784). Monozygotic or identical twins arise from splitting of a fertilized egg (zygote) during the first 14 days after fertilization. They have the same genetic make-up and therefore sex. Dizygotic, non-identical twins, result from the fertilization of two independently released ova by two different sperm. They are no more alike than are any two siblings. About one third of twins in the UK are monozygotic.

Special considerations

- Pregnancy can be more tiring; anaemia (➲ Anaemia in adults p. 652) and fluid retention more common; and may need extra prenatal care and monitoring (➲ Antenatal care and screening p. 426).
- Babies are often born premature (➲ Pre-term infants p. 176) or of ↓ birthweight; this may result in death of one or more babies.
- Coping with two or more newborn babies can seem an overwhelming task and financially problematic.
- Multiples may experience language delay (➲ Speech and language acquisition p. 218), behavioural disorders (➲ Behavioural disorders in children p. 326), excessive rivalry, or dependency.

Extra help

Extra help is usually needed at first, not just to cope with physical demands but also to give time to each baby and to the parents' own needs. Health visitors (➲ Health visiting p. 46) are able to provide local information on childcare support (➲ Support for parenting p. 172).

Feeding and sleeping

Breastfeeding should be encouraged (➲ Breastfeeding p. 182), particularly in premature babies and because two babies can be fed and held close at once. Twins, particularly premature twins, placed in the same cot are often more contented than when alone. Usual advice is given on sleeping (➲ Babies, children, and sleeping p. 200; ➲ Sudden infant death syndrome p. 278).

Development and treating each baby and child as an individual

Parents should be encouraged to remember that each baby has their own needs and they need to create time to spend with each. Identical twins need to be treated as individuals (different clothes, feeding equipment, and bed clothes) and will have different developmental progress.

Further information

Multiple Births Foundation (*Information for both professionals and parents*). Available at: ℘ www. multiplebirths.org.uk

Twins and Multiple Birth Association (*Parenting*). Available at: ℘ https://www.tamba.org.uk/ parenting

Breastfeeding

Exclusive breastfeeding is the optimum method for the first 6mths of life and thereafter alongside other foods for around 2yrs.[19] The UK has some of the ↓ breastfeeding rates in the world (with 8 out of 10 ♀ stopping before they want to.[20] Only 34% of ♀ maintain any breastfeeding to 6mths compared to 49% in the USA and 71% in Norway (➲ UK health profile p. 2). The UNICEF UK Baby Friendly Initiative supports maternity, neonatal, health visiting (HV) (➲ Health visiting p. 46) and children's centre services to transform their care to better support families with feeding and with developing close, loving relationships, ensuring that all babies get the best possible start in life[21] (➲ Promoting the health of children p. 152).

Health and well-being outcomes

- ↓ incidence of ear, chest, and gut infections (➲ Infections in children p. 288), of necrotising enterocolitis, and of sudden infant death syndrome (➲ Sudden infant death syndrome p. 278)
- Supports close and loving relationships which helps attachment and the baby's brain development (➲ Emotional development in babies and children p. 210)
- ↓ tooth decay and dental malocclusion (➲ Development and care of teeth for young children p. 196), ↓ overweight and obesity (➲ Overweight children and adolescents p. 302), and ↑ intelligence score and educational attainment
- ↓ incidence of breast cancer (➲ Breast cancer p. 774) and protective effect against ovarian cancer in mother (➲ Gynaecological cancers p. 776)
- Supports close and loving relationships, ↑ mental health, and ↓ risk of postnatal depression (➲ Postnatal depression p. 440)

Caution

Certain diseases can be transferred in breast milk, e.g. Hepatitis B (➲ Viral hepatitis p. 724), HIV (➲ Human immunodeficiency virus p. 462). In the UK, mothers with HIV are advised not to breastfeed. Some drugs/medicines can pass from mother through breast milk to baby (➲ Prescribing for special groups p. 138), e.g. combined oral contraceptive (➲ Combined hormonal contraceptive methods p. 402) contraindicated in breastfeeding mothers.

Getting breastfeeding off to a good start

- Skin-to-skin contact between a mother and baby stimulates powerful surges of milk-producing and mothering hormones, encouraging the mother to instinctively respond to her baby for food, love, and comfort.
- In response to touch and suckling, the release of the hormone prolactin switches on the milk-producing cells; the hormone oxytocin works on the muscle cells, causing them to contract and squeeze milk down to the baby.
- Feedback inhibitor of lactation (FIL) is a protein in the milk, which alerts the milk-producing cells to stop making milk if the breast become full. As milk is removed, FIL levels ↓ and milk production ↑. Therefore, the more milk removed, the more milk made.
- Responsive breastfeeding involves a mother responding to her baby's cues, as well as her own desire to satisfy her baby's needs. A breastfed baby cannot be overfed or spoilt.

Supporting a mother to breastfeed

Positioning is the term used to describe how a mother holds her baby to enable the infant to attach effectively to the breast. There are many different positions a mother will adopt, depending on where she is and what she is doing: cross cradle, lying down, laid back. Using the CHIN acronym:

- Close: baby needs to be close to their mother so that s/he can take enough breast into their mouth.
- Head free: their head should be able to tilt back freely to allow the chin to lead as the baby comes onto the breast.
- In line: the head and body should be in alignment, so the baby does not twist their neck, which will make feeding and swallowing difficult.
- Nose to nipple: mother's nipple should rest just below the baby's nose; the infant will root and tilt their head backwards; the nipple will slip under the top lip, upwards and backwards into the mouth, coming to rest at the junction of the hard and soft palate.

Signs of effective attachment: feeding is pain-free, chin indenting breast, mouth wide open, cheeks full and rounded, more areola may be visible above top lip, rhythmic suck/swallow.

Early breastfeeding challenges

A full breastfeeding assessment should be carried out by the HV at the new birth visit. This can help to prevent problems and promote the mother's confidence. Key points include:

- How it feels for the mother: discomfort, nipple damage, breast engorgement, often caused by ineffective positioning and attachment
- Baby's appearance, behaviour, and tone: unsettled, distressed, lethargic, jaundiced, breast refusal
- Baby's urine and stool output: after day 3 and before 6wks, there should be a minimum of two soft yellow stools and five or six wet nappies daily
- Number of feeds in 24hrs: no fewer than 8–10 feeds in 24hrs, but preferably more
- Revisit key principles of positioning and attachment. Reassure the mother and support skin-to-skin contact to promote instinctive behaviour. If necessary, try hand expression of breast milk.

Expressing breast milk

Hand expressing is useful skill for mothers to learn. It can help mothers to soften the breasts by removing a little milk if they become full, and to self-manage blocked ducts and prevent engorgement and mastitis. Breast milk can be stored for up to 5 days in the fridge at 4°C and up to 6mths in a freezer. Breast milk can also be expressed by pump when a mother is separated from her baby, e.g. when infant is in the neonatal unit or mother is returning to work. Bottles and milk should be treated as for bottle feeding (→ Bottle feeding p. 186). See government guidelines on vitamin D requirements for babies from birth to 1yr.[22]

Breastfeeding support organizations

- National Breastfeeding Helpline:
  - ☎ 0300 100 0212
- Association of Breastfeeding Mothers:
  - ℗ https://abm.me.uk/
- The Breastfeeding Network:
  - ℗ https://www.breastfeedingnetwork.org.uk/
- La Leche League GB:
  - ℗ https://www.laleche.org.uk/
- National Childbirth Trust Breastfeeding Line:
  - ☎ 0300 330 0700

References

19. Rollins, N., et al. (2016) Why invest, and what it will take to improve breastfeeding practices? *Lancet*, 387 (10017), 491–504
20. NHS Digital (2012) *Infant Feeding Survey 2010*. Available at: https://digital.nhs.uk/data-and-information/publications/statistical/infant-feeding-survey/infant-feeding-survey-uk-2010
21. UNICEF UK (2018) *The Baby Friendly Initiative*. Available at: https://www.unicef.org.uk/babyfriendly/
22. Scientific Advisory Committee on Nutrition (2016) *Vitamin D and health report*. Available at: www.gov.uk/government/publications/sacn-vitamin-d-and-health-report

Bottle feeding

In the UK, there is a strong bottle-feeding culture; by 1wk of age over half of all babies will have received formula milk via a bottle, and by 6wks this rises to three quarters of all babies. Many breastfed (➔ Breastfeeding p. 182) babies also receive breast milk in a bottle.

Formula feeding

Parents need to know: how to minimize the risks of giving formula; how to make up feeds; how to bottle feed; and what formulas to use and to know the costs involved.[23,24] The UNICEF UK Baby Friendly Initiative includes standards for infants who are formula-fed and for parents who are bottle feeding, and provides evidence-based information for health professionals on how best to support parents to responsively bottle feed and what infant formula to choose. Families on ↓ incomes may be entitled to Healthy Start vouchers to purchase formula for their babies

Preparation of equipment

There are several ways to sterilize equipment; cold-water solution, steam, and boiling. Wash hands first. All feeding items should be thoroughly washed and rinsed before they are sterilized. Sterilize according to manufacturer's instructions until >6mths of age.

How to make up a feed

• Support parents to make up formula exactly to the manufacturer's instructions and not to add extra powder. Formula milk is available ready-made in cartons (↑ expensive) and in powder form.
• Even when tins and packets of powdered infant formula are sealed, they can sometimes contain harmful bacteria that could make baby ill. Although these bacteria are rare, the infections they cause can be life-threatening.
• Feeds should be made up one at a time, as the baby needs them (to ↓ risk of infection).
• Boiled water, at a temperature of 70°C, should be used (will kill any harmful bacteria). Feed should then be allowed to cool before being given to baby.
• Any infant formula left in the bottle after a feed should be thrown away; also unused feed that has been kept at room temperature for >2hrs.

What infant formula to choose

• There is no evidence that any one brand is superior to another or to support the use of 'follow-on formulas'; babies should be fed 'first-stage milks' for the 'first year' (➔ Evidence-based healthcare p. 72). It does not matter if the mother chooses cow's or goat's milk-based formula.
• Soya formula is made from soya, not cow's milk. Soya formula contains ↑ levels of a chemical called phytoestrogen which may have negative effects on babies, and so should only be used in exceptional circumstances and only under the recommendation of a doctor.
• Other artificial formulas are available for babies intolerant of cow's milk. Such babies are usually under the care of a paediatric consultant and formula milk is prescribed as advised.

Introduction of full-fat, pasteurized cow's milk

Not recommended until the baby is >1yr old as this is less digestible and deficient in vitamins A, C, D, and iron. Breast or first-formula milk should be used until 1yr, then switched to full-fat cow's milk. A 'follow-on' formula is not necessary.

Responsive bottle feeding

Although true responsive feeding is not possible when bottle feeding, as this risks overfeeding, the mother–baby relationship will be helped if mothers are supported to tune in to feeding cues and to hold their babies close during feeds. Offering the bottle in response to feeding cues, gently inviting the baby to take the teat, pacing the feeds, and avoiding forcing the baby to finish the feed can all help the experience, as well as ↓ the risk of overfeeding. Supporting parents to give most of the feeds themselves (particularly in the early days and weeks) will help them to build a close and loving relationship with their baby, and help their baby to feel safe and secure (➲ Emotional development in babies and children p. 210).

References

23. Renfrew, M., Ansell, P., & Macleod, K. (2003) Formula feed preparation: helping reduce the risks. A systematic review. *Archives of Disease in Childhood*, 88(1), 855–8
24. Renfrew, M., McLoughlin, M., & McFadden, A. (2008) Cleaning and sterilisation of infant feeding equipment: a systematic review. *Public Health Nutrition*, 11(11), 1188–99

Further information

First Steps Nutrition Trust (*Infant milks*). Available at: ℘ https://www.firststepsnutrition.org/infant-milks-overview/

UNICEF UK (*Guidelines on providing information for parents about formula feeding*). Available at: ℘ https://www.unicef.org.uk/babyfriendly/wp-content/uploads/sites/2/2018/02/Guidelines-on-providing-information-for-parents-about-formula-feeding.pdf

UNICEF UK (*Responsive feeding: supporting close and loving relationships*). Available at: ℘ https://www.unicef.org.uk/babyfriendly/baby-friendly-resources/relationship-building-resources/responsive-feeding-infosheet/

Weaning

Weaning (also known as 'complementary feeding') is the gradual shift from a milk-based diet to family food (➲ Bottle feeding p. 186; ➲ Breastfeeding p. 182). The WHO recommend that milk only is sufficient until 6mths.[25] The child is likely to be ready for mixed feeding when they can sit up, wants to chew (putting objects in mouth, rather than pushing out), and reaches and grabs accurately. Weaning prior to 6mths should be discouraged and, if started early, advise sterilizing bowls and spoons (➲ Home food safety and hygiene p. 352), and avoid foods likely to cause allergies (e.g. wheat-based foods and others containing gluten, eggs, fish, shellfish, nuts, seeds, and soft and unpasteurised cheeses) (➲ Allergies p. 694).

How to start weaning

Offer just a few teaspoons of food, once a day. Use a little of usual milk to mix food to desired consistency. Give baby a range of foods and textures to taste, trying new foods one at a time. Allow them to touch food in the bowl or spoon. Encourage the baby to feed themselves, using their fingers as soon as they show an interest. Use bibs and covers to catch the mess. If baby does not want solids, then wait and try again later. Do not add any foods (including rusks, cereal, or sugar) to infant formula feeds.

Suitable weaning foods

• Blended, mashed, or soft-cooked sticks of parsnip, broccoli, potato, yam, sweet potato, carrot, apple
• Finger foods such as carrot sticks, cooked and cooled green beans, cubes of cheese, chopped peeled fruit (⚠ risk of choking with whole grapes (➲ Child choking p. 806)), all types of breads

Foods to avoid

• Salt should not be added to any food and avoid salty foods like bacon, sausages, crisps, ready-meals, takeaways, and gravy made with stock cubes
• Do not add sugar to foods; try naturally sweet foods (e.g. bananas)
• Honey until >1yr, as some contain bacteria that causes infant botulism and contributes to dental caries (➲ Development and care of teeth for young children p. 196)
• Raw eggs; they should be cooked well (➲ Food-borne disease p. 730)
• Whole nuts until >5yrs in case of choking; they can be crushed or ground
• Low-fat foods are not suitable for <2yrs as fat needed for calories and vitamins
• Soft cheeses which can contain listeria, including mould-ripened soft cheese (e.g. brie and camembert), ripened goat's milk cheese (e.g. chevre), and soft blue-veined cheese (e.g. roquefort)
• Unpasteurized cheeses, due to the risk of listeria
• Raw shellfish, due to ↑ risk of food poisoning
• Shark, swordfish, or marlin, which have ↑ levels of mercury affecting the growing nervous system.

Allergies

A family history of allergies may make a baby more prone to allergies. Advise to: breastfeed to 6mths, and introduce foods that commonly cause allergies one at a time (e.g. foods such as eggs, wheat, nuts, seeds, fish, and shellfish).

Established meals

Eating family foods together at meal times promotes good eating habits, offers opportunities for interaction, and seems to develop less 'fussy' eaters. Keeping meal times free of arguments about eating contributes to this. Commercially produced foods in jars and packets should not replace family food altogether.

By 9mths, the baby should be eating three meals a day, which include protein, carbohydrates, and fruit and vegetables (vitamin C is important for absorption of iron). Intake of milk is reduced as solid food increases, but child still needs at least 600mL/day of milk. However, cow's milk is not suitable as a drink until 1yr old, but can be used in cooking and mixing foods (❺ Food and the under-fives p. 212).

Vitamin supplements

All children should take vitamin drops with vitamins A, C, and D from the age of 6mths to 5yrs old. Breastfed babies should be given a daily vitamin D supplement from birth. Vitamins should be available via schemes such as Healthy Start for low-income parents.

Reference

25. WHO (2018) *Infant and young child feeding*. Available at: ℘ https://www.who.int/news-room/fact-sheets/detail/infant-and-young-child-feeding

Further information

Baby Led Weaning (*Getting started*). Available at: ℘ www.babyledweaning.com/
NHS (*Start for life: weaning*) Available at: ℘ https://www.nhs.uk/start4life/weaning
NHS Scotland (*Ready steady baby: weaning your baby*). Available at: ℘ www.readysteadybaby.org.uk/growing-together/looking-after-your-growing-baby/weaning-your-baby/index.aspx
NICE (*Maternal and child nutrition [PH11]*). Available at: ℘ http://www.nice.org.uk/PH11

Growth 0–2 years

Growth starts *in utero* and ends after puberty (→ Puberty and adolescence p. 228).

Infant growth

Dependent on nutrition, good health, happiness, pituitary growth hormone, thyroid hormone, and vitamin D. All babies lose weight in first week of life and 80% reach birthweight by 2wks. Growth measurement should only be undertaken by those trained to do so or others supervised by them. Definitions:
- Low birthweight: <2.5kg
- Very low birthweight: <1.5kg
- Small for gestational age: length or weight at birth <2nd centile
- Large for gestational age: birthweight >90th centile

When to weigh and measure

Babies are weighed in first week to help assess feeding and thereafter as needed. If parents wish, or there is professional concern, babies can be weighed at 6–8, 12, and 16wks, 12–13mths at time of routine immunizations (→ Childhood immunization p. 164). If there is concern, weigh more often but no more frequently than: once a month from 2wks to 6mths; once every 2mths from 6 to 12mths; and once every 3mths from >1yr. Length is measured if there are any worries about a child's weight gain, growth, or general health. Head circumference is measured at birth, at 6–8wk check, and any time after, if concerns about child's head growth or development.

How to measure

- Weight: remove baby's clothes and nappy; weigh only on Class III clinical electronic scales
- Length (until 2yrs): supine, without clothes, nappy, or shoes; use approved measuring board or mat and two people measuring
- Head circumference: remove all headwear; use narrow plastic or disposable paper tape measure where head circumference is greatest

Recording and interpretation

Plotted as single dot on UK–WHO 0–4yrs boy's or girl's growth charts[26,27] and parent-held child health record (→ Client- and patient-held records p. 90).
- Full-term infants (37–42wks): birthweight (and, if measured, length and head circumference) plotted at age 0 on the 0–1yr chart (Fig. 6.2).
- Healthy infants born after 32wks and before 37wks: all measurements plotted in pre-term section until 2wks after the expected date of delivery, then on the 0–1yr chart using gestational correction (plot at actual age with arrow back to weeks since birth).
- Pre-term born before 32wks or hospitalized neonate: a separate low birthweight chart is used (→ Pre-term infants p. 176).

The charts show the growth range of children in the UK. The centile indicates the expected number of children below (e.g. 50% below the 50th

Newborn term infants

Plotting in the first 2 weeks

Plot all term infants (37 or more weeks) at age 0 weeks

You will also see the 2 week gap in the 0 to x 1 year weight chart, and in the 0 to 1 year head circumference chart.

Some degree of weight loss is common after birth. Calculating the percentage weight loss is a useful way to identify babies who need assessment.

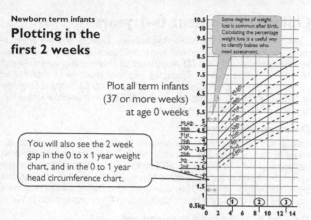

Fig. 6.2 Plotting in the first two weeks.

© Royal College of Paediatrics and Child Health (2009) *Plotting and assessing newborn infants* (UK–WHO growth charts: fact sheet 4). Available at: https://www.rcpch.ac.uk/sites/default/files/Plotting_newborn_infants.pdf. Reproduced with permission from the Royal College of Paediatrics and Child Health.

centile). Plotting a weight or length within 25% of the space above or below a centile is described as 'on the centile', otherwise it is described as between two centiles (e.g. 50th–75th). Weight usually tracks within one centile. The term 'faltering weight gain' refers to slow weight gain and may indicate a feeding problem. Rates of growth vary, but review by GP or child health doctor if:

• Birthweight not regained by 2wks (possible illness)
• Weight graph sustained downwards or crossing down two centile lines
• <0.4th centile or >99.6th centile

Poor weight gain may be due to either organic causes or from psychosocial factors (➲ Identifying the child in need of protection p. 250; ➲ Growth disorders p. 298). A full assessment and care plan will address more than just improved nutrition.

References

26. Royal College of Paediatrics and Child Health (2009) *Boy's UK–WHO growth chart 0–4 years.* Available at: https://www.rcpch.ac.uk/sites/default/files/Boys_0-4_years_growth_chart.pdf
27. Royal College of Paediatrics and Child Health (2009) *Girl's UK–WHO growth chart 0–4 years.* Available at: https://www.rcpch.ac.uk/sites/default/files/Girls_0-4_years_growth_chart.pdf

Child development 0–1 years

Child development is the interaction between heredity and the environment. In assessing development as part of the assessment of children, young people, and families (➲ Assessment of children, young people, and families p. 156), it is often subdivided into four areas: gross motor; fine motor and vision; speech, language, and hearing (➲ Speech and language acquisition p. 218); and social, emotional (➲ Emotional development in babies and children p. 210), and behaviour.

Developmental progress

This is about the sequential acquisition of skills. It is important to remember: there is a wide timescale within normal range, e.g. children walking unaided 25% by 11mths, 90% by 15mths, 97.5% by 18mths; median ages indicate when half a standard population should have acquired the skill (Table 6.3 for children 0–1yrs); and pre-term babies are assessed from expected date of delivery up until 2yrs of age (➲ Pre-term infants p. 176).

Delayed or suboptimal development

Indirect causes of delayed or suboptimal development include adverse environmental factors or ill health, and direct causes include neurological or neurodevelopmental problems. Refer for more in-depth assessment and investigation by community or hospital paediatrician if there is a failure to meet acquisition by upper limits of age, e.g. no responsive smile by 8wks; good eye contact not achieved by 3mths; and not sitting unsupported by 9mths. Also refer if: parents concerned; discordant levels of development between areas; regression of previously acquired skills; and development plateaus.

Table 6.3 Overview of median age of development in children 0–1 years

Gross motor	
Newborn	Limbs flexed, symmetrical postures; marked head lag on pulling up; primitive reflex Moro and stepping
6–8wks	Raises head to 45°
3–4mths	Holds head up while lying prone
6–7mths	Sits without support, with rounded back
8–10mths	8mths: crawling; sits without support, with straight back. 10mths: furniture walking
11–12mths	Walking unsteadily, broad gait, hands apart

Fine motor and vision	
Newborn	Reflex grasp; follows face in midline
6–8wks	Follows moving object by turning head
3–4mths	Reaches out for objects
6–7mths	Palmar grasp; transfers objects from one hand to other
8–10mths	Pincer grip
11–12mths	Walking unsteadily, broad gait, hands apart

Language, speech, and hearing	
Newborn	Startles and blinks to loud noises
6–8wks	Gurgles in response; notices sudden sounds and pauses to listen
3–4mths	Vocalizes alone or when spoken to; laughs, squeals, blows between lips; quietens or smiles to voice of parent
6–7mths	Coos and babbles; uses syllables—da, ba, ka; turns immediately to parent's voice; turns to soft sounds out of sight if not preoccupied
8–10mths	Two-syllable babble; sounds used discriminately, e.g. dada, mama
11–12mths	At least one word with meaning and understands some words

Social, emotional, and behavioural	
Newborn	Soon after birth flickers eyes when spoken to; after 2wks recognizes parent
6–8wks	Smiles responsively; responds to conversation through movements
3–4mths	Responds in conversations with smiles, gurgles, movements
6–7mths	Curious about all sights, sounds, people. 6mths: puts arms out to be picked up; may be shy of strangers; finger feeds. 7mths: looks for dropped items
8–10mths	8mths: separation anxiety; familiar with routines. 10mths: waves bye-bye, plays peek-a-boo; looks for hidden items
11–12mths	Drinks from cup; gives kisses

Further information

Edmond A. (2019) *Health for all children* (5th edn). Oxford: Oxford University Press

Sharma, A. & Cockerill, H. (2014) Mary Sheridan's 'From birth to five years: children's developmental progress'. Oxford: Routledge

Baby hygiene and skin care

Many new parents need reassurance and advice about hygiene and skin care. Parents can be reminded that these activities create good opportunities for talking and playing with the baby and for creating a good attachment.

Skin cleaning

A daily bath is not essential, although with an older baby it is helpful as part of an evening routine. Face, hands, and neck creases need washing as necessary, but at least once a day. Eyes should be washed in the newborn with wet cotton wool balls. Avoid poking around in ears and nostrils.

Skin in the nappy area needs protecting at every nappy change by washing (or use of a baby wipe) and by the application of a barrier cream to protect against nappy rash. Nappy changing should happen at least after every feed and more frequently as necessary. In girls, nappy area cleaning should be from front to back (i.e. towards the anus), without opening the vulva. In boys, it is not necessary to pull back the foreskin. Skincare products should be non-perfumed to avoid irritation and dryness. If nappy rash is suspected:
- More frequent changing and cleaning will be indicated
- Expose the area to air by leaving the nappy off as long as possible
- Try a different barrier cream
- If associated with fungal infection, refer to a prescriber (➔ Fungal infections p. 686)

Bathing babies

Key principles involve concern for safety (➔ Accident prevention p. 168), maintaining body temperature, and having a pleasurably interactive time together. Bath in warm room with no draughts. Make sure all equipment is to hand before starting. Add hot water to cold, to shallow depth (5–8cm for new baby). Temperature should always be checked with elbow, inner wrist, or bath thermometer (37–38°C). A non-perfumed bath lotion can be used. Talk, smile, and reassure baby through whole process. Introduce water toys as child gets older. Wrap baby in towel; wash and dry face before placing in bath. In young babies, also wash and dry hair/top of head before lowering baby in. Always support a young baby in water, with adult's arm under their back and grasping baby's arm that is furthest away. Bath seats are available for older babies, but babies should never be left alone in them. On lifting out, immediately wrap in towel and dry to maintain body heat.

Hair care

Hair washing is easiest as part of bath routine. After about 3–4mths, hair is thicker and a small amount of baby shampoo (i.e. non-stinging if gets in eyes) is better at cleaning. Soft baby hair brushes are available. Cradle cap (a form of seborrhoeic dermatitis) is common in young babies, producing thick, yellow scales over the scalp. Daily gentle shampooing may help. Also, rubbing olive oil into the scalp, leaving overnight to soften scales, then shampooing out and rubbing scales off with fingers. ⚠ Only use olive oil on cradle cap; not routinely on dry skin. If becomes inflamed, refer to a prescriber.

Nail care

Best trimmed after a bath when soft. Blunt-ended baby scissors are available.

Nappies

Parents choose disposable (including biodegradable) or cloth nappies according to their circumstances, finances, and available information. New types of cloth nappies are both cheaper and more environmentally friendly than disposables. Cloth nappies now come in much easier designs (e.g. using Velcro™) that use disposable or washable liners. They do not need soaking if machine washed at 60°C. Should be washed using a non-irritant powder.

Related topics

➔ Eczema in childhood p. 284

Further information

UK Nappy Network (*Resources*). Available at ℛ: http://www.uknappynetwork.org/

Development and care of teeth for young children

The age at which teeth cut through the gum varies. Most start ~6mths, but very occasionally babies are born with a tooth (sometimes removed if loose or badly positioned) and some do not cut teeth until >12mths. 1° teeth are important as they guide adult teeth into the correct position. Twenty 1° teeth cut through the gum in the same order: lower then upper two incisors (6–12mths); lower then upper canines (6–18mths); first molars (12–20mths); and second molars (18–24mths).

Teething

Signs of teething include: dribbling, wanting to chew or gnaw, irritability, and red cheeks. Interventions include giving the baby something hard to gnaw on (e.g. carrot, teething ring) and the use of over-the-counter teething gels or granules.

Toothbrushing

Teeth need to be cleaned twice a day as soon as they appear with a smear of fluoride baby toothpaste on a soft brush. Encourage toothbrushing as a game or copycat activity. The British Dental Association recommends all children <3yrs old should use a smear of toothpaste with a fluoride level of at least 1,000ppm (parts per million), both morning and night. From 3yrs old, they should use a pea-sized amount that contains 1,350–1,500ppm.[28]

Children need help and supervision in cleaning their teeth until ~7yrs. Clean a baby's teeth with them sat on lap or in chair, and head slightly tilted for a good view inside the mouth. Adults need to stand behind older children to clean their teeth. Children should spit out after cleaning their teeth with fluoride toothpaste (advise not to rinse as the fluoride will not work). See Box 6.1.

Dental check-ups

Babies should be registered with a dentist from birth if possible. Initial appointment should be when first teeth break thorough. Country-specific advice on frequency of check-ups varies. Usually, 6-mthly in <18yrs, but may be more or less frequently according to individual assessment. <18yrs

---

Box 6.1 General care of teeth
Encourage
- Water and milk-only drinks
- Savoury and calcium-rich diet
- Use of cup rather than bottle when weaning, to promote good alignment of teeth
- Sugar-free medications

Discourage
- Sweetened drinks
- Dummies and sucking on thumb, to avoid misalignment of teeth
- Putting baby to bed with a bottle

exempt from payment for NHS dental check-ups and treatment. Dentists may advise pit and fissure sealants (plastic coating) for adult molars and pre-molars to prevent caries.[29] Parents should look for early signs of tooth decay at least every 4wks. If parents are unsure of signs of tooth decay, they can be supported by their health visitor (→ Health visiting p. 46) or dentist.

Use of fluoride supplements

Each area will have a policy on the need for fluoride supplements in view of levels of fluoride in drinking water. Only a few places have enough natural fluoride to benefit dental health. In some places, it is added to water. Water suppliers will be able to outline the local situation. Use of fluoride supplements should be on the advice of a dentist and at recommended dosage. Dental fluorosis can occur when too much fluoride is taken (e.g. when water supply is already fluoridated and supplements are taken, or when children 'eat' toothpaste). Fluorosis can lead to pitting or flecking of tooth enamel.

Fluoride varnish

Fluoride varnishes are effective in preventing dental caries.[30] Prescribed by dentists and applied by dental staff 2–4 times a year to children aged >2yrs (→ Prescribing p. 136). May be part of NHS dental public health programme.

Dental health promotion programmes

Some countries and LA areas have targeted dental health programmes, which may include distribution of toothbrushes, fluoride toothpaste, and leaflets at fixed times for children <5yrs, plus supervised toothbrushing in nurseries (e.g. Childsmile in Scotland).

Related topics

→ Dental health in older children p. 226

References

28. Oral Health Foundation (undated) *Fluoride*. Available at: https://www.dentalhealth.org/fluoride
29. Oral Health Foundation (undated) *Pit and fissure sealants*. Available at: https://www.dentalhealth.org/pit-and-fissure-sealants
30. Marinho, V., Higgins, J., Logan, S., & Sheiham, A. (2008) *Fluoride varnishes for preventing dental caries in children and adolescents*. Available at: https://www.cochrane.org/CD002279/ORAL_fluoride-varnishes-for-preventing-dental-caries-in-children-and-adolescents

Further information

Childsmile (*Dental health promotion programme for children in Scotland*). Available at: ℘ www.childsmile.org.uk/index.aspx
PHE (*Water fluoridation health monitoring report for England 2018*). Available at: ℘ https://assets.publishing.service.gov.uk/government/uploads/system/uploads/attachment_data/file/692754/Water_Fluoridation_Health_monitoring_report_for_England_2018_final.pdf

Crying babies

All babies cry, and some a great deal. Some parents need support to recognize that this is babies' way of alerting them to the need for attention, comfort, or care (➲ Support for parenting p. 172). Early evening is the most common time for this to happen. Parents, particularly first timers, may need help recognizing the causes and developing strategies that work for them and the baby. Dealing with babies that cry a lot can be stressful and frustrating, and parents and carers need to be aware that shaking a baby is particularly dangerous (➲ Safeguarding children p. 248). While crying is normal, there is usually a reason for excessive crying.

Soothing babies

As a general rule, most babies are soothed by movement, contact, and sound, e.g. rocking, mobile over cot, cuddling and walking, holding them at the same time as talking or crooning. Having babies in baby slings or closely wrapped on the parent's back creates contact and movement. Some babies are quite 'sucky' and might calm with a feed, or a thumb or dummy in the mouth. Parents learn to recognize causes of crying in their baby and address them:

- Hunger or thirst: check if he/she needs a feed
- Tired, but fighting sleep: lay them down either in a quiet darkened place or in a buggy to go out for a walk (➲ Babies, children, and sleeping p. 200)
- Discomfort with wet or dirty nappy: change it
- Discomfort as too hot or cold: remove or add clothes or covering
- Lack of contact: lift and cuddle, stroke, talking
- Pain: through a physical cause, e.g. wind after feeding, colic, or teething (➲ Development and care of teeth for young children p. 196)

Parents need to be alert that the crying and associated behaviour may be unusual for their baby, and it is a sign of illness or infection that requires medical attention.

Colic

Colic affects ~one in four babies in first 3–4mths. Inconsolable crying and/or drawing up of knees can last for hours and occurs mostly in the evenings. Cause is unknown. It is benign but distressing for parents. No evidence that gripe water, herbal remedies (➲ Complementary and alternative therapies p. 838), or changing mother's diet are beneficial (➲ Evidence-based healthcare p. 72). Reassure parents, work through possible list of causes, and suggest soothing strategies.

Older babies

As babies get older, the causes change, and can include:

- Boredom: needs company and distractions, such as rattles, toys, talking to, playing with
- Frustration: as they start to crawl and cruise, items have to be put out of the way, leading to great frustration; distraction tactics become important

- Fear of separation and strangers: usually between 6–8mths. Give lots of reassurance, cuddling, comfort, gradual periods of separation, help with ongoing familiarity with new surroundings (➔ Emotional development in babies and children p. 210).

When the crying becomes too much

Sometimes parents feel overwhelmed and frustrated by a baby who will not stop crying. Any health professional working with parents (➔ Working with parents p. 170) who say that their babies cry a lot should help them work through coping strategies to ensure they do not overreact, lose their temper, or become rough with the baby. These coping mechanisms include:

- Having another adult look after the baby for an hour or so
- Creating time to think through strategies by putting the baby down safely and leaving the room
- Talking to a health visitor (➔ Health visiting p. 46)
- Using a helpline such as Cry-sis ☎ 08451 228 669
- Remembering that the difficult time will not last forever.

Further information

Cry-sis (*Support for crying and sleepless babies*). Available at: ℗ https://www.cry-sis.org.uk/
National Childbirth Trust (*Crying*). Available at: ℗ https://www.nct.org.uk/baby-toddler/crying
Institute of Health Visiting Practice (*When your baby cries during feeds or has colic*). Available at: ℗
    https://ihv.org.uk/for-health-visitors/resources-for-members/resource/ihv-tips-for-parents/
    breastfeeding-2/when-your-baby-cries-during-feeds-or-has-colic/

Babies, children, and sleeping

A newborn baby's sleep pattern is determined by their weight and feeding requirements (➲ Growth 0–2 years p. 190). When they are not feeding, most babies are asleep, although some are active and alert for long periods. However, every baby is individual and patterns will vary. Some sleep for long periods, some in short snatches. Most babies are able to sleep for longer periods through the night without feeds by 6wks. The periods of wakefulness during the day extend as they get older. Older babies need morning and afternoon naps during the first year.

Safe sleeping

The safest place for a baby to sleep is in a cot beside the parents' bed for the first 6mths. To reduce the incidence of sudden infant death syndrome (SIDS) (➲ Sudden infant death syndrome p. 278), the baby put down to sleep should: be on their back; have their head uncovered; have their feet to foot of the cot; and not get too hot or too cold (Box 6.2). Other advice to prevent SIDS includes that parents should stop smoking (➲ Smoking cessation p. 356) and should never smoke in the same room as the baby.

Co-sleeping

While some parents choose to share beds with their baby, this involves real risks. Those who do should ensure: pillows, blankets, and any objects that could obstruct the baby's breathing or cause them to overheat are kept away from the baby; pets and other children are not allowed in the bed; and that baby cannot fall from the bed or get trapped between the mattress and the wall.

⚠ Parents should never share a bed or bring the baby into the bed if:
• Either parent smokes
• They have been drinking (➲ Alcohol p. 360) or taking illegal drugs
  (➲ Substance use p. 476) or medication that increases drowsiness
• They are unwell or extra tired so it might affect their ability to arouse or respond to the baby
• Baby was premature (born <37wks) or ↓ birthweight (< 2.5kg) (➲ Pre-term infants p. 176)

⚠ Parents or carers should never fall asleep with a baby whilst on an armchair or sofa, as there are real dangers of the person shifting and suffocating the baby.

Sleeping and settling routines

Bedtime sleep routines help babies and parents establish good patterns of separating to sleep. Around 6wks is a good time to start, and they are

> **Box 6.2 Ensuring a safe sleeping temperature**
> • Cotton sheets and blankets not duvets, baby nests, or sheepskins
> • No pillows, wedges, or cot bumpers
> • Never placed with hot water bottles or electric blankets, or next to radiators or fires, or in direct sunshine
> • Ideal room temperature is between 16°C and 20°C (61–68°F)
> • Only need to wear nappy, vest, and sleep suit

usually established by 3–6mths. Most routines tend to include some or most of the following: bathing; feeding; quiet time; placing in bed and singing a lullaby (or a story for older children); cuddle and kiss goodnight; and leaving them in a darkened room, with a night light, baby listener switched on, and gentle music playing (e.g. part of a mobile).

Night-waking babies 0–6mths
Any night feeds still required should be very low-key, with little eye contact or words; all signals that this is not the time to be awake. Check for all causes of crying, and settle.

Night-waking babies 6–12mths
Babies who wake at night or only go back to sleep with lots of parental attention/feeds can usually be persuaded to change their behaviour by the checking routine (also used for older children). Over a 2-wk period, when the baby wakes: leave to cry for 5mins; parent goes in and checks them, tucks them in, and leaves; and parent does not cuddle, give drink, or 'reward' in any way. This process is repeated with ↑ intervals until baby recognizes that night-time waking produces no results, and stays or quickly returns to sleep. Parents need to be convinced of the value of this process and not undermine their own efforts by restarting to 'reward' night waking.

Older children
↑ number of sleep problems reported in older children. Sleep deprivation and ↓ sleep quality may impact on growth, learning (➔ Communication and learning problems p. 224), attention, and behaviour (➔ Behavioural disorders in children p. 326). Healthy sleep habits for children include: a regular wake-up time and bedtime, even at the weekend; a bedroom that is a calm, non-stimulating environment; calm activities and no screen time in the hour before bed; limits on sugar, particularly after lunchtime; and avoidance of caffeine and energy drinks.

Further information
Cry-sis (*Help with sleepless babies*). Available at: ℅ https://www.cry-sis.org.uk/help-with-sleepless-babies

Lullaby Trust (*Safer sleep*). Available at: ℅ https://www.lullabytrust.org.uk/safer-sleep-advice/

Sleep Scotland (*Supporting families of children and young people with additional support needs and sleep problems*). Available at: ℅ http://www.sleepscotland.org/

The Children's Sleep Charity (*Sheep Dreams Campaign*). Available at: ℅ https://www.thechildrenssleepcharity.org.uk/

Promoting baby development safely 0–1 years

Health professionals, particularly health visiting (HV) (➔ Health visiting p. 46) teams, are in a good position to advise parents on how to help their babies develop (➔ Promoting the health of children p. 152). From birth, parents are encouraged to support their child's communication, personal/ social, problem-solving, gross motor, and fine motor skills. In addition to this, health promotion, including accident prevention in the home (➔ Accident prevention p. 168) and common childhood illness, is discussed.

Key principles to promote with parents and carers

Babies are learning from the first day and their abilities quickly develop. New parents need to learn to play and talk to their babies to stimulate them and support cognitive development. Interacting with the baby in every activity promotes attachment or bonding, learning, and speech development (➔ Emotional development in babies and children p. 210; ➔ Speech and language acquisition p. 218; ➔ Communication and learning problems p. 224). This interaction includes: talking to them, with eye-to-eye contact and with the face up close when newborn; responding early and appropriately to cues; holding them to feed; holding on the lap; carrying; cuddling; singing nursery rhymes; and playing games like peek-a-boo. Babies should be helped to find out about the world around them, e.g. allowing supervised tummy time. Parents should have realistic expectations of the developmental stage; toys should be age-appropriate and stimulating.

Encouraging movement safely
- Learning to crawl: needs opportunities on tummy on the floor.
  ⚠ Supervision is required at all times. ⚠ Once independently moving by rolling, crawling, furniture cruising, it is essential to remove poisonous substances from reach level (➔ Poisoning and overdoses p. 822), fit safety gates, remove glass-topped items, and protect from sharp-edged furniture.
- Discourage parents from using baby walkers since prolonged periods in them affects positioning of feet, with children learning to walk on their toes and not with feet flat on the surface to allow them to weight bare and balance.

Resources to support development

Many HVs and children's centre teams have produced resource packs or have drop-in sessions to support parents in helping the development of their babies (➔ Support for parenting p. 172). HV teams in many areas (England, Wales, and Northern Ireland) distribute book packs via Bookstart (see ℘ https://www.booktrust.org.uk/). Toy libraries often provide packs and ideas for 0–1yrs.

Promoting accident prevention

All baby equipment should be to British or European Standards.

Baby car seats

New babies should be in rear-facing car seats. ⚠ Car seats should never be placed in the front seat if the car has air bags. For further advice regarding car seats, see ℘ www.childcarseats.org.uk/

Accident prevention for babies

- Falls (e.g. rolling off changing mats): promote strapping in buggies, changing nappies on the floor, and never leaving baby unattended on a bed or changing table
- Sleep (➔ Babies, children, and sleeping p. 200; ➔ Sudden infant death syndrome p. 278)
- Burns and scalds (e.g. bath water too hot, spilt hot drinks): promote cold water, then hot, in the bath, testing bath water, not having hot drinks near baby (➔ Burns and scalds p. 816)
- Fires in the home (e.g. distracted parent leaves chip pan over heat): promote smoke alarms
- Drowning (e.g. in bath): highlight danger in leaving baby alone in, or near, water. Children can drown where the depth of water is as little as 2cm.
- Choking: highlight danger of prop feeding and small items sticking in trachea (➔ Child choking p. 806)
- Mobile phones: encourage parents not to use mobile phones when handling babies/children to prevent distraction and accidents

Encourage parents to attend basic life support and first aid classes (➔ Child basic life support p. 800).

Further information

British Association for Early Childhood Education (*Babies–learning starts from the first day*). Available at: ℘ https://www.early-education.org.uk/babies-learning-starts-first-day

Child Accident Prevention Trust (*Safety advice*). Available at: ℘ https://www.capt.org.uk/capt-safety-advice

National Literacy Trust (*Early years resources*). Available at: ℘ https://literacytrust.org.uk/resources/?phase=early-years

The 1001 Critical Days (*Manifesto*). Available at: ℘ https://www.1001criticaldays.co.uk

Child development 1–5 years

Child development is the interaction between heredity and the environment. Development is assessed as part of the Healthy Child Programme (➔ Overview of the Healthy Child Programme p. 154; ➔ Assessment of children, young people, and families p. 156).

Developmental progress

This is about the sequential acquisition of skills. It is important to remember: there is a wide timescale within the normal range (e.g. children walking unaided—25% by 11mths, 90% by 15mths, 97.5% by 18mths); median ages indicate when half a standard population should have acquired the skill (Table 6.4); and pre-term babies (➔ Pre-term infants p. 176) are assessed from expected delivery date up until 2yrs of age only.

Delayed or suboptimal development

Indirect causes of delayed or suboptimal development include adverse environmental factors or ill health, and direct causes include neurological or neurodevelopmental problems. Refer for more in-depth assessment and investigation by community or hospital paediatrician if there is a failure to meet acquisition by upper limits of age. For example: not walking unaided by 18mths; no pincer grip by 18mths; not saying single words with meaning by 18mths; and no two- or three-word sentences by 30mths (➔ Speech and language acquisition p. 218). Also refer if: parents concerned about an aspect of development; discordant levels of development between areas; regression of previously acquired skills; and development plateaus.

Table 6.4 Overview of median age of development in children 1–5 years

Gross motor	
15mths	Walks alone steadily
18mths	Bends to pick up without toppling
2yrs	Kicks a ball without toppling; runs 2.5yrs: jumps with both feet off the ground
3yrs	Up and down stairs without holding on; pedals trikes
4–5yrs	Hops; skips; catches ball

Fine motor and vision	
15mths	Scribbles with pencil
18mths	Turns pages in books; feeds him/herself with spoon; able to put on some clothes; builds tower of 3 bricks
2yrs	Builds tower of 6 bricks; able to take off most clothes and put some on
3yrs	Builds bridge with 3 bricks; draws • (copies 6mths earlier); does up buttons
4–5yrs	Builds copy of 6 bricks in steps 4yrs: draws × 4.5yrs: draws Δ 5yrs: uses scissors

Language, speech, and hearing	
15mths	Shows 2 parts of body; follows simple instructions; single words
18mths	10–20 words, usually nouns; hums
2yrs	Uses 2 or more phrases to make simple sentences 2.5yrs: talks constantly, in 3- or 4-word phrases
3yrs	Vocab 200–300 words; starts asking 'why?' frequently; begins to grasp concept of numbers; knows age and a few colours
4–5yrs	Talks a great deal; boasts; tells stories

Social, emotional, and behavioural	
15mths	Imagination appears in doll play
18mths	Symbolic play; imitates adults; plays alongside (parallel) others
2yrs	Learning to play with others but often rivalries; dry by day and bowel control; starts saying 'no' often
3yrs	Interactive play with other children; takes turns; dry by night
4–5yrs	Expanding sense of self; growing confidence; wants to be grown up

Further information

Edmond, A. (2019) *Health for all children* (5th edn) Oxford: Oxford University Press
Sharma, A. & Cockerill, H. (2014) Mary Sheridan's 'From birth to five years: children's developmental progress'. Oxford: Routledge

Growth 2–4 years

Growth starts *in utero* and ends after puberty (➔ Puberty and adolescence p. 228). It is good practice to record height and weight in any child about whom there is concern, who has chronic ill health, or requires prolonged follow-up for any reason (➔ Growth disorders p. 298).

Growth

Dependent on nutrition, good health, happiness, pituitary growth hormone, thyroid hormone, and vitamin D. Growth measurement should only be undertaken by those trained to do so.

When to weigh and measure

Children should be weighed at routine visits for review or immunization (i.e. 24mths, between 3–4yrs) (➔ Childhood immunizations p. 164). If there is a concern, weigh more often, but no more frequently than 3mthly as can be misleading. Height should be measured, if requested by parent, whenever: there are concerns about weight gain, growth, or general health; when weight is <0.4th centile or >99.6th centile; and there is rapid weight gain. Growth charts have adult height prediction sections. Head circumference should be measured if there are concerns about growth or development.

How to measure

• Weight: toddlers in vest and pants; older children in light clothing only, on Class III clinical electronic scales.
• Height: without footwear, using correctly installed stadiometer or appropriate portable measuring device. Child should stand with heels, bottom, back, and head touching apparatus, and ears and eyes at 90° to the apparatus. Measure on expiration.
• Head circumference: remove all headwear; use plastic or disposable paper tape measure where head circumference is greatest.

Recording and interpretation

Plotted as a single dot on UK–WHO 0–4yrs boy's or girl's growth charts[31,32] and parent-held child health record (➔ Client- and patient-held records p. 90). Also plotted on body mass index (BMI) conversion section of chart if concern about growth.

Most children will have a BMI between the 25th and 75th centiles, whatever their height centile. BMI is a measure of bone and muscle, as well as fat. The higher BMI is indicative of excess fat. Referral is indicated when: BMI >91st centile, as suggests overweight (>98th centile is clinically obese) (➔ Overweight children and adolescents p. 302); BMI <2nd centile, as may reflect lack of nutrition.

Acute illness may cause weight loss, but usually regained within 2–3wks. Prolonged failure to gain weight or continuing weight loss may indicate other illness or non-organic failure to thrive (➔ Safeguarding children p. 248).

References

31. Royal College of Paediatrics and Child Health (2009) *Boy's UK–WHO growth chart 0–4 years*. Available at: ℘ https://www.rcpch.ac.uk/sites/default/files/Boys_0-4_years_growth_chart.pdf
32. Royal College of Paediatrics and Child Health (2009) *Girl's UK–WHO growth chart 0–4 years*. Available at: ℘ https://www.rcpch.ac.uk/sites/default/files/Girls_0-4_years_growth_chart.pdf

Further information

E-Learning for Healthcare (*Healthy Child Programme: Module 8 Growth and Nutrition*). Available at: ℘ https://www.e-lfh.org.uk/programmes/healthy-child-programme/

NICE (*Faltering growth: recognition and management of faltering growth in children [NG75]*). Available at: ℘ https://www.nice.org.uk/guidance/ng75

Wright, C. (2019) Growth monitoring. In: Edmond, A. (ed.) *Health for all children* (5th edn). Oxford: Oxford University Press, pp. 208–23

Promoting development in the under-fives

Health professionals, particularly health visiting (HV) (➔ Health visiting p. 46) teams, are in a good position to advise parents on how to help their young children develop, at the same time as providing health promotion advice on child injury prevention (➔ Accident prevention p. 168; ➔ Promoting the health of children p. 152). They are encouraged to work in partnership with parents, and with early years' providers of childcare and education (➔ Working with parents p. 170; ➔ Teamwork p. 58). All UK countries have policies emphasizing support for early years and child development in the under-fives in readiness for 1° school. This includes frameworks for activities and the curriculum in pre-school childcare and education providers, part-time places at nursery schools for 3–4yr olds, and early years' providers statements of individual child development at 2yrs given to parents (➔ Services for children, young people, and families p. 24).

Key principles to promote with parents and carers

Young children are curious and learning about life, their family, and their home all the time. They learn by being part of everyday family life and asking questions. Parents, family, and carers help children develop by:

• Encouraging and rewarding all efforts, attempts, new achievements, and good behaviour with touching, smiling, words of praise, listening, cuddles
• Including them in daily activities, e.g. shopping and family events
• Talking to them, singing with them, reading together
• Playing games and providing opportunities for different types of games, e.g. outdoor running games, wet play in the bath, imaginative play with dressing-up clothes, manipulation games with puzzles

Social skills are developed through opportunities to meet other children and adults, e.g. drop-ins and play groups. Children need the opportunity to be outside—to run about, let off steam, and get fresh air—every day.

Resources to support development

Many HV and children's centre teams have produced resource packs or have drop-in sessions to support parents. Book and toy libraries often provide packs and ideas for under-fives. Local children's or early years' services may provide a range of resources about play groups, drop-ins, and more.

Promoting injury prevention

With ↑ mobility, there is ↑ risk of accidental injuries (➔ Accident prevention p. 168). Young children need constant supervision as they are very curious. Think about:

• Falls: consider window safety catches, safety gates
• Poisoning: keep household cleaning products and medicines away from children and in a locked cabinet. Be careful not to leave handbags containing packets of medication unattended (➔ Poisoning and overdoses p. 822)
• Burns and scalds: keep hot drinks and saucepans out of reach (➔ Burns and scalds p. 816)

- Drowning: never leave <4yrs in bath alone; fill in or fence off ponds; empty paddling pools
- Cuts and bruises: protect sharp edges in the home; fit safety glass; use door guards to prevent trapped fingers
- Road traffic accidents: teach road safety to children; use age-appropriate car seats
- Think sun safety (➲ Skin cancer prevention p. 374)

Further information

British Literacy Association (*Tips for talking to your baby and young child*). Available at: ℘ https://literacytrust.org.uk/resources/tips-talking-your-baby-and-young-child/

Department of Education (*Statutory Framework for the Early Years' Foundation Stage*). Available at: ℘ https://assets.publishing.service.gov.uk/government/uploads/system/uploads/attachment_data/file/596629/EYFS_STATUTORY_FRAMEWORK_2017.pdf

Department of Transport (*Road safety resources for teachers, pupils, and parents*). Available at: ℘ https://www.think.gov.uk/

Scottish Government (*Early education and care*). Available at: https://www.gov.scot/policies/early-education-and-care/early-learning-and-childcare/

The Foundation Years from Pregnancy to 5 (*Information and resources for parents and early years and health practitioners*). Available at: ℘ www.foundationyears.org.uk

Emotional development in babies and children

Significant and critical brain and intellectual development occurs during the first 3yrs of life. It is influenced by nutritional and health status, and also by interactions developed with people and objects.

Key points

Highly dependent on adequate nutrition, stimulation, and optimal care. During first years, key brain pathways for lifelong capabilities are established. Once developed, the brain is much harder to modify. Dual relationship created by caregiver, and baby builds and strengthens brain architecture and creates relationship in which experiences are affirmed and new abilities nurtured. By school age, a lot of key language abilities (➌ Speech and language acquisition p. 218), physical capabilities, and cognitive foundations have been set in place. While a focus on first education is important, 5yrs is too late to start paying attention to children's emotional development needs.

Sensitive and responsive parent–child relationships are also associated with stronger cognitive skills in young children and enhanced social competence and work skills later in school.

Developmental guidelines

Think in terms of stages, not ages. The following ages are guidelines only:
- 1mth: voice recognition, expresses interest (e.g. attend to pictures), visual focus
- 6mths: senses pleasure, smiling, mouthing objects important, different communication methods (e.g. pointing, vocalizing, responding to words and pictures)
- 9mths: facial expressions reflecting emotions (e.g. fear), comfort objects
- ~2yrs: attachment vital, self-centred, gaining personal identity, change-resistant
- 3yrs: conforms, more secure, adventurous, enjoys music, imaginative play, regulation of emotions and self-distraction beginning
- 4yrs: sure of self, tests self, often negative, needs controlled freedom
- 5yrs: self-assured, stable, self-adjusted, enjoys responsibilities, capable of self-criticism, likes to follow rules
- By 6yrs: learnt which emotions are socially (un)acceptable
- Middle childhood: aware actions lead to (dis)approval, internalizes standards of conduct

Basics for positive emotional health

- Unconditional love from family
- Safe and secure surroundings
- Supportive caregivers, encouraging teachers
- Self-confidence and self-esteem
- Appropriate discipline
- Make time for play
- Set good example/role model
- Opportunity to play with other children

Key principles for parents

Social and emotional milestones harder to pinpoint than signs of physical development. Early support and intervention may prevent damaging patterns being established within families. Significant events in adult carer and family life impact on children too, e.g. deaths of grandparents, birth/illness of siblings, family break-up.

Related topics

◆ Emotional problems in children p. 330; ◆ Behavioural disorders in children p. 326

Further information

Association of Infant Mental Health (*Getting to know your baby*). Available at: ℛ https://aimh.org. uk/getting-to-know-your-baby/

Child Psychotherapy Trust (*Understanding childhood*). Available at: ℛ http://www. understandingchildhood.net/

Zero to Three (*Early connections last a lifetime*). Available at: ℛ www.zerotothree.org

Food and the under-fives

Good nutrition in preschool children is important. It ensures optimum growth and functional development, impacts on health in the present and in adulthood, and encourages a taste for healthy foods in preference to fatty, salty, and sugary foods. Under- and over-nourishment are public health issues, influenced by factors such as poverty and inappropriate feeding practices (➲ Overweight children and adolescents p. 302). By 5yrs, children should be eating family food that is a balanced healthy diet

Nutritional requirements

1–5yr olds have ↑ energy and nutrient requirements relative to their size. They need nutritious snacks between meals as part of a fixed routine (not constant snacking). Estimated average requirements:
• Boys 1–3yrs: 1230 kcal/day, 4–6yrs 1715 kcal/day
• Girls 1–3yrs: 1165 kcal/day, 4–6yrs 1545 kcal/day

The developing body, in particular bones and teeth, need a good supply of protein, calcium, iron, and vitamins A and D.

Diets of preschool children

Parents should be encouraged to offer children the family meals, containing food from all four food groups (e.g. cereals, fruit and vegetables, meat, egg and pulses, and milk and milk products). Use full-fat cow's milk until 2yrs, when semi-skimmed can be substituted provided the diet is otherwise nutritionally adequate. Skimmed milk is not suitable <5yrs. Encourage plenty of fluids, preferably plain tap water, to prevent constipation (➲ Constipation and encopresis p. 286). Promote dental health by keeping sugary foods and drinks to meal times only (➲ Development and care of teeth for young children p. 196. No more than 10% of dietary energy should be in sugars. Supplement with vitamins A, C, and D from 6mths, unless adequate vitamins through diverse diet and moderate exposure to sunlight. Avoid:
• Salty foods and the addition of salt at table
• Excessive fibre intake—compromises energy and mineral intake
• Tea and coffee to ensure mineral (especially iron) bioavailability

Vegetarians and vegans

Children need to be offered a mixture of plant proteins (e.g. cereals, pulses, seeds, ground-up nuts) to ensure the combinations complement each other in forming high-quality protein ≥ animal protein. Iron from plant sources is better absorbed with vitamin C, e.g. fruit juice. Children on vegan diets may need supplements or fortified foods to achieve enough calcium, vitamins D and B12, and riboflavin.

State-provided nutrition support for children

• Healthy Start schemes for families on low incomes provide vouchers for milk, fruit, and vegetables as well as vitamin drops
• Day-care providers can claim for a third of a pint of milk for each child attending >2hrs each day through the nursery milk scheme
• School fruit and vegetable scheme gives all children aged 4–6yrs in LA schools a free piece of fruit or vegetable each school day

Eating as a social skill

Food and eating offers opportunities for learning and interaction with adults, such as helping to shop, cooking, laying the table, washing up. Specific skills include:

- How to feed themselves more skilfully in accordance with family practices, including using utensils
- How to participate in a social occasion that requires certain ways of behaving

Children have to be given opportunities to feed themselves, to sit at a table to eat with others, and to enjoy mealtimes. Parents need to be:

- Prepared for messy mealtimes with toddlers
- Consistent about the expected behaviour at the meal table and realistic in what is manageable for the child's age

Food problems

Food preferences and refusal are common <5yrs. They are part of growing up and asserting independence, but are also often a source of tension at mealtimes. Parents may need advice on positive behaviour management. Key advice: children will not harm themselves if they do not eat for a short while; do not allow child to stop eating an entire food group (e.g. fruit and vegetables); if a food is rejected, try another from the same group or presenting it in a different way (including in a more fun way); and if child refuses to eat, do not insist, and do not substitute with snacking.

Foods for children to avoid

- Whole nuts in case of choking (➲ Child choking p. 806)
- Shark, swordfish, and marlin because levels of mercury may affect development of nervous system
- Raw shellfish and, in infants and toddlers, runny eggs to avoid risk of food poisoning (➲ Food-borne disease p. 730)

Further information

British Nutrition (*Nutrition through life: toddlers and pre-school children*). Available at: ᘔ https://ihv. org.uk/families/top-tips/

Toilet training

Most children can do without nappies by day from 2–3yrs and by night from 3–5yrs. How to approach toilet training will vary from child to child. If the child does not succeed within a few days, then either try training pants or revert to nappies and try again at a later date.

Key principles

Wait until the child is ready

The child can indicate that they are going to the toilet and has shown an interest in using a potty or toilet. It is helpful to have a potty or child's toilet seat (to put on a normal toilet) for the child to become familiar with before starting toilet training.

Pick a good time

When the child can have a few days at home without nappies, where accidents do not matter. Make sure plenty of spare clothes are available.

Keep the potty handy or stay within easy reach of the toilet

When the child says they wish to go, sit them immediately on the toilet. Reward any result with praise. Do not punish the child for any accidents. Advise the parent to ask the child to help clear up any mess and reinforce that it would be better to use the potty/toilet next time.

Until confident, continue using nappies when out and at night

Take the child to the toilet at night before bedtime. When dry nappies are consistently noted in the mornings, try the child without nappies at night—a plastic sheet on the mattress is useful. Even when a child has been dry for some time, accidents are common if the child is tired, unwell, etc.

Teach to wipe

Teach wiping from front to back (girls) and hand hygiene (Baby hygiene and skin care p. 194).

Toilet training for children with developmental delay

The same basic principles apply, only at a later chronological age. Parents usually advised to watch for signs of the child becoming aware of a need to go to the toilet (e.g. fidgeting) and for signs of physical readiness (e.g. dry for 1–2hrs and during naps). Parents may be advised to institute a toileting programme, i.e. a structured daily programme around that child's toileting habits, supported by visual signs to indicate each activity (e.g. take down pants, flush toilet) and reinforced with rewards.

Related topics

 Constipation and encopresis p. 286; Nocturnal enuresis p. 296.

Further information

ERIC: The Children's Bowel and Bladder Charity (*Potty training*). Available at: ℅ https://www.eric.org.uk/Pages/Category/potty-training

Understanding behaviour 1–5 years

Developing from a helpless baby to a relatively independent 4yr old is a time of great learning and emotion that can often feel very difficult for parents and carers. Toddlers and children are at an egocentric stage in their development, seeing themselves at the centre of the world, ready to be involved in everything, but often overwhelmed with feelings that they cannot yet manage. Children react individually and very differently to the triumphs and setbacks of each day, needing different types of support and understanding from parents and carers.

Behaviours

Bossy

This is one way of covering up that they are still small and there are things they cannot do. Often irritating to other children and adults, but they still need love and support.

Fussy

Including fads and rituals, this is one way of asserting independence against adults. Adults need to demonstrate how to give in gracefully over things that are less important (e.g. wearing odd clothes). Sometimes, a child is anxious or worried, but unable to talk about it, so it is easier to control what goes on their dinner plate than control the anxious feeling. These feelings come and go, but if behaviour becomes particularly difficult, consider if there is a particular stress and address that.

Clingy and fearful

This is one way of saying they still feel small, but it can be trying for parents and carers. Like all children, they need support, love, and encouragement, but also more time to take those steps to independence. Important to take new things slowly (e.g. settling into an early years setting, meeting new people).

Key principles for parents

- Give positive attention (e.g. active listening, smiling, talking to, hugging) to the child so they feel encouraged, supported, loved.
- Reward efforts, attempts, and good behaviour with smiles, words of praise, cuddles, etc.
- Help build self-esteem by letting children have a go at things.
- Relax and enjoy your children; do fun activities together.
- ↓ your own stress, e.g. create time away.

  When things get tense over behaviour:
- Do not reward poor behaviour or encourage its continuation with lots of attention.
- Make sure you stay in control of your own behaviour; leave the room if you are not (⮕ Safeguarding children p. 248).

Temper tantrums

Children are coping with strong feelings all day. A temper tantrum is a display of how it feels on the inside at a point when they can no longer cope, are feeling exhausted, and have not got the words to describe or deal with the feelings. In dealing with a tantrum, parents should be advised to:

- Count to 10 before doing anything, unless the child is in danger.
- Stay calm and acknowledge the child's feelings.
- Recognize the child is beyond reasoning and do not get into an argument.
- Do not ask more of them than they can manage.
- Try to avoid saying hurtful things that you do not mean.
- Trying to hold or hug the child may make it worse. After it subsides, cuddling may help reassure, while explaining it was not acceptable behaviour.

New siblings

More than one child brings additional complexities to family life. A new baby is the choice of the parents, not the siblings. Key principles:

- Prepare other child(ren) during the pregnancy (➔ Pregnancy p. 424).
- Recognize that the older child may feel sad, angry, or upset as they are no longer the centre of attention.
- The older child needs attention, reassurance, expressions of love, and time alone with parents.
- Find small, manageable ways for the older child to help with the new baby.

Related topics

➔ Behavioural disorders in children p. 326; ➔ Emotional development in babies and children p. 210; ➔ Emotional problems in children p. 330

Further information

Child Psychotherapy Trust Information (*Series of leaflets on understanding childhood*). Available at: ℘ www.understandingchildhood.net/

Family Lives (*Advice*). Available at: ℘ https://www.familylives.org.uk/advice/

Speech and language acquisition

Children follow a systematic path to the effective use of language and communication skills. Speech and language development is multidimensional, including speech, vocabulary, syntax, expression, and verbal comprehension. Speech, language, and communication difficulties can affect future learning and achievement (⊃ Communication and learning problems p. 224), literacy, behaviour and social emotional functioning (⊃ Emotional development in babies and children p. 210), confidence, and independence. Speech and language is developed through parents and carers talking and listening to babies and young children. 1° care nurses and health visiting (HV) (⊃ Health visiting p. 46) teams promote good interactive practice by advising parents to:

- Talk to the child when playing or doing things together
- Have fun with nursery rhymes and songs
- Encourage the child to listen to different sounds (e.g. birds, animals)
- Gain the child's attention when you want to talk together
- Encourage the child to communicate in any way, not just through words
- ↑ vocabulary by giving choices, e.g. 'Do you want an apple or banana?'
- Talk about things as they happen (e.g. when bathing, shopping)
- Listen carefully and give the child time to finish talking
- Take turns to speak
- Always respond in some way when the child says something
- Help the child to use more words by adding to what is said, e.g. if they say 'car', adult responds 'Yes, it's a red car driving down the road'
- If the child says something incorrectly, repeat it correctly, e.g. if they say 'Doggy bited it', adult responds 'Yes, the dog bit it, didn't he?'
- Try and have a special time with the child each day to play with toys and look at picture books together

Every child in England and Wales is entitled to a free Bookstart, with books and guidance materials for parents and carers, before they are 12mths old and again aged 3–4yrs (27mths in Wales). These may be given out by HV teams, children's centres, or libraries (⊃ Services for children, young people, and families p. 24).

Interactive practice skills are also promoted in parenting skills programmes as well as in other types of group settings for parents and babies, e.g. mother and baby groups, postnatal groups, infant massage groups (⊃ Support for parenting p. 172).

Babies and young children in bilingual families should be encouraged to speak both family language and English. Bilingualism does not delay speech and language acquisition.

Speech and language delay

1° speech and language delays are those not attributed to other conditions such as hearing loss or other more general developmental disabilities. Difficulties may arise with receptive language, expressive language, social communication, speech, fluency, or voice. Such delays are important as:

- They cause concern to parents
- They are often associated with behavioural and other difficulties in the preschool period (⊃ Behavioural disorders in children p. 326)

- They constitute a risk factor for subsequent poor school performance, and for a wide range of personal and social difficulties
- Children with untreated speech and language difficulties may go on to have mental health problems (→ Child and adolescent mental health p. 246)

Up to 60% of speech and language delays may resolve without treatment between 2–3yrs old. However, it is not possible to predict which children will spontaneously resolve at the time of identification.

Identification and action

No universal screening test, but nurses and HV teams should be alert to parental concerns and observe children's communication behaviours for evidence of delay. On identification of speech or language delay, HVs should: check no other related problem (e.g. hearing); refer to speech and language therapy according to local policy; offer advice on improving inter-active communication; and suggest or introduce parent/carer and child to socializing and play opportunities (e.g. one o'clock club, playgroup, mother and children group, childminder group).

Further information

Book Trust (*Bookstart*). Available at: ℛ www.bookstart.org.uk
Talking Point: the first stop for information on children's communication (*Ages and stages*). Available at: ℛ http://www.talkingpoint.org.uk/

Child development 5–11 years

Child development is the interaction between heredity and the environment. Development is assessed (⊃ Assessment of children, young people, and families p. 156) as part of the child assessment framework. Developmental progress is about the sequential acquisition of skills, and there is a range of time within which children acquire these skills (Table 6.5).

Children are expected to achieve nationally defined skills and knowledge in a range of subjects specified in the national curricula for state schools. In England and Wales: Key Stage 1 by age 7yrs and Key Stage 2 by age 11yrs. Standard Assessment Tests (SATs) are taken in reading, writing, and mathematics in school year 2 (age 6–7yrs) and school year 6 (age 10–11yrs).

Table 6.5 Overview of median age of development in children 5–11 years

	5–7 years	7–11 years
Gross motor	↑ strength, e.g. running faster, jumping higher. ↑ agility, e.g. stand on one leg longer, walk a narrow beam. ↑ co-ordination, e.g. learns to ride a 2-wheel bike, learns to swim.	Strength, agility, stamina, and co-ordination continue to develop. ↑ ability to play in team sports.
Fine motor and vision	Fine motor skills further developed in manipulating smaller objects with more precision. Able to dress and undress.	Fine motor skills ↑ developed. Dressing, undressing. and self-care skills much more developed.
Cognitive development	↑ linguistic skills. Conversations more complicated. Learning to read, write, and problem solve. Dominant mode of thought is tied to immediate circumstances and specific experiences. Beginning to grasp more abstract ideas like numbers, time, and distance.	Abilities described in 5–7yrs continue to develop. Egocentrism ↓—greater ability with language leads to greater socialization. More objective view of world and causes of physical events and their relationships.
Social, emotional, and behavioural	↑ independence from adults and personal confidence. Able to wash and bath with less supervision. Still needs help in brushing teeth properly. Plays games with simple rules and many fantasy games. Identifies with same-sex friends. Peer acceptance and approval begins to become important.	↑ desire for independence at the same time as a continued need for parental support. Friends still primarily of the same gender, but interest in opposite gender beginning. ↑ joining into groups and sometimes cliques. Exclusion can feel devastating. ↑ competitive and self-conscious. Peer approval and acceptance continues to grow in importance. Growing influence of social media – both positive and negative

In Scotland, each subject is described at six levels, starting at Level A. The majority of children are expected to reach Level B by the end of 1° year 4.

Puberty follows a well-defined set of stages starting between 8.5yrs and 12.5yrs in girls and between 10yrs and 14yrs in boys (**➲** Puberty and adolescence p. 228). The first stage is breast development in girls and testicular development in boys. Girls with early onset of puberty while in 1° school may need particular support in dealing with their difference from their peers (**➲** Working in schools p. 44; **➲** School nursing p. 42).

Further information

Cowie, H. (2012) *From birth to sixteen: children's health, social, emotional and linguistic development.* London: Routledge

Growth and nutrition 5–11 years

Growth is dependent on nutrition, good health, emotional health and well-being, pituitary growth hormone, thyroid hormone, and vitamin D. 2–12yrs contributes ~40% of adult height, often in rapid growth spurts during puberty (→ Puberty and adolescence p. 228). Obesity is a major public health issue with an estimated fifth of children (22.6%) in England aged 4–5yrs overweight or obese, rising to ~third of children overweight or obese (34.3%) by age 10–11yrs[33] (→ UK health profile p. 2; → Overweight children and adolescents p. 302)

All those involved in measuring children should receive training, and understand local policies and guidance.

Reasons for measuring school-aged children

- Indicator of health
- Identify disorders in growth (→ Growth disorders p. 298)
- Identify individual overweight and obesity, and underweight
- Monitor population levels of obesity in children as part of public health programmes (e.g. National Child Measurement Programme (NCMP) in England)

When to weigh and measure height

- At school entry, age 4–5yrs, as part of child health promotion programme) (→ Working in schools p. 44; → School nursing p. 42)
- National policies then apply, e.g. as part of NCMP in England, in reception year (4–5yrs) and year 6 (10–11yrs)
- Good practice as part of reviews of children with chronic illness (→ Children with complex health needs and disabilities p. 238), concerns about growth, safeguarding issues (→ Safeguarding children p. 248), or children with special educational needs (→ Children with special educational needs p. 242)

How to measure

Weight

Remove heavy clothing and shoes; use Class III clinical electronic scales.

Height

- Without footwear, using a rigid rule with T piece or stadiometer
- Bottom, back, and heels touching apparatus; ears and eyes at 90° to apparatus
- Measure on expiration

Recording

- Plotted as a small dot on UK–WHO 2–18yrs boy's or girl's growth charts and parent-held child health record
- Also plotted on body mass index (BMI) conversion and parental height comparator sections of chart if concern about growth
- Adult height predictor can be plotted if child or parent wishes

Interpretation

- A child whose weight is average for their height will have a BMI between the 25th and 75th centiles, whatever their height centile.
- Most children are within two centile spaces of the mid-parental height centile.
- BMI >91st centile suggests overweight.

Review by GP or community paediatrician

- BMI >98th centile (clinically obese)
- BMI <2nd centile may reflect poor nutrition, but may also simply reflect a small frame or low muscle mass
- Child height centile more than three centile spaces below mid-parental centile

Overweight

Overweight children should be encouraged to remain at a constant or slow increase, while their height increases through healthy eating and increased exercise (→ Exercise p. 354).

Underweight

Underweight children should also be monitored for any underlying medical conditions, mental health problems (→ Child and adolescent mental health p. 246), or safeguarding issues.

Nutrition

Estimated average requirements for energy:

- Boys 7–10yrs: 1970kcal/day
- Girls 7–10yrs: 1740kcal/day

All children should be eating family food in a balanced healthy diet: 47–50% carbohydrates (preferably complex), 15% protein, 5+ portions of fruit and vegetables a day, some fats, and low in salty and sugary foods. Vegetarian diets need to ensure adequate protein, iron, and selenium, as well as ad-equate B12 for vegans.

Food in schools

Parents can buy reduced-cost milk daily for children in 1° schools via the European Union school milk subsidy scheme. Children whose parents re-ceive low-income benefits are eligible for free school meals and sometimes free milk. Government set standards for nutrition in school-provided meals.

Reference

33. NHS Digital (2017) *Obesity prevalence increases in reception age primary school children.* Available at: https://digital.nhs.uk/news-and-events/news-archive/2017-news-archive/obesity-prevalence-increases-in-reception-age-primary-school-children

Further information

NHS Digital (*National Child Measurement Programme*). Available at: ℘ https://digital.nhs.uk/services/national-child-measurement-programme/

Royal College of Paediatrics and Child Health (*Growth charts*). Available at: ℘ https://www.rcpch.ac.uk/resources/growth-charts

Communication and learning problems

Some children will require extra help at some point in their schooling, ♂ > ♀ (● Working in schools p. 44; ● School nursing p. 42). Poor progress at school can be caused by a range of physical, social, and emotional problems (● Emotional problems in children p. 330), as well as problems in school or the home environment. Children may also have specific communication and learning problems that require individual assessment (● Assessment of children, young people, and families p. 156) and support, that may include special educational needs statements (● Children with special educational needs p. 242).

Dyslexia

Dyslexia is a combination of abilities and difficulties that affect the learning process in one or more of reading, spelling, and writing. It does not reflect the intelligence of the individual and the term is often used interchangeably with 'specific learning difficulties'. Approximately one in ten of the population has some degree of dyslexia, ♂ > ♀. It is a persistent condition, affecting children (and adults) across the ability range. Accompanying difficulties, often in areas of: spoken language (● Speech and language acquisition p. 218) and motor skills; speed of processing information and short-term memory; and organization and sequencing of items. If suspected, teachers consider specific educational support and involve the Special Educational Needs and Disability Co-ordinator (SENDCO). May require assessment and recommendations for educational support by educational psychologist.

Dyscalculia

Dyscalculia is the mathematical equivalent of dyslexia (i.e. difficulty in conceptualizing numbers, number relationships, outcomes of numerical operations, and estimation). If suspected, teachers consider specific educational support and involve SENDCO. The child may require assessment and recommendations for educational support by educational psychologist. Speech and language therapy (SALT) may be required.

Dyspraxia

Dyspraxia is the impairment of the organization of movement, and may be associated with other problems of language, perception, and thought. It used to be known as 'clumsy child' syndrome, developmental co-ordination disorder, or motor learning difficulties. ♂ > ♀. Common features include: late in reaching preschool milestones (e.g. rolling over, sitting, standing, walking, and speaking) (● Child development 1–5 years p. 204); clumsiness, poor body awareness, poor posture, awkward gait; difficulty hopping, skipping, riding bike, catching things; reading and writing difficulties; unable to remember or follow instructions, poorly organized; better in 1:1 than group teaching situations; and speech production difficulties (developmental verbal dyspraxia). If suspected, teachers consider specific educational support and involve SENDCO. The child may require assessment and recommendations for educational support by educational psychologist. Also may require SALT, physiotherapy, and occupational therapy support (● Teamwork p. 58).

Dysfluency (stammering)

About 5% of all children will have some difficulty with fluency during the development of their speech. About 80% of these will achieve normal fluency. Causes are multifactorial. The problem can fluctuate from mild to severe depending on the situation, the time of day, or for some other unidentifiable reason. Often embarrassing or distressing for the speaker, so the child will often adopt strategies to minimize or hide problems (e.g. not speaking in class or avoiding words they stammer on).

General advice for adults: do not say the word or finish the sentence for the child; be patient—do not ask multiple questions, and give time for the child to talk; do not tell the child to slow down or take a deep breath (becomes part of the struggle to speak); and praise the child for things that they are doing well. General advice for the child/young person: take time, rather than rushing, and speak a bit more slowly; pause for a moment before starting to speak; and remember to think well done for having a go.

If parent and child agree there is a cause for concern, then refer to SALT according to local policy.

Further information

British Dyslexia Association. Available at: ℘ https://www.bdadyslexia.org.uk/parent

Department of Education Statutory Guidance (SEND code of practice: 0–25 years). Available at: ℘ https://www.gov.uk/government/publications/send-code-of-practice-0-to-25

Dyspraxia Foundation (What is dyspraxia?). Available at: ℘ https://dyspraxiafoundation.org.uk/about-dyspraxia/

Dental health in older children

Most children start to lose their 1° teeth and gain their adult teeth at about 6yrs (❸ Development and care of teeth for young children p. 196). By 12yrs, most children will have 28 adult teeth. The four molars or wisdom teeth usually appear at 16–22yrs.

Dental health promotion programmes such as Childsmile (Scotland)[34] and Designed to Smile (Wales)[35] have had an impact on the incidence of dental caries. Although oral health is improving in England, around a quarter of 5yr olds have tooth decay (❸ UK health profile p. 2). Each child with tooth decay will have on average three or four teeth affected.[36] In Scotland, over the last decade the number of children with tooth decay has ↓: 2016 figures show that 69.4% of 1° school children had no decay compared with 54.1% in 2006. In Wales, there has also been a ↓ in the number of children with tooth decay from 46.6% in 2008 to 34.2% in 2016. In Northern Ireland, a 20% ↓ in tooth decay in children was reported in 2015. In each country, children from disadvantaged groups have the poorest dental health and are more likely to have dental caries. There are country-specific dental public health programmes.[34,35]

Sports injuries and accidents

Dentists can make mouth guards to protect teeth during contact sports (e.g. rugby) (❸ Accident prevention p. 168). Advice for knocked-out teeth: hold by tooth not root; if dirty, rinse in milk or water; and push gently back into socket or keep moist (in milk, water, or inside of mouth) until they can get to a dentist.

Orthodontic treatment

Common dental problems include protruding upper front teeth, crowding, asymmetrical alignment, bite problems, and impacted teeth. This may start in 1° school years, but more commonly in teenagers. Children are referred by their dentist to a specialist for orthodontic treatment. NHS-funded if the need for treatment is sufficient.

Treatment
- May include: removable, fixed, and functional braces; removal of teeth; use of orthodontic headgear; retainers (for ensuring teeth remain in place after treatment)
- Takes between 18–24mths with appointments every 4–6wks

Day-to-day management
- Orthodontists give advice on managing discomfort when appliances altered (painkillers and soft diet for a day or two) and on dental hygiene (special toothbrushes and mouthwash).
- It is recommended that removable appliances are removed for contact sports, and that mouth guards should be worn over fixed appliances.
- Teenagers often feel self-conscious about having to wear an appliance (❸ Working with teenagers p. 232). Adults need to be very supportive and encouraging not to become shy or withdrawn. Be alert to signs of teasing or bullying.

References

34. NHS Scotland (2018) *Childsmile—Improving the oral health of children in Scotland*. Available at: http://www.child-smile.org.uk/

35. NHS Wales (2018) *Designed to Smile (Wales)*. Available at: http://www.designedtosmile.org/

36. PHE (2018) *Child oral health: applying All Our Health*. Available at: https://www.gov.uk/government/publications/child-oral-health-applying-all-our-health/child-oral-health-applying-all-our-health

Further information

British Orthodontic Association (*FAQ for schools*). Available at: ℘ https://www.bos.org.uk/Information-for-Schools/FAQ-for-Schools

British Orthodontic Association (*Orthodontics and contact sports*) Available at: ℘ https://www.bos.org.uk/Public-Patients/Orthodontics-for-Children-Teens/Fact-File-FAQ/Orthodontics-Contact-Sports

Puberty and adolescence

Adolescence

The period between childhood and adulthood broadly corresponds with the teenage years, a time of rapid physical development and deep emotional changes. These are exciting times, but can be confusing and uncomfortable for the child and parents. Young people:

- Become more independent, learn how to get on with other people, and gain a sense of identity that is distinct from that of the family
- Make close relationships outside family, with friends of their own age. Friends and peer-group identity is very important to most.
- Find that parents become ↓ important in their eyes as their life outside the family develops. They develop views of their own that are often not shared by their parents.

Puberty

The period when 2° sexual characteristics develop and sexual organs mature. In healthy children, starts 9–14yrs in ♂; 8–13yrs in ♀.

Girls

Oestrogens stimulate growth and development of reproductive organs, deposition of fat (to produce narrow shoulders, broad hips, breasts, external genitalia), body hair, and softer texture skin. Sequence of changes:

- Breast development: is the first sign. Breast buds are the initial phase; followed by breast growth, with smooth contoured areola; then areola projects above the breast and breast tissue grows to adult shape.
- Pubic hair growth and rapid height spurt: occur almost immediately after breast buds appear. Then axillary hair.
- Menarche (first menstruation): occurs between 9–16yrs, on average 2.5yrs after start of puberty, and signals end of growing (on average, another 5cm of height remains).

Boys

Androgens, primarily testosterone, stimulate growth and development of the reproductive organs, body hair pattern, enlargement of the larynx, and muscles. Boys will begin to experience erections, often unconsciously, as soon as they start to mature sexually. Sequence of changes:

- Testicular enlargement: the first sign. Accompanied by growth in length then circumference of penis, darkening of scrotal skin.
- Pubic hair growth: follows testicular growth.
- Husky voice: often first indicator of larynx enlargement that lowers pitch of voice by an octave.
- Sequence of hair growth: pubic, axillary, facial, thoracic, scapular, ear, and nasal.
- Height spurt: occurs later and of greater magnitude than in girls.

Up to a third of boys around 12–14yrs will start to develop breasts that disappear later on. This is caused by lag in production of testosterone allowing female hormones to act, and can be a great worry and embarrassment. As soon as testosterone increases, the breast growth goes.

Most experience unconscious erections and ejaculation during their sleep ('wet dreams'). For the first time, sexual feelings become strong urges, which require conscious control.

Both sexes

Body odour

Two types of sweat glands: eccrine glands produce sweat used to control body temperature; and apocrine glands. The latter only start working at puberty. Secrete a different type of odourless sweat in response to stress, excitement, and sexual excitement. When bacteria start decomposing it, a strong distinct smell is released, thus causing body odour.

Sleep

Sleep patterns changed by both behaviour and hormonal changes. Enough sleep essential because the hormone to stimulate growth spurt is released during sleep. Lack of sleep contributes to moodiness, impulsiveness, and depression (➔ Babies, children, and sleeping p. 200)

Spots

~80% of teens suffer to some degree. Boys more than girls because testosterone increases spots, whereas oestrogen prevents them. The face is the most common area, but can appear on the neck, upper back, shoulders, and chest. The cause is overactive sebaceous glands.

Mood changes

Teenagers experience mood swings (➔ Working with teenagers p. 232). This could be the effect of raging hormones (particularly for girls in premenstrual hormone fluctuations), but also response to physical and emotional changes that leave them feeling uncertain and self-conscious. Moodiness changes as teenagers become more confident.

Vulnerability

Young people may be at risk of child sexual exploitation (➔ Safeguarding children p. 248) and mental health problems (➔ Child and adolescent mental health p. 246) as they become more independent from their parents or carers. Self-harming behaviours may also manifest during early adolescence (➔ Suicidal intent and deliberate self-harm p. 494). Professionals and parents need to be alert to changes in mood, behaviour, or school attendance, and appropriate action taken.

Related topics

➔ Growth and nutrition 12–18 years p. 234; ➔ Acne vulgaris p. 300; ➔ Growth disorders p. 298

Further information

Department for Education (*Child sexual exploitation*). Available at: ℅ https://www.gov.uk/government/publications/child-sexual-exploitation-definition-and-guide-for-practitioners

National Society for the Prevention of Cruelty to Children (NSPCC) (*Child sexual exploitation*). Available at: ℅ https://www.nspcc.org.uk/preventing-abuse/child-abuse-and-neglect/child-sexual-exploitation/

NSPCC (*Self-harm*). Available at: ℅ https://www.nspcc.org.uk/preventing-abuse/keeping-children-safe/self-harm/

Royal College of Paediatrics and Child Health. Available at: ℅ https://www.rcpch.ac.uk/topic/adolescent-health

Young Minds (*Fighting for young people's mental health*). Available at: M https://youngminds.org.uk/

Health promotion in schools

Promoting health is part of the school curriculum in each country of the UK, although the emphasis varies in local areas (→ Working in schools p. 44; → School nursing p. 42). The science curriculum, which is a statutory requirement, includes a range of topics such as sexual health (→ Sex and relationship education p. 236) and substance abuse (→ Substance use p. 476). Substance abuse includes the abuse of alcohol (→ Alcohol p. 360), tobacco, cannabis and other drugs, and solvent and volatile substance abuse. Sexual health includes issues related to contraception (→ Contraception: general p. 400), pregnancy (→ Pregnancy p. 424), and sexually transmitted infections (→ Sexual health: general issues p. 760; → Sexually transmitted infections p. 764). School health services may contribute to this and healthy schools programmes, as requested by the school.[37] In England and Wales (but not Scotland), Sex and Relationship Education (SRE) is statutory.

In England, Personal, Social, and Health Education (PSHE) brings together personal, social, health education, work-related learning, careers, enterprise, and financial capability. There are two non-statutory programmes of study at Key Stages 3 and 4: personal well-being, economic well-being, and financial capability based on policy aims specified in the Children Act 2004. In Wales and Scotland, themes are similar, but there are differences to the PSHE programmes.

PSHE health objectives for children 5–7yrs

- How to make simple choices that improve their health and well-being
- To maintain personal hygiene
- Process of growing from young to old, and how people's needs change
- Names of the main parts of the body
- That all household products, including medicines, can be harmful (→ Accident prevention p. 168; → Poisoning and overdoses p. 822)
- Rules and ways for keeping safe, including basic road safety and people who can help them to stay safe

PSHE health objectives for children 7–11yrs

- The components of a healthy lifestyle, including the benefits of exercise (→ Exercise p. 354) and healthy eating
- The importance of hygiene in stopping the spread of diseases (→ Infectious diseases in childhood p. 290)
- How the body changes approaching puberty (→ Puberty and adolescence p. 228)
- Substances and drugs that are legal and illegal, their effects and risks
- To recognize the different risks in different situations and then decide how to behave responsibly, including sensible road use
- How to recognize and resist pressures to behave in an unacceptable or risky way, and how to ask for help
- Basic emergency aid procedures (→ Child basic life support p. 800; → Adult basic life support and automated external defibrillation p. 792)

PSHE health objectives for children 11–14yrs

- To recognize and manage the physical and emotional changes that take place at puberty
- How to keep healthy and what influences health, including the media
- That good relationships and a balance between work, leisure, and exercise can promote physical and mental health
- Basic facts and laws about alcohol, tobacco (by 15yrs, 24% are regular smokers), illegal substances (experimentation starts around 13–14yrs), and the risks of misusing prescribed drugs
- SRE links with strategies to reduce teenage conceptions (➔ Pregnancy p. 424)
- To recognize and manage risk, and make safer choices about healthy lifestyles, different environments, and travel
- How to recognize and resist pressures to behave in an unacceptable or risky way, and how to ask for help
- Basic emergency aid procedures

PSHE health objectives for children 14–16yrs

- To think about the alternatives, and long- and short-term consequences when making decisions about personal health
- The causes, symptoms, and treatments for stress and depression, and to identify strategies for prevention and management (➔ Child and adolescent mental health p. 246)
- About the link between eating patterns and self-image, including eating disorders (➔ People with eating disorders p. 474)
- About the health risks of alcohol and other substances
- Making safer choices/understanding risk-taking behaviours
- SRE links with strategies to reduce teenage conceptions and sexually transmitted infections
- To seek professional advice confidently and find information about health (➔ Confidentiality p. 89)
- Develop the skills to cope with emergency situations that require basic aid procedures, including resuscitation techniques

Reference

37. Department for Education (2012) *Healthy schools*. Available at: https://webarchive. nationalarchives.gov.uk/20130104132539/https://www.education.gov.uk/schools/ pupilsupport/pastoralcare/a0075278/healthy-schools

Further information

PSHE Association (*A whole-school approach to promoting health in schools*). Available at: ℳ https://www.pshe-association.org.uk/news-and-blog/blog-entry/whole-school-approach-promoting-health-schools

Working with teenagers

Teenagers are coping with the ambiguity of not being a child or an adult. Professionals need to assess their biological, psychological, and social development so they interact relevantly and give appropriate responsibility without unacceptable risk. This is reflected in what they can do at particular ages:

- Be held criminally responsible: aged 10yrs (England, Wales, and Northern Ireland). Currently 8yrs in Scotland but Bill raised in 2018 to ↑ to 12yrs
- Buy cigarettes: aged 16yrs in UK
- Drive a moped: aged 16yrs in UK
- Join the armed forces: aged 16yrs in UK
- Drive a car: aged 17yrs in UK (or 16yrs if eligible for the enhanced rate of the mobility component of Personal Independence Payment)
- Vote in an election: aged 18yrs in UK
- Order alcohol (➔ Alcohol p. 360) in a public house: aged 18yrs in UK

Teenage healthcare

- Health indicators for age group have changed little in the past 20yrs
- Patterns of behaviour and use of services acquired at this point carry on into adult life
- Teenagers are represented in key target areas of sexually-transmitted disease (➔ Sexually transmitted infections p. 764) and teenage pregnancy
- Adolescents assess risk differently from health professionals; peer pressure is more significant than long-term consequences

Services

Services should be age-appropriate, and responsive to the needs of teenagers (➔ Services for children, young people, and families p. 24). Teenagers use general services in hospitals, surgeries, and health centres, and those designed specifically for them, e.g. school nurse drop-ins, (➔ Working in schools p. 44, ➔ School nursing p. 42) child and adolescent mental health services (➔ Child and adolescent mental health p. 246), and young people's sexual health clinics. In encouraging teenagers to take responsibility for their own health, professionals face the challenge of urging them to use mainstream services. Peer educators (teenagers who work alongside those of a similar age and background) may facilitate this. They appreciate different health services together in one relaxed setting, without appointment systems.

Key principles of contact with teenagers

- Foster a spirit of partnership, identifying needs of the young person (e.g. stress, body piercing, menstruation), as well other ↑ profile issues (nutrition (➔ Growth and nutrition 12–18 years p. 234), sexual health (➔ Sexual health: general issues p. 760), mental health, and substance misuse (➔ Substance use p. 476).
- Have confidentiality (➔ Confidentiality p. 89) explained and guaranteed, except in case of child protection issues, when it might be broken (➔ Child protection processes p. 252).

- Let the young person increasingly take decisions appropriate to his/her age and development. Consenting to health interventions (Fraser competencies) is dependent on age and understanding of the issues (➲ Consent p. 82).
- Focus on communication, establishing rapport and an honest open relationship by listening, questioning, understanding, responding, explaining, and summarizing. Teenagers value staff being approachable and positive in attitude.
- Empower young people to set and achieve their own goals.

Individual contact with teenagers needs to go alongside national and community approaches (➲ Community approaches to health p. 338). This might include banning of smoking in public places, the wider availability of contraception (➲ Contraception: general p. 400), and whole-school approaches impacting on nutrition in the school canteen.

Consider vulnerability

Young people may be at risk of child sexual exploitation (➲ Safeguarding children p. 248) and mental health problems as they become more independent from their parents or carers. Self-harming behaviours (➲ Suicidal intent and deliberate self-harm p. 494) may also manifest during early adolescence. Professionals and parents need to be alert to changes in mood, behaviour. or school attendance, and appropriate action taken to support young people (➲ Identifying the child in need of protection p. 250).

Further information

National Society for the Prevention of Cruelty to Children (NSPCC) (*Child sexual exploitation*). Available at: https://www.nspcc.org.uk/preventing-abuse/child-abuse-and-neglect/child-sexual-exploitation/

NSPCC (*Self-harm*). Available at: https://www.nspcc.org.uk/preventing-abuse/keeping-children-safe/self-harm/

NSPCC (*Gillick Competency and Fraser Guidelines*). Available at: https://learning.nspcc.org.uk/research-resources/briefings/gillick-competency-and-fraser-guidelines/

Growth and nutrition 12–18 years

The pubertal growth spurt is the fourth phase of human growth (⮕ Puberty and adolescence p. 228). Sex hormones cause the back to lengthen, adding 15% to final height, and fuse the epiphyseal growth plates. If puberty is early (not uncommon in girls), the final height is reduced because of early fusion of epiphyses.

Nutrition

All young people should eat a balanced healthy diet. Short term, this helps appearance (shiny hair, healthy skin) and, in the long term, protects against cardiovascular disease (⮕ Coronary heart disease p. 624) and osteoporosis.
↑ energy requirements:

- Boys: 11–14yrs 2220kcal/day; 15–18yrs 2755kcal/day
- Girls: 11–14yrs 1845kcal/day; 15–18yrs 2110kcal/day

Protein requirements ↑ by approximately 50%. Calcium requirements higher than adults, as skeletal development is rapid: boys 1000mg; girls 800mg a day. Once menstruation starts, girls need 14.8mg of iron a day compared to 8.7mg for boys.

Key issues in teenagers

- About 60% regularly skip breakfast (breakfast cereals and breads are fortified with vitamins and minerals).
- Inadequate nutrients (particularly vitamins and minerals) in diet and fats feature ↑ for energy sources. About 50% girls aged 15–18yrs do not have adequate nutrients (especially iron and calcium) in diet.
- 46% boys and 69% girls 15–18yrs spending less than recommended 1hr/ day in activities of moderate intensity (⮕ Exercise p. 354).
- ↑ use of unsuitable methods to control weight, e.g. skipping meals, very ↓ energy dieting, and smoking (⮕ Smoking cessation p. 356).
- Vegetarianism more common among teenagers (more girls), but with a poor understanding of how to achieve a balanced diet with adequate protein, iron, and selenium.

Monitoring

Routine monitoring of weight and height beyond reception class entry (4–5yrs) and year 6 (England only) is not recommended (⮕ Working in schools p. 44; ⮕ School nursing p. 42). Good practice to record height and weight in any young person over whom there is a concern or who has chronic ill health. Use UK–WHO 2–18yrs growth charts to assess growth and any problem[38,39] (⮕ Growth disorders p. 298; ⮕ Overweight children and adolescents p. 302).

Key nutrition and obesity prevention messages

Best delivered through media that reach young people, in peer settings, through PSHE curriculum and healthy schools initiatives:

- Base your meals on starchy foods.
- Eat lots of fruit and vegetables (at least five portions a day).
- Eat moderate amounts of protein, iron-rich foods, low-fat dairy produce, and more fish.

- Do not skip breakfast.
- Get active and minimize sitting activities.
- Cut down on saturated fat and sugar.
- Try to eat less salt: no more than 6g/day.
- Drink plenty of water.

Foods for young people to avoid

- Shark, swordfish, and marlin because levels of mercury may affect development of nervous system.
- Girls should limit portions of oily fish to twice a week because of the potential build-up of dioxins that may affect the development of any fetus in later life.[40]

Food in schools

<16yrs whose parents receive state benefits for ↓ income are eligible for free school meals. Many schools have whole-school food policies, incorporating a range of activities throughout the curriculum and school day (➔ Health promotion in schools p. 230).

References

38. Royal College of Paediatrics and Child Health (2012) Boys: UK growth chart 2–18 years. Available at: https://www.rcpch.ac.uk/sites/default/files/Boys_2-18_years_growth_chart.pdf
39. Royal College of Paediatrics and Child Health (2012) Girls: UK growth chart 2–18 years. Available at: https://www.rcpch.ac.uk/sites/default/files/Girls_2-18_years_growth_chart.pdf
40 British Nutrition Foundation (2018) School children. Available at: https://www.nutrition.org.uk/nutritionscience/life/school-children.html?start=1

Further information

British Nutrition Foundation (Food in schools). Available at: ℳ https://www.nutrition.org.uk/foodinschools.html
NICE (Obesity prevention [CG43]). Available at: ℳ www.nice.org.uk/CG43
Vegetarian Society (Young veggie). Available at: ℳ www.youngveggie.org

Sex and relationship education

Sex and relationship education (SRE) takes place in schools and may involve health professionals, particularly school nurses (➲ School nursing p. 42) and sexual health outreach nurses (➲ Working in schools p. 44). Given that some children are not in school because of exclusion or truancy, or are withdrawn by parents from this potentially sensitive subject, educational input in other settings (e.g. home, youth group, community group) is to be encouraged. Government guidance states that SRE should be part of PSHE and citizenship. All schools (1° and 2°) must have a written policy on sex education, developed with parents and agreed by the school governors. Opinions are often strongly held as to how SRE should be taught or if it should be taught at all. Any SRE has to be as stated within the school policy. Most agree that SRE should begin before children reach puberty (➲ Puberty and adolescence p. 228). Discussion of relationships in their widest sense is appropriate from school entry and before.

SRE seeks to help and support young people through their physical, emotional (➲ Emotional development in babies and children p. 210), and moral development. SRE is about the importance of stable and loving relationships, respect, love, and care, as well as teaching about sex, sexuality, and sexual health (➲ Sexual health: general issues p. 760). SRE is seen as important in contributing to a ↓ in the number of teenage conceptions (➲ Pregnancy p. 424).

Elements of SRE

Attitudes and values
- Issues of individual conscience
- Value of family life
- Nurturing of children

Personal and social skills
- How to manage emotions
- Developing respect for self and others
- Realizing the consequences of own choices
- Recognizing and avoiding exploitation and abuse (➲ Safeguarding children p. 248)

Knowledge and understanding
- Physical development at particular stages
- Understanding human sexuality, reproduction, sexual health, emotions, and relationships
- Contraception (➲ Contraception: general p. 400), avoidance of pregnancy, and protection from sexually transmitted infections (➲ Sexually transmitted infections p. 764)
- Reasons for choosing to delay or commence a sexual relationship

Delivery of SRE

Whoever is involved in providing SRE, the following contribute to positive evaluations:
- Established skills in facilitating groups
- Relevant and up-to-date knowledge

- Motivation to lead the session
- Positive attitudes and values in relation to sexual behaviour
- The use of discussion as a teaching strategy. Young people do not like the emphasis on physical aspects of reproduction, preferring the opportunity to discuss feelings, relationships, and values.
- A safe environment facilitated by agreed ground rules and de-personalization of the issues

Issues to consider

- Single-sex groups: more appropriate for some issues at some points
- Confidentiality: a statement of confidentiality needs to be discussed with the whole class, exhibited, and adhered to by all involved (→ Confidentiality p. 89)
- Age of consent: sexual activity with <16yrs is illegal, yet ~20% of teenagers will commence sexual activity before 16yrs. Concerns will be raised by sexual activity involving a young person <13yrs or a young person with a significantly older partner (→ Identifying the child in need of protection p. 250)
- Sexual orientation: good practice requires that questions are dealt with honestly and sensitively, but there should not be direct promotion of any sexual orientation

Continuing professional development

School nursing and health visiting education programmes will have prepared staff to work with groups of young people. Continuing professional development (CPD) programmes in PHSE are available to nurses (→ Continuing professional development p. 53).

Related topics

→ Health promotion in schools p. 230

Further information

PSHE Association (*Sex and relationship education for the 21st century*). Available at: ℅ https://www.pshe-association.org.uk/curriculum-and-resources/resources/sex-and-relationship-education-sre-21st-century

Sex Education Forum (*What we do*). Available at: ℅ http://www.sexeducationforum.org.uk/about/what-we-do

Children with complex health needs and disabilities

Children with disabilities are among the most stigmatized and excluded groups of children around the world. They are likely to have poorer health, ↓ education, and ↓ economic opportunity than their peers without disabilities[41] (➔ Promoting the health of children p. 152).

About 8% of children are disabled, and the prevalence of severe disability is increasing.[42] Advances in assistive technology have improved the functioning of children with disabilities; supporting communication, mobility, self-care, household tasks, family relationships, education, and engagement in play and recreation; enhancing both the quality of life for both children and their families (➔ Assistive technology and home adaptations p. 834).

The term 'disabled children' is used here to include children and young people with learning disabilities (➔ People with learning disabilities p. 456), autistic spectrum disorders (➔ Autistic spectrum disorders p. 322), sensory impairments (➔ Deafness in children p. 268; ➔ Blindness and partial sight p. 748), physical impairments, and emotional/behavioural disorders (➔ Emotional problems in children p. 330; ➔ Behavioural disorders in children p. 326).

Health and education policies explain that the role of health practitioners in supporting children with complex needs should include: encouragement to participate fully in family and community life; integrated multi-agency assessments (➔ Assessment of children, young people, and families p. 156; ➔ Teamwork p. 58), leading to timely, responsive care plans that support the child to reach their full potential; involving children, young people, and their families in important decisions regarding their care; and collaborative multi-agency working in order to safeguard and protect children and young people with disabilities (➔ Safeguarding children p. 248; ➔ Suicidal intent and deliberate self-harm p. 494; ➔ Child protection processes p. 252).

The Children and Families Act 2014[43] states that LAs and clinical commissioning groups (CCGs) must make joint commissioning arrangements for education, healthcare, and care provision for children and young people with disabilities (➔ Commissioning of services p. 12). These services should include specialist children's services, child development centres (multidisciplinary assessment and treatment centres), and child development teams (community-based multidisciplinary teams). The rationale is to provide co-ordinated assessment and a consistent care plan.

Child development teams commonly include:
- Community paediatrician specializing in child development
- Specialist health visitors (➔ Health visiting p. 46)
- Speech and language therapists (➔ Speech and language acquisition p. 218), occupational therapists, and physiotherapists
- Home-based learning support teachers and nursery nurses, e.g. Portage (see ℘ https://www.portage.org.uk/about/what-portage)
- Orthoptists
- Educational psychologists
- Social workers
- School nurses (➔ School nursing p. 42)

Key principles for working with children and families

- Early identification through antenatal screening (➲ Antenatal care and screening p. 426), child health promotion programme (➲ Overview of the Healthy Child Programme p. 154; ➲ Health promotion in schools p. 230), response to parental concern, follow-up of high-risk newborn babies (➲ Pre-term infants p. 176)
- Integrated diagnosis and assessment processes
- Early interventions through home-based learning services (e.g. Portage), as well as interventions to support optimal physical and cognitive development, while promoting child and family's inclusion in community
- Co-ordination between 1° and 2° healthcare
- Provision of a key worker/care manager, recognized by others in multidisciplinary service environment, to ensure delivery of services is co-ordinated; family has access to all services, and key worker/care manager becomes first point of contact if problems arise
- Supporting parents and families as carers (➲ Carers p. 458)

Promote social inclusion

- Ensure family has knowledge about all benefits and charities that can help (e.g. the Family Fund: see 🔊 https://www.familyfund.org.uk/)
- Access to mainstream public services and children's services including social services, therapy services, and child and adolescent mental health services as these children are more vulnerable to mental health difficulties than children without disabilities (➲ Child and adolescent mental health p. 246)
- ↓ impact of multiple healthcare appointments on schooling and family
- Access to suitable housing (➲ Homes and housing p. 26), equipment, and assistive technology
- Access to play, sport, leisure, and holiday facilities
- Access to appropriate educational opportunities

Additional considerations

All professionals need to be aware that these children are at ↑ risk of abuse than other children, particularly if they live away from home. Transition from child to adult services needs particular care in planning as, in many cases, it is poorly co-ordinated, resulting in a decline in support and deterioration in health and social inclusion (➲ Transition of young people to adult services p. 468).

For some children, their condition may require adequate consideration of palliative care needs and additional support to family and carers through this period and on a child's death (➲ Coping with bereavement p. 574).

Under the Children Act 2004, the LA must keep a register of all children with disabilities in its area.

References

41. WHO (2015) *Assistive technology for children with disabilities: creating opportunities for education, inclusion and participation.* Available at: https://www.unicef.org/disabilities/files/Assistive-Tech-Web.pdf

42. Department for Work and Pensions (2018) *Family Resources Survey 2016/2017.* Available at: https://assets.publishing.service.gov.uk/government/uploads/system/uploads/attachment_data/file/692771/family-resources-survey-2016-17.pdf

43. HM Government (2014) *Children and Families Act.* Available at: http://www.legislation.gov.uk/ukpga/2014/6/contents/enacted

Further information

Contact for Families with Disabled Children (*About us*). Available at: ℰ https://contact.org.uk/about-us/

Disabled Living Foundation (*Children*). Available at: ℰ www.livingmadeeasy.org.uk/children/

Scope (*Advice for families with disabled children and young people*). Available at: ℰ https://www.scope.org.uk/support/families

Children with special educational needs

A child or young person is considered to have special educational needs (SEN) if they have a learning difficulty or disability (➲ People with learning disabilities p. 456) which calls for special educational provision to be made for him or her. SEN are explained as when a child has ↑ difficulty in learning, compared with the majority of others of the same age, which prevents him or her from making use of facilities of a kind generally provided for their peers in mainstream schools or mainstream post-16yrs institutions[45] (➲ Working in schools p. 44).

Codes of practice (UK)

Guidance published in 2015[44] outlines changes regarding the SEN code of practice as introduced by the Children and Families Act (2014). These include:

- The code of practice now covers the 0–25yrs age range and includes guidance relating to disabled children and young people with SEN
- Emphasis on the participation of children and young people (CYP) and parents in decision making
- Strong focus on ↑ aspirations and improving outcomes for CYP in order to make a successful transition to adulthood
- Joint planning and commissioning of services to ensure close co-operation between education, health, and social care (➲ Commissioning of services p. 12)
- A graduated approach to identifying and supporting students with SEN (to replace school action and school action plus)
- A co-ordinated assessment process and implementation of education, health, and care plan which replaces statements and learning difficulty assessments
- Information is provided on relevant duties under the Equality Act (2010) and Mental Capacity Act (2005)
- New guidance on supporting CYP with SEN who are in youth custody

Involvement of health services

- In early years, child health services must alert the parents and the LA to the child's potential difficulties. A child development centre or team may provide a multi-professional view at an early stage.
- All educational settings need to know how, with parental consent (➲ Consent p. 82), to obtain information and advice on health-related matters, using school health service (➲ School nursing p. 42), GP (➲ General practice p. 18), or a relevant member of child development centre or team.
- Each health area has to designate a medical officer (usually a community paediatrician) to work with the LA on behalf of children with SEN and to lead the health services contribution to the statutory assessment process.

Graduated educational assessments for children over 2 years old

All early years' providers are required to have arrangements in place to identify and support children with SEN or disabilities and to promote the equality of opportunity for children in their care. These requirements are detailed in the Early Years' Foundation Stage Framework (England only).[45]

- When a child is aged 2–3yrs, early years' practitioners must review progress and provide parents with a summary of their child's development, focusing on communication and language, physical development, and personal, social, and emotional development (⊘ Emotional development in babies and children p. 210).
- If there are any significant emerging concerns (or identified SEN or disability), practitioners should develop a targeted plan to support the child, involving other professionals such as the SENDCO.
- Early Years Action and Early Years Action Plus have been replaced by SEN support, a graduated approach to supporting children with SEN.
- When despite the setting having taken relevant and purposeful action to identify, assess, and meet the SEN needs of the CYP, the CYP has not made the expected progress, the setting should request an education, health, and care needs assessment.
- The code applies equally to maintained schools, academies, and free schools.
- The code does not distinguish between 1° and 2° phases.

Special educational needs assessment

The SEN assessment process should:
- Focus on the needs of the CYP
- Be easy to navigate and avoid jargon
- Highlight the CYP's strengths and capacities
- Organize assessments to minimize demands on the family
- Involve all professionals involved in the family (⊘ Teamwork p. 58)
- Deliver an outcomes-focused and co-ordinated plan for the CYP

Duties on mainstream schools

- Ensure that a child with SEN gets the support he/she needs.
- Integrate CYP with SEN with pupils who do not have SEN.
- Designate a teacher to be responsible for co-ordinating SEN.
- Inform parents when they are making special educational provision for a CYP.
- When a CYP with SEN is identified, a cycle of assess, plan, do, and review is adopted.

Assessments and education, health, and care plans

If a LA considers it necessary for a child to have an education and healthcare (EHC) plan, it must conduct an assessment of educational and healthcare needs. EHC plans should be forward-looking, help ↑ aspirations, and outline the provision required to meet the pupil's needs and support them in their ambitions. EHC plans should specify how services will be delivered as part of a whole package and how to achieve the outcomes across education, health, and social care for the CYP.

The code explains that young people without an EHC plan continue to have the right to request an assessment of their SEN at any point prior to their 25th birthday (unless an assessment has been carried out in the previous 6mths).

Local offer

LAs must publish a local offer detailing, in one place, information about SEN provision available for CYP in their area. Arrangements for resolving disagreements, mediation, and parents' and young people's rights to appeal a decision of the LA should be sent to the SEN tribunal.

References

44. Department of Health and Department of Education (2015) Special educational needs and disability code of practice: 0–25 years. Statutory guidance for organisations which work with and support children and young people who have special educational needs or disabilities. Available at: https://assets.publishing.service.gov.uk/government/uploads/system/uploads/attachment_data/file/398815/SEND_Code_of_Practice_January_2015.pdf

45. Department of Education (2017) Statutory framework for the early years' foundation stage. Setting the standards for learning, development and care for children from birth to five. Available at: https://www.gov.uk/government/publications/early-years-foundation-stage-framework--2

Further information

Mencap (*Advice and support for children and young people*). Available at: ℘ https://www.mencap.org.uk/advice-and-support/children-and-young-people

National Portage Association (*What is Portage?*). Available at: ℘ https://www.portage.org.uk/about/what-portage

Child and adolescent mental health

Psychological well-being in children and young people is well recognized as essential for health, development, and resilience. Mental health problems can be observed in difficulties in play and learning, personal relationships, psychological development, and in distress and maladaptive behaviour (◆ Emotional problems in children p. 330). One in eight children and young people aged between 5–19yrs, surveyed in England in 2017, had a mental disorder.[46] It is important to be especially aware of these problems in three groups:

- Looked-after children (◆ Looked-after children p. 254)
- Children and young people with learning disabilities (◆ People with learning disabilities p. 456; ◆ Children with complex health needs and disabilities p. 238)
- Young offenders

It is recognized that everyone has a role in ensuring the environment in which children grow up promotes their mental health. Policies encourage health, education, and public services to:

- Tackle bullying and racism
- ↑ awareness of mental health issues
- Improve the recognition of children's emerging needs
- Provide support for those children with particular needs
- Address online sexting and bullying (◆ Safeguarding children p. 248)

Child health promotion policies make it explicit how health visitors (HV) (◆ Health visiting p. 46), school nurses (SN) (◆ School nursing p. 42), and 1° care services should promote child mental health and link to specialist services (◆ Promoting the health of children p. 152).

Primary level of care (tier 1)

Includes all services contributing to mental healthcare of CYP, e.g. GPs, HVs, SNs, social workers, teachers, juvenile justice workers, and voluntary agencies. Focus on the initial assessment and identification of difficulties (◆ Assessment of children, young people, and families p. 156). May include advice or the provision of therapeutic help not requiring specialist training.

Specialist individuals, teams, and inpatient services (tiers 2–4)

Likely to include child and adolescent psychiatrists, clinical psychologists, nurses, psychotherapists, occupational therapists, speech and language therapists, art, music, and drama therapists, and family therapists (◆ Teamwork p. 58). These teams will be part of Child and Adolescent Mental Health Services (CAMHS) that assess and treat young people with emotional, behavioural, or mental health difficulties. CAMHS support covers: anxiety and depression (◆ People with anxiety and depression p. 478); problems with food (◆ People with eating disorders p. 474); self-harm (◆ Suicidal intent and deliberate self-harm p. 494); abuse; violence, or anger; bipolar disorder (◆ People with bipolar affective disorder p. 482); and schizophrenia (◆ People with psychosis p. 486).

Key points

All policies emphasize the need for clear, co-ordinated care pathways for referrals, as well as training and support for 1° care professionals. The Green Paper 'Transforming children and young people's mental health provision'[47] sets out the need for:

- A mental health lead in every school and college
- Mental health support teams working with schools and colleges and alongside others who provide mental health support including SNs, educational psychologists, school counsellors, voluntary and community organizations, and social workers (→ Working in schools p. 44)
- Shorter waiting times to get treatment from CYP mental health services
- Improving understanding of mental health; looking at how social media affects the health of CYP
- Research on how to support families, including how parents and carers can bond better with their children, which helps their mental health
- Research on how to prevent mental health problems

References

46. NHS Digital (2018) *Mental health of children and young people in England 2017*. Available at: https://digital.nhs.uk/data-and-information/publications/statistical/mental-health-of-children-and-young-people-in-england/2017/2017

47. Department of Education, Department of Health and Social Care (2018) *Transforming children and young people's mental health provision: a green paper*. Available at: https://www.gov.uk/government/consultations/transforming-children-and-young-peoples-mental-health-provision-a-green-paper/quick-read-transforming-children-and-young-peoples-mental-health-provision#contents

Further information

Anti-Bullying Alliance (*Tools and information*). Available at: https://www.anti-bullyingalliance.org.uk/tools-information

Child and Adolescent Mental Health (*Problems and disorders*). Available at: http://www.camh.org.uk/

ChildLine (*Information and advice*). Available at: https://www.childline.org.uk/info-advice/

Royal College of Psychiatrists (*Young people's mental health*). Available at: https://www.rcpsych.ac.uk/mental-health/parents-and-young-people

Safeguarding children

Safeguarding and promoting the welfare of children is defined for the purposes of this guidance as:

- Protecting children from maltreatment
- Preventing impairment of children's health or development
  (➔ Promoting the health of children p. 152)
- Ensuring that children grow up in circumstances consistent with the provision of safe and effective care
- Taking action to enable all children to have the best outcomes
  (➔ Identifying the child in need of protection p. 250; ➔ Child protection processes p. 252)

Protecting (or safeguarding) children is a duty of care for all organizations who are required to have criminal records checks, through the Disclosure and Barring Service (DBS), on all volunteers and employees coming into contact with children.

Child protection

Is part of safeguarding and promoting welfare; it is the activity that is undertaken to protect specific children who are suffering, or are likely to suffer, significant harm.

In the UK, inquiries into child deaths from abuse and neglect show that most occur in what is perceived to be a context of ↓ level need. They also show that the agency most likely to be involved is a healthcare agency. Common professional failings include: inadequate sharing of information (➔ Teamwork p. 58); poor assessment processes (➔ Assessment of children, young people, and families p. 156); lack of clarity about roles and responsibilities; poor recording of information (➔ Record keeping p. 86); and failure to keep the child in focus.

National frameworks: Working Together to Safeguard Children (England)

This document[48] sets out the parameters of good practice: be alert to indicators of abuse or neglect; be alert to the risks that individuals may pose to children; and share information that relates to concerns about child safety and welfare.

> ⚠ Familiarize yourself with guidelines and procedures that detail exactly what individuals and agencies must do when abuse is suspected: government guidance; and local child protection procedures agreed through the local safeguarding partners (the LA, a CCG for the area, and the chief officer of police or Area Child Protection Committee).

Sources of advice and support

Every health provider has to have a safeguarding team, named doctor, and nurse to offer advice and support to employees with regard to children about whom they have concerns.

Every Local Safeguarding Children Board (LSCB)/LA area has a designated doctor and nurse to give advice and support regarding children at risk of harm, and to support commissioning services.

⚠ Find out the names of the nurse and designated doctor for child protection, and how to contact them.

What nurses should do in cases where abuse is suspected

First, discuss the case with senior colleagues as appropriate. Second, decide whether the child needs immediate protection and/or urgent medical attention.

If protection and/or medical attention required

Contact LA children's social care service (➲ Social services p. 30) or the police, and relevant medical service. Discuss concern with parent/carer and child, unless it is unsafe to do so (be aware that in some cases it could ↑ risk to child). Record all relevant information and action taken.

If protection and/or medical attention not required

Discuss concern with parent/carer. Listen carefully to the child. Consult colleagues who know the child/family, such as social worker, GP (➲ General practice p. 18), health visitor (➲ Health visiting p. 46), or teacher (➲ Working in schools p. 44). There may be earlier or ongoing concerns. Record suspicions and evidence that supports them. Decide whether to refer to social services. Seek advice, if necessary, from one of the named or designated child protection nurses or doctors or another experienced colleague.

Referral to children's social care

LA children's social care have the statutory responsibility for making enquiries into child protection referrals and co-ordinating the inter-agency response.

When making a referral to social services

Discuss concerns with social worker and confirm referral in writing within 48hrs. Record whether parent has been informed and, if not, why not. Follow up outcome to referral to establish that it has been understood and responded to appropriately.

Reference

48. HM Government (2018) Working together to safeguard children: March 2018. A guide to inter-agency working to safeguard and promote the welfare of children. London: Crown Publications. Available at: https://www.gov.uk/government/publications/working-together-to-safeguard-children--2

Further information

Centre for Excellence for Looked-After Children in Scotland (*Protecting children*). Available at: ℅ https://www.celcis.org/our-work/protecting-children/

Department of Health Northern Ireland (*Child protection*). Available at: ℅ https://www.health-ni.gov.uk/topics/social-services/child-protection#toc-9

NSPCC (*Child protection in the UK*). Available at: ℅ https://www.nspcc.org.uk/preventing-abuse/child-protection-system/

Scottish Government (*Child protection*). Available at: ℅ https://www.gov.scot/policies/child-protection/

Welsh Government (*Safeguarding*). Available at: ℅ https://gov.wales/topics/health/socialcare/safeguarding/?lang=en

Identifying the child in need of protection

Sustained abuse or neglect can have a major impact on all aspects of a child's health, well-being, and development (⊃ Safeguarding children p. 248). Assessment should be made within the Child Assessment Framework (⊃ Assessment of children, young people, and families p. 156).

Factors that increase risk of abuse or neglect

If parent/carer has a history of any of the following:
- Drug and/or alcohol misuse (⊃ Substance use p. 476; ⊃ Alcohol p. 360)
- Domestic violence (⊃ Domestic violence p. 450)
- Mental health problems (⊃ People with anxiety and depression p. 478; ⊃ People with psychosis p. 486; ⊃ People with bipolar affective disorder p. 482; ⊃ Post-traumatic stress disorder p. 490)
- Learning difficulties (⊃ People with learning disabilities p. 456)
- Abuse in their own childhood

The risk is further increased if:
- Poor attachment to child, e.g. intolerant and/or indifferent
- Non-compliance, e.g. parent denies there is a problem and/or refuses to engage with professional network

And if the child is:
- Premature or low birthweight infant (⊃ Pre-term infants p. 176)
- A multiple birth (e.g. twins) or <18mths between siblings (⊃ Twins and multiple births p. 180)
- A child with a disability (⊃ Children with complex health needs and disabilities p. 238)
- Born unwanted and/or unplanned
- A child not attending school
- A looked-after child (⊃ Looked-after children p. 254)

Evidence of harm

Harm means ill-treatment or the impairment of health or development. Ill-treatment is classified under four categories of abuse and neglect. Evidence that a child is being harmed is obtained by observation, allegation, and/or disclosure.

Observation of signs in child

Unexplained bruising or bruising in unusual places. Injuries with inconsistent explanations or inappropriate to developmental age. Appears afraid, quiet, withdrawn. Appears constantly tired, hungry, or dirty.

Observation of perpetrator

Acting aggressively, violently, or in a sexual manner to child or young person.

Allegation

From a child or another person.

Disclosure

From a child or someone who says they are harming a child.

Ill-treatment

Physical abuse

Physical abuse is violence directed towards children, including hitting, shaking, suffocating, burning (➲ Burns and scalds p. 816), and poisoning (➲ Poisoning and overdoses p. 822). Points to remember: the younger the child, the ↑ risk from physical abuse; sometimes minor injuries signal something more serious; and domestic violence and child abuse coexist in most cases and can begin in pregnancy (➲ Pregnancy p. 424).

Child sexual abuse

Child sexual abuse is sexual molestation of children by adults or older children. It involves forcing or enticing a child or young person to take part in activities that lead to the sexual arousal of the perpetrator. Points to remember: it is an abuse of power that often relates to age difference; perpetrator is usually known to the child, and probably a family member; and most perpetrators deny abuse and refuse treatment programmes.

Emotional abuse

Emotional abuse is a relationship between a child and parent that is characterized by harmful interactions that convey to the child that they are worthless or unloved. Integral to all forms of abuse and neglect, but also occurs alone. Points to remember: under-reported, despite easily identifiable negative parent/child interactions; and sustained abuse has impact on long-term mental health (➲ Child and adolescent mental health p. 246), self-esteem, and behaviour (➲ Behavioural disorders in children p. 326).

Neglect

Neglect is the persistent failure to meet a child's basic physical and emotional needs, and the failure to provide or respond to the changing needs of a growing child. Points to remember: neglect is the most prevalent form of child maltreatment; neglect is usually chronic and rarely a single incident; and mental health problems, learning difficulties, and substance misuse are common in the histories of the parent.

Further information

ChildLine (*Abuse and safety.*) Available at: ℘ https://www.childline.org.uk/info-advice/bullying-abuse-safety/abuse-safety/

HM Government (*What to do if you're worried a child is being abused Advice for practitioners*). Available at: ℘ https://assets.publishing.service.gov.uk/government/uploads/system/uploads/attachment_data/file/419604/What_to_do_if_you_re_worried_a_child_is_being_abused.pdf

NSPCC (*Preventing abuse*). Available at: ℘ https://www.nspcc.org.uk/preventing-abuse/

Child protection processes

All countries have legislation and agreed frameworks for these processes. Following a referral reporting a concern about a child, social services will carry out an initial enquiry and assessment, and decide whether to hold a child protection conference (➲ Safeguarding children p. 248; ➲ Identifying the child in need of protection p. 250).

Child protection conference

Convened by LA children's social care, it is a confidential meeting of parents, social workers, health and other professionals involved with the family, and the police (➲ Teamwork p. 58). Its purpose is:

• To share information and assess risk to the child.
• To decide whether to place child's name on the child protection register. If the decision is 'yes', then a review conference has to be held within 6mths.
• To draw up a protection plan to safeguard the child, including: support and services to be provided to the child and family; changes required to ↓ risk; and how social services will monitor the child's welfare.

Information sharing and confidentiality

Sharing confidential information (➲ Confidentiality p. 89) is essential. In many cases, it is only when information is shared that it becomes clear that a child is at risk. Points to remember:

• Disclose information relevant to safeguarding the child. This will be about: health and development of a child, and her/his exposure to harm; parent/carer who is unable to care adequately for a child; and other individuals who may present a risk to the child.
• Share information on a 'need-to-know' basis.
• If in doubt, consult one of the named or designated nurses or other experienced colleague.

Further information

Department of Health Northern Ireland (*Child protection*). Available at: ℘: www.dhsspsni.gov.uk/index/hss/child_care/child_protection.htm

HM Government (2018) Working together to safeguard children: March 2018. A guide to inter-agency working to safeguard and promote the welfare of children. London: Crown Publications. Available at: ℘ https://www.gov.uk/government/publications/working-together-to-safeguard-children--2

NSPCC (*Recognising and responding to abuse*). Available at: ℘ https://learning.nspcc.org.uk/child-abuse-and-neglect/recognising-and-responding-to-abuse/

Scottish Government (*Child protection*). Available at: ℘ https://www.gov.scot/policies/child-protection/

Welsh Government (*Safeguarding*). Available at: ℘ https://gov.wales/topics/health/socialcare/safeguarding/?lang=en

Looked-after children

Children in the care of LAs are described as 'looked-after children'. They live in a variety of settings including foster care, residential care homes, kinship care, residential school, or young offender units. Many will have become looked after as a result of abuse or neglect, whilst others are looked after because of family dysfunction or distress (➔ Safeguarding children p. 248; ➔ Child protection processes p. 252). They are among the most vulnerable children in the UK: ↑ number have mental health problems (➔ Child and adolescent mental health p. 246) and ↑ number are parents by 20yrs.

The aim is to support children back into the care of families where possible. About 40% return home within 6mths, but 60% are looked after for longer. Recent substantial criticism that public authorities are failing these children. Current policy aims to: improve the stability of placements and continuity of at least one carer; ↑ adoption orders and special guardianship orders; improve educational attainments of those looked after >6mths; and improve health and access to health care, particularly Child and Adolescent Mental Health Services.

Health needs

Many of these children have ↑ health needs in comparison to those with families from comparable socioeconomic backgrounds. These needs may arise from: living in families affected by alcohol (➔ Alcohol p. 360), domestic violence (➔ Domestic violence p. 450), or drugs (➔ Substance use p. 476); a disability or special needs; having a highly mobile family; poorer access to universal services, such as dental services (➔ Dental health in older children p. 226; ➔ Development and care of teeth for young children p. 196), immunizations (➔ Childhood immunizations p. 164), routine child health surveillance, and health promotion; and grief and loss through experience of leaving family and being placed in care.

Improving healthcare

The LA should notify the relevant health organization of each child moving in or leaving area. Each area has a designated community paediatrician(s) and designated nurse(s) for looked-after children. They are responsible for ensuring:

- A holistic health assessment (including health promotion) by a doctor as soon as practicable after a child starts to be looked after (➔ Assessment of children, young people. and families p. 156).
- The health assessment is recorded, and a health plan is included in the care plan for the child; child and/or carer holds a personal health record (➔ Client- and patient-held records p. 90).
- Subsequent health reviews are undertaken by nurse: 2–5yrs, at least every 6mths; >5yrs, at least annually.
- Children/carers are able to access universal health (e.g. GP (➔ General practice p. 18)), and health promotion services and records are 'fast tracked' if moving placement.

All young people leaving care should have access to a leaving care health service, which includes access to a GP and dental services. Issues of particular risk in this group, i.e. unsafe sex (➲ Sexual health: general issues p. 760), self-harming (➲ Suicidal intent and deliberate self-harm p. 494), and substance and alcohol misuse, are addressed for each young person. Each health professional who comes into contact with children or young people in this situation is expected to consider the widest range of health and health promotion needs of the young person.

Adoption

In the UK, up to 5,000 children are waiting for permanent new families at any time. Fostering is a temporary arrangement, although sometimes it may be the plan until the child grows up. An adoption order severs all legal ties with the birth family and confers parental rights and responsibilities onto the new adoptive family (can be married, single, unmarried couple of any sexuality). Adoption is through an adoption agency, usually social services, and also voluntary agencies (e.g. Barnardos). Applicants are screened for suitability (including requesting information from GP) and matched to children (via the Adoption Register in England and Wales). Proposed matches are presented to an adoption panel, which decides whether to proceed with the placement. The child moves to live with new parent/s after planned period of introductions, with the support of a social worker. Court cannot make an adoption order until the child has lived with adopters for ≥13wks (19wks if newborn). A number of organizations provide support for new adoptive parents and children (e.g. British Association of Fostering and Adoption). All adopted children receive the usual child health promotion programme and any additional services in response to particular needs. Note: international adoption has different regulations.[49]

References

49. Intercountry Adoption Centre (2019). *Intercountry adoption*. Available at: http://www.icacentre.org.uk/

Further information

CoramBAAF (*Fostering and adoption*). Available at: ℘ https://corambaaf.org.uk/fostering-adoption
Department of Education (*Looked after children*). Available at: ℘ https://www.gov.uk/topic/schools-colleges-childrens-services/looked-after-children
NICE (2015) *Looked after children and young people [PH28]*. Available at: https://www.nice.org.uk/guidance/PH28
NSPCC (*Looked after children*). Available at: ℘ https://learning.nspcc.org.uk/children-and-families-at-risk/looked-after-children/

Child and adolescent health

Birth injuries 258
Cleft lip and palate 259
Congenital heart defects 260
Congenital impairments 262
Bone and joint problems 264
Deafness in children 268
Genetic problems 270
Neural tube defects 274
The sick baby and child 276
Sudden infant death syndrome 278
Febrile convulsions and epilepsy 280
Vomiting and diarrhoea in children 282
Eczema in childhood 284
Constipation and encopresis 286
Infections in children 288
Infectious diseases in childhood 290
Insects and infestations 294
Nocturnal enuresis 296
Growth disorders 298
Acne vulgaris 300
Overweight children and adolescents 302
Endocrine problems 304
Asthma in children 306
Sickle cell disorders 308
Thalassaemia 312
Cancer in childhood 314
Cystic fibrosis 318
Cerebral palsy 320
Autistic spectrum disorder 322
Behavioural disorders in children 326
Depressive behaviours 328
Emotional problems in children 330

Birth injuries

Babies may be injured at birth if they are too large for the pelvic outlet or malpositioned. Rarer are injuries from assisted vaginal deliveries (e.g. using forceps) (➔ Complicated labour p. 436).

Soft-tissue injuries

- Bruising and swelling to face after face delivery, or to buttocks after breech delivery—resolves in a few days
- Caput succedaneum: bruising and oedema of the presenting part of the body—resolves in a few days
- Cephalhaematoma: rare haemorrhage beneath the periosteum—resolves over a few weeks

Parents need reassurance as their child can look very alarming.

Nerve injuries

Nerve injuries can occur during breech deliveries or with shoulder dystocia (shoulder trapped behind pelvic bone) during birth. Damage is to cervical nerve roots in the brachial plexus. Palsy (loss of control of muscles) according to which cervical nerve damaged. Most common types:

- Erb's palsy: upper nerve root injury; one arm abducted, rotated in and fingers flexed
- Klumpke's palsy: lower nerve root injury causing hand weakness;fingers do not move
- Complete brachial plexus palsy: entire arm is paralysed, with sensory loss
- Facial palsy: causes facial asymmetry

Most offered paediatric physiotherapy and followed up by paediatrician. Most resolve within a few weeks. In some rare cases, injury may not resolve, and referred to paediatric neurologist. Nerve or tendon release surgery may be considered. Parents need support and reassurance.

Bone injuries

- Clavicle fracture: occurs in some births from shoulder dystocia—heals rapidly without treatment
- Humerus or femur fractures: can occur in breech deliveries—requires immobilization and heals rapidly (parents will need support, reassurance, and advice on care of baby while limb is immobilized)

Related topics

➔ New birth visits p. 174; ➔ New babies p. 178; ➔ Bone and joint problems p. 264

Cleft lip and palate

Cleft lip is the failure of fusion of fronto-nasal and maxillary processes. Cleft palate is the failure of fusion of palatine processes. Affects about 1 per 700 children. Most is inherited (➲ Congenital impairments p. 262), but may be part of a syndrome. Usually referred to regional specialist cleft lip and palate multidisciplinary team (➲ Teamwork p. 58) at diagnosis.

Surgical repair

- Lip: surgical repair may be performed in first weeks or first 2–3mths
- Palate: usually repaired by 1yr

Feeding

Babies may have difficulty combining reflex actions, creating vacuum, and correctly positioning tongue. Regional team provides specialist advice. Parents need lots of reassurance as milk and foods may pass into nose and cause sneezing.

Babies with cleft lip

- Can breastfeed but may need to try different positions and holding breast differently (➲ Breastfeeding p. 182)
- If bottle fed, may need larger hole in soft teat (➲ Bottle feeding p. 186)
- May be fed with cup and spoon after repair and until healed

Babies with cleft lip and palate

- May be given an orthodontic plate to help feeding
- Many can breastfeed—if breast held in area where palate is complete, will be well latched-on, with good supply of milk
- Some babies may need nasogastric tubes to feed, or be fed by cup and spoon
- After repair, depends on age, but may be asked to use cup and spoon rather than bottle

Other issues

Specialist team will monitor speech development (➲ Speech and language acquisition p. 218) and provide therapy if any difficulties. Hearing is also monitored as middle-ear infections common (➲ Hearing screening p. 163). If the gum is affected by the cleft, then teeth may also be missing, twisted, or be misaligned (➲ Development and care of teeth for young children p. 196). Orthodontic referral may be required when adult teeth coming in.

Further information

Cleft Lip and Palate Association (CLAPA) (*What is cleft lip and palate?*). Available at: M https://www.clapa.com/what-is-cleft-lip-palate/

Congenital heart defects

Congenital heart defects affect ~1 in 133 births (◆ Congenital impairments p. 262; ◆ Children with complex health needs and disabilities p. 238). ↑ defects detected at antenatal ultrasound (◆ Antenatal care and screening p. 426). ↑ diagnosed by non-invasive echocardiography. ↑ number of defects can be treated non-invasively. The most common congenital heart defects are as follows.

Non-cyanotic
- Ventriculoseptal defect (VSD)—a hole connects the two ventricles
- Patent ductus arteriosus—ductus arteriosus fails to close after birth
- Pulmonary valve stenosis
- Atrial septal defect—a hole connects the two atria
- Coarctation of the aorta—localized narrowing of the descending aorta
- Aortic valve stenosis

Cyanotic
- Tetralogy of Fallot—large VSD and pulmonary stenosis
- Transposition of the aorta and pulmonary artery

Signs and symptoms
- Heart murmur, but only 54% of murmurs heard at neonatal examination are due to cardiac defects; most are innocent
- Heart failure includes: breathlessness, particularly when crying/feeding; cyanosis; ↑ respiratory and pulse rates; failure to thrive or weight ↑ due to fluid retention; recurrent chest infection; heart and/or liver enlargement; and cool peripheries

Treatment
Refer for specialist paediatric and/or cardiology opinion. Specialist treatment of valve lesions depends on the size. Most congenital cardiac lesions require medical treatment plus surgery. May have O$_2$ therapy at home.

Care management issues
Feeding
Slow feeding is a common problem. Long feeds ↑ tiredness in babies and mothers. Vomiting after feeds often a problem. Encourage ↓ amount given at any one time, whilst ↑ frequency. If bottle fed (◆ Bottle feeding p. 186), then may need to experiment with teats and bottles to aid feeding. Night feeds often take longer than other babies. Weight gain may also be a problem. Usually seen by dietitian in specialist team. May need ↑ calorie formula feed (in addition if breastfeeding (◆ Breastfeeding p. 182)). Introduction of ↑ calorie weaning foods often aids weight gain. Some babies at home may have nasogastric tube or percutaneous endoscopic gastronomy (PEG) (◆ Enteral and tube feeding p. 594).

Immunization

Usual programme (including annual flu vaccine from the age of 6mths) (→ Childhood immunization p. 164; → Childhood immunization schedule UK p. 166). Vaccinations against pneumonia and bronchiolitis may also be recommended by cardiologist.

General

Most children recover quickly after surgery and are back at nursery, early years setting, or school within a month. Exercise tolerance varies and each child is encouraged to find own limits. Antibiotic prophylaxis for dental and surgical procedures given as ↑ risk of developing bacterial endocarditis. Many adolescents and adults require revision of surgery performed in early life (e.g. replacement of artificial valves).

Further information

British Heart Foundation (*Congenital heart disease*). Available at: ℬ https://www.bhf.org.uk/informationsupport/conditions/congenital-heart-disease

Children's Heart Federation (*Information service*). Available at: ℬ http://www.chfed.org.uk/how-we-help/information-service/

Congenital impairments

Congenital impairments are present in approximately 1 in 49 of live births and stillbirths[1] (➋ UK health profile p. 2). Causes may be genetic, chromosomal, teratogenic (viral, bacterial, medications, alcohol (➋ Alcohol p. 360), drugs (➋ Substance use p. 476)), multiple other causes, or unknown. Individual child and family needs should be identified and addressed accordingly (➋ Assessment of children, young people, and families p. 156; ➋ Children with complex health needs and disabilities p. 238).

Congenital adrenal hyperplasia

Congenital adrenal hyperplasia is caused by autosomal recessive disorders. Cortisol deficiencies cause overproduction of adrenal androgens. Results in: virilization of external genitalia of girls, for which reconstructive surgery may be considered; penis enlargement and precocious puberty in some boys (➋ Puberty and adolescence p. 228); and adrenal crisis in some male babies within first 3wks requiring emergency treatment. All require long-term glucocorticoid therapy and monitoring of growth by specialists.

Congenital infections

Cytomegalovirus (CMV)

Affects 5 per 1,000 births. 90% of affected children develop normally. The remainder have neurological problems, e.g. cerebral palsy (➋ Cerebral palsy p. 320), epilepsy (➋ Febrile convulsions and epilepsy p. 280), and developmental delay.

Rubella

Usually intrauterine <18wks' gestation from infected mother (➋ Pregnancy p. 424). Preventable. May cause deafness (➋ Deafness in children p. 268), congenital heart defects (➋ Congenital heart defects p. 260), cataracts, and other problems.

Toxoplasmosis

0.1 per 1,000 births. About 10% of affected have problems, usually neurological (e.g. hydrocephalus and retinopathy).

Urogenital problems

Babies with ambiguous genitalia

Require full biochemical and sometimes surgical (laparoscopic) investigation prior to assigning sex. Decision and time to correctly assign often causes additional distress to parents, but important to consider as has potential lifelong social, psychological, medical, and legal consequences. Caused by chromosomal or adrenal problems. Parents, and later the child, need psychological support as well as information at different stages. Surgery may be required at different stages of development, as well as long-term glucocorticoid therapy and hormone therapy.

Male genitourinary problems

- Hypospadias: urethral opening on the underside of the penis. 1 in 300 boys. Corrected surgically <2yrs.
- Undescended testes: occurs in 5% full-term boys. Most descend by 3mths; if not, corrected surgically (orchidopexy) at about 2yrs.

Urological malformations

Increasingly diagnosed by antenatal ultrasound scan (USS). Horseshoe kidney or double elements in the system are common and in themselves are not a problem. However, predispose to reflux and recurrent urinary tract infections (UTIs) and cause renal damage. Often prophylactic antibiotics started at birth to prevent renal damage. USS again within first 6wks; some malformations may have resolved. Prophylactic antibiotics continue if malformation remains. Obstructions such as posterior urethral valve require surgical intervention.

Related topics

→ Antenatal care and screening p. 426

Reference

1. PHE (2018) National Congenital Anomaly and Rare Disease Registration Service statistics: 2016 summary report. Available at: https://www.gov.uk/government/publications/ncardrs-congenital-anomaly-annual-data/national-congenital-anomaly-and-rare-disease-registration-service-statistics-2016-summary-report

Further Information

Great Ormond Street Hospital (*Medical conditions*). Available at: ℬ https://www.gosh.nhs.uk/medical-information/search-medical-conditions

Great Ormond Street Hospital (*Congenital adrenal hyperplasia*). Available at: ℬ https://www.gosh.nhs.uk/conditions-and-treatments/conditions-we-treat/congenital-adrenal-hyperplasia-cah

Great Ormond Street Hospital (*Hypospadias*) Available at: ℬ https://www.gosh.nhs.uk/conditions-and-treatments/conditions-we-treat/hypospadias

NICE (*Undescended testes*). Available at: ℬ https://cks.nice.org.uk/undescended-testes

WHO (*Congenital anomalies*). Available at: ℬ https://www.who.int/news-room/fact-sheets/detail/congenital-anomalies

Bone and joint problems

Variations of normal posture

These are common and most resolve without any treatment, but any that are severe, painful, or asymmetrical are referred for specialist opinion.

Bow legs (genu varum)

Bowing of tibiae. Common up to age 3yrs and resolves spontaneously. Other causes include rickets (usually caused by vitamin D and calcium deficiency and treatable with oral supplements or injections).

Knock knees

Seen in children 2–7yrs. Usually resolves spontaneously.

Flat feet (pes planum)

All babies and toddlers have flat feet. The arch develops after 2–3yrs of walking. Persistent flat feet may be familial or due to joint laxity. If painful, referred for specialist advice.

Disorders of the hip, knee, and foot

Developmental dysplasia of the hip

Previously known as congenital dislocation of the hip. Describes a spectrum of disorders from dysplasia through to dislocation of the hip. One or two per 1,000 live births. May be detected at routine neonatal and 6-wk screening but if not, it should be suspected if an infant seems unwilling to take weight on leg or does not learn to walk. Referred for specialist opinion. Treatment depends on when the condition is diagnosed: young babies, with splinting (where the hips are held in partial abduction using slings under each thigh); and older babies and toddlers, with surgery.

Irritable hip

Most common cause of acute hip pain in 2–12yrs. Cause is unknown. Usually resolves in 7 days.

Slipped capital femoral epiphysis

Affects older children. A displacement of the femoral head epiphysis causes pain and difficulty walking. Treatment is surgical. It is more common in overweight children (➔ Overweight children and adolescents p. 302).

Talipes (clubfoot)

This is treated with the Ponseti method, involving recurrent manipulation of the foot into splints over a period of perhaps 8wks, with then a possible operation on the Achilles tendon.

Disorders of the back and spine

Back pain

Uncommon pre-adolescence. A young child with back pain should be medically assessed. In adolescents, common cause is muscle spasm, often from sports-related injuries and poor posture.

Scoliosis

Lateral curvature of the spine, which may lead to pain and limitation of activities, and respiratory restriction. Causes can be idiopathic, congenital (➲ Congenital impairments p. 262) or 2° to another disorder. Early-onset idiopathic scoliosis usually resolves. Late-onset idiopathic scoliosis (most common) mainly affects ♀ at pubertal growth spurt (➲ Puberty and adolescence p. 228). Treatment of severe scoliosis is with spinal braces and sometimes surgery.

Torticollis (wry neck)

Sudden restriction of head turning due to a mobile nodule in muscle. Resolves in 2–6mths.

Painful limbs

Growing pains

Also known as nocturnal idiopathic pain. Common in preschool children. Children with hypermobility in joints often also complain of pain in limbs. Cause unknown. Often wakes child at night but settles with massage and comforting.

Osteomyelitis

Painful bone infection. Usually caused by bacterial infection. Often affects the long bones of the arms and legs. Needs early treatment with antibiotics (➲ Sepsis p. 826).

Arthritis

Rare in children. Presents with well-localized joint pains +/- hot, tender, swollen joints. Two types: septic arthritis and juvenile idiopathic arthritis.

Septic arthritis is a serious infection of the joint space that can lead to bone destruction. Most common <2yrs. The child is usually systemically unwell and the joint may be swollen, hot, and tender. Often in the hip and picked up when changing nappies. ⚠ Requires urgent medical assessment, admission to hospital, and IV antibiotics.

Juvenile idiopathic (chronic) arthritis (JIA) is a group of conditions which last >6wks. It is an autoimmune condition in which the immune system attacks the body's own tissues. There are several different types. Oligoarticular JIA is the most common type. Treatment can include medication, physiotherapy, and occupational therapy. Child may be identified as having special needs according to severity and effect.

Osteogenesis imperfecta

Autosomal dominant inheritance. A group of disorders of collagen metabolism resulting in fragile bones which fracture easily. Other features include lax joints, thin skin, blue sclerae, hypoplastic teeth, and deafness (➲ Deafness in children p. 268). Severe forms present with fractures at birth (many stillborn). Less severe cases present later and may be mistaken for non-accidental injury. Management is supportive, with treatment of fractures as they occur. Child may be identified as having special needs according to severity and effect.

Osteopetrosis
Marble bone disease, in which bones are dense but brittle. Rare. Autosomal dominant form presents in childhood with fractures, osteomyelitis +/− facial paralysis. Recessive form is more severe, causing bone marrow failure (bone marrow transplantation can be curative) and death.

Marfan's disease
Autosomal dominant disorder of connective tissue associated with altered body proportions, tall stature, hyper-extensible joints, long thin digits, scoliosis, cardiovascular problems, and dislocation of the eye lenses and severe myopia.

Related topics
→ Bone and connective tissue disorders p. 738

Further information
Arthritis Research UK (*Juvenile idiopathic arthritis*). Available at: ⅍ https://www.arthritisresearchuk.org/arthritis-information/young-people/juvenile-idiopathic-arthritis.aspx
Brittle Bone Society (*What is osteogenesis imperfecta?*). Available at: ⅍ https://brittlebone.org/what-is-oi/
Great Ormond Street Hospital (*Factsheets*). Available at: ⅍ www.gosh.nhs.uk/medical-information-0
Scoliosis Association (UK) (*Scoliosis information*). Available at: ⅍ https://www.sauk.org.uk/scoliosis-information/scoliosis-information
Steps (*Hip dysplasia*). Available at: ⅍ https://www.steps-charity.org.uk/conditions/hip-dysplasia-ddh/

Deafness in children

Deafness

The prevalence of confirmed childhood hearing impairment of >40 decibel hearing loss (Db HL) in the UK is 1.3 children per 1,000 live births at age of 5yrs.

Causes

Prenatal
- 50% genetic
- Infections in pregnancy, e.g. cytomegalovirus, measles, toxoplasmosis (● Pregnancy p. 424)
- Ototoxic medications in pregnancy (● Prescribing for special groups p. 138)

Postnatal
- Prematurity, sequelae of prematurity (e.g. jaundice) (● Pre-term infants p. 176)
- Infections, e.g. measles, meningitis, mumps (● Infections in children p. 288)
- Ototoxic medications for other infections

Types

- Conductive: also known as glue ear; sound cannot pass through outer and middle ear to cochlea and auditory nerve
- Sensorineural: fault in inner ear of auditory nerve
- Mixed: e.g. problem with glue ear and auditory nerve

Management

Hearing loss/deafness is identified through screening (● Hearing screening p. 163). Children are referred to specialists, including audiology, according to local care pathways and protocols. As in all situations where special needs are identified, the parents and child need support, services, and information from a multidisciplinary team (● Teamwork p. 58). Very few deaf children have no useful hearing and most children can hear some sounds at certain frequencies and volume, so with the use of hearing aids or implants they may be able to hear more sounds. Management depends on type, severity of loss, and impact.

Hearing aids

Acoustic aids come in a range of shapes and sizes and may be analogue or digital. Some children may use radio transmitter systems to ↓ background noise (e.g. in classrooms). When a child gains no benefit from acoustic aids, a cochlear implant may be considered. The electrodes are inserted surgically and directly stimulate the auditory nerve.

Communication

Deaf children, like hearing children, need lots of attention and interaction to learn and develop communication skills. Special needs teams advise on learning additional communication methods, e.g. oral–auditory systems, lip reading, sign bilingualism, British Sign Language, and total communication (➔ Adults and children with additional communication needs p. 122).

Further information

National Deaf Children's Society (*First diagnosis*) Available at: ℬ https://www.ndcs.org.uk/information-and-support/first-diagnosis/

PHE (*NHS newborn hearing screening programme*) Available at: ℬ https://www.gov.uk/topic/population-screening-programmes/newborn-hearing

Genetic problems

There are 46 chromosomes: 22 are matching pairs with matching genes (autosomes); the remaining pair are sex chromosomes that may match (XX = ♀) or differ (XY = ♂). Parents of any child affected by a genetic problem are offered genetic counselling and prenatal diagnosis (➔ Antenatal care and screening p. 426), if available, for any subsequent pregnancies. Care, support, and treatment depends on specific problems of each child and family. The 1° healthcare team, specialist healthcare services, social services, community paediatric services, education services, and voluntary organizations are involved as necessary (➔ Teamwork p. 58; ➔ Children with complex health needs and disabilities p. 238). Each child and family should be reviewed regularly.

Down's syndrome

Trisomy 21 (an extra chromosome number 21). Commonest chromosomal abnormality affecting 1 in 600 births (➔ UK health profile p. 2). Incidence ↑ with maternal age at conception. Life expectancy is ↓, but ~ half live to 60yrs. Clinical features:
- Facial abnormalities: flat occiput, oval face; low-set eyes with prominent epicanthic folds
- Single palmar crease
- Hypotonia
- Developmental delay
- Congenital heart disease (➔ Congenital heart defects p. 260)

Edward's syndrome

Trisomy 18. Affecting 1 in 8,000 births. Life expectancy is ~10mths (♀ > ♂). Clinical features:
- Facial abnormalities: low-set malformed ears, receding chin, protruding eyes, cleft lip or palate (➔ Cleft lip and palate p. 259)
- A short sternum makes the nipples appear too widely separated
- Fingers cannot be extended and the index finger overlaps the third digit
- Developmental delay
- Umbilical or inguinal hernias
- Rocker-bottom feet
- Rigid baby with flexion of the limbs

Patau's syndrome

Trisomy 13. Affecting 1 in 7,500 births. 50% die <1mth. Usually fatal in the first year. Multiple abnormalities including:
- Small head and eyes
- Brain malformation
- Heart malformations
- Polycystic kidneys
- Cleft lip/palate
- Skeletal abnormalities, e.g. flexion contractures of hands +/− polydactyly with narrow fingernails

Cri du chat syndrome

Deletion of the short arm of chromosome 5 is the most common deletion syndrome. Affects 1 in 25,000–50,000 births. Life expectancy unpredictable. Presents with:

- Abnormal cry (cat-like)
- Microcephaly
- Developmental delay
- Marked epicanthic folds
- Moon-shaped face
- Alert expression

Sex chromosome abnormalities

Turner's syndrome

XO: deletion of one X chromosome. Affects 1 in 2,500 live births. Mosaicism may occur (XO, XX). Lifespan is normal. Clinical features:

- ♀ appearance
- Short stature (<130cm)
- Hyperconvex nails
- Wide carrying angle (cubitus valgus)
- Inverted nipples
- Broad chest
- Ptosis
- Nystagmus
- Webbed neck
- Coarctation of the aorta
- Left heart defects
- Lymphoedema of the legs
- Ovaries are rudimentary or absent

Specialist management: human growth hormone may be considered for short stature.

Klinefelter's syndrome

XXY or XXYY polysomy. Affects 1 in 1,000 live births. Life span is normal. Clinical features:

- ♂ appearance
- Often undetected until presentation with infertility in adult life
- May present at adolescence with psychopathy, ↓ libido, sparse facial hair, gynaecomastia, and small firm testes (➔ Puberty and adolescence p. 228)

Associations: hypothyroidism (➔ Thyroid p. 702), diabetes mellitus (➔ Endocrine problems p. 304), and asthma (➔ Asthma in children p. 306). Specialist management: androgens and surgery may be used for gynaecomastia.

Autosomal dominant inheritance

>1,000 diseases are known to be inherited in this way. Individually, they are rare and together account for <1% of all disease. Heterozygotes demonstrate the disease. One in two pregnancies of an affected individual will be affected; usually ♂ = ♀. Expression of the gene in a given individual may vary (e.g. Marfan's syndrome).

Autosomal recessive inheritance

>700 known diseases. Only manifest in the homozygote. Heterozygotes may be asymptomatic or show milder abnormalities. To develop severe disease, the affected gene must be inherited from both parents who must both be heterozygotes. The risk of an affected pregnancy (◆ Pregnancy p. 424) is one in four; usually ♂ = ♀. Affected individuals have unaffected children, unless their partner is a heterozygote.

Glycogen storage diseases

Incidence ~1 in 25,000. A group of hereditary disorders caused by enzyme deficiencies involved in glycogen synthesis or breakdown and characterized by deposition of abnormal amounts or types of glycogen in tissues. Inheritance is autosomal recessive for all forms except type VI, which follows an X-linked inheritance. Symptoms and age of onset vary considerably:
• Predominantly liver involvement (types I, III, IV, VI) → hepatomegaly, hypoglycaemia, metabolic acidosis
• Predominantly muscle involvement (types V, VII) → weakness, lethargy, poor feeding, heart failure

Treatment involves frequent, small, carbohydrate meals; allopurinol (to prevent renal urate stone formation and/or gout) +/− limiting anaerobic exercise. A high-protein diet is also helpful for some patients.

Other examples

Phenylketonuria (PKU) (◆ Endocrine problems p. 304); sickle cell (◆ Sickle cell disorders p. 308); thalassaemia (◆ Thalassaemia p. 312); and cystic fibrosis (◆ Cystic fibrosis p. 318).

Sex-linked disorders

Around ~100 are recognized. Most are recessively inherited from the mother and affect only ♂ offspring:
• A ♂ child of a heterozygote mother has a one in two chance of developing the disease.
• A ♀ child of a heterozygote mother has a one in two chance of carrying the disease.
• A ♀ child can only be affected by the disease if father has the disease and mother is a carrier, when she has a one in two chance of being affected and, if not affected, will be a carrier.

Fragile X syndrome

Affects 1 per 1,250 ♂ births and 1 per 2,500 ♀ births. Genetic abnormality carried on the X chromosome comprising:
• Low IQ (20–70)
• Large testes
• High forehead
• Large jaw
• Facial asymmetry
• Long ears
• Short temper (◆ Behavioural disorders in children p. 326)

Half of carrier ♀ have a normal IQ; half are affected. Fragile X syndrome should be considered in any child with developmental delay of unknown cause (◐ Child development 0–1 years p. 192).

There is some evidence that folic acid supplements ↓ hyperactive and disruptive behaviour tendencies in children with Fragile X. Antenatal testing is possible for future pregnancies.

Other examples

Haemophilia, Duchenne's muscular dystrophy

Polygenic inheritance

Familial trends of disease are commonly seen, but there is often no simple inheritance pattern. Usually due to the combination of genes inherited (polygenic inheritance).

Further information

Association for Glycogen Storage Disease (UK) (*What is GSD?*) Available at: ℘ https://agsd.org.uk/all-about-gsd/what-is-gsd/

Down's Syndrome Association (*For new parents*). Available at: ℘ https://www.downs-syndrome.org.uk/for-new-parents/

Fragile X Society (*Information about Fragile X*). Available at: ℘ https://www.fragilex.org.uk/fragilexsyndrome

Genetics Alliance UK (*Information*) Available at: ℘ https://www.geneticalliance.org.uk/information/

National Society for Phenylketonuria (*What is PKU?*). Available at: ℘ http://www.nspku.org/information/whatispku

Turner's Syndrome Support Society (*What Is TS?*). Available at: ℘ https://tss.org.uk/ts/what

Neural tube defects

The neural tube fuses in the first 28 days after conception (➔ Pregnancy p. 424). Incomplete fusion leads to four types of malformation. Prevention is through folic acid supplements in ♀ planning pregnancy and in first 12wks. Most defects are detected antenatally (➔ Antenatal care and screening p. 426). Prevalence of neural tube defect pregnancies in the past 20yrs was 1.28 per 1,000 total births of which 19% led to live births[2] (➔ UK health profile p. 2). Mothers who have had one fetus with a neural tube defect have a very ↑ risk of a second and should take ↑ dose of folic acid preconceptually and for first 12wks (➔ Preconceptual care p. 422).

Malformations

Anencephaly
Absence of most of cranium and skull. Stillborn or die shortly after birth. Antenatal termination offered if detected.

Encephalocoele
Midline skull defect, and brain and meninges herniated through. Corrected by surgery, but may be underlying malformations.

Spina bifida occulta
Failure of fusion of the vertebral arch. May be associated with skin lesion or tuft of hair. Usually asymptomatic.

Spina bifida
Two types:
- Meninges only protrude (meningocoele) and repaired surgically, with a good prognosis
- Myelomeningocoele (meninges and spinal cord) protrude. 80% of spina bifida cases. Surgically treated soon after birth. Problems can include hydrocephalus, scoliosis, paralysis of legs, sensory loss, neuropathic bladder and bowel. Hydrocephalus may be treated by endoscopic surgery or introduction of ventricular shunt to drain cerebrospinal fluid.

Long-term care for the parents and child with spina bifida

These children will be treated and managed by specialist multidisciplinary paediatric teams, with long-term follow-up as needs change with age and they become adults (➔ Children with complex health needs and disabilities p. 238). 1° care professionals provide long-term support and services as with all children with special needs. Need for emotional support, as well as physical care and information, important for parents and child (➔ Emotional problems in children p. 330).

Prevention of renal problems
Many parents are taught intermittent catheterization when child is very young, to ensure bladder emptying. More require support at school (➔ Working in schools p. 44).

Recognition of shunt blockage or infection problems

Onset may be gradual including headaches, irritability, vomiting, and general malaise (➲ The sick baby and child p. 276). Schools and other child carers need to be informed of signs. Needs assessment and attention at specialist centre, not local hospitals.

Reference

2. Morris, J., et al. (2016) Prevention of neural tube defects in the UK: a missed opportunity. *Archives of Disease in Childhood*, 101, 604–7

Further information

Shine (Providing specialist advice and support for spina bifida and hydrocephalus across England, Wales, and Northern Ireland). Available at: ℜ https://www.shinecharity.org.uk/
Spina Bifida Hydrocephalus (SBH) Scotland (*About SBH Scotland*). Available at: ℜ www.ssba.org.uk/

The sick baby and child

Minor illnesses (e.g. viral upper respiratory tract infections (URTIs)) are commonplace (➲ Infections in children p. 288). Most <5yrs have at least five viral URTIs a year (➲ Viral infections p. 720). Parents need to be re-assured, as well as informed, on how to manage minor illness and recognize signs for seeking medical attention. Ill babies and children become pale, list-less, and do not want to eat.

Advice for parents on managing minor illness

- Ensure plenty of fluids and wake babies to offer feed if sleeping a lot.
- Babies and children with fever should not be underdressed or over-wrapped.
- Use paediatric liquid paracetamol to address discomfort and keep temperature down.
- Use a digital thermometer in the armpit to monitor temperature (37°C normal).
- Keep monitoring how they look, their breathing, how much they are drinking, and how much fluid they lose (e.g. how often they vomit or have wet nappies).

⚠ Ill babies <6mths may deteriorate rapidly. Parents should be encouraged to seek medical advice promptly.

Advice on when to seek medical attention promptly for a baby

- ↑ pitched or weak cry
- Much less active or more floppy than usual
- Looks very pale all over
- Grunts with each breath or has dips in upper abdomen or between ribs when breathes
- Has not taken fluids in 8hrs; has fewer wet nappies than usual
- Repeated vomiting or vomits bile (green fluid)
- Passes blood in stool
- ↑ fever or sweating a lot
- Temperature >38°C for a baby <3mths or >39°C for a baby >3mths
- Fontanelles bulging or sunken
- Neck stiffness
- Spotty, purple-red rash anywhere on the body (may be meningitis)

Any practitioner consulted about a sick baby or child should refer for med-ical opinion if significant signs as listed.

Advice for parents on when to seek urgent medical attention

☏ 999 for an ambulance if:
- Stops breathing or goes blue
- Is unresponsive
- Has glazed eyes and does not focus on anything

- Cannot be woken
- Has a fit, even if recovers without medical attention (⊕ Febrile convulsions and epilepsy p. 280)

Any practitioner consulted or first on scene when a baby or child has these symptoms should request an ambulance is called; if in surgery or clinic, call for medical help, and then assess and commence CPR if required (⊕ Child basic life support p. 800).

Related topics

⊕ Sudden infant death syndrome p. 278; ⊕ Sepsis p. 826; ⊕ Cancer in childhood p. 314

Further information

NICE (*Fever in under 5s: assessment and initial management*). Available at: ℜ https://www.nice.org.uk/guidance/ng143

Sudden infant death syndrome

Sudden infant death syndrome (SIDS) is the sudden, unexpected death of an apparently well baby (also known as cot death). It affects <200 babies in UK each year (→ UK health profile p. 2). Most are <1yr, but the majority <3mths and more ♂ than ♀.

Risk factors

It is more common in socioeconomically deprived groups and associated with parental smoking. Risk factors include: ↓ birthweight, prematurity (→ Pre-term infants p. 176), young maternal age, higher parity, multiple births (→ Twins and multiple births p. 180), baby placed face down to sleep (→ Babies, children, and sleeping p. 200), and overheating.

Approaches after a death

All sudden, unexpected deaths are under the jurisdiction of the coroner and post-mortems have to be carried out. The police investigate if there is any suspicion it may have been unnatural (→ Death confirmation and certification p. 840). Protocols likely to include:

- Ambulance staff will attempt resuscitation and always take to A&E (→ Child basic life support p. 800).
- Immediate notification to coroner's office, GP (→ General practice p. 18), police team, and responsible paediatrician.
- Home visit by paediatrician and police within 24hrs to talk with parents and see the place where the child died.
- Paediatrician collates all medical records and liaises with children's social services (→ Social services p. 30), keeping in close contact with police and coroner—consideration of need for Section 47 strategy meeting (→ Child protection processes p. 252).
- Post-mortem carried out and findings reported to parents as soon as possible by pathologist, paediatrician, and/or GP.
- Case discussion, as per agreed guidelines, usually within 6wks, involving all professionals involved with family to scrutinize all aspects of death and contributory factors, and to plan ongoing support for family at that point and when they plan another pregnancy (→ Preconceptual care p. 422). Paediatrician and/or GP and/or health visitor (HV) (→ Health visiting p. 46) meet with parents to share conclusions and offer ongoing support.
- Child Death Overview Panel, under local child protection, subsequently reviews the case to identify any actions to prevent future child deaths.

Best practice guidance for health visitors and primary care nurses

If first to visit home when SIDS discovered: check that an ambulance has been called; if in doubt, resuscitation should always be attempted; ensure parents and siblings have support from friends and family; and spend time listening to the parents.

If you learn later that a baby has died, HV team should liaise with GP to avoid duplication and to visit as close to death as possible to: offer condolences and an opportunity for the parents to talk (→ Talking therapies

p. 472); provide information and support through post-mortem, coroner procedures, funeral (➲ Registration of births, marriages and deaths p. 842), and bereavement (➲ Coping with bereavement p. 574); discuss methods of suppression of lactation if the mother was breastfeeding (➲ Breastfeeding p. 182); ensure the parents have information from The Lullaby Trust and its befriender scheme; and confirm parents have been given (and content discussed) leaflets on post-mortems of a baby or child ordered by a coroner (consent not required (➲ Consent p. 82)) and retention of human tissue (consent required).

Check the following agencies have been informed of the baby's death: medical records departments of maternity/children's hospitals to avoid follow-up appointments being sent; child health records system to avoid letters being sent about immunizations and development checks; and the school, if there are school-age children in the family.

Later revisit, following funeral and follow-up to case discussion, to offer further time to talk and information about local bereavement services. Remember to talk about the deceased baby by name, at anniversaries, and during subsequent pregnancies and births. Offer information about local Care of Next Infant (CONI) Scheme.

Care of next infant

CONI is a programme available in many areas of the UK, where a local co-ordinator supports parents and professionals through subsequent pregnancies and first year of child's life. Programme includes additional visits from a HV, symptom diary, loan of apnoea monitors, basic life-support training, room thermometer, and additional advice.

Further information

Blair, P.S. & Pease, A. (2019) Prevention of sudden infant death syndrome (SIDs). In: Edmond, A. (ed.) *Health for all children* (5th edn). Oxford: Oxford University Press, pp. 181–9

Lullaby Trust (*Befriending scheme*). Available at: ℘ https://www.lullabytrust.org.uk/bereavement-support/how-we-can-support-you/befrienders/

Royal College of Pathologists/Royal College of Paediatrics and Child Health (*Sudden unexpected death in infancy and childhood. Multi-agency guidelines for care and investigation*). Available at: ℘ https://www.rcpath.org/uploads/assets/uploaded/af879a1b-1974-4692-9e002c20f09dc14c.pdf

Febrile convulsions and epilepsy

A seizure or fit is when there is a sudden disturbance of neurological function associated with an abnormal neuronal discharge. The child is referred for paediatric assessment.

Febrile convulsions

A febrile convulsion is defined as an event in infancy or childhood, usually occurring between 3mths and 5yrs of age, associated with fever but without evidence of intracranial infection or defined cause. Seizures with fever in children who have experienced a previous non-febrile seizure are excluded. Febrile seizures should be distinguished from epilepsy, which is characterized by recurrent non-febrile seizures.[3] Febrile convulsions present as tonic-clonic seizures, which are usually generalized with widespread muscle contraction, muscular rigidity, intense jerking movements, and accumulation of saliva in the mouth.[4] 1 in 50 children will have had a febrile convulsion by the time they are 5yrs old.[5]

Febrile seizures are defined as being 'simple' if lasting less than 10mins, resolve spontaneously, and do not recur in the next 24hrs. 'Complex' febrile seizures last more than 10mins and occur multiple times in 24hrs. The child may not regain full consciousness within 1hr after seizure has terminated and there is a brief period of paralysis after the seizure.[6] The risk of subsequent epilepsy is low.

Management

- Most children do not need hospital admission.
- Parent reassurance and education are important.
- The trend of using combination antipyretics is common in children; however this is not in line with NICE guidelines[7] and not proven to prevent febrile convulsions occurring.
- Parents should have education on how to safely manage a febrile convulsion, when to call for medical assistance, and appropriate follow-up.
- Those with recurrent or complex febrile convulsions are referred to paediatrician and are sometimes treated with anti-seizure medication.

Epilepsy

Epilepsy is recurrent seizures other than febrile convulsions, and not due to intracranial infection. Surgery is increasingly being used for some types of childhood epilepsy. Every child is reviewed at least annually by specialist paediatric services (➲ Seizures and epilepsy p. 740)

Support and education for parents and children

Epilepsy is a diagnosis that can cause great alarm and fear. Education is very important. Parents, children, and young people need clear information on:

- What to expect about living with this condition
- What to do during a seizure and how to brief other people (e.g. school staff (➲ Working in schools p. 44))
- Avoiding risks (e.g. swimming or cycling alone) but not being over-protective

- Importance of concordance with medication, particularly with teenagers (⊃ Medicine concordance and adherence p. 132)
- When drug withdrawal may be considered if fit-free
- How adolescent girls in particular may need specific advice around contraception (⊃ Contraception: general p. 400) and pregnancy (⊃ Pregnancy p. 424)

School health staff may have a particular role in helping educate school staff and other children about the condition.

References

3. BMJ Best Practice (2018) *Febrile seizure*. Available at: ℛ https://bestpractice.bmj.com/topics/en-gb/566#referencePop1

4. Innes, R. (2015) Understanding the pathophysiology behind febrile convulsions. *Nursing Children and Young People*, 27(2), 20–23

5. Great Ormond Street Hospital (2014) *Febrile convulsions*. Available at: https://www.gosh.nhs.uk/file/1716/download?token=1LZnVj67

6. Paul, S. (2015) Febrile convulsions in children. *Nursing Children and Young People*, 27(5), 14–15

7. NICE (2013) *Feverish illness in children*. Available at: https://www.nice.org.uk/donotdo/antipyretic-agents-do-not-prevent-febrile-convulsions-and-should-not-be-usedspecifically-for-this-purpose

Further information

Epilepsy Action (*Advice and information*). Available at: ℛ www.epilepsy.org.uk
Young Epilepsy (*About epilepsy*). Available at: ℛ www.youngepilepsy.org.uk/

Vomiting and diarrhoea in children

Most children experience vomiting in childhood. In most instances, the symptoms are mild and transient. Advice is given to parents on nursing a sick child and identifying signs as to when to seek medical advice (➲ The sick baby and child p. 276).

Posseting and regurgitation

Terms used to describe non-forceful return of milk. It usually resolves with the introduction of solid food and by 1yr.

Vomiting

The forceful ejection of gastric contents. It may be linked to specific events (e.g. travel sickness or a symptom of an infection (➲ Infections in children p. 288)).

Projectile vomiting

A symptom of pyloric stenosis: infantile hypertrophic pyloric stenosis usually develops in the first 3–6wks of life (rare after 12wks). Failure of the pyloric sphincter to relax and hypertrophy of the adjacent pyloric muscle. Requires paediatric assessment. If the condition is not treated, the baby will become dehydrated and not gain weight. Signs of dehydration include lethargy, less frequent wet nappies than normal, and possible sunken soft spot (fontanelle) on the top of the head.[8] Treated with surgery, with no long-term effects.

Vomiting and diarrhoea

Parent information important to determine nature and seriousness of problem, including:
- Nature and duration of symptoms
- Presence of green bile in vomit
- Presence of blood in the stool
- Other accompanying symptoms (e.g. fever)
- Contact with anyone else with similar symptoms
- History of recent foreign travel

Possible causes

Breastfed (➲ Breastfeeding p. 182) babies have loose, often explosive 'mustard grain' stools. Toddlers often have intermittent loose stools related to diet. Usually resolves by 5yrs. Gastrointestinal infection an important cause: child may have diarrhoea, vomiting, or combination of the two. Usually viral in origin (e.g. Norovirus) and common in winter (➲ Viral infections p. 720). Parents advised: to ensure adequate fluids to prevent dehydration; to eat normally, especially in cases of diarrhoea, or reintroduce as soon as possible; and, in cases of diarrhoea, to avoid giving fruit juice and carbonated drinks until diarrhoea has stopped. Seek medical attention if condition deteriorates or fails to improve.

Actions to prevent spread

Advice on preventing spread of gastrointestinal viruses:[9]

- All household members should wash hands frequently with liquid soap, in warm running water, and dry carefully; in particular, after going to the toilet or changing nappies, and before preparing, serving, or eating food (**➔** Home food safety and hygiene p. 352)
- Individual towels and no sharing infected child towels
- While child/infant has vomiting or diarrhoea, they should not attend any school or childcare facility until after 48hrs of last episode
- Children should not swim in swimming pools for 2wks after the last episode of diarrhoea

A vaccine for infants against the most common strains of rotavirus was introduced into the childhood immunization schedule in July 2013 (**➔** Childhood immunization p. 164; **➔** Childhood immunization schedule (UK) p. 166). Rotavirus is the most common cause of gastroenteritis among children and results in a significant number of young children being admitted to hospital each year.[10]

References

8. Great Ormond Street Hospital (2018) *Pyloric stenosis*. Available at: https://www.gosh.nhs.uk/conditions-and-treatments/conditions-we-treat/pyloric-stenosis
9. NICE (2009) *Management of acute diarrhoea and vomiting due to gastroenteritis in children under 5s [CG84]*. Available at: www.nice.org.uk/CG84
10. PHE (2013) *Rotavirus vaccination programme for infants*. Available at: https://www.gov.uk/government/collections/rotavirus-vaccination-progarmme-for-infants

Eczema in childhood

Atopic eczema is an inflammatory skin condition characterized by dry, itchy, red and inflamed skin. A genetically determined disorder with hypersensitivity to certain antigens such as pollen, house dust, household pets, so these patients often have asthma (→ Asthma in children p. 306) and hay fever as well (→ Allergies p. 694). It affects ~15% of the child population. Usually starts <6mths and 90% are in remission by 15yrs. <10% eczema is result of food and inhalant allergies. Can affect self-esteem in children and young people and affect the whole family (e.g. through infant sleep disturbance). Signs and symptoms include:

- Dry skin and itchiness
- Erythema, papules, vesicles
- Exudation, crusting, scaling, fissures
- Hyper- or hypopigmentation on some areas

In the acute stages, the skin is red and inflamed leading to vesicles, exudations, and crusting. In the chronic stages, the skin is dry and thickened from repeated scratching. Food allergies considered if reacting to certain foods and inhalant allergies if seasonal flare-ups.

Care and support

Eczema in a family can cause an increase of stress for other family members. Explain condition and overall good prognosis. Advise:

- Avoid the use of soaps and detergents on the skin
- Loose cotton clothing next to the skin
- Nails kept short to reduce damaging the skin if scratching
- Avoid and minimize irritants, e.g. dust mites (damp dusting, vacuuming the room and bed, changing the bedding regularly, wash soft toys frequently), and keep pets separate

Food allergies and eczema

Breastfeeding (→ Breastfeeding p. 182) should be encouraged in all babies <6mths. If food allergy is confirmed, then specialist advice about food adaptation should be obtained. Babies allergic to cow's milk should be referred to specialist allergy services and dietician for specialist testing and advice on dietary manipulation.

Specific treatment

Treatment aims to replace moisture loss on skin and provide a waterproof barrier to prevent further moisture loss and to protect skin. It aims to ↓ inflammation and relieve the intense itch. A stepped up and down approach is used according to severity of eczema. Referral to dermatologists if the eczema is not responding to treatment or severe presentations.

Emollients therapy

- Emollients help to repair the broken skin barrier by acting like an artificial fat, filling the cracks and allowing water to be retained by the skin cells.
- All soaps and detergents (and shampoo in <12yrs) should be replaced with emollient soap substitute and emollient bath oil. A daily soak for

at least 15mins hydrates the skin and provides a good base for the applications of emollients.
- Emollient creams and ointment should be applied three or four times a day, even when the skin is clear.

Topical corticosteroids

Topical steroids are effective to control inflammation and stop itchiness. Benefits of correct usage outweigh potential harms. A stepped approach to usage in response to severity of the eczema.

Wet wrapping

Wet wrapping used, but little evidence about its effectiveness. Aims to: re-hydrate and cool the skin; treat inflammation and promote skin healing; ↓ itching and protection against scratching; and ↑ comfort and ↑ sleep if applied before bed. The wet wrap technique involves the following: bath the child with emollients added; pat dry; apply generous amounts of emollient ointment; apply wet layer of tubifast garment and a dry layer. It should not be used if child's skin is infected. The community children's nurse, dermatology nurse, or health visitor can teach the parents how to apply the wet wrap garments.

Paste bandaging and other treatments

Paste bandages are used at night over steroids for licenification caused by rubbing or scratching. Contain emollient, coal tar, or calamine. Usually prescribed by dermatologists. Other treatments include:
- Antihistamines: to stop the itching and scratching. Short-term use in acute phases only. They are used an hour before bedtime, and daytime use should be avoided.
- Antibiotic therapy: to treat any 2° infection.
- Complementary therapies (➔ Complementary and alternative therapies p. 838) and diets: many parents want to try diets but should get nutritional advice before embarking on prolonged dietary changes.

Dermatologists treating severe eczema may prescribe topical calcineurin inhibitors, phototherapy, and oral steroids.

Related topics
➔ Eczema/dermatitis p. 684

Further information
National Eczema Society (*Information, advice and fact sheets*). Available at: ✍ www.eczema.org
NICE (*Management of atopic eczema in children from birth up to the age of 12 years*). Available at: ✍ www.nice.org.uk/guidance/cg57

Constipation and encopresis

Constipation

The painful passage of hard, infrequent stools. It is common in childhood, being prevalent in around 5–30% of the child population, with more ♂ than ♀.[11]

Babies show considerable variation in bowel habit according to diet (and if breastfed (◗ Breastfeeding p. 182)). Babies can change colour when passing a stool and look as if they are straining, even when passing a liquid stool. Changing from breastfeeding to formula feeds (◗ Bottle feeding p. 186) and/or solids results in a change of stool colour and consistency (◗ Weaning p. 188).

Causes of constipation in babies

May occur from hunger, over-strength feeds, and poor hydration. Rare causes include congenital abnormalities (e.g. spinal cord lesions, Hirschsprung's disease).

Causes in older children

- Poor or chaotic diet, inadequate fluid intake, and activity
- Failure to establish toileting routine during toilet training (◗ Toilet training p. 214)
- Resistance to potty training and desire to defecate into nappy
- Withholding faeces
- Behavioural or psychological problems (◗ Behavioural disorders in children p. 326), anxiety (◗ Child and adolescent mental health p. 246), and emotional upset (◗ Emotional problems in children p. 330)
- Developmental problems (learning disability (◗ People with learning disabilities p. 456), autism (◗ Autistic spectrum disorder p. 322))
- Fear of toilets, especially school toilets
- Sedentary lifestyle
- Vicious cycle created of ignoring sensation, hard stool, anal pain, deferring defecation as long as possible
- Severe loading, i.e. rectum and colon filled with faeces; may also have faecal incontinence or staining

Management of short-lived or mild constipation

Explanation of reasons for problems is important, as is engaging the child and parents in promotion of healthy diet, ↑ fluids, and ↑ exercise (◗ Growth and nutrition 5–11 years p. 222; ◗ Growth and nutrition 12–18 years p. 234; ◗ Food and the under-fives p. 212). Ascertain if afraid of the toilet; suggest ways to make toilet appealing. Advice to include:

- Ensure adequate fibre and fluid intake.
- Allow sufficient time and privacy for morning bowel emptying.
- Eat breakfast and try 20–30min later.
- Sit comfortably on toilet with feet supported (footstool may help).
- Avoid holding breath and straining.
- Push using abdominal muscles, and relax anus.
- Consider simple rewards (e.g. star chart).

- Avoid punishments/reprimands.
- Always respond to 'urge'; do not defer (arrange with teacher).

Laxative might be indicated; liaise with GP.

Management of severely constipated child

These children are referred for medical review. May have painful anal conditions, e.g. anal fissure.

Encopresis

Most children are continent of faeces by 2.5–3yrs. Faecal soiling during daytime after this age usually occurs when:

- Child has bowel control, but passes stool in socially unacceptable places. Cause is often emotional. Consider referral to CAMHS and/or via GP, as per local policy.
- Firm stool passed occasionally in the toilet, but usually in the pants; try a consistent training programme similar to those used for nocturnal enuresis.
- Soft stool causes child to soil themselves and smell of faeces; consider possibility of overflow faecal incontinence due to underlying chronic constipation.

Reference

11. NICE (2017) *Constipation in children and young people: diagnosis and management* [CG 99]. Available at: www.nice.org.uk/guidance/CG99

Further information

ERIC (*How to prevent constipation*). Available at: https://www.eric.org.uk/how-to-prevent-constipation-in-children

ERIC (*What is encopresis?*). Available at: https://www.eric.org.uk/Blog/what-is-encopresis

Infections in children

Viral infections (➔ Viral infections p. 720) are very common in childhood. Advice to parents on caring for a sick child and when to seek medical advice is important

Respiratory tract infections

Most are viral in origin and will resolve spontaneously. Evidence suggests (➔ Evidence-based healthcare p. 72) there should be no or delayed antibiotic prescribing for self-limiting respiratory tract infections unless systemically un-well, have symptoms suggestive of serious illness, at high risk of serious complications because of comorbidity (e.g. cystic fibrosis (➔ Cystic fibrosis p. 318), young children born prematurely (➔ Pre-term infants p. 176), children <2yrs with bilateral acute otitis media, and children with otorrhoea who have acute otitis media[12] (➔ Antimicrobial stewardship p. 146)).

Upper respiratory tract infections (URTIs)

Are extremely common and usually viral in origin. URTIs include the common cold (coryza), which presents with discharging or blocked nose, malaise, cough, and sometimes mild pyrexia. Resolves in a few days with paracetamol suspension and fluids. May cause exacerbation of asthma (➔ Asthma in children p. 306) and, in infants, difficulty in feeding and febrile convulsions (➔ Febrile convulsions and epilepsy p. 280). Purulent sputum indicates infection and may require antibiotics.

Acute otitis media

Infection (bacterial or viral) of the middle ear. 20% of <4yrs experience at least one episode per yr. Average total illness length = 4 days. Presents with pain and fever. On visual inspection with auroscope, red bulging drum. Many will resolve spontaneously within 24hrs; >80% resolve in <3 days without treatment. Many local policies advocate conservative approaches to prescribing antibiotics, e.g. manage with paracetamol and fluids, antibiotics reserved for unresolved infections after 3 days. Recurrent ear infections can lead to chronic secretory otitis media (known as glue ear)—most common cause of conductive hearing loss (➔ Deafness in children p. 268). May be referred for paediatric assessment and insertion of grommets into tympanic membrane. Current debates on effectiveness of this procedure.

Sore throat/tonsillitis

Pharyngitis (infection of throat, usually viral) with intense inflammation of tonsils, often with purulent exudates. May be treated with antibiotics. Children with recurrent infections of tonsils and adenoids referred for paediatric assessment. May have adenotonsillectomy if interfering with development/schooling or has abscess.

Bronchiolitis

Serious respiratory infection; usually viral. In <1yr characterized by cold symptoms, followed by dry cough and increasing breathlessness. Requires medical assessment and often hospital admission for humidified O_2.

Croup

A viral URTI characterized by a barking cough and inspiratory stridor. Steam may help. Requires medical review and may be admitted to hospital in acute phase.

Pneumonia

May be viral or bacterial. Child has fever, malaise, cough, often purulent sputum. Requires medical review and may need hospital admission (➲ Pneumonia p. 750).

Urinary tract infections (UTIs)

8% ♀ and 2% ♂ experience UTIs; most <1yr. Most caused by normal bowel flora. UTIs may be more common in children with renal abnormalities. Consequences can include renal scarring. Infants and toddlers may present with non-specific symptoms (e.g. fever and vomiting). Older children may present with dysuria, frequency, abdominal pain, and enuresis (➲ Nocturnal enuresis p. 296). Diagnosis by microscopy, culture, and sensitivity of clean-catch urine sample. Treated with antibiotics as per local guidelines. Referred to paediatrician if <3mths and UTI suspected or if recurrent infections, as may have renal abnormality.

Other common infections

Conjunctivitis

Infection (bacterial or viral) of the conjunctiva. Young children are very susceptible to repeated episodes and severe forms. Presents with red eye(s), swollen eyelid(s), and discharge which often sticks lids together. 64% resolve in 5 days without treatment. Antibiotic treatment (eye drops or ointment) may be indicated. Up to 25% physical transmission in household, so advise to avoid sharing towels etc. No need for exclusion from day care or school. Swab if presenting with these symptoms <1mth (different from newborn sticky eye), as potentially contracted sexually transmitted infection (➲ Sexually transmitted infections p. 764) through the birth canal (ophthalmic neonatorum).

Impetigo

See ➲ Bacterial skin infections p. 680.

Reference

12. NICE (2008) *Respiratory tract infections (self-limiting): prescribing antibiotics [CG69]*. Available at: www.nice.org.uk/CG069

Further information

NICE (*Urinary tract infection in under 16s: diagnosis and management*). Available at: ℘ https://www.nice.org.uk/guidance/cg54

PHE (*Health protection in schools and other childcare facilities*). Available at: ℘ https://www.gov.uk/government/publications/health-protection-in-schools-and-other-childcare-facilities

Infectious diseases in childhood

1° immunization has virtually eliminated all traditional childhood diseases with the exception of chickenpox and measles (◆ Childhood immunization p. 164; ◆ Childhood immunization schedule (UK) p. 166). Key aspects of these diseases are summarized in Table 7.1. Parents should be advised on caring for a sick child and reminded of key indicators when to seek medical advice (◆ The sick baby and child p. 276; ◆ Sepsis p. 826). See Table 7.2 for infectious disease exclusion times.

Table 7.1 Infectious disease in childhood

Disease	Transmission/ incubation	Presentation	Treatment	Complications	Infectious
Chickenpox	Physical contact, droplet, airborne 11–20 days	Rash +/– fever. Spots progress from macule to papule to vesicle. Crops appear for 5–7 days. Vesicles dry out and scab over (usually in <14 days)	Supportive: paracetamol, fluids, topical calamine lotion to lesions	Eczema herpeticum, encephalitis, pneumonia	Until 5 days after skin eruption
Diphtheria (very rare in UK)	Droplet 2–5 days	Inflammatory exudate that forms a greyish membrane in respiratory tract	Hospital admission for antitoxin and antibiotics	Respiratory obstruction	
Haemophilus influenzae (very rare in UK)	Respiratory droplet; nasal secretions	Meningitis: 60%	Antibiotics	Permanent neurological sequelae: mortality 5%	Until antibiotic treatment for 24hrs
Erthema infectiosum (5th disease)	Respiratory droplet 4–7 days	Erthematous maculo-papular rash starting on face; then lacy rash on trunk and limbs. Mild fever	Paracetamol and fluids		Probably only during prodome. Important for pregnant ♀ to report contact to GP
Measles	Respiratory droplet 10–14 days	Early: fever, conjunctivitis, cough, colic Later: Koplik's spots (white spots on bright red background inside mouth); red maculopapular rash appears after 4 days Lasts 8–10 days	Paracetamol and fluids	Broncho pneumonia, otitis media, gastroenteritis, encephalitis	Highly contagious for up to 18 days to non-immune

(Continued)

Table 7.1 (contd.)

Mumps	Respiratory droplet 16–21 days	Fever, malaise, tender enlargement of one or both parotids +/– submandibular glands	Paracetamol and fluids	Aseptic meningitis, epididymo-orchitis, pancreatitis	Up to 29 days
Poliomyelitis (rare in UK)	Droplet or faeco-oral 7 days	Flu-like prodrome; then fever, tachycardia, headache, vomiting, neck stiffness and unilateral tremor, paralysis	Hospital admission	Permanent disability may result. <10% of those developing paralysis die	
Rubella (German measles)	Respiratory droplet 14–21 days	Pink maculopapular rash for 3 days, mild fever	Paracetamol and fluids	Birth defects if infected in pregnancy, arthritis (adolescents), thrombo cytopoenia (rare)	15–23 days
Roseola infantum (<2yrs)	Oral secretions 4–7 days	High fever, sore throat, macular rash appears after 3 or 4 days as fever drops	Paracetamol and fluids		5–15 days
Scarlet fever	Respiratory droplet 2–4 days	Fever, malaise, headache, tonsillitis, rash, 'scarlet' facial flushing	Penicillin	Rheumatic fever	Not known
Whooping cough (Pertussis)	Respiratory droplet 7 days	Catarrhal stage: as URTI; coughing stage: paroxysmal cough with spasms of coughing followed by a 'whoop'. Lasts 4–6wks	Antibiotics in catarrhal stage	Pneumonia, bronchiectasis, convulsions	Up to 5 days after start of antibiotics

Table 7.2 Infectious diseases exclusion times

Disease	Exclusion period from early years care/schools
Chickenpox (varicella)	5days from start of skin eruption; all lesions should be crusted over before the children return to nursery or school
Conjunctivitis	None
Diarrhoea and vomiting (gastroenteritis)	Usually 48hrs after last episode of diarrhoea or vomiting
Glandular fever	None
Head lice	None
Hepatitis A	While unwell or 7 days after onset of jaundice
Hepatitis B, C, HIV/AIDs	None
Herpes simplex	None
Impetigo	Until lesions healed/crusted or 48hrs from starting antibiotics
Infectious mononucleosis	None
Influenza	Until recovered
Measles	4days from onset of rash
Meningococcal disease	Bacterial—duration of illness. Viral–none
Mumps	5days from onset of swelling
Rubella	5days from onset of rash
Scabies	Return after first treated
Scarlet fever	24hrs from start of antibiotic treatment
Shingles	Only if rash weeping and cannot be covered
Tinea (ring worm)	None
Threadworms	None
Tuberculosis	Smear positive: 2wks after starting treatment, as long as responsive to anti-TB therapy. Non-pulmonary TB: no exclusion
Typhoid and paratyphoid	Follow advice of Health Protection Team
Warts and verrucas	None
Whooping cough (pertussis)	5days from starting antibiotics, otherwise 48hrs of appropriate treatments with antibiotics and if person feels well enough or >3wk from onset of illness if no antibiotic treatment

Insects and infestations

Insect bites and stings

Response depends on the insect involved and the individual's response to the bite. The response ranges from blisters, through papules, to urticarial wheals. Stings should be removed if still embedded. Itching resulting from bites from fleas, flies, and mosquitoes can be treated with topical antihistamine, although greater allergic reactions (→ Allergies p. 694) may need oral antihistamines. Potential for anaphylactic reaction (→ Anaphylaxis p. 810).

Animal flea infestation in homes needs treatment of animals and carpets; sprays available OTC but severe infestations may need widespread spraying by a commercial company or local environmental health department (→ Environmental health services p. 27). Use a mosquito deterrent when travelling to parts of the world where mosquitos live (→ Malaria prevention p. 398).

Tick bites can cause Lyme disease if they transmit a bacterial infection. Carefully remove the tick with its mouth parts. The bacterial infection is uncommon after tick bite but might be suggested by a flu-like illness or a typical skin rash at the bite site.

Head lice (Pediculus capitis)

These are wingless insects. Most commonly found on children age 4–16yrs (♀ > ♂), but can infest anyone. Spread by lice walking from head to head. Eggs are known as 'nits' and laid at base of hair shaft; hatch within 7–10 days. Empty white shells remain 'glued' to hair. Nymph stage is 7–10 days to adult and then able to reproduce. Lice pierce the scalp to feed on blood.

Prevention

No evidence of effectiveness of prophylactic treatment or use of herbal-based lotions (→ Evidence-based healthcare p. 72). Health promotion schemes with children and parents (e.g. Bug Busters), particularly in early years facilities and schools, encourages: hair management strategies; early detection by weekly combing of wet, conditioner-covered hair with light-coloured, bevel-edged, louse-detection (fine-tooth) comb; and early treatment to prevent spread.

Symptoms

Itchy scalp and scratching. Detection of a moving louse, not old egg shells, confirms infestation. It is difficult to detect moving louse on dry or damp hair unless very severe infestation. Experts continue to debate effectiveness of wet combing and insecticides.

Treatment by mechanical removal (wet combing)

- After washing hair, apply conditioner and systematically comb all hair with fine-tooth detector comb (available from local pharmacies).
- Rinse comb after each stroke to remove trapped lice and to prevent combing lice back into hair.
- Repeat on days 5, 9, 13 to remove nymphs.

Detailed instruction on sites such as NHS Choices and Bug Busters. Bug Buster™ kit can be prescribed on NHS.

Chemical treatments with insecticides
- Available OTC and on NHS prescription.
- Malathion, phenothrin, permethrin, and carbaryl are mostly effective against lice.
- To overcome the development of resistance, a mosaic strategy is used, rotating to different insecticide if treatment fails.
- Application as per instructions for contact time of 12hrs, repeated 7 days later.
- Aqueous formulations preferred for small children and those with severe eczema or asthma.

Some community concerns about using pesticides including organophosphates on children (see Pesticide Action Network[13]).

All close contacts should be examined and treated as necessary.

Scabies (Sarcoptes scabie)

The scabies mite is 7.5mm long and spread by direct physical contact.

Symptoms

Appear 4–6wks after infection. Red burrows, tracking in irregular lines, commonly between fingers and toes. Intense itching. Scratching results in excoriations.

Treatment

Treated with permethrin 5% aqueous preparation over whole body including the face, neck, scalp, and ears. Washed off after 8–12hrs, and repeated one week later. If the hands are washed within 12hrs of application, retreat the hands with cream. All close contacts need treatment. All worn clothing and bedding should be washed. Itching may persist for some time after elimination; often alleviated by topical antihistamines.

Threadworm (Enterobulus vermicularis)

Threadworm is common among children. Worm lives about 6wks. Causes anal itch as it leaves the bowel to lay eggs on the perineum. Often seen as silvery thread-like worms in stools or at the anus. Scratching transfers eggs to nails and hands, then ingested. Child >2yrs and household members treated with mebendazole. OTC piperazine for children <6mths. Prevention includes promoting good hand washing before meals and after going to the toilet, and ensuring short and clean nails.

Reference

13. Pesticide Action Network (2017) *Impacts of pesticides on women and children*. Available at: ◌ http://www.pan-uk.org/effects-pesticides-women-children/

Further information

Bug Busting (*What is bug busting?*). Available at: ◌ www.chc.org
NICE (*Head lice*). Available at: ◌ https://cks.nice.org.uk/head-lice#!topicSummary
NICE (*Lyme disease*). Available at: ◌ https://cks.nice.org.uk/lyme-disease#!topicSummary
NICE (*Scabies*). Available at: ◌ https://cks.nice.org.uk/scabies#!topicSummary
NICE (*Threadworms*). Available at: ◌ https://cks.nice.org.uk/threadworm#!topicSummary

Nocturnal enuresis

Bedwetting is considered normal up to the age of 5yrs, and is common up to the age of 10yrs (€ Toilet training p. 214). It ↓ to ~15% at 5yrs, 10% at 7yrs, and 5% at 10yrs. More ♂ than ♀. Major impact on self-esteem. Causes are unclear, but may be associated with bladder dysfunction, sleep arousal difficulties, polyuria, and runs in families.

Principles of care

- Ensure child, young person, and family understands it is not their fault and punitive measures will not help.
- Involve child (irrespective of age) in discussions and planning.
- Discuss with parents if they need additional support in coping.

Assessment

Includes history, current symptoms, toileting patterns, fluid intake, assessment for triggers (e.g. constipation (€ Constipation and encopresis p. 286), UTI (€ Infections in children p. 288)), developmental problems, neurological or congenital conditions, soiling (double incontinence suggests neurological causes or developmental delay), sleeping arrangements, family dynamics, and possible maltreatment (€ Assessment of children, young people, and families p. 156; € Safeguarding children p. 248). Urinalysis not required unless recent start or other indications of ill health. Invasive tests and examination not usually indicated initially.

Management

Engage the child and family. Support for the child and family. <5yrs, advice only as usually resolves spontaneously. >5yrs, more actively managed in stepwise fashion:

- Review fluid and diet intake
- Fluid intake recommendations (Table 7.3)[14]
- Advise on reward system (e.g. star chart for dry nights)
- Enuresis alarms offered (often via enuresis clinics): may take 4wks for response; used until 2wks of dry nights
- Desmopressin, given by tablet or melting wafer, tops up the hormone vasopressin, which tells the kidneys to produce less urine at night-time
- Incontinence nappies/pants may be needed for neurogenic incontinence and if laundry is causing an intolerable burden

Table 7.3 Daily fluid intake recommendations for children

4–8 years	9–13 years	14–18 years
~1280ml	♀ ~1520ml	♀ ~1600ml
	♂ ~1680ml	♂ ~2000ml

Reference

14. Association of British Dieticians (2017) *Food fact sheet: fluid.* Available at: https://www.bda. uk.com/foodfacts/fluid.pdf

Further information

ERIC (*What is bedwetting?*) Available at: ℘ https://www.eric.org.uk/what-is-bedwetting
ERIC (*Night-time wetting*) Available at: ℘ https://www.eric.org.uk/flowchart-nighttime-wetting
NICE (*Bedwetting in children and young people*). Available at: ℘ https://pathways.nice.org.uk/pathways/bedwetting-in-children-and-young-people
NICE (*Bedwetting in under 19s*). Available at: ℘ www.nice.org.uk/guidance/CG111

Growth disorders

Growth starts *in utero* and ends after puberty (➔ Puberty and adolescence p. 228).

Measurement

Details of national policies on weight, height, and head circumference measurement are given in Chapter 6: Child Health Promotion. Good practice is to also record height and weight if there are concerns about a child either because of chronic ill health or requires prolonged follow-up.

Interpretation

Interpretation of measurements for stage of puberty, including predicting child's adult height and comparison with parental height is done with use of UK–WHO growth charts.[15] Review by GP (➔ General practice p. 18) or community paediatrician indicated if: weight or height or BMI is below the 0.4th centile, unless already fully investigated at an earlier age; the height centile is more than three centile spaces below the mid-parental centile; there is a drop in height centile position of more than two centiles; and smaller centile seen in combination with other concerns about the child's growth.

Short stature

Usually defined as height below 2nd centile. Most of these will be normal, but short. Most short children are well adjusted to their size; however, there may be issues at school with bullying (➔ Child and adolescent mental health p. 246), low self-esteem, and disadvantages at sport. Also, may be treated inappropriately by others as younger than their age.

Causes
- Psychosocial deprivation: children subjected to physical and emotional deprivation (➔ Emotional development in babies and children p. 210; ➔ Identifying the child in need of protection p. 250) may be short, underweight, with delayed puberty (➔ Puberty and adolescence p. 228)
- Intrauterine growth disorders
- Chronic illness associated with nutritional problems (e.g. coeliac disease (➔ Coeliac disease p. 714)) and cystic fibrosis (➔ Cystic fibrosis p. 318)
- Chromosomal disorders, e.g. Down's syndrome, Turner's syndrome, and achondroplasia (➔ Genetic problems p. 270)
- Endocrine problems, e.g. hypothyroidism treated with thyroxine (➔ Thyroid p. 702) and growth hormone deficiency

Tall stature

Most tall stature is inherited from parents. Some adolescents become concerned about excessive height during pubertal growth spurt. Tall children may be disadvantaged by being treated older than their chronological age. 2° endocrine causes are rare (e.g. pituitary adenoma (gigantism) (➔ Pituitary disorders p. 701)). Some long-legged tall stature seen in children with chromosome syndromes, e.g. Marfan's and Klinefelter's (XXY) syndromes (➔ Genetic problems p. 270).

Abnormal head growth

Most head growth occurs <2yrs, and 80% of adult head size achieved by age 5yrs, reflecting brain growth. Posterior fontanelle closes by 8wks; anterior by 12–18mths. Small or large heads may be familial. Children with head circumference <3rd or >97th centile referred for paediatric assessment. Abnormal head growth includes:

- Skull asymmetry: may be due to an imbalance in growth, or in pre-terms lying on sides in incubators for a long time, and usually resolves
- Craniosynostosis: premature fusion of skull sutures—referred urgently to specialist
- Microcephaly: circumference <2nd centile; small head out of proportion with the body. Associated with developmental delay. Causes include genetic, intrauterine infection (e.g. rubella, cytomegalovirus), and hypoxia
- Macrocephaly: circumference >98th centile. Most are normal children with familial large heads; however, rapidly rising head circumference may be due to hydrocephalus, subdural haematoma, or brain tumour—refer urgently to specialist (➔ Cancer in childhood p. 314)

Premature sexual development

Development of 2° sexual characteristics before 8yrs ♀ and 9yrs ♂ is outside the normal range. Usually referred to specialist for assessment and investigation:

- Precocious puberty: usually familial and organic causes rare (e.g. congenital adrenal hyperplasia, androgen-secreting tumour)
- Premature breast development only (thelarche): usually 6mth–2yrs ♀ and self-limiting
- Premature pubic hair only (adrenarche): usually self-limiting

Delayed puberty

Delayed puberty is the absence of pubertal development by 14yrs ♀ and 15yrs ♂. Common in boys with familial history of delayed puberty. May be a source of problems at school and cause low self-esteem. Often referred for specialist assessment to identify any underlying chronic systemic disorders, e.g. Crohn's disease or hormonal problems. May be treated with weak androgenic anabolic steroids, and testosterone (♂) or oestradiol (♀).

Reference

15. Royal College of Paediatrics and Child Health (2009) UK–WHO growth charts: 2–18 years. Available at: https://www.rcpch.ac.uk/resources/uk-who-growth-charts-2-18-years

Further information

Child Growth Foundation (Information and support). Available at: 🔊 http://childgrowthfoundation. org/supportforfamilies/

Great Ormond Street Hospital (Medical conditions: achondroplasia). Available at: 🔊 https://www. gosh.nhs.uk/conditions-and-treatments/conditions-we-treat/achondroplasia

Restricted Growth Association (About restricted growth). Available at: 🔊 https://rgauk.org/ about-restricted-growth

Acne vulgaris

A disease of the pilo-sebaceous units that can occur on the face, chest, or back. Most commonly occurs between 13–20yrs (➔ Puberty and adolescence p. 228). Everyone gets some acne. May continue into the 20s or 30s and, occasionally, into later life. Often has an emotional impact on confidence and self-esteem (➔ Child and adolescent mental health p. 246). Genetic factors are important in the severity, duration, and clinical pattern. Rarer causes include endocrine problems (➔ Endocrine problems p. 304), chemicals, and steroids.

Factors

1° pathogenic factors in the development of acne include:
- ↑ sebum production
- Presence of proprionibacterium acne bacteria
- Abnormal keratinization
- Inflammation

Stress, heavy sweating, and premenstrual hormonal changes may have an impact (➔ Menstrual problems p. 778). Some beauty products (e.g. pomades, defrizzing agents, suntan oils) may also impact. Limited evidence to support the argument that poor diet or poor hygiene has an impact on the development or severity of acne.

Clinical features

- Comedones (or blackheads): plug of keratin and sebum extrudes from pilo-sebaceous orifice
- Whiteheads, papules, pustules, nodules, cysts, and scars may also be present

General advice on management

- Wash twice daily with soap and water, and apply moisturizer.
- Do not squeeze red or yellow pustules.
- OTC preparations: use lowest concentrations and consult health professional if no improvement within 2mths.
- Avoid using thick, oil-based types of make-up.
- Maintain a healthy diet (➔ Growth and nutrition 12–18 years p. 234).

Treatment

Treatment is commenced early to prevent scarring:
- Comedonal acne: azelaic acid or benzoyl peroxide (OTC)
- Mild inflammatory acne: topical retinoid (contraindicated in pregnancy (➔ Pregnancy p. 424) and breastfeeding (➔ Breastfeeding p. 182)) and topical antibiotic or benzoyl peroxide plus topical antibiotic
- Moderate inflammatory acne: long-term tetracycline plus topical retinoid or other antibiotic (doxycycline, erythromycin, lymecycline, minocycline). For ♀ oral anti-androgen plus topical retinoid
- Severe inflammatory acne: referred to dermatology specialist. Treated with oral isotretinoin or high-dose oral antibiotic plus topical retinoid

Refer to dermatology specialist

If severe, any scarring, or associated with fever or arthritis (◒ Bone and joint problems p. 264), or no improvements with treatments.

Related topics

◒ Bacterial skin infections p. 680

Further information

NICE (*Acne vulgaris scenario: management of acne vulgaris in primary care*). Available at: ℛ https://
   cks.nice.org.uk/acne-vulgaris#!scenarioRecommendation
Teenage Health Freak (*Spots*). Available at: ℛ www.teenagehealthfreak.org/spots

Overweight children and adolescents

Obesity in children is major public health concern. Approximately 30% of those aged 2–10yrs, and 35% of those aged 11–15yrs, are overweight or obese (➲ UK health profile p. 2).

Measurement and interpretation

- Detail of national policies on weight, height, and head circumference measurement is given in Chapter 6: Child Health Promotion.
- Interpretations of weight and height measurements are done with use of UK–WHO growth and BMI charts.
- A child whose weight is average for their height will have a BMI between the 25th and 75th centiles, whatever their height centile.
- BMI >91st centile suggests overweight and advice/actions according to local guidelines.
- Review by GP (➲ General practice p. 18) or community paediatrician indicated if >98th centile is clinically obese.

Advice for overweight children and families

- Children are growing, so need to maintain their current weight (not lose weight) while they continue to grow in height.
- Eat well as a family, including healthy meals eaten together (➲ Food and the under-fives p. 212).
- Get active as a family (➲ Exercise p. 354).
- Parents need to help build self-esteem of overweight children, so positive encouragement for all attempts/small steps of the earlier listed points (➲ Emotional development in babies and children p. 210).
- Engage school support through joining in activities and supporting healthy eating opportunities (e.g. healthy lunch boxes).

Weight management programmes for children

A number of programmes tailored to children and young people of different ages may be available through the NHS and LA public health departments.

Further information

My Time Active (*Child weight management*). Available at: ℅ https://www.mytimeactive.co.uk/ health/health-service/child-weight-management
NHS (*Change4life*). Available at: ℅ https://www.nhs.uk/change4life#
Royal College of Paediatrics and Child Health (*UK–WHO growth charts: 2–18 years*). Available at: ℅ https://www.rcpch.ac.uk/resources/uk-who-growth-charts-2-18-years

Endocrine problems

Endocrine problems

Diabetes

Incidence is ↑ and now affects 2 in 1,000 children <16yrs. Almost all have Type 1 diabetes, with peak years of presentation at 12–13yrs with polyuria, polydipsia, and weight loss. Type 2 is rare in children but ↑, and is mostly obesity-related (➋ Overweight children and adolescents p. 302). Symptoms of polydipsia, polyuria, tiredness, and weight loss or looking thinner. ⚠ Currently one in four diagnosed when in diabetic ketoacidosis (➋ Diabetes: overview p. 660; ➋ Principles of diabetes management p. 664).

On diagnosis, the child is referred to specialist diabetes team. Commenced on insulin by subcutaneous (SC) injection. Young children usually given insulin twice a day. Older children and teenagers often have three or four injections a day, relating insulin more closely to food and exercise; diet and insulin have to be closely matched. NHS funding for delivery via pumps may be available for those >12yrs if multiple injections is impractical or inappropriate. Parents and children need intensive education and support to cover:
• Nature of diabetes
• Injecting insulin
• Diet
• Sick-day rules during illness to prevent ketoacidosis
• Blood glucose and HbA1c monitoring
• Recognition and treatment of hypoglycaemia
• How to get help and advice 24h/day
• Emotions and coming to terms with the diagnosis.

Children have special needs and schools need to be included in addressing specific needs through the day (e.g. a snack and what to do if child becomes hypoglycaemic) (➋ Working in schools p. 44).

Hypoglycaemia

Most complain of hunger, dizziness, wobbly feeling in legs, irritability. Treated with easily absorbed glucose (e.g. glucose tablets and gels). Parents and schools should be provided with and taught how to use intramuscular glucagon injection kit for hypoglycaemia if child is not responding.

Screening offered for complications and associated conditions
• Coeliac disease at time of diagnosis (➋ Coeliac disease p. 714)
• Thyroid disease at diagnosis and annually until transfer to adult services (➋ Thyroid p. 702)
• >12yrs retinopathy, microalbuminuria, and blood pressure (BP)

Neonatal (congenital) hypothyroidism

Affects 71 per 4,000 live births. Due to congenital absence of the thyroid gland. One of few preventable causes of severe learning difficulties (➋ People with learning disabilities p. 456). Normally detected by blood spot/heel prick testing (➋ Child screening tests p. 160). Child is referred for specialist advice. Treatment is with lifelong thyroxine replacement. In most treated infants, development is normal.

Hyperthyroidism

Usually the result of Graves' disease. Characterized by anxiety, restlessness, weight loss, thyrotoxicosis, and exophthalmos. The child is referred to specialist for drug therapy lasting up to 2yrs and then possible surgery if relapse.

Inborn errors of metabolism

Many hundreds of enzyme defects have been identified, mostly with an autosomal recessive inheritance. Very rare and consequently managed at specialist centres.

Phenylketonuria (PKU)

Deficiency of the enzyme phenylalaninehydroxylase. Affects 1 in 10,000–20,000 live births. Detected by blood spot/heel prick test. Treated with lifelong restriction of dietary phenylaline and particularly during pregnancy (➔ Pregnancy p. 424). With treatment, growth and development are normal.

Galactosaemia

Rare deficiency of galactose-1-phosphate uridyl transferase. Inability to mobilize glucose from galactose, resulting in hypoglycaemia and accumulation of galactose. Lactose in milk is a disaccharide containing glucose and galactose, so when milk is introduced it results in vomiting, jaundice, hepatic failure. Management is by lactose- and galactose-free diet. Even if treated early, severe learning difficulties are common.

Further information

NICE (Diabetes (Type 1 and Type 2) in children and young people: diagnosis and management). Available at: ℛ www.nice.org.uk/guidance/ng18

NICE (*Quality standards for diabetes in children and young people*). Available at: ℛ www.nice.org.uk/guidance/qs125

Asthma in children

Asthma is a lung disease, with intermittent narrowing of the bronchi, causing shortness of breath, noisy breathing, recurrent wheeze, dry cough (particularly at night), and tightness in the chest (● Asthma in adults p. 608). During an asthma attack, the muscles in the bronchi contract and the lining swells, becomes inflamed, and produces excess mucus (● Acute asthma in adults (asthma attacks) p. 612). Affects one in eleven children. Breastfeeding has preventative effect (● Breastfeeding p. 182). The majority of children who present with asthma aged <2yrs are free of symptoms by age 6–11yrs. Although detection and treatment are improving, it is still a major cause of school absenteeism and a major anxiety in children and families. About 20 children die from asthma in the UK each year.

Predisposing factors and common precipitating factors

Predisposing factors include both genetic predisposition and environmental factors: family history of atopy (i.e. allergies, eczema, rhinitis, hay fever (● Allergies p. 694)); coexistence of atopic disease; bronchiolitis in infancy; parental smoking; and prematurity (● Pre-term infants p. 176). Common precipitating factors include: infection; exercise; heightened emotion; household allergens (including house mites, fur, and feathered pets); adverse weather (e.g. fog, cold air, thunderstorms); and air pollutants (smoke, traffic, and dust).

Diagnosis

Diagnosis made on history and clinical examination. In children >5yrs: bronchodilator responsiveness, peak flow variability, and spirometry are used to confirm diagnosis, as for adults (● Measuring lung function p. 606). Height of children is the only determinant of peak exploratory flow rate (PEFR). Often referred to specialists for diagnosis and establishment of treatment. Often also referred for skin allergy testing.

Management and treatment

The aim of treatment and management is to: allow child to lead as normal life as possible; minimize need for relieving medication; and prevent severe attacks or exacerbations. Treatment is by a stepwise approach that includes short-acting inhaled bronchodilator therapy (relievers) (e.g. salbutamol) and prophylactic therapy (preventers) (e.g. inhaled steroids). As the severity and frequency of symptoms ↑ so do the addition of therapies until good control reached. Then treatment is stepped down (● Drugs commonly used in the treatment of respiratory conditions p. 620). Advice on other measures is also given (e.g. parental smoking cessation (● Smoking cessation p. 356)).

Types of chronic asthma and management

- Infrequent episodic: symptom-free for at least 6wks at a time; flare ups but need no regular treatment, only inhaled bronchodilators as required
- Frequent episodic: symptoms every 4–6wks; need regular inhaled prophylactic therapy, initially with low-dose steroid, plus an inhaled bronchodilator as required
- Persistent asthma: need prophylaxis with inhaled steroids; also may need long-acting bronchodilator and oral steroids. Usually treated and monitored in specialist clinics.

Structured proactive review and monitoring

Regular, structured patient review of symptoms, level of symptom control, and use of medications should be organized and delivered by nurse or doctor with asthma management training in 1° care. Review should include the childhood asthma control test, asthma education, parent/child self-management, and action plans, as well as use of symptom diaries. Adolescents in particular are ↑ users of A&E with acute asthma. Encourage parents and young people to seek review if: needing more and more reliever treatment; waking at night coughing, wheezing, with shortness of breath; non-attendance at day care or nursery/school because of asthma; and unable to do usual physical activities and sports.

Inhalers

Inadequate technique may be mistaken for drug failure. Children <15yrs should have a pressurized metered-dose inhaler and spacer device, or a dry-powder inhaler. <5yrs, with face mask if necessary; if not effective, nebulizer therapy is considered (➔ Nebulizers p. 623). Advice on pressurized metered-dose inhalers and spacers includes:

- Shake inhaler well before fitting to spacer. Press inhaler once and without delay allow child to take five slow breaths in and out of the spacer (tidal breathing).
- Remove inhaler, shake well, and repeat as prescribed.
- Spacers should be cleaned monthly in mild detergent as per manufacturer's instructions, and replaced every 6–12mths.

With a dry-powder inhaler, there is a need to breathe in quickly and deeply until the lungs feel full, to be sure all the medicine is inhaled.

Further information

NICE (*Asthma*). Available at: ℬ https://cks.nice.org.uk/asthma
Scottish Intercollegiate Guidelines Network (SIGN) (*SIGN 158 British guideline on the management of asthma*). Available at: ℬ https://www.sign.ac.uk/assets/sign158.pdf

Sickle cell disorders

Haemoglobinopathies refers to a range of genetically inherited disorders of red blood cell haemoglobin (Hb) (◉ Genetic problems p. 270). Sickle cell disorders (SCD) refer to an inherited sickle Hb disorder including sickle cell anaemia. Sickle cell anaemia (Hb SS) is an autosomal recessive genetic condition in which two Hb S genes are inherited from both parents. Hb S refers to haemoglobin that is deformed, rigid, 'sickle' shaped, and unable to transport O_2 effectively. Sickle cells have a ↓ life span, and block small capillaries, ↓ O_2 transportation, and → thrombosis and ischaemia. This is made worse by factors such as dehydration and cold, or situations of ↓ O_2 availability (e.g. anaesthesia and high altitudes).

Around 350 children a year in the UK are born with sickle cell anaemia[16] (◉ UK health profile p. 2). Mainly affects people of African or Caribbean descent, but also affects people from Asia, the Middle East, and the eastern Mediterranean. The UK has antenatal (◉ Antenatal care and screening p. 426) and newborn screening programmes (◉ Child screening tests p. 160).

Those with one HbA gene and one HbS gene have sickle cell trait and are therefore carriers of sickle cell anaemia. They have enough normal HbA to not experience the problems of those with sickle cell anaemia.

Children identified with HbSS are referred to a named paediatrician. Children (and adults) with sickle cell anaemia will vary in the severity of symptoms and problems. Symptoms include: anaemia (◉ Anaemia in adults p. 652); infections, due to splenic dysfunction causing increased susceptibility; and jaundice due to chronic haemolysis.

Importantly, they also experience pain as a result of vaso-occlusive crises. Pain can vary in frequency and severity. Can occur anywhere in the body, but often occurs in the limbs, back, and abdomen. Also presents as dactylitis. This hand/foot syndrome is a painful swelling of the hands, feet, or both and affects children <3yrs old. Often the pain is excruciating. ♂ can also experience priapism.

Types of vaso-occlusive crisis that may require blood transfusions include:
- Sequestration crisis: a sudden ↓ Hb concentration due to pooling of a large volume of blood in the spleen, liver, or lungs. Painful swelling of the organ with worsening anaemia. Can affect children within the first 5yrs, and in rare instances can result in death from circulatory collapse, anaemia, and hypovolaemic shock.
- Haemolytic crisis: when events such as infections cause a serious ↓ in the number of red blood cells
- Aplastic crisis: occurs at any age as a result of a ↓ of bone marrow activity; may be life-threatening
- Megaloblastic changes/crisis: rare and due to folic acid deficiency

Long-term problems may include: cardiac problems from chronic anaemia; and gall stones due to chronic haemolysis of red blood cells, cerebrovascular accident (◉ Recognizing and responding to a stroke p. 830), and ulcerated legs (◉ Leg ulcer assessment p. 536).

Advice and management

Specific treatment for sickle cell disease includes prophylactic antibiotics and the full child immunization schedule, plus annual influenza vaccination (● Childhood immunization p. 164); ● Childhood immunization schedule (UK) p. 166). Some children will require regular blood transfusions. Hydroxyurea is a medicine that can decrease several complications of SCD. Hydroxyurea ↑ production of fetal Hb, that then ↓ the tendency of sickle cells to sickle, as well as ↓ white blood cells that contribute to the general inflammatory state in sickle cell patients.

Another treatment to consider is a stem-cell transplant, which infuses healthy cells into the body to replace damaged or diseased bone marrow. Although transplants of bone marrow or blood from healthy donors are increasingly being used to successfully cure SCD, there are significant risks involved, and should therefore be considered carefully by the child/young person, their family, and healthcare professionals involved in the child's care.[17]

Key areas of advice

- As normal lifestyle as possible, but act early in any illness
- Ensure a healthy lifestyle and good nutrition (including folic acid)
- Avoid triggers to crisis (e.g. dehydration, cold, strenuous exercise in damp or wet conditions)
- Seek medical advice early for any infections (● Infections in children p. 288)
- Travel advice: ensure adequate malaria prophylaxis—sickle cell disease offers no protection (● Malaria prevention p. 398). ⚠ Crisis can be precipitated by antimalarials
- Recommend wearing a medic alert bracelet
- Important to ensure childcare and school staff understand the condition and support the active management to avoid triggers (● Working in schools p. 44).

Management of crises

Minor ones are managed at home with support of GP (● General practice p. 18) and 1° care team. Key management elements are analgesia, ↑ fluid intake, and warmth. Pain can be helped by:

- Careful assessment; diaries provide useful insight into patient's pain experience and coping strategies
- Warmth, massaging, and rubbing, and by heat (e.g. hot water bottles)
- Bandaging to support the painful region
- Resting the body, deep breathing exercises, and distraction techniques
- Pain relief prescribed according to severity (see BNF/BNF Online for Children)

Children with more severe crisis will be admitted to hospital (e.g. severe pain, high fever, or other symptoms such as dyspnoea or neurological signs requiring intravenous fluids and opiate analgesia).[18]

Related topics

→ Children with complex health needs and disabilities p. 238; → Thalassaemia p. 312

References

16. Sickle Cell Society (2018) *About sickle cell.* Available at: https://www.sicklecellsociety.org/about-sickle-cell/
17. Centers for Disease Control and Prevention (2018) *Complications and treatment of sickle cell disease.* Available at: https://www.cdc.gov/ncbddd/sicklecell/treatments.html
18. NICE (2012) *Sickle cell disease: managing acute painful episodes in hospital.* Available at: https://www.nice.org.uk/guidance/cg143

Thalassaemia

Thalassaemia is a less common haemoglobinopathy than sickle cell (→ Sickle cell disorders p. 308) in the UK. There were about 1,300 people with the most severe form of thalassaemia in 2019[19] (→ UK health profile p. 2). ↑ prevalence in Cypriot, Italian, Greek, Indian, Pakistani, Bangladeshi, Chinese, and South Asian populations. Also (less common), Northern European population. The UK has antenatal and newborn screening programmes (→ Antenatal care and screening p. 426; → Child screening tests p. 160). Any child identified with thalassaemia is referred to a named paediatrican.

B thalassaemia major

Children (and adults) with this condition are unable to produce Hb, resulting in life-threatening anaemia (→ Anaemia in adults p. 652) and jaundice from ~6mths. They require regular blood transfusions for life, accompanied by regular chelation therapy to prevent iron deposition. Even with treatment, these children often have complex problems including: growth and sexual development problems, enlarged spleen, diabetes (→ Endocrine problems p. 304), and heart problems (→ Children with complex health needs and disabilities p. 238). A bone marrow transplant can offer a cure but carries significant risks also.

Thalassaemia intermedia is another less severe form and may require less frequent transfusions.

Management of care

These children and their families are primarily supported by specialist services. Families and children need continual support and recognition of problems being faced over a lifetime.

Reference

19. National Haemoglobinopathy Registry (2019) *Data*. Available at: http://nhr.mdsas.com/

Further information

NHS (*Sickle cell and thalassaemia screening programme*). Available at: ℘ www.nhs.uk/conditions/pregnancy-and-baby/screening-sickle-cell-thalassaemia-pregnant/
UK Thalassaemia Society (*About thalassaemia*). Available at: ℘ www.ukts.org

Cancer in childhood

Cancer in children is rare: <2,000 cases per year in the UK[20] (**⊃** UK health profile p. 2; **⊃** Children with complex health needs and disabilities p. 238). Most cancers occur as a result of mutations in cellular genes, which may be inherited or sporadic. Emphasis with all cancers is on early diagnosis and treatment, e.g. a maximum of 2wks from GP (**⊃** General practice p. 18) urgent referral of suspected cancer to first hospital assessment. Most children with cancer in the UK are initially treated in regional centres, and then returned to the care of local specialists and 1° care, including support from specialist outreach nurses from regional centres or children's community nursing teams. Survival rate for many cancers has ↑ dramatically.

In the early days:

• Parents need opportunities to discuss diagnosis and feelings, as well as written information on the disease, implications, and treatments.

• The child and siblings need age-appropriate explanations and opportunities to discuss their feelings.

• Family may need help with practical issues such as transport, accommodation, finance, and care of siblings while attending tertiary centre.

• Once treatment is established and the disease is under control, families are encouraged to return to as normal a life as possible:
  • Early return to school is encouraged.
  • Child and family should be offered ongoing opportunities to discuss feelings and find ways of coping with unknown long-term outcome.
  • Parents should be supported in having time out from caring to focus on themselves and their own needs (**⊃** Talking therapies p. 472).

General overview of treatment and management

Treatment

May involve chemotherapy, surgery, and radiotherapy. Bone marrow transplantation may be used to treat patients after administering very ↑ doses of chemotherapy and/or radiotherapy that damages normal tissue and particularly bone marrow.

Long-term follow-up

Monitors residual problems, risks of second tumours, and specific problems as a result of the treatment (e.g. poor growth, sexual dysfunction).

Palliative care

Despite treatment, some children progress to the terminal stages of their cancers. Specialist palliative care or hospice teams may be involved. General principles of palliative care at home (**⊃** Palliative care in the home p. 550) apply:

• Address pain relief and symptom control (**⊃** Pain assessment and management in palliative care p. 554).

• Provide emotional support for child and family.

- Ensure continuity with as few professionals as possible (➲ Continuity of care p. 598).
- Provide ongoing support to family members after the child has died (➲ Coping with bereavement p. 574).

Main types

Leukaemia, brain, other central nervous system (CNS) and intracranial tumours, and lymphomas account for more than two thirds of all cancers diagnosed in children. Leukaemia is the most commonly diagnosed cancer in children.

Acute leukaemia

Peak presentation at age 2–4yrs. 80%: acute lymphoblastic leukaemia; others, acute myeloid or acute non-lymphocytic. Usually presents with a short history (weeks) of pallor, fatigue, irritability, fever, bone pain, and/or bruising/petechiae.

Lymphomas

Malignancies of the cells of the immune system. Peak presentation is at age 10–14yrs. Two main types: Hodgkin's disease (usually presents as painless lymphadenopathy, often in the neck, and may also have a long history of weight loss, sweating, priutius, and fever); and non-Hodgkin's lymphoma (usually presents with painless lymphadenopathy, often in the neck, and/or disease in the abdomen, with an often rapid progression of symptoms).

Brain tumours

Almost always 1° tumours and present with signs of raised intracranial pressure, e.g. headache (worse when lying down), vomiting, squint, nystagmus, personality or behaviour change. Tumour identified on computerized tomography (CT)/positron emission tomography (PET)/magnetic resonance imaging (MRI) scans. Outcome influenced by position and size. Survivors may have very complex problems.

Neuroblastoma

Derived from neural crest tissue in adrenal medulla and sympathetic nervous system. Tends to affect children <5yrs. Most present with abdominal mass. Children with extra-abdominal tumours and those who are <1yr at diagnosis have better prognosis.

Wilms' tumour (nephroblastoma)

Kidney tumour from embryonal renal tissue. Usually affects children <5yrs old. Presents with fever, weight loss, anaemia, abdominal mass, and pain.

Retinoblastoma

Rare tumour of the eye. Usually affects children <5yrs. Usually detected by a white pupillary reflex found at routine developmental screening, or with squint or inflammation of the eye.

Rhabdomyosarcoma

Presents with a mass at any age. May be at any site.

Osteosarcoma (bone tumour)

10–14yrs. Presents with persistent bony pain, most commonly in a limb.

Reference

20. Cancer Research UK (undated) *Childhood cancer incidence statistics*. Available at: www. cancerresearchuk.org/cancer-info/cancerstats/childhoodcancer/incidence/ childhood-cancer-incidence-statistics

Further information

Macmillan Cancer Support (*Cancer in children and young people*). Available at: ℘ https://www. macmillan.org.uk/information-and-support/audience/childrens-cancer/about-childrens-cancer/ cancer-in-children.html

Together for Short Lives (*Making a lifetime of difference for children expected to have short lives*). Available at: ℘ https://www.togetherforshortlives.org.uk/

Young Lives vs Cancer (*Lives with cancer*). Available at: ℘ https://www.clicsargent.org.uk/ life-with-cancer/

Cystic fibrosis

Cystic fibrosis (CF) is a common, serious pulmonary and genetic disease, affecting 1 in 2,500 children (UK) (➲ UK health profile p. 2). ~1 in 25 of the UK white population are carriers of a copy of the CF gene. Rare in children of African or Asian descent.

Diagnosis

Identified through neonatal screening (➲ Child screening tests p. 160) or antenatal test if thought to be at high risk (➲ Antenatal care and screening p. 426). Pre-conceptual screening also available (➲ Preconceptual care p. 422). If the screening test suggests a child may have CF, they will need additional tests to confirm they have the condition including:[21]

- A sweat test: to measure the amount of salt in sweat, which will be abnormally high in someone with CF
- A genetic test: where a sample of blood or saliva is checked for the faulty gene that causes CF

CF affects movement of salt and water across cell membranes and causes sticky mucous. CF is a multi-system disease characterized by life-threatening pulmonary and gastrointestinal problems. No cure for CF but treatments can control symptoms, prevent or ↓ complications, and make life easier for people affected by the disease. Life expectancy for people with CF has improved in recent years, and is now ~47yrs.[22]

Care and management

Children with CF should be linked to a specialist centre with aims of:
- Promoting independence, improving quality of life, and ↑ life expectancy
- Working in partnership with child and family for long-term support
- Good multidisciplinary team working (➲ Teamwork p. 58), especially with school as child grows older (➲ Working in schools p. 44)

Care for lung-associated problems

- Twice daily chest physiotherapy and autogenic drainage to loosen thick mucus. Parents are taught how to do this by hospital staff, and ongoing support from community paediatric nurses. Patients can do this themselves as they become adult.
- Immunizations and flu vaccination.
- Rapid treatment with antibiotics with any sign of chest infection. IV antibiotic therapy in the community offered in many areas. Some children are prescribed prophylactic antibiotics.
- Some children will have inhalers for asthma and inhaled medication to reduce stickiness of secretions, as well as corticosteroids.
- Home O_2 to aid breathing and, in severe cases, candidates for heart–lung transplants (➲ Long-term oxygen therapy p. 622).

Care for gastrointestinal associated problems

- Pancreatic enzymes with each meal to aid digestion
- Vitamin supplements, especially A and D
- Medicines to relieve constipation (➲ Constipation and encopresis p. 286)
- ↑ protein and high ↑ calorie diet

Complications and associated issues

Behavioural and psychological problems arising from having life-threatening disease (⊃ Behavioural disorders in children p. 326; ⊃ Child and adolescent mental health p. 246); CF-related diabetes (⊃ Endocrine problems p. 304); fertility problems (⊃ Problems with fertility p. 784); and genetic counselling.

References

21. NICE (2017) *Cystic fibrosis diagnosis and management [NG78]*. Available at: https://www.nice.org.uk/guidance/ng78
22. Cystic Fibrosis Trust (2018) *What is cystic fibrosis?* Available at: ℜ https://www.cysticfibrosis.org.uk/what-is-cystic-fibrosis/faqs

Cerebral palsy

Cerebral palsy (CP) is the most common cause of motor disability in child-hood, characterized by impaired movement and posture[23] (➔ Children with complex health needs and disabilities p. 238). 'Cerebral' refers to the brain's cerebrum, which is the part of the brain that regulates motor function. 'Palsy' describes the paralysis of voluntary movement in muscles within the body. It affects about 1:400 live births in the UK[24] (➔ UK health profile p. 2). Causes:

- Antenatal: periventricular leukomalacia, cerebral malformation, stroke, and infections such as rubella, cytomegalovirus, chickenpox, and toxoplasmosis (➔ Antenatal care and screening p. 426; ➔ Pregnancy p. 424)
- Intrapartum: birth asphyxia/trauma (➔ Complicated labour p. 436)
- Postnatal: head trauma (➔ Safeguarding children p. 248) and brain infections (e.g. meningitis, hydrocephalus)

Increased risk

There are some factors that can ↑ a baby's risk of being born with CP. These include: premature birth babies born ≤32ks (➔ Pre-term infants p. 176); ↓ birthweight; a twin or multiple pregnancy (➔ Twins and multiple births p. 180); the mother being ≥35yrs of age; and the mother having un-usually ↓ or ↑ BP (➔ Common problems in pregnancy p. 432).

Associated problems

- Intellectual impairment
- Epilepsy (➔ Febrile convulsions and epilepsy p. 280; ➔ Seizures and epilepsy p. 740)
- Visual impairment and squints
- Hearing loss (➔ Deafness in children p. 268)
- Speech and language disorders (➔ Speech and language acquisition p. 218)
- Feeding, drooling, and swallowing difficulties
- Gastro-oesophageal reflux disease (GORD)
- Constipation and urinary incontinence (➔ Constipation and encopresis p. 286)
- Scoliosis (➔ Bone and joint problems p. 264)

Classification

Three main types, but mixed forms are common.[25]

Spastic CP

Damage to upper motor neurone pathway. Affects motor function, and muscles are stiff and tight (especially when trying to move them quickly) making it difficult to move and ↓ the range of movement that's possible. Affected limbs are underdeveloped and muscle tone is tight. Spasticity can be very painful with muscles often going into spasm. It can affect many dif-ferent areas of the body.

Athetoid and dyskinetic syndromes

Damage is to basal ganglia. Constant involuntary movements, poor postural control, and unsteadiness in walking and sitting. The person may find it difficult to control the tongue, vocal chords, and breathing. This may affect speech and language.

Ataxic CP

Damage is to the cerebellum. Poor co-ordination, ↓ muscle tone, poor balance, unsteady gait, tremor, and difficulty with fine movements. Most people with ataxic CP can walk but they will be unsteady, with shaky movements. Ataxia can also affect speech and language.

Diagnosis

Often abnormalities in tone, reflexes, and posture are noted during routine developmental screening and referred to paediatrician.

Care management

There is no cure for CP. The aim is to enable children to develop maximum independence and support the family in achieving this. A range of health and social care problems have to be identified and addressed through co-ordinated and multidisciplinary (◆ Teamwork p. 58) care plans involving physiotherapists, occupational therapists, speech and language therapists, community paediatricians, GPs (◆ General practice p. 18), health visitors (◆ Health visiting p. 46), social workers, and early years' care staff and teachers, in liaison with the child and parents.

Medications can be given to relieve symptoms of CP including: oral muscle relaxants; botulinum toxin injections that relax certain muscles or groups of muscles for a few months at a time; melatonin for sleeping difficulties; anti-seizure medication for epilepsy; laxatives for constipation; and painkillers for any pain or discomfort.

References

23. Centers for Disease Control and Prevention (2018) *Basics about cerebral palsy*. Available at: ℘ https://www.cdc.gov/ncbddd/cp/index.html
24. Cerebral Palsy Organization UK (2018) *What is cerebral palsy?* Available at: ℘ https://www.cerebralpalsy.org.uk/cerebral-palsy.html#
25. Scope (2018) *(Family services)*. Available at: ℘ https://www.scope.org.uk/family-services

Autistic spectrum disorder

Autistic spectrum disorder (ASD) is a lifelong developmental disorder with no known cause. There are ~700,000 people on the autism spectrum in the UK.[26] Autism is used here to describe all diagnostic profiles including Asperger syndrome and pathological diagnostic profiles. It presents in early childhood, usually <3yrs, and can be challenging to successfully transition children and young people with autism to live independently in adulthood. Children with developmental difficulties associated with autistic spectrum disorders are identified during the child health programme (➲ Overview of the Healthy Child Programme p. 154). Some professionals use the Modified Checklist for Autism in Toddlers (M-CHAT) as a screening tool to assess for possible indicators of autism, but not to diagnose.[27]

Diagnosis of autistic spectrum disorder

Diagnosis of autism is based on a multidisciplinary team (➲ Teamwork p. 58) assessment involving speech and language therapist (➲ Speech and language acquisition p. 218), paediatrician, educational psychologist, psychiatrist, and occupational therapist.[28] The characteristics of autism vary from one person to another, but in order for a diagnosis to be made a person will usually be assessed as having had persistent difficulties with social communication and social interaction, and restricted and repetitive patterns of behaviours, activities, or interests since early childhood, to the extent that these limit and impair everyday functioning.

Indicators of autism

Indicators of autism in early infancy include no baby babble or use of other vocal sounds (➲ Child development 0–1 years p. 192). Older children have problems using non-verbal behaviours to interact with others (e.g. they have difficulty with eye contact, facial expressions, body language and gestures) (➲ Child development 1–5 years p. 204). They may give no or brief eye contact and ignore familiar or unfamiliar people. Children with ASD are often attracted to older or younger children, rather than interacting with their peers, and they often play alone. They find it difficult to understand emotions and feelings, and find starting conversations challenging (➲ Emotional development in babies and children p. 210). Language development is often delayed. Children often present with atypical physical patterns such as flapping hands and walking on tiptoes. Some have hypersensitivity (e.g. to noise or light). About two thirds have a general learning disability (➲ People with learning disabilities p. 456). About a quarter have epilepsy (➲ Febrile convulsions and epilepsy p. 280; ➲ Seizures and epilepsy p. 740). Many children with autism have very challenging behaviour (➲ Behavioural disorders in children p. 326).

Management

There are many approaches, therapies, and interventions for improving the lives of children and young people with autism. These include referral to specialist services and assessment for special educational needs (➲ Children with special educational needs p. 242). Parents need a great deal of support. Approaches to teaching social skills and ↓ difficult behaviour include: SPELL (structure, positive approaches and expectations, empathy, low arousal, links); TEACCH (teaching, expanding, appreciating, collaborating and co-operating, and holistic); and social stories. Some children will need highly specialized education, whilst others will follow a more mainstream path. Children and young people with moderate symptoms of autism usually grow up to live independent lives, but those with severe symptoms usually need to be supported in adulthood.

Advice on communication

➔ Adults and children with additional communication needs p. 122)

- Always use the child's name at the beginning of the communication so that they know you are talking to them.
- Make sure the child is paying attention before asking a question or giving an instruction.
- Use their special interest, or the activity they are currently doing, to engage them.
- Say less and say it slowly.
- Use specific key words, repeating and stressing them.
- Pause between words and phrases to give the child or young person time to process what has been said.
- Do not use too many questions.
- Use less non-verbal communication (e.g. eye contact, facial expressions, gestures, body language) when the child or young person is showing signs of anxiety.
- Use visual supports.
- Ask only the most necessary questions.
- Take time to structure questions, e.g. offer options or choices.
- Be specific (e.g. ask 'Did you enjoy your lunch?' and 'Did you enjoy your English lesson?' rather than 'How was your day?').
- Avoid using irony, sarcasm, figurative language, rhetorical questions, idioms, or exaggeration.

Advice on behaviour management

Be consistent and keep your word. Try to develop routines through the day and help your child understand what will happen next (e.g. through pictures). Try to recognize patterns or events that are upsetting for the child and trigger tantrums, and move in early to distract from or remove these. Encourage the child to go somewhere safe when they become upset or angry. Find ways of positive encouragement for good behaviour.

Asperger syndrome

Asperger syndrome is a mild form of the social impairments of autism in the presence of near-normal speech development. It manifests in difficulties in social encounters, stilted language, and narrow interests often not shared with others.

References

26. National Autistic Society (2016) *What is autism?* Available at: https://www.autism.org.uk/about/what-is/asd.aspx
27. M-CHAT (2018) *M-CHAT revised with follow up.* Available at: https://m-chat.org/en-us/page/take-m-chat-test/print-version
28. NICE (2011) *Autistic spectrum disorder in under 19s: recognition, referral and diagnosis [CG128].* Available at: https://www.nice.org.uk/guidance/cg128

Further information

National Autistic Society (*Supporting autistic people using the SPELL framework*). Available at: ℬ https://www.autism.org.uk/SPELLintervention
National Autistic Society (*TEACCH*). Available at: ℬ https://www.autism.org.uk/about/strategies/teacch.aspx

Behavioural disorders in children

Behavioural disorders are also known as 'externalizing' disorders. They include attention-deficit hyperactivity disorder (ADHD), oppositional defiant disorder (ODD), and conduct disorder (CDD). Behaviours are usually noticeable by others: aggression, hyperactivity, distractibility, and defiance.

Attention-deficit hyperactivity disorder

Prevalence

- ~2–5% of school-age children can suffer from ADHD
- ♂ more commonly affected than ♀

Presentation

All children can be overactive, behave impulsively, and find it hard to concentrate sometimes. With ADHD, this behaviour is persistent and occurs wherever the child is, not just in one place (e.g. school or at home). Varying degrees of severity. Sometimes found together with other conditions, e.g. dyslexia. ADHD is a distinct condition associated with:

- Impairment in social and/or academic functioning compared to individuals at a comparative level of development
- Developmentally inappropriate degrees of inattention
- Impulsivity
- Hyperactivity
- Presentation before 7yrs
- Presentation in two or more settings
- Not being better accounted for by another disorder

Need to ensure behaviours are not due to other problems, e.g. hearing loss (Э Deafness in children p. 268), epilepsy (Э Febrile convulsions and epilepsy p. 280; Э Seizures and epilepsy p. 740), or Tourette syndrome.

Aetiology

- Strong evidence of genetic contribution
- ↑ maternal consumption of alcohol (Э Alcohol p. 360) during pregnancy (Э Pregnancy p. 424)
- More likely in children who have significant traumatic experiences as a child

Treatment/management

Early identification important. Identify and address any other medical or social problems. Important that all involved with the child work together to assess and agree on ways of managing. Referral to specialists or child and adolescent mental health services (CAMHS) for: parental education; behavioural management; parenting skills work; cognitive behavioural therapy (CBT) (Э Talking therapies p. 472) for school-age or psychological therapies for teenagers; and medication.

Outcome

Family disturbance contributes to continuity of childhood ADHD into adolescence. For many, hyperactivity decreases after adolescence; and for about one in seven children, their ADHD will continue into adulthood, with half having some problems as adults, although not full ADHD.

Associated problems

Difficult interaction with peers, delayed social and educational development (➔ Children with special educational needs p. 242), other psychological problems (➔ Child and adolescent mental health p. 246), and low self-esteem. Can evoke cycle of 'negative parenting'.

Conduct disorders

Conduct disorders are characterized by excessive levels of fighting, bullying, cruelty, destructiveness, stealing, lying, truancy, temper tantrums, and disobedience. They are severe and persistent (>6mths). Delinquency is antisocial law-breaking behaviour. ODD is the term usually reserved for less severe, but equally persistent conduct problems in younger children.

Prevalence

~5% with a strong social class gradient and an excess of ♂

Aetiology

- Adverse psychosocial environments
- Child's temperament
- Poor physical health

Treatment/management

Referral to specialists or CAMHS for: problem-solving skills training; CBT; and family therapy, including parent management training.

Outcome if not 'treated'

- Delinquency, offending, and criminality
- Emotional disorders (➔ Emotional problems in children p. 330)
- Substance misuse (➔ Substance use p. 476)
- Teenage pregnancy
- Early violent deaths

Most antisocial disorders do not progress to adulthood, but many aggressive antisocial adults had the pattern of behaviour in childhood.

Further information

National Attention Deficit Disorder Information Services (*Information centre*). Available at: ℬ http://www.addiss.co.uk/allabout.htm

NICE (*Attention deficit hyperactivity disorder: diagnosis and management*). Available at: ℬ https://www.nice.org.uk/guidance/ng87

NICE (*Antisocial behaviour and conduct disorders in children and young people: recognition and management*). Available at: ℬ https://www.nice.org.uk/guidance/cg158

Royal College of Psychiatrists (*ADHD and hyperkinetic disorder: for parents and carers*). Available at: ℬ https://www.rcpsych.ac.uk/mental-health/parents-and-young-people/information-for-parents-and-carers/attention-deficit-hyperactivity-disorder-and-hyperkinetic-disorder-information-for-parents-carers-and-anyone-working-with-young-people?searchTerms=ADHD

Royal College of Psychiatrists (*Behavioural problems and conduct disorder: for parents, carers and anyone who works with young people*). Available at: ℬ https://www.rcpsych.ac.uk/mental-health/parents-and-young-people/information-for-parents-and-carers/behavioural-problems-and-conduct-disorder-for-parents-carers-and-anyone-who-works-with-young-people?searchTerms=conduct%20disorder

Young Minds (*ADHD and mental health*). Available at: ℬ https://youngminds.org.uk/find-help/conditions/adhd-and-mental-health/#what-is-adhd

Depressive behaviours

This includes depressive feelings, depressive behaviour, depressive cognitions or beliefs, as well as depressive disorders (→ Child and adolescent mental health p. 246). Depression is thought to occur in 1–3% children and young people, with an ↑ in prevalence as children get older. ♀ outnumber ♂ in diagnosed problems in adolescence. Predisposing factors include: genetic, temperament, biological, chronic life adversity. Factors associated with an ↑ risk of depression include:

- Psychosocial: family discord, bullying, all forms of abuse
- Other disorders: including drug and alcohol use (→ Alcohol p. 360; → Substance use p. 476), and a history of parental depression (→ People with anxiety and depression p. 478)
- Social problems: including homelessness (→ Homeless people p. 446) and living in institutional settings (→ Looked-after children p. 254)
- Single life-event losses (→ Coping with bereavement p. 574)

Presentation

Common to suffer > one internalizing disorder, e.g. anxiety, social withdrawal, loneliness.

Preschool

- Apathy and food refusal, miserable, irritable, cries, and rocks
- Growth failure may occur (→ Growth 0–2 years p. 190)

5–12yrs

- Use language of emotional affect
- Psychosomatic symptoms
- Poor concentration, failure to progress at school
- Irritability, social withdrawal, temper outbursts (→ Behavioural disorders in children p. 326)
- Usually complain of being bored

Adolescence

- Alike to adulthood depression
- Complaints of boredom, sadness, apathy, lacking energy
- Appetite and sleep disorders more common

Assessment in primary care

- Identify if one of following key symptoms present most days, most of the time >2wks: persistent sadness or low (irritable) mood; loss of interests and/or pleasure; and fatigue or low energy.
- If any key symptoms present, ask about associated symptoms: poor or increased sleep; poor concentration or indecisiveness; ↓ self-confidence; poor or increased appetite; suicidal thoughts or acts; self-harm thoughts; agitation or slowing of movements; and guilt or self-blame (→ Suicidal intent and deliberate self-harm p. 494).
- Find out about past history of depression, life events, family history, associated disability, school contexts, quality of family and peer relationships, and availability of social support.

Action on assessment

If seen as mild depression with few of these symptoms, no family history, social support present, not actively suicidal, then general advice and watchful waiting. Reiterate advice on good nutrition, good sleep patterns, and need for exercise. Offer emotional support/active listening or referral to self-help groups or other forms of support (e.g. youth groups). Respond to identified adverse events/problems such as action in instances of bullying.

If five or more symptoms, past or family history, ↓ level of social support, associated social disability, child or relative requests, self-neglect (➲ Safeguarding children p. 248), then see as moderate or severe depression with more active 1° care intervention and/or referral to Child and Adolescent Mental Health Services (CAMHS). ⚠ Urgent referral to CAMHS psychiatrist if active suicidal ideas, psychotic symptoms, severe agitation, severe self-neglect.

Mental health treatments

Depends on severity of depression:

- Ongoing mild depression beyond 4wks: non-directive supportive therapy, group CBT, or guided self-help (➲ Talking therapies p. 472)
- Moderate to severe depression: specific psychological therapy, e.g. individual CBT, interpersonal therapy, or shorter-term family therapy. If unresponsive, different and combined therapies considered, including the use of medication.

Inpatient care considered when child or young person at significant risk of self-harm.

Advice for family members

- Encourage child to talk about worries; listen and offer help
- If suspect more than passing phase, contact GP/get professional help

Outcomes

- Most children (two out of three) improve, but full recovery may take years
- Liability to further episodes
- Increased risk of depression in adulthood

Further information

NICE (*Depression in children and young people*). Available at: ℘ www.nice.org.uk/CG28

Royal College of Psychiatrists (*Depression in children and young people: for young people*). Available at: ℘ https://www.rcpsych.ac.uk/mental-health/parents-and-young-people/young-people/depression-in-children-and-young-people-for-young-people

Young Minds (*Depression*). Available at: ℘ https://youngminds.org.uk/find-help/conditions/depression/#what-is-depression?

Young Minds (*Suicidal feelings*). Available at: ℘ https://youngminds.org.uk/find-help/feelings-and-symptoms/suicidal-feelings/

Emotional problems in children

This includes a range of internalizing disorders including fear, anxiety, and phobias. Management and treatment approaches are similar.

Fear and anxiety

Fear focuses on a specific object or situation. Anxiety is diffuse and anticipatory (has developmental variations):

- Both fear and anxiety result in the same physiological manifestations: unhappiness, irritability, tantrums, sleep disruption
- Age and sex trends: no consistent sex differences during infancy and preschool years; however, in school years it is suggested that ♀ have more specific fears than ♂

Anxiety in infants as part of normal development

- ➔ Child development 1–5 years p. 204
- Stranger anxiety: by 4–5mths, peaks 12mths
- Separation anxiety: related to stranger anxiety, from 8–24mths, peaks 9–13mths, decreases from 30mths

Anxiety in childhood and adolescence

- ➔ Child development 5–11 years p. 220; ➔ Working with teenagers p. 232
- Separation and stranger anxiety diminish as capacity to anticipate events develops
- Stranger fear may manifest itself as shyness
- At school age, most common fears are for harm coming to others
- May start to exhibit anxiety about personal adequacy and achievement (e.g. test anxiety)
- Adolescents may show anxieties relating to social situations (e.g. rejection, may develop phobias or sexual fears)

Generalized anxiety disorder

Characterized as 'worriers'; affects ~2% of children. Not related to environmental circumstances. Five broad features: worries; restlessness, nervousness, and inability to relax; physical symptoms; difficulty concentrating; and irritability.

Separation anxiety disorder

Anxiety related to separation from people to whom child is attached. Affects ~3% of children. Onset occurs before adolescence; may continue into early adulthood. May result in school refusal—peak occurs at time of transition, also in adolescence and at 5yrs, 11yrs, 14–15yrs is most common.

Specific phobias

These are fears that result in avoidance behaviour to the point of interfering with daily functioning. These may involve certain objects or situations. The child may develop anticipatory anxiety for phobic situation. Prevalence is unknown.

Aetiology
- Genetic and constitutional: runs in families
- Temperament
- Parental behaviour (e.g. overprotection and criticism)
- Specific experiences and life events
- Cognitive appraisal of stressful events (e.g. abuse (➲ Safeguarding children p. 248))
- Social adversity

Treatment/management
Referred to local CAMHS as per local guidance (➲ Child and adolescent mental health p. 246). Interventions dependent on type of anxiety:
- Generalized anxiety: remove/↓ stresses; enhance coping mechanisms; psychotherapy (➲ Talking therapies p. 472); medication may help
- Separation anxiety: brief, focused counselling; improve understanding of anxiety; behavioural treatment (e.g. behavioural control skills)
- Other specific phobias: behavioural methods
- Panic disorder: behavioural methods; medication may help
- Social phobia: behavioural methods

Behavioural methods
Modification of acceptable and unacceptable behaviours. Reinforcement of good/wanted behaviour, ignore/distract from unacceptable/bad behaviour. May use training procedures—rewards (reinforcement) and punishments. Generally, children with anxiety disorders have reasonably good prognosis, but may experience some remissions and some exacerbations throughout childhood and into adulthood.

Advice for parents
Follow guidance on basics for emotional support, as well as specifics as provided by CAMHS.

Related topics
➲ Emotional development in babies and children p. 210; ➲ Understanding behaviour 1–5 years p. 216; ➲ Behavioural disorders in children p. 326

Further information
Association for Infant Mental Health (AIMH) (*Why does AIMH exist?*). Available at: ℛ https://aimh. org.uk/about/

Mental Health Foundation Children and Young People (*Children and young people*). Available at: ℛ https://www.mentalhealth.org.uk/a-to-z/c/children-and-young-people

Royal College of Psychiatrists (*Young people's mental health*). Available at: ℛ https://www.rcpsych. ac.uk/mental-health/parents-and-young-people

Adult health promotion

Models and approaches to health promotion *334*

Group health promotion *336*

Community approaches to health *338*

Expert patients and self-management programmes *340*

Nutrition and healthy eating *342*

Adult body mass index chart *346*

Overweight and obesity *348*

Malnutrition *350*

Home food safety and hygiene *352*

Exercise *354*

Smoking cessation *356*

Managing stress *358*

Alcohol *360*

UK screening programmes *362*

Menopause *364*

Healthy ageing *366*

Falls prevention *368*

Weather extremes *370*

Cancer prevention *372*

Skin cancer prevention *374*

Bowel cancer screening *376*

Breast cancer awareness and screening *378*

Cervical cancer screening *380*

Cervical sample taking *384*

Testicular self-examination *386*

New patient health check *387*

Abdominal aortic aneurysm screening *388*

Immunization administration *390*

Targeted adult immunization *392*

Travel healthcare *394*

Travel health promotion *396*

Malaria prevention *398*

Travel vaccinations *399*

Contraception: general *400*

Combined hormonal contraceptive methods *402*

Incorrect use of combined hormonal contraceptive methods *406*

Contraception: progestogen-only methods *410*

Contraception: intrauterine devices and systems *414*

Barrier contraceptive methods *416*

Natural family planning and sterilization *418*

Emergency contraception *420*

Preconceptual care *422*

Pregnancy *424*

Antenatal education and preparation for parenthood *425*

Antenatal care and screening *426*

Maternity rights and benefits *430*

Common problems in pregnancy *432*

Birth options and labour *434*

Complicated labour *436*

Postnatal care *438*

Postnatal depression *440*

Models and approaches to health promotion

Health promotion aims to enable people to ↑ control over and to improve their health. It involves a wide range of individual, social, and environmental interventions. The Ottawa Charter[1] incorporates three strategies to enable, mediate, and advocate for health by: building healthy public policy; creating supportive environments; strengthening community actions; developing personal skills; and reorientating health services. There is no universally accepted model of health promotion. There are three main types of approaches: individual-focused, group-focused, community-focused. Table 8.1 summarizes the main theories and key concepts within these approaches.

Table 8.1 Summary of theories: focus and key concepts of health promotion

Theory	Focus	Key concepts
Stages of change model	Individual's readiness to change or attempt to change toward healthy behaviours	• Pre-contemplation • Contemplation • Decision/determination • Action • Maintenance
Health belief model	Person's perception of the threat of a health problem and the appraisal of recommended behaviour(s) for preventing or managing the problem	• Perceived susceptibility • Perceived severity • Perceived benefits of action • Cues to actions • Self-efficacy
Social learning theory	Behaviour explained via a 3-way, reciprocal theory = personal factors, environmental influences, and behaviour continually interact	• Behaviour capability • Reciprocal determinism • Expectations of self-efficacy • Observational learning • Reinforcement
Community organization theories	Emphasizes active participation and development of communities that can better evaluate and solve health and social problems	• Empowerment • Community competence • Participation and relevance • Issue selection • Critical consciousness
Organizational change theory	Strategies for ↑ chances that healthy policies and programmes will be adopted and maintained in formal organizations, e.g. NHS	• Problem definition • Initiation of action • Implementation of change • Institutionalization of change
Diffusion of innovation theory	How new ideas, products, and social practices spread within a society or from one society to another	• Relative advantage • Compatibility • Complexity • Trialability • Observability

Individual-focused approaches

Making behavioural changes such as improving diet (◆ Nutrition and healthy eating p. 342) or reducing alcohol consumption (◆ Alcohol p. 360) can considerably reduce the risk of poor health. Making Every Contact Count[2] emphasizes that every interaction between healthcare professionals and service users/patients is an opportunity to promote health. Practitioners may use a range of interventions with an individual to improve their health, but they will usually include a behaviour change technique as it is important to sustain the changes.[3]

Group-focused approaches

Normally a combination of educational and behavioural change approaches (◆ Group health promotion p. 336), although can also be community development focused. Requires an understanding of group dynamics.

Community-focused approaches to health promotion

Involves one or a combination of approaches.

Epidemiological-focused approaches

Based on information on prevalence and/or incidence of condition in geographical area (◆ Health needs assessment p. 15). Use standardized statistical information to introduce health promotion initiatives (e.g. tuberculosis (◆ Tuberculosis p. 728) prevention).

Social/societal change

Initiating or lobbying for change involving policy or legislation change or innovation. Often based on epidemiological evidence, but may be instigated by expressed need of community or policy initiative (e.g. physical activity promotion).

Community development

Interventions are identified by the community (◆ Community approaches to health p. 338). They may involve health and other professionals working with communities to empower them to identify their own health promotion and health improvement needs. These may differ radically from the agenda of health and social care professionals.

Related topics

◆ Public health in the NHS and beyond p. 14; ◆ Key definitions of primary care and public health p. 4

References

1. WHO (1986) *Ottawa Charter for Health Promotion.* Available at: http://www.who.int/healthpromotion/conferences/previous/ottawa/en/
2. NHS Health Education England (2018). Available at: http://www.makingeverycontactcount.co.uk/
3. NICE (2014) *Behaviour change: individual approaches [PH49].* Available at: https://www.nice.org.uk/guidance/ph49

Further information

NHS Scotland (*Improve policy and practice*). Available at: ℘ http://www.healthscotland.scot/improve-policy-and-practice
PHE (*Health and wellbeing: introduction to the directorate*). Available at: ℘ https://www.gov.uk/government/publications/health-and-wellbeing-introduction-to-the-directorate
Public Health Northern Ireland (*About us*). Available at: ℘ http://www.publichealth.hscni.net/about-us
Public Health Wales (*About us*). Available at: ℘ http://www.publichealthwales.wales.nhs.uk/
WHO (*Healthy settings*). Available at: ℘ http://www.who.int/healthy_settings/en/

Group health promotion

Group work can be an effective method of health promotion (➋ Models and approaches to health promotion p. 334), although there is little evidence to show that it is more effective than individual health promotion[1] (➋ Evidence-based healthcare p. 72). Health visitors (➋ Health visiting p. 46) and other public health nurses (➋ Public health in the NHS and beyond p. 14) are often more involved in group health promotion work than other nurses in 1° care, but all nurses can use these techniques. Group health promotion could include:

- Teaching about health topics to a small group (e.g. antenatal education classes (➋ Antenatal education and preparation for parenthood p. 425), a class in a school (➋ Health promotion in schools p. 230), a leg ulcer club (➋ Leg ulcer assessment p. 536)
- Using techniques from participatory adult learning in community group situations (e.g. session on contraception (➋ Contraception: general p. 400) in youth group)
- Forming and/or supporting groups for self-help, mutual support, and health information (e.g. carers' (➋ Carers p. 458) support group)
- Becoming part of a group made up of local people/professionals to influence policy and/or services (e.g. estate action group or campaigning group on housing problems (➋ Homes and housing p. 26))

In each case, it is important to consider how the outcomes of the group may be determined by leadership style (➋ Leadership p. 60), personality, participant characteristics, or the more complex interactions that occur in groups.

Principles of health promotion in small groups

Setting

- Consider how the setting will impact on the group processes and outcomes (e.g. access issues, comfort, temperature, or meaning attributed to the setting by participants).
- Plan how the environment will help group work (e.g. seats in circles, separate crèche for small children).

Intervention

- Consider what the intervention is going to be and what quantity will be delivered.
- Consider what outcomes are required (e.g. to initiate behaviours or to sustain change in behaviour).
- Decide what the target population will be and how they will become group members.
- Plan how you will use your time with the group and plan the appropriate materials.

In the session

- Involve everyone from the beginning by getting them to introduce themselves and saying what they would like to get out of session.

Consider icebreaking activities that encourage each member to speak briefly.

- Establish any ground rules the group think are necessary (e.g. listen to each other, discussion confidential (→ Confidentiality p. 89) to the group).
- Use activities that include active participation and sharing by the members such as: brainstorming (e.g. what are the different types of contraception?); problem solving (e.g. what would you advise mum to do if 3yr-old John has a full-blown temper tantrum in the supermarket?); discussions (e.g. sharing experiences of health behaviour); and exercises (e.g. completing puzzles or practical exercises to learn about healthy options).
- Break up time and change activities using additional inputs/health promotion materials.
- Summarize activity at the end of the session. Offer time for participants to summarize/raise any issues. Provide back-up written materials or detailed information (e.g. local directory of services aimed at carers).

Principles for helping to establish and run a group

- Identify the need for the group; make sure a similar group does not already exist that you could support or refer to instead.
- Clarify the purpose of the group (e.g. support/social opportunity (→ Social support p. 28) for carers, with 'sitting' facilities for person cared for).
- Consider any finance required and possible local sources.
- Identify a suitable local venue for the purpose of the group.
- Identify the target participants for the group and send out personal invitations plus wider local publicity.
- Consider the relationship between the leader and the participants in the group and who will carry out organizational tasks.
- Plan first meeting and tasks for facilitators, e.g. arranging space, greeting people, starting and ending the meeting.
- Consider how to involve others in group roles to share workload and increase commitment.
- Consider how the group could become self-sustaining.
- Recognize that many groups have their own life cycle, and ending a group or watching it change into something completely different is often appropriate and healthy.

Reference

4. Hoddinott, P., Allan, K., Avenell, A., & Britten., J. (2010) Group interventions to improve health outcomes: a framework for their design and delivery. *BMC Public Health*, 10, 800

Further information

Scriven, A. (2010) *Promoting health: a practical guide* (6th edn). Edinburgh: Baillière Tindall Elsevier, pp. 177–90 (Working with groups)

Community approaches to health

Despite advances in healthcare, avoidable health inequalities persist (➲ UK health profile p. 2). Communities have an important role to play in improving health.[5] Healthy communities are characterized by social cohesion and civic engagement. The family of community-centred approaches is a framework of evidence-based interventions (➲ Evidence-based healthcare p. 72) to strengthen communities and improve community health.[6]

Strengthening communities

Developing community capacities and assets to take action on health and the social determinants of health, without relying on healthcare services. Examples include programmes tackling: social isolation (➲ Social support p. 28) (e.g. Buddy Hub (🔗 https://www.buddyhub.co.uk/) and Men's Sheds (🔗 https://menssheds.org.uk/)); recovery communities for people with a history of drug (➲ Substance use p. 476) or alcohol misuse (➲ Alcohol p. 360) (e.g. Alcoholics Anonymous (🔗 https://www.alcoholics-anonymous. org.uk/)); and time banking (a reciprocity-based work-trading system in which hours are the currency).

Volunteer and peer roles

Enhancing individuals' capabilities to provide advice, information, and support, or to organize activities around health in their communities: health trainer roles (e.g. gypsy traveller (➲ Gypsies and travellers p. 448) health workers); peer support roles (e.g. breastfeeding (➲ Breastfeeding p. 182) support workers); peer trainer roles (e.g. trainers on self-management programmes (➲ Expert patients and self-management programmes p. 340)); and volunteer health roles (e.g. walking for health scheme leaders (➲ Exercise p. 354)).

Collaborations and partnership

Encouraging communities and local services to work together (➲ Teamwork p. 58) in the planning, design, commissioning (➲ Commissioning of services p. 12), and delivery of healthcare services.

Access to community resources

Connecting people to community resources, practical help, group activities, and volunteering opportunities to meet health needs and increase social participation:

- Social prescribing: referrals to a range of local, non-clinical services (e.g. prescription for learning, an arts prescription, books on prescription, or exercise on prescription)
- Community hubs: providing facilities to foster community activity and bring residents, local businesses, and organizations together to improve quality of life (see Bromley by Bow Centre (🔗 https://www.bbbc.org.uk/))

Related topics

➲ Health needs assessment p. 15; ➲ Public health in the NHS and beyond p. 14; ➲ Models and approaches to health promotion p. 334

References

5. King's Fund (2018) *Communities and health*. Available at: https://www.kingsfund.org.uk/publications/communities-and-health
6. PHE (2015) *A guide to community-centred approaches to health and wellbeing*. Available at: https://assets.publishing.service.gov.uk/government/uploads/system/uploads/attachment_data/file/417515/A_guide_to_community-centred_approaches_for_health_and_wellbeing__full_report_.pdf

Expert patients and self-management programmes

Expert patients are people living with a long-term condition (LTC) who are able to take more control over their health by understanding and managing their condition.

Benefits of patient engagement

Patient engagement is critical to managing health spending and improving patient outcomes. Expert patients may: demonstrate ↑ confidence and control of their lives; manage their condition in partnership with healthcare professionals; communicate effectively with healthcare professions and share responsibility for treatment; be realistic about the impact of their disease on themselves and their family (➲ Carers p. 458); and use their skills and knowledge to lead full lives. Leading healthcare providers, commissioners, and entrepreneurs are harnessing the expert patient. For example: incentivizing healthier lives through the Vitality Insurance Programme; patient-led commissioning (➲ Commissioning of services p. 12) through Personal Health Budgets; online and remote healthcare support through HealthConnect at Kaiser Permanente; and peer to peer support through the PatientsLikeMe online community.[7]

Self-Management UK

Formerly called the Expert Patient Programme, Self-Management UK was an NHS initiative launched to help patients with LTCs to develop new skills to self-manage their condition better and take control of their lives. It recognizes that people with all kinds of LTCs are dealing with similar issues on a daily basis, including pain, stress (➲ Managing stress p. 358), and low self-esteem.

Self-Management UK is a charitable organization commissioned to deliver self-management courses in local community venues as well as online. These courses are free to patients and carers, and provide tools and techniques to develop the confidence, skills, and knowledge to manage any LTC. The focus is on five core skills: problem solving; decision making; making the best use of resources; developing effective partnerships with healthcare providers; and taking appropriate action. The majority of courses are delivered by trained tutors who have personal experience of living with a LTC. Courses usually run over six weekly sessions and include topics such as: dealing with pain; extreme tiredness; coping with feelings of depression (➲ People with anxiety and depression p. 478); relaxation techniques; exercise (➲ Exercise p. 354); healthy eating (➲ Nutrition and healthy eating p. 342); communicating with family, friends, and healthcare professionals; and planning for the future (➲ Mental capacity p. 470).

Other programmes

In addition to programmes provided by Self-Management UK, other self-management programmes are available and sometimes commissioned, e.g. DESMOND (Diabetes Education and Self-Management for Ongoing and Newly Diagnosed Diabetes) (➲ Principles of diabetes management p. 664).

Reference

7. Corrie, C. & Finch, A. (2015) *Expert patients*. Available at: http://www.reform.uk/wp-content/uploads/2015/02/Expert-patients.pdf

Further information

DESMOND (*General enquiries*). Available at: ℜ http://www.desmond-project.org.uk/about/contact/

Self-Management UK (*Contact us*). Available at: ℜ https://www.selfmanagementuk.org/contact-us

Nutrition and healthy eating

Energy is needed to stay alive, grow, keep warm, and be active. Carbohydrates, proteins, and fat provide energy. Estimated average requirements for energy in the UK:

- ♂ 19–54yrs: 74kg, 2682kcal/day
- ♀ 19–54yrs: 61–63kg, 2139kcal/day

Energy requirements ↓ gradually >50yrs in ♀ and >60yrs in ♂ as typically activity levels ↓. Energy requirements for pregnancy (➔ Pregnancy p. 424) increase by 0.8MJ/day or 200kcal/day, but only in the final 3mths. To maintain body weight, it is necessary to expend as much energy as is derived from food (➔ Malnutrition p. 350); to lose weight, energy must exceed intake[8] (➔ Overweight and obesity p. 348).

Body mass index (BMI)

BMI is a tool for calculating healthy weight for height. BMI = weight/height.[9] Normal BMI = 18.5–24.9; <18.5 = underweight; 25–30 = overweight; >30 = obese; >40 = severely obese (➔ Adult body mass index chart p. 346).

Waist circumference

Also used to assess obesity and associated health risk. Measured mid-point between lowest rib and top of right iliac crest. ♂ >94cm (37 inches) and ♀ >80cm (31.5 inches) associated with ↑ visceral fat mass and comorbidities. Increased risk for people of Asian origin at ≥90cm (35 inches) for ♂ and ≥80cm (31 inches) for ♀.

Nutritional requirements

Carbohydrates

Recommended as 50% of daily intake, with not more than 5% free sugars. Complex (plant-derived) (e.g. bread, potatoes, rice) are slower to break down and release energy.

Protein

Recommended as 15% of daily intake. Needed for growth and repair, and energy (e.g. fish, meat, legumes). Protein requirements ↓ for ♂ >50yrs, but increase slightly for ♀. Calculate as 0.75g protein per kg body weight per day in adults.

Fibre

Recommended average 18g/day for an adult. Keeps gut healthy and helps prevent constipation (e.g. fruit and vegetables) (➔ Constipation in adults p. 512).

Fats

Total recommended as up to 35% of daily intake, with not more than 11% saturated fat. Unsaturated fats include nuts, oily fish, vegetable oils. Saturated fats include meat products, hard cheese, and butter. Required for absorption of vitamins, energy, and essential fatty acids omega-3 and omega-6.

Vitamins

Government recommended daily allowance includes:
- A: for growth, development, and eyesight
- B group: help body use energy
- B12: for blood cells and nerve function
- C: for skin and tissue growth, also absorption of iron
- D: for bone metabolism and calcium absorption

Minerals
- Calcium: for development and maintenance of bones. i ♀ requirement for calcium after menopause (➔ Menopause p. 364)
- Iron: for red blood cells. After menopause, ♀ requirement for iron is reduced to same level as that for ♂.
- Phytonutrients: plant compounds that act as antioxidants against free radicals (substances implicated in cancer and heart disease)

Hydration

Intake of 1.5–2L of fluids/day recommended in temperate climates

A healthy balanced diet

Encourage a diverse diet from the five food groups, eating more from groups 1 and 2 than 3 or 4

Group 1: fruit and vegetables

Five or more portions a day. Portion = 80g (e.g. one medium apple, a bowl of salad, three heaped tablespoons of peas). Fruit juice, smoothies, beans, and pulses only count as one portion per day.

Group 2: bread, other cereals, and potatoes

A third of total food intake. At least one food from this group at each meal.

Group 3: milk and dairy foods

Two or three servings a day. A serving = milk 200mL glass, yogurt small pot (150g), cheese 30g (matchbox size).

Group 4: meat, fish, and alternatives

Moderate amounts recommended, as well as two portions of fish (two oily fish) each week. Vegetarians and vegans should ensure adequate protein, iron, selenium, and vitamin B12 (especially vegans) in diet.

Group 5: foods containing fat or sugar

Sparingly (e.g. butter, spreads, sweets, crisps) or not eaten too often.

The amounts that should be consumed will vary depending on energy needs (based on age, sex, and physical activity levels) and appetite. See Box 8.1 for healthy eating guidelines.

Box 8.1 Eight guidelines for healthy eating
- Base your meals on starchy foods.
- Eat lots of fruit and vegetables.
- Eat more fish.
- Cut down on saturated fat and sugar.
- Eat ↓ salt (<6g/day).
- Get active and try to be a healthy weight.
- Drink plenty of water.
- Do not skip breakfast.

Reference

8. British Nutrition Foundation (2016) *Nutrition requirements*, Available at: www.nutrition.org.uk

Further information

Food Standards Agency (*Nutrition*). Available at: ℘ https://www.food.gov.uk/topic/nutrition

Adult body mass index chart

⚠ Assessing growth and BMI of children and young people is undertaken differently (Chapter 3: Child Health Promotion). Adult BMI charts (Fig. 8.1) are not accurate for pregnant women (➲ Pregnancy p. 424), athletes, or older people.

Related topics

➲ Overweight and obesity p. 348; ➲ Malnutrition p. 350

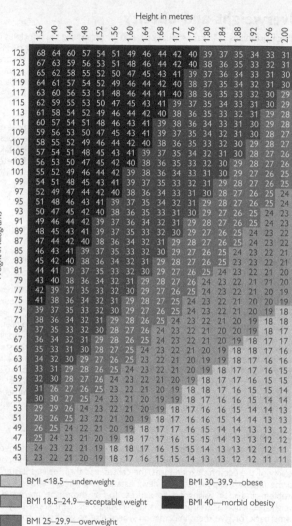

Height in metres

	1.36	1.40	1.44	1.48	1.52	1.56	1.60	1.64	1.68	1.72	1.76	1.80	1.84	1.88	1.92	1.96	2.00
125	68	64	60	57	54	51	49	46	44	42	40	39	37	35	34	33	31
123	67	63	59	56	53	51	48	46	44	42	40	38	36	35	33	32	31
121	65	62	58	55	52	50	47	45	43	41	39	37	36	34	33	31	30
119	64	61	57	54	52	49	46	44	42	40	38	37	35	34	32	31	30
117	63	60	56	53	51	48	46	44	41	40	38	36	35	33	32	30	29
115	62	59	55	53	50	47	45	43	41	39	37	35	34	33	31	30	29
113	61	58	54	52	49	46	44	42	40	38	36	35	33	32	31	29	28
111	60	57	54	51	48	46	43	41	39	38	36	34	33	31	30	29	28
109	59	56	53	50	47	45	43	41	39	37	35	34	32	31	30	28	27
107	58	55	52	49	46	44	42	40	38	36	35	33	32	30	29	28	27
105	57	54	51	48	45	43	41	39	37	35	34	32	31	30	28	27	26
103	56	53	50	47	45	42	40	38	36	35	33	32	30	29	28	27	26
101	55	52	49	46	44	42	39	38	36	34	33	31	30	29	27	26	25
99	54	51	48	45	43	41	39	37	35	33	32	31	29	28	27	26	25
97	52	49	47	44	42	40	38	36	34	33	31	30	28	27	26	25	24
95	51	48	46	43	41	39	37	35	34	32	31	29	28	27	26	25	24
93	50	47	45	42	40	38	36	35	33	31	30	29	27	26	25	24	23
91	49	46	44	42	39	37	36	34	32	31	29	28	27	26	25	24	23
89	48	45	43	41	39	37	35	33	32	30	29	27	26	25	24	23	22
87	47	44	42	40	38	36	34	32	31	29	28	27	26	25	24	23	22
85	46	43	41	39	37	35	33	32	30	29	27	26	25	24	23	22	21
83	45	42	40	38	36	34	32	31	29	28	27	26	25	23	23	22	21
81	44	41	39	37	35	33	32	30	29	27	26	25	24	23	22	21	20
79	43	40	38	36	34	32	31	29	28	27	26	24	23	22	21	21	20
77	42	39	37	35	33	32	30	29	27	26	25	24	23	22	21	20	19
75	41	38	36	34	32	31	29	28	27	25	24	23	22	21	20	20	19
73	39	37	35	33	32	30	29	27	26	25	24	23	22	21	20	19	18
71	38	36	34	32	31	29	28	26	25	24	23	22	21	20	19	18	18
69	37	35	33	32	30	28	27	26	24	23	22	21	20	20	19	18	17
67	36	34	32	31	29	28	26	25	24	23	22	21	20	19	18	17	17
65	35	33	31	30	28	27	25	24	23	22	21	20	19	18	18	17	16
63	34	32	30	29	27	26	25	23	22	21	20	19	19	18	17	16	16
61	33	31	29	28	26	25	24	23	22	21	20	19	18	17	17	16	15
59	32	30	28	27	26	24	23	22	21	20	19	18	17	17	16	15	15
57	31	26	27	26	25	23	22	21	20	19	18	18	17	16	15	15	14
55	30	30	27	25	24	23	21	20	19	19	18	17	16	16	15	14	14
53	29	29	26	24	23	22	21	20	19	18	17	16	16	15	14	14	13
51	28	26	25	23	22	21	20	19	18	17	16	16	15	14	14	13	13
49	26	25	24	22	21	20	19	18	17	17	16	15	14	14	13	13	12
47	25	24	23	21	20	19	18	17	17	16	15	15	14	13	13	12	12
45	24	23	22	21	19	18	18	17	16	15	15	14	13	13	12	12	11
43	23	22	21	20	19	18	17	16	15	15	14	13	13	12	12	11	11

Weight in kilograms

BMI <18.5—underweight

BMI 18.5–24.9—acceptable weight

BMI 25–29.9—overweight

BMI 30–39.9—obese

BMI 40—morbid obesity

Fig. 8.1 BMI ready reckoner.

Reproduced from Simon, C., Everitt, H., & Van Dorp, F. (2010) Oxford Handbook of General Practice (3rd edn). Oxford: Oxford University Press. By permission of Oxford University Press.

Overweight and obesity

All opportunities in 1° care should be taken for promoting the principles of good nutrition and healthy eating (**◆** Nutrition and healthy eating p. 342) and exercise (**◆** Exercise p. 354). Particularly important to teach children and young people these principles, as eating patterns continue into adulthood (**◆** Overweight children and adolescents p. 302). In 2014, 64% of adults in England were obese[9] (**◆** UK health profile p. 2).

Overweight

People who take in more energy than they require, store the energy as excess fat and become overweight, and if this continues will become obese. The main contributory factors are sedentary lifestyle and ↑ energy intake. Obesity is directly linked to increased risks of morbidity, e.g. diabetes, coronary heart disease (CHD), and hypertension. Classification of BMI (**◆** Adult body mass index charts p. 346):

• 18.5–24.9 = healthy weight
• 25–29.9 = overweight
• 30–34.9 = obese Class I
• 35–39.9 = obese Class II
• >40 = morbid obesity

⚠ People of Asian origins at ↑ risk of morbidity at lower BMI levels.

Obesity

Obesity is a major public health issue (**◆** Public health in the NHS and beyond p. 14). Many factors interact to cause weight gain (e.g. behavioural, genetic predisposition, lifestyle). Weight gain increases with age; ♀ gain weight more easily; ↑ risk in lower socioeconomic groups; ↑ prevalence in some minority ethnic groups (e.g. ♀ of Caribbean and Pakistani origin). 80% of ex-smokers ↑ weight, but benefits of cessation outweigh not stopping (**◆** Smoking cessation p. 356). People who are obese have a ↓ life expectancy, ↑ risk of developing CHD (**◆** Coronary heart disease p. 624) and Type 2 diabetes (**◆** Diabetes: overview p. 660), as well as ↑ risk of respiratory and musculoskeletal (MSK) problems (**◆** Common musculoskeletal problems p. 734) and stress incontinence (**◆** Urinary incontinence p. 504).

Raising the issue

Assess willingness to change. Overweight and obesity is an issue that needs to be raised in an open, empathetic manner that acknowledges the complexity of the person's experiences, the causes, and their feelings. Listening to the patient's experience and views establishes their perception of the problem and their willingness to address it. For those not interested in weight reduction at this point, it is important to let them know they can come back, or give them information where else to go if they choose to address the issue later.

Supporting those interested in weight reduction

In general, aim to promote good nutrition and healthy eating, ↑ physical activity and ↓ sedentary behaviour, and ↑ self-awareness about day-to-day behaviours. Make time to clarify patient expectations and ability to engage. Discuss the options on how to support weight reduction. This may be inside the NHS (e.g. community dieticians, GP practice (➔ General practice p. 18) may have a weight management protocol, weight management clinic, or health visitors (➔ Health visiting p. 46) may have a weight management group) or outside of the NHS (e.g. Weight Watchers (🖱 https://www. weightwatchers.com/uk/)).

Supporting weight reduction in primary care

The aim is for a realistic, modest weight loss. Some local areas are supported by community dietician programmes and protocols. Protocols usually include:

- Agreement between person and professional on goals and means of achieving them
- Structured assessment, recording, and regular follow-up
- Specific dietary advice and menu sheets for weight loss: ↓ calorific intake by about 600kcal/day to total of 1200–1600kcal will usually achieve target weight loss; ↓ fat intake with accompanying ↑ in fruit and vegetables
- Advice supported with weight management leaflets, activity and eating diaries, information on local organizations, and increasing exercise
- Group activities have higher success rates in reducing and maintaining weight loss than one-on-one consultations

Obese people with attendant health problems and difficulties in losing weight may be considered by GPs for drug therapies or, as a last resort, surgical intervention.

Reference

9. NHS Digital (2018) *Statistics on obesity, physical activity and diet, England 2018*. Available at: https:// www.gov.uk/government/statistics/statistics-on-obesity-physical-activity-and-diet-england-2018

Further information

Food Standards Agency (*Nutrition*). Available at: 🖱 https://www.food.gov.uk/topic/nutrition
National Obesity Forum (*About the National Obesity Forum*). Available at: 🖱 http://www. nationalobesityforum.org.uk/index.php/about-the-nof.html
NICE (*Obesity prevention [CG43]*). Available at: 🖱 https://www.nice.org.uk/guidance/CG43

Malnutrition

Malnutrition can refer to either over- or undernutrition. This section focuses specifically on undernutrition in adults: a deficiency of energy, protein, and other nutrients. The impact of undernutrition includes:[10]

- ↑ risk of falls (⊃ Falls prevention p. 368)
- ↓ recovery from illness and surgery
- ↓ clinical outcomes (including ↑ mortality)
- ↓ immune response
- ↓ muscle strength and frailty (⊃ Frailty p. 678)
- ↓ wound healing (⊃ Wound assessment p. 522)
- ↓ psychosocial functioning

At-risk groups

- People with LTCs (e.g. COPD (⊃ Chronic obstructive pulmonary disease p. 614), cancer, gastrointestinal disease (⊃ Coeliac disease p. 714); ⊃ Inflammatory bowel disease p. 712))
- Progressive neurological disease (e.g. dementia, (⊃ People with dementia p. 498), motor neurone disease (⊃ Motor neurone disease p. 672))
- Acute illness (where adequate food is not consumed ≥5 days)
- Debility (including frailty, immobility, depression (⊃ People with anxiety and depression p. 478))
- Social issues (e.g. social isolation (⊃ Social support p. 28), housebound, poverty)
- Rehabilitation post stroke, injury, or cancer treatment
- End-of-life care (⊃ Palliative care in the home p. 550)
- Older people, particularly those living in care homes (⊃ Care homes p. 32)
- People who misuse drugs (⊃ Substance use p. 476) or alcohol (⊃ Alcohol p. 360)
- People with eating disorders (⊃ People with eating disorders p. 474)

Screening

Identify opportunistically (e.g. first contact with a new service) or upon clinical concern. Use a validated screening tool. Malnutrition Universal Screening Tool (MUST) is widely used in clinical settings (Table 8.2).[11]

Management

Management should be linked to the level of risk. For all those at risk, a care plan should be provided, and interventions monitored and evaluated. ⚠ Difficulty in swallowing should always be referred for medical assessment.

Low risk

- Provide verbal and written information on eating well.
- Determine frequency of rescreening (e.g. annually according to patient's condition/circumstances, or more frequently per local policy).
- If obese, treat according to local policy (⊃ Overweight and obesity p. 348).

Table 8.2 Malnutrition Universal Screening Tool

Step 1: Measure height and weight to get a BMI score	BMI >20 = 0 BMI 18.5–20 = 1 BMI <18.5 = 2
Step 2: Note % unplanned weight loss in past 3–6 months	<5% = 0 5–10% = 1 >10% = 2
Step 3: Establish acute disease effect and score	If patient is acutely ill and there has been or is likely to be no nutritional intake for >5 days = 2
Step 4: Add scores from steps 1, 2, and 3 to get overall risk score	Low risk = 0 Medium risk = 1 High risk = 2+

Medium risk

- Provide verbal and written advice to maximize nutritional intake.
- Eat little and often.
- Eat/drink ↑ energy and protein food/fluids.
- Add powdered nutritional supplements to water/milk.
- Determine frequency of rescreening (e.g. 1–3mths according to patient's condition/circumstances, or more frequently per local policy).

High risk

- Provide verbal and written advice to maximize nutritional intake.
- Prescribe oral nutritional supplements and monitor (see local guidelines and formularies on prescribing adult oral nutritional supplements in the community).
- Rescreening should occur 4–6wks after prescription. If no improvement, refer to dietician.

Related topics

→ Adult body mass index chart p. 346

References

10. Managing Adult Malnutrition, Multi-Professional Consensus Panel (2017) *A guide to managing adult malnutrition in the community.* Available at: https://www.malnutritionpathway.co.uk/contact

11. British Association for Parenteral and Enteral Nutrition (2003/2011) *The MUST explanatory booklet: a guide to the MUST for adults (revised 2011).* Available at: https://www.bapen.org.uk/pdfs/must/must_full.pdf

Home food safety and hygiene

Food poisoning is a significant issue in the UK with all countries having food-borne disease-reduction strategies (➲ Food-borne disease p. 730).

Key principles for food safety and hygiene

Hand washing

Before starting, after touching any meat or raw fish, after going to the toilet, or touching pets.

Cleaning up

Wash all chopping boards and surfaces before and after cooking. Wash and replace tea towels, cloths, sponges frequently.

Separate raw meat

Contains harmful bacteria. Store in fridge at the bottom so it cannot drip on ready-to-eat food. Avoid cross-contamination with other ready-to-eat foods by using different cutting boards, cleaning surfaces, cleaning utensils after using on raw meat. Do not place raw meat next to cooked foods, e.g. on barbeques. Always wash hands after handling.

Raw fish

May contain microbes that can cause food poisoning. To prevent this store fish in fridge. Treat raw fish as raw meat. Elderly or sick people, young children, and pregnant women should not eat raw, or partially-cooked fish and shellfish (➲ Food and the under-fives p. 212; ➲ Pregnancy p. 424).

Fruit and vegetables

Always wash before use to remove any bacteria. Scrap or peel skin off root vegetables to remove earth not removed by washing.

Cook through

Ensure items are cooked all the way through, i.e. piping hot so steam is rising from centre of dish if pierced with knife or skewer. Fully cook (i.e. no pink flesh) poultry, rolled meat joints, kebabs, burgers, and chicken nuggets to ensure all harmful bacteria are killed.

Leftovers and reheating food

Should be cooled and placed in fridge within 90min and used within 2 days. This includes rice and grains because if they are cooked and then left at room temperature longer than 90min, spores germinate, which produce toxins that cause vomiting and diarrhoea. These toxins are not killed by re-heating. Foods should only be reheated once and cooked through.

Eggs

Some eggs contain salmonella bacteria. Eggs with a 'Lion Mark' are from hens vaccinated against salmonella. Eating raw eggs, or eggs with runny yolks, or any food containing these, can cause food poisoning. Care is required in preparation in order not to spread bacteria on work surfaces, utensils, etc. Advise to cook eggs until the yolk and the white are solid, especially for the very young (i.e. babies to toddlers) and those who are older, pregnant, or unwell.

Freezing at home

Cooked foods should be cooled quickly, placed in clean containers/bags, labelled, and stored according to freezer or cookery guide. Uncooked and chilled foods should be frozen and used according to the instructions on retailers' labels.

Defrosting foods

Foods that require defrosting throughout should be left at a temperature (e.g. in the fridge) that will not allow bacteria or toxins to multiple during process. Cook within 24hrs. Do not refreeze.

Laundry

- ↑ risk items that are visibly soiled or might excrete pathogens of the body (e.g. bed linen and underwear) should be washed at 40–60°C with a bleach-based laundry product.
- ↓ risk items that are not in contact with the body or in ↓ risk areas of soiling (e.g. shirts, socks, and trousers) should be washed at ≤40°C with non-bleach-based products.
- Do not leave laundry in the washing machine, as germs multiply.

⚠ Treat healthcare workers' uniforms as high-risk items.

Hygienic cleaning

- Hand-to-hand contact surfaces and food contact surfaces can be hygienically cleaned with soapy water, and then rinsed.
- Where a surface cannot be adequately rinsed (e.g. large food surfaces, handles, toilet seats), and is likely to leave behind pathogens, then a disinfectant should be used.
- Use separate chopping boards for uncooked food (e.g. raw meat) and food that does not need cooking (e.g. salad leaves).

Further information

Community Infection Control Nurses Network (*Prevention of infection in the home: a training resource for carers and their trainers*). Available at: ℘ http://www.nhs.uk/Livewell/homehygiene/Documents/ICNA-TRAINING-RESOURCE-BOOKLET[1].pdf

Food Standards Agency (*Food safety and hygiene*). Available at: ℘ https://www.food.gov.uk/food-safety

Home Hygiene and Health (*Resources*). Available at: ℘ http://www.ifh-homehygiene.org/resources

Exercise

Physical activity ↓ the risk of morbidity and improves many conditions including CHD (◆ Coronary heart disease p. 624), hypertension (◆ Hypertension p. 628), Type 2 Diabetes (◆ Diabetes: overview p. 660), and COPD (◆ Chronic obstructive pulmonary disease p. 614). It ↓ risk of some cancers (colon, breast, prostate (◆ Cancer prevention p. 372) and prevents osteoporosis (and thus risk of fractures). It also improves mental health (◆ People with anxiety and depression p. 478) and helps in weight management (◆ Overweight and obesity p. 348). It is a government priority to encourage the population to become ↑ active and ↓ sedentary. Physical activity levels ↓ dramatically with age. They also vary between people of different social class, gender, and ethnicity.

Definitions

Aerobic fitness
Ability of cardiovascular system to supply O_2 to muscles. Achieved through moderate-intensity activity (e.g. brisk walking and cycling), which causes breathing and heart rate to increase, and vigorous-intensity exercise (e.g. running and climbing stairs), which causes rapid breathing and heart rate.

Muscular strength and muscular endurance
Muscular strength is the maximum force a muscle can exert ↑ with exercise such as lifting. Muscular endurance is the ability of muscles to work for longer before feeling fatigued. Weak muscles need to ↑ strength before endurance.

Flexibility and motor fitness
Flexibility is the maximum range of movement in a joint. Motor fitness relates to speed, reaction time, balance, and co-ordination.

Recommended physical activity levels

19–64 years
Moderate-intensity activity for 150min or vigorous activity for 75min over a week. Activities to improve muscle strength undertaken on at least 2 days/wk. Minimize time spent being sedentary.

Over 65 years
Moderate-intensity activity for 150min or, if already active, vigorous activity for 75min over a week. Activities to improve muscle strength on at least 2 days (e.g. chair exercises). If at risk of falls, incorporate activities to improve balance and co-ordination on at least 2 days (e.g. tai chi, yoga) (◆ Falls prevention p. 368). Minimize time spent being sedentary.

People with specific health problems
For example, COPD. Require specific advice, tailored to them, from qualified health or fitness professionals.

Evidence-based interventions for promoting exercise

No one health discipline or model has been shown to be more effective than others in delivering exercise promotion (◆ Evidence-based healthcare p. 72). Advice-only strategies to ↑ exercise result in ↑ exercise, but it is not sustained for longer than a year. ↓ intensity exercise incorporated into daily routine is more successfully sustained than commitments to new ↑ intensity exercise, e.g. going to a gym. There is some evidence that activity/exercise in groups is more successfully sustained than exercise on an individual basis, and that support from family, peers, community, and healthcare professionals is beneficial.

Community/environmental strategies and partners for exercise include:
- Walking and cycling to work in partnership with employers
- Preserving and encouraging use of playing fields and open spaces in partnership with LAs
- Local walking groups including health walks

Individual exercise promotion strategies should include:
- Identification of patient/client's current daily/weekly activity levels as opportunities present (e.g. consultation for contraception (⊕ Contraception: general p. 400)
- Routine advice given in 1° care, including written materials, on recommended levels of physical exercise and how to ↑ levels of physical activity in daily routines (e.g. use stairs, cut down on watching television/screen time, walk faster, do household chores/garden more energetically and on most days)
- Use of client-centred, individualized action plans, based on agreed, targeted behaviour change
- Use of exercise referral schemes to LA exercise groups (sometimes known as prescription for exercise schemes)

Older people: special considerations
For frail older people, strength should be built up before progressing to dynamic exercise (e.g. through chair-based exercises). Moderate physical activity results in physical and emotional health improvements, as well as modifies risks/impacts of falls. Training specifically in balance, strength, co-ordination, and reaction time leads to reduction of injurious falls. Weight-bearing exercise, plus the earlier mentioned points, leads to decrease in fractures.

Further information
Department of Health (*UK physical activity guidelines*). Available at: ℘ www.gov.uk/government/publications/uk-physical-activity-guidelines
NICE (*Physical activity*). Available at: ℘ https://www.nice.org.uk/Guidance/Lifestyle-and-wellbeing/Physical-activity#panel-pathways

Smoking cessation

Smoking is the leading cause of preventable disease and death in the UK. Cigarette smoke contains 50 known carcinogens and metabolic poisons, as well as nicotine. Half of all regular smokers will die as a result of smoking. Rates are higher in people in lower social class groups, in younger people, and in vulnerable groups (e.g. those with mental health problems). Nicotine is addictive, and has psychological and physiological effects. The majority of smoking-related deaths in UK are from lung cancer (➔ Lung cancer p. 751), COPD (➔ Chronic obstructive pulmonary disease p. 614), and CHD (➔ Coronary heart disease p. 624).

Passive smoking is associated with increased risk of CHD and lung cancer. In children, ↑ risk of cot death (➔ Sudden infant death syndrome p. 278), bronchitis, and otitis media (➔ Infections in children p. 288). Health promotion for young people is aimed at preventing them starting smoking.

Helping people to stop smoking

It is an NHS priority to help smokers quit. Ceasing smoking at any age brings health benefits. About 4 million smokers try each year, but only 3–6% succeed. There are smoking status recording standards for general practice (➔ General practice p. 18) in the Quality and Outcomes Framework (➔ Quality and Outcomes Framework p. 74). National 'No Smoking Day' is always the second Wednesday in March in the UK.

Brief smoking-cessation advice
In 1° care, this should include:
- Asking about smoking status at each contact, including intention to quit, and recording it (at least annually in general practice)
- Giving advice about the benefits of stopping, particularly if a link can be made to the person's ill health or the effects on children, fetus, etc., and providing leaflets
- Assessing motivation to stop, e.g. are you ready to give up for good?

If person is not ready to quit, then provide information for future, e.g. Smokefree National Helpline (☎ 0800 123 1044). If person is ready to quit, then refer to local smoking-cessation service and/or offer nicotine replacement therapy (NRT) prescription and stop-smoking support, as follows. Most cessation services offer specific stop-smoking training for 1° care professionals.

Supporting a smoker to quit
- Help smoker set a date to quit and advise seeking support of friends and family.
- Identify triggers to smoking (e.g. alcohol, coffee) and advise on plan to reduce these during the first days.
- Encourage smokers to persist, as it can take three or four attempts to stop.
- Explain about nicotine withdrawal symptoms (includes irritability, dizziness, increased appetite) and craving (symptoms are most intense within 24–48hrs after cessation and decline over 2–4wks).

- Explain about availability of NRT and other smoking-cessation medication and encourage those smoking >10/day to consider it.
- Identify if person is likely to experience high levels of withdrawal symptoms (e.g. from previous experience, smokes within 30min of waking, smokes >15/day (this group may benefit from NRT)).
- Offer review, follow-up, and motivational support (➲ Motivational interviewing in consultations p. 126).

Aids to smoking cessation

OTC nicotine gum, patches, inhalers, etc., are available to those who are committed to stopping smoking. For further information, see NICE.[12] For available preparations, see BNF/BNF Online, with special attention to contraindications. Complementary therapies are unproven, but some evidence for hypnotherapy (➲ Complementary and alternative therapies p. 838). E-cigarettes are the most popular quitting tool in England, with almost ten times as many people using them as using stop-smoking services. However, stop-smoking services are the most effective way to quit.[13]

References

12. NICE (2018) *Stop smoking interventions and services*. Available at: ᐅ https://www.nice.org.uk/guidance/ng92
13. PHE (2016) *Consensus on E-cigarettes*. Available at: https://www.gov.uk/government/publications/e-cigarettes-a-developing-public-health-consensus

Further information

Action on Smoking and Health (ASH) (*About ASH*). Available at: ᐅ http://ash.org.uk/home/

Managing stress

Stress is the feeling of being under too much mental or emotional pressure. A normal body response to stress is to ↑ the production of adrenaline and cortisol, which ↑ heart rate, BP, and metabolism to improve performance.

People react differently to stress. Some respond by ↑ behaviours likely to cause other health problems (e.g. ↑ smoking, ↑ eating comfort food, ↑ drinking alcohol). Continued exposure to stress can lead to mental and physical symptoms (e.g. mood swings, anxiety, depression, sleep disturbances, indigestion, and diarrhoea) (➔ People with anxiety and depression p. 478; ➔ Dyspepsia, gastro-oesophageal reflux disease, and peptic ulceration p. 708). Chronic stress can ↑ risk of CHD (➔ Coronary heart disease p. 624). Common sources of stress-related ill health include:
- Relationship problems
- Work problems
- Financial problems
- Bereavement (➔ Coping with bereavement p. 574)
- Exams
- Change or loss of work
- Being an informal carer (➔ Carers p. 458)

Early recognitions of signs and symptoms of stress can help ↓ their impact. Stress can affect feelings, behaviour, and physical health. Individuals may notice ↑ irritability, anxiety, pessimism, racing thoughts, low self-esteem, or mood. May experience headaches, muscle tension, sweating, dry mouth, loss of libido (➔ Sexual problems p. 768). Many people benefit from simple advice and support, while others find one of the talking therapies beneficial (➔ Talking therapies p. 472).

Managing mind set

Setting realistic goals; thinking about achievements as successes, not belittling them or taking them down. Thinking of stressful events as something to be managed and planned, not as overwhelming events that leave patient powerless.

Health promotion

- Make use of people around patient in coping; delegate tasks to others and talk to others about how feeling.
- Actively relax.
- Learn to express anger in an assertive not aggressive way (e.g. speaking in strong, steady voice not shouting).
- Have enough uninterrupted sleep. Actively address sleep problems (e.g. create a bedtime routine that helps relax, cut out late-night alcohol, make bedroom as dark as possible, do not read in bed).
- Do things you enjoy; have fun and plan treats; escape to a world of movies, books, music, etc.
- Create time for regular exercise (➔ Exercise p. 354). Exercise helps release physical tension, can be sociable, and releases mood-enhancing endorphins in the brain. Smiling and laughter also release endorphins.

Simple relaxation technique

Can be practised on own or in groups with one person talking through the steps. Steps for simple relaxation:

- Find a quiet place where you will not be interrupted.
- Make yourself comfortable, lying or sitting, with eyes closed.
- Breathe slowly, deeply, effortlessly.
- Working from your feet to head, tense, then relax each part of the body: starting with the feet, tense them for a count of five, then release and count to five; repeat with small areas of the body (including face) until every part of the body has been tensed and released
- Finally, tense all parts of body, count five, release, then remain in that position, breathing slowly and deeply for at least 5–20min.

There are many different types of guided relaxation exercises. Self-help tapes and books are available at most bookstores.

Further information

Health and Safety Executive (*Information on workplace stress*). Available at: ℘ www.hse.gov.uk/stress/

Mental Health Foundation (*How to manage and reduce stress*). Available at: ℘ https://www.mentalhealth.org.uk/publications/how-manage-and-reduce-stress

Alcohol

Alcohol misuse is a significant public health concern (➔ Public health in the NHS and beyond p. 14; ➔ Substance use p. 476). Most health-related harm is caused by non-dependent drinkers. Sensible drinking limits are defined as:

- <14 units of alcohol a week for both ♀ and ♂, spread over three or more days
- Plus two alcohol-free days a week

One unit of alcohol

- Half pint of ordinary strength beer, lager, or cider
- Quarter pint of extra strength beer, lager, or cider
- One small glass of white (8 or 9% ABV (alcohol by volume)) wine
- Two thirds small glass of red (11 or 12% ABV) wine
- One single measure of spirits (30mL)

Alcohol should be avoided in pregnancy (➔ Pregnancy p. 424), before driving, operating machinery, swimming, or working at heights, or whilst using electrical equipment.

Harmful/hazardous drinking is associated with hypertension (➔ Hypertension p. 628), cirrhosis of the liver (➔ Problems of liver, gallbladder, and pancreas p. 718), injuries and accidents (e.g. falls), depression (➔ People with anxiety and depression p. 478), loss of work, family break-up (➔ Domestic violence p. 450), homelessness (➔ Homeless people p. 446), and offending behaviours.

Promoting sensible drinking

Nurses in 1° care have a wide range of opportunities to promote sensible drinking. These include as part of: other clinic/surgery consultations (e.g. for travel advice (➔ Travel healthcare p. 394); specific health-promoting care (e.g. preconceptual or antenatal care (➔ Preconceptual care p. 422; ➔ Antenatal education and preparation for parenthood p. 425)), and in group health promotion (e.g. parenting groups).

NICE guidance recommends Alcohol Use Disorders Identification Test (AUDIT) to help to identify individuals with harmful and hazardous patterns of alcohol consumption. Scores provide guidance on level of intervention from alcohol education to referral for specialist help.[14]

Harmful/hazardous drinking

Signs and symptoms of harmful/hazardous drinking include:

- Feeling depressed
- Feeling nervous or on edge
- Having difficulty in sleeping
- Physical symptoms (e.g. gastritis)
- History of accidents or injuries due to alcohol
- Poor concentration or memory
- Self-neglect (e.g. poor hygiene)

Interventions and management

Strategies to help people ↓ drinking at harmful levels include:
- Give information on sensible drinking levels and risks of harmful drinking, and encourage the person to consider ways to cut down.
- Encourage patient/client to keep a drinking diary and feedback on the number of units of alcohol s/he drinks a week.
- Discuss how and why patient/client believes s/he benefits from drinking, and consider willingness to change.
- Discuss how much drinking costs patient/client each week.
- Discuss how to avoid situations where patient/client feels need to drink (e.g. social situations and stressful situations).
- Discuss strategies for ↓ intake, e.g. low-alcohol beer; water to quench thirst for in between drinks, and to drink with food;, switch to half pints; avoid buying rounds; avoid friends who drink heavily.
- Discuss benefits of ↓ alcohol intake (e.g. sleep better, ↑ energy, ↓ loss of weight, ↑ money).

Dependent drinking

Defined as when three of the following are present:
- Patient/client has difficulty in controlling drinking.
- There is a very strong urge to drink.
- Patient/client can drink large amounts of alcohol without feeling intoxicated.
- Drinking continues despite harm it causes.
- Day-to-day activities are neglected due to alcohol use.
- If drinking is stopped, withdrawal symptoms (e.g. tremors, anxiety, and sweating) occur.

Patients who are drinking at high levels and are dependent drinkers need longer and more detailed interventions, determined by whether patient/client wishes to change their drinking behaviour. These patients need to be referred to GP and/or NHS specialist alcohol services.

Reference

14. NICE (2011) *Alcohol-use disorders [CG115]*. Available at: http://guidance.nice.org.uk/CG115

Further information

Adfam (*Improving life for families affected by drugs and alcohol*). Available at: ℘ https://adfam.org.uk
Alcoholics Anonymous (*About AA*). Available at: ℘ https://www.alcoholics-anonymous.org.uk/

UK screening programmes

There are internationally agreed criteria for appraising the viability, effectiveness, and appropriateness of screening before a condition screening programme is initiated, including the condition, the test, the intervention, the screening programme, and the implementation criteria.

The UK has a committee that appraises the evidence and advises the central health department on implementation of screening programmes. It also lists conditions which are not recommended for screening because insufficient evidence exists or evidence shows that screening does more harm than good.

Current national screening programmes

Antenatal

➔ Antenatal care and screening p. 426

Newborn and child health

➔ Child screening tests p. 160; ➔ Overview of the healthy child programme p. 154

Young person and adult

- Abdominal aortic aneurysm (➔ Abdominal aortic aneurysm screening p. 388)
- Bowel cancer (➔ Bowel cancer screening p. 376)
- Breast cancer (➔ Breast cancer awareness and screening p. 378)
- Cervical cancer (➔ Cervical cancer screening p. 380)
- Diabetic retinopathy (➔ Principles of diabetes management p. 664; ➔ Common problems affecting eyes p. 746)
- Sexually transmitted infections (e.g. Chlamydia) (➔ Sexually transmitted infections p. 764)

Further information

PHE (*Population screening programmes*). Available at: ℜ https://www.gov.uk/topic/population-screening-programmes

UK National Screening Committee (NSC) (*Role of the group*). Available at: ℜ https://www.gov.uk/government/groups/uk-national-screening-committee-uk-nsc#role-of-the-group

UK NSC (*Current UK NSC recommendations*). Available at: ℜ https://legacyscreening.phe.org.uk/screening-recommendations.php

Menopause

Menopause

The cessation of menstruation usually occurs between 45 and 55yrs. Peri-menopause is the time from when the ovaries start to produce less oestrogen and symptoms may be experienced, until 12mths after the last period and beyond. ♀ experience menopause in many different ways. Most experience peri-menopause over 4–5yrs; some experience abrupt cessation. Contraception (➔ Contraception: general p. 400) advised for 2yrs after last period if <50yrs and 1yr if >50yrs.

Premature menopause

Cessation of menstruation <45yrs. Occurs in some syndromes, e.g. Turner's (➔ Genetic problems p. 270), and as a result of some gynaecological surgery or radiotherapy (➔ Hysterectomy p. 782). Lack of oestrogen is associated with ↑ risk of osteoporosis and cardiovascular disease (➔ Coronary heart disease p. 624). Premature menopause may be treated with hormone replacement therapy (HRT).

Signs and symptoms

- Menstruation changes: cycle may shorten or lengthen to many months; often ↑ in menstrual loss (➔ Menstrual problems p. 778)
- Hot flushes and night sweats: experienced by about 80% of women
- Thinning of the skin, brittle nails, hair loss, headaches, and generalized aches and pains
- Urinary symptoms: urinary stress incontinence (➔ Urinary incontinence p. 504); recurrent lower urinary tract infection (UTI) (➔ Urinary tract infection p. 756)
- Vaginal discomfort and dryness: leading to dyspareunia, possible cause of UTI symptoms (➔ Vaginal and vulval problems p. 786)

In addition, some ♀ may experience a range of emotional changes, although these may be related to other life events and not only sequelae of menopause. Some mood changes such as irritability and difficulties in concentration may be a result of disturbed sleep through night sweats. Loss of libido may occur (➔ Sexual problems p. 768), but non-hormonal factors, such as inadequate stimulation, depression, and life stresses may be contributing factors.

Consequences of the menopause

Many women experience the end of menstruation as very liberating. Reduction in oestrogen causes ↑ risk of osteoporosis, urogenital atrophy, cardiovascular disease, and stroke. ↑ weight, at or around menopause, to central abdominal area is an additional risk factor for cardiovascular disease.

General advice

- Osteoporosis prevention
- ↓ cardiovascular risk through exercise, nutrition, and healthy eating (➔ Nutrition and healthy eating p. 342), weight management, smoking cessation (➔ Smoking cessation p. 356)
- Pelvic floor exercises
- Stress management through ↑ exercise and relaxation techniques (➔ Managing stress p. 358)

Managing symptoms

Many ♀ experience very mild symptoms and manage them easily. ~40% experience symptoms that are distressing at some point. Key symptoms include hot flushes and night sweats, urinary symptoms, and vaginal dryness. May be helped by ⇄ exercise, ↓ stress, avoiding triggers (such as caffeine, smoking, and alcohol), wearing lighter clothes, and sleeping in cooler room, etc. Herbal therapies (e.g. red clover, black cohosh, isoflavones, soya products) are used by many women to some benefit, but research evidence is inconclusive (➋ Complementary and alternative therapies p. 838; ➋ Evidence-based healthcare p. 72). HRT may be indicated. The type of HRT will be dependent on whether the woman has a uterus. It is important to be aware of the ♀ for whom HRT is contraindicated. You need also be aware of side effects. Ensure familiarity with current best practice guidance (e.g. guidance on duration of treatment).

Further information

British Menopause Society (*Our work*). Available at: ♫ https://thebms.org.uk/about-the-charity/our-work/

Menopause Matters (*What to do at menopause*). Available at: ♫ https://www.menopausematters.co.uk/what_to_do_at_menopause.php

NICE (*Menopause guidance*). Available at: ♫ http://cks.nice.org/menopause

Royal College of General Practitioners (*Menstrual wellbeing toolkit*). Available at: ♫ http://www.rcgp.org.uk/menstrualwellbeingtoolkit

Healthy ageing

Everyone should have the opportunity to live a long and healthy life. In 2001, the National Service Framework for Older People[15] set out to extend the healthy life expectancy of older people. In the UK, life expectancy at birth is 79.5yrs for ♂ and 83.1yrs for ♀ (➲ UK health profile p. 2). The number of years lived in self-assessed good health is 63.4yrs for ♂ and 64.1yrs for ♀.[16] The WHO defines healthy ageing as the process of developing and maintaining the functional ability that enables well-being in older age.[17] They focus on the following five domains.

Ability to meet basic needs

Financial security
- Social pension provision
- Protection from the costs of healthcare and long-term care
- Schemes to enable older people to stay in the workforce longer

Prevent crime and reduce fear of crime
- Security equipment in the home (e.g. door chains)
- Designing well-lit and accessible neighbourhoods
- Encouraging older people to participate in community activities
- Dispelling myths about the amount of crime against older people
- Avoiding sensationalist reporting of crimes against older people

➲ Victims of crime p. 452

Prevent the abuse of older people
- Inter-agency responses to allegations of abuse
- Helplines to provide information and referrals for victims
- Monitoring of account patterns by banking/financial institutions
- Provision of emergency shelter

➲ Adults at risk from harm and abuse p. 454

Improve access to adequate and affordable housing
- Provision of social housing, supported housing, and care homes
- Supporting housing modifications
- Investment in assistive technologies
- Schemes to maintain optimal housing temperatures
- Programmes to ↓ hazards in the home (e.g. pollutants and mould)

➲ Homes and housing p. 26; ➲ Assistive technology and home adaptations p. 834; ➲ Care homes p. 32

Ability to learn, grow, and make decisions

- Challenging negative attitudes and stereotypes of older people
- Improve literacy in older people (including health literacy)
- Invest in lifelong learning opportunities (e.g. University of the Third Age)
- Facilitate choice and control (e.g. personal health budgets)

Ability to be mobile

- Rehabilitation following stroke, cardiac events, or injury
- Provision of physical activity guidelines and programmes (➲ Exercise p. 354)
- Provision of mobility aids
- Support for older drivers
- Addressing barriers in the built environment (e.g. ↑ visibility of road crossings)
- Improving availability and accessibility of transport (e.g. ↓ price fares)

Ability to build and grow relationships

- Identifying and tackling social isolation (➲ Social support p. 28)
- Creating opportunities for reciprocal relationships (e.g. time banking) (➲ Community approaches to health p. 338)
- Improving access to information and communication technologies (e.g. Zoom, Skype and Facetime)

Ability to contribute to society

- Opportunities to mentor younger people
- Creating environments that embrace diversity
- Reform pension systems that encourage early retirement
- Support flexible working arrangements
- Help older people plan for retirement
- Encourage volunteering

References

15. Department of Health (2001) *National service framework for older people.* Available at: https://www.gov.uk/government/publications/quality-standards-for-care-services-for-older-people
16. PHE (2017) *Research and analysis: health profile for England.* Available at: https://www.gov.uk/government/publications/health-profile-for-england
17. WHO (2015) *World report on ageing and health.* Available at: http://apps.who.int/iris/bitstream/handle/10665/186463/9789240694811_eng.pdf;jsessionid=C872F69CB8F71304246 1D567065D7FDD?sequence=1

Falls prevention

A fall is an unintended event that results in a person coming to rest on the ground, floor, or lower level. While accident prevention is a public health issue for all ages, falls and their sequelae are a particular issue for older people. Studies of people ≥65yrs suggest that 20–30% fall each year and the rate ↑ with age.[18] Falls are under-reported.

Consequences

It is estimated that 40–60% of falls result in no injury, 30–50% in minor injury, 5% in fractures, and 5–6% in other major injury[18] (◑ Sprains, strains, and fractures p. 824). The inability to get up after a fall → hypothermia (◑ Hypothermia p. 820), pneumonia (◑ Pneumonia p. 750), dehydration, and pressure ulceration (◑ Pressure ulcer prevention p. 520). Other consequences include increased fear of falling, loss of confidence, and restriction of activities.

Risk factors

Physical factors

- Age >75yrs, ♀ (◑ Frailty p. 678)
- Cognitive impairment (◑ People with dementia p. 498)
- Depression (◑ People with anxiety and depression p. 478)
- Parkinson's disease (◑ Parkinson's disease 674)
- Dizziness and vertigo
- History of stroke
- Rheumatic disease (◑ Rheumatoid arthritis p. 602)
- Urinary incontinence (◑ Urinary incontinence p. 504)
- Hypotension
- Diabetes (◑ Diabetes: overview p. 660)
- Pain
- History of falls
- Walking aid use
- Gait problems
- Physical disability
- Vision impairment (◑ Blindness and partial sight p. 748) or hearing impairment (◑ Deafness p. 696)

Medication factors

- Number of medications (polypharmacy)
- Use of anti-epileptics or sedatives or anti-hypertensives

Environmental factors

- In the home: bed or chair too low, poor lighting, or loose rugs
- Outside the home: public transport, uneven pavements

Risk identification

Older people should be asked about falls when they have routine reviews or health checks. For example: In the past year have you had any fall including a slip or a trip in which you lost your balance and landed on the floor or ground or lower level?

Multifactorial risk assessment

Older people who have fallen in the last year or who are at risk of falls should be offered a multifactorial falls risk assessment. This should be performed by a healthcare professional with appropriate skills and experience, and will usually take place within a specialist falls service.[19] This may include:
- Identification of falls history
- Neurological examination
- Cardiovascular examination
- Medication review (➔ Principles of medication reviews p. 142)
- Assessment relating to: gait, balance, mobility, and muscle weakness; osteoporosis risk; functional ability and fear of falling; visual impairment; cognitive impairment; urinary incontinence; and home hazards

Multifactorial intervention

Older people who are assessed at risk of falls should receive an individualized multifactorial intervention. This may include:[19]
- Strength and balance training (➔ Exercise p. 354)
- Home hazard intervention (➔ Assistive technology and home adaptations p. 834)
- Vision referral (➔ Common problems affecting the eyes p. 746)
- Medication review with modification and/or withdrawal

Fall alarm systems

Home alarm systems (e.g. wireless devices worn as a wristband or pendant) may reduce rescue time following a fall (➔ Telehealth and telecare p. 832).

References

18. Becker, C., Woo, J., & Todd, C. (2017) Falls. In: Michel, J.P., Beattie, L., Martin, F., & Walston, J. (eds) *Oxford Textbook of Geriatric Medicine* (3rd edn). Oxford: Oxford University Press
19. NICE (2013) *Falls in older people: assessing risk and prevention.* Available at: https://www.nice.org.uk/guidance/cg161

Weather extremes

Older people, very young children, pregnant women (◆ Pregnancy p. 424), homeless people (◆ Homeless people p. 446), and people with LTCs are particularly vulnerable to the effects of weather extremes.

Hot weather

Key public health messages for hot weather are summarized in Box 8.2.[20]

Heat exhaustion

Heat exhaustion can occur after exposure to ↑ temperatures. It usually gets better when the person is helped to cool down. Signs and symptoms include:
- Headache or dizziness and confusion
- Loss of appetite and feeling sick
- Excessive sweating and pale, clammy skin
- Cramps in arms, legs, and stomach
- Fast breathing and fast pulse
- Temperature of ≥38°C
- Intense thirst

Treatment should include:
- Moving to a cool place
- Lying down with feet raised
- Drinking plenty of water
- Cooling the skin with cool water and a fan
- Monitoring for relief of symptoms
- If no improvement within 30mins, seek emergency treatment

⚠: Untreated heat exhaustion can lead to heatstroke, which is a medical emergency.

Heatstroke

⚠: Heatstroke requires emergency treatment. It can result in organ failure, brain damage, or death. Signs and symptoms of heatstroke include:
- Skin feels hot and dry
- Absence of sweating

Box 8.2 Key public health messages in hot weather

- When outside, stay in the shade and wear a hat.
- Drink plenty of cold drinks.
- Take cool baths or showers.
- Wear light-coloured, loose clothing.
- Sprinkle water over skin or clothing.
- Avoid the sun (especially between 11.00–15.00 (British Summer Time)).
- Avoid excess alcohol and extreme exercise.
- Remember to keep medicines <25°C.
- Keep internal environment cool.
- Keep curtains in windows exposed to the sun closed.
- Turn off non-essential lights and electrical equipment.
- Electric fan may help if temperatures are <35°C.

- Temperature ≥40°C
- Rapid breathing or shortness of breath
- Confusion
- Seizures
- Loss of consciousness

Cold weather

Cold weather ↑ the risk of heart attacks, stroke (➔ Recognizing and responding to a stroke p. 830), respiratory illness (➔ Acute asthma in adults (asthma attacks) p. 612; ➔ Management of chronic obstructive pulmonary disease exacerbation p. 618), influenza, falls and injuries (➔ Falls prevention p. 368), and hypothermia (➔ Hypothermia p. 820). Key advice should include:[21]

- Eligible groups should receive free flu vaccination (➔ Targeted adult immunization p. 392)
- Heat home to ≥18°C
- Wear suitable clothing, including layers
- Eat plenty of hot food and consume hot drinks
- Stay active and wear appropriate footwear both indoors and out (➔ Exercise p. 354)
- Gas heating and cooking appliances should be checked by a Gas Safe registered engineer (➔ Poisoning and overdoses p. 822)

Grants, benefits, and sources of advice may be available to make residential properties more energy-efficient and for help paying bills (➔ Homes and housing p. 26).

Related topics

➔ Skin cancer prevention p. 374

References

20. PHE (2018) *Heatwave plan for England: protecting health and reducing harm from severe heat and heatwaves.* Available at: https://assets.publishing.service.gov.uk/government/uploads/system/uploads/attachment_data/file/711503/Heatwave_plan_for_England_2018.pdf
21. HM Government (2017) *Keep warm, keep well.* Available at: https://assets.publishing.service.gov.uk/government/uploads/system/uploads/attachment_data/file/653267/Keep_Warm_Keep_Well_2017.pdf

Further information

UK Meteorological Office (*Weather warnings*). Available online, ➔ https://www.metoffice.gov.uk/

Cancer prevention

One person in two in the UK is diagnosed with cancer at some time in their life. Only two or three in every 100 cancer cases are genetically inherited (e.g. the BRCA genes are linked with breast (➲ Breast cancer p. 774), ovarian (➲ Gynaecological cancers p. 776), prostate (➲ Prostate problems p. 758) and other cancers). Experts estimate that four in ten cancer cases could be prevented, largely through lifestyle changes such as: not smoking (➲ Smoking cessation p. 356); keeping to a healthy body weight (➲ Adult body mass index chart p. 346); undertaking brisk physical activity each day (➲ Exercise p. 354); ↑ daily intake and variety of fruit and vegetables to five or more portions daily and ↓ foods containing animal fats (➲ Nutrition and healthy eating p. 342); cutting back on alcohol (➲ Alcohol p. 360); avoiding excessive exposure to sunlight especially children, adolescents, and those with tendency to burn (➲ Skin cancer prevention p. 374); and adhering to safety regulations about exposure to known carcinogens.

Early signs of cancer

Cancer is not just one disease, but at least 200 different types, with a wide range of possible symptoms. Early detection is aided by knowing what is normal for the individual and acting on changes. Professionals should be consulted about the following signs and symptoms:

- Ongoing chest or throat problems: coughing or hoarseness that lasts >3wks, haemoptysis (➲ Lung cancer p. 751)
- Changes in bowel function: unexplained changes such as chronic constipation (➲ Constipation in adults p. 512), diarrhoea or a change in the size of the stool, blood in the stool, melaena, occult blood, and frank blood (➲ Colorectal cancer p. 715)
- Changes in bladder function: dysuria, haematuria, or unexplained changes in micturition (➲ Prostate problems p. 758)
- Unexplained intermenstrual bleeding or discharge (➲ Gynaecological cancers p. 776)
- Skin changes: skin changes can occur in internal cancers as well as skin cancers (➲ Skin cancer p. 682). These can include: hyperpigmentation, erythema, pruritus, hirsutism, and ulceration
- Changes in skin moles: in colour, shape, size, or sensation, i.e. pain or itching; bleeding or crusting; moles that have multiple colours; moles with irregular edges, uneven or raised surfaces

Other signs include: lumps or thickening that does not go away; ongoing indigestion or swallowing problems; and unexplained fatigue, pain, and/or weight loss

Related topics

➲ UK screening programmes p. 362; ➲ Cervical cancer screening p. 380; ➲ Bowel cancer screening p. 376

Skin cancer prevention

Skin cancer is the most commonly diagnosed cancer in the UK (➜ Skin cancer p. 682). It includes: non-melanoma skin cancer (NMSC) such as basal cell skin cancer (BCC), squamous cell skin cancer (SCC), and malignant melanoma (MM). MM are 2° to exposure to sunlight or artificial UV light. They are uncommon on areas protected from sun exposure and are most common in ♂ on the back and in ♀ on the legs. UV rays from the sun classified into: UVA and UVB. Majority of UV radiation is UVA. UV light is natural in sunlight or artificial (e.g. sunbeds). UV penetrates cloud and water, and UVA penetrates glass, sand, snow, and concrete. The majority of skin cancers are preventable (➜ Cancer prevention p. 372).

Risk factors

- UV radiation is most intense between 11.00–15.00 (British Summer Time (BST)) or 10.00–14.00 hours (Greenwich Mean Time (GMT)).
- Burning from over-exposure to UV light doubles the risk of MM.
- Repeated intense exposure to UV light ↑ risk of development of MM.
- UV damage to skin in the first 15yrs linked to risk of MM in later life.
- Those with naturally fair skin are ↑ risk of DNA damage.
- Those with fair skin which burns and freckles easily, light eye colour, and red or fair hair
- Large number of moles (e.g. >50)
- Family history of skin cancer
- Previous melanoma and some other cancers, e.g. breast, non-Hodgkin lymphoma, renal cell, prostate, thyroid, and leukaemia
- Other medical conditions and treatments (e.g. organ transplant, possibly through the use of immunosuppressant drugs (➜ Principles of working with someone with compromised immunity p. 466))

Prevention

Exposure to sunlight

Avoid time in the sun when sun is at its strongest: in the UK, between 11.00–15.00 from March to October (➜ Weather extremes p. 370). Avoid sunburn and cover up with suitable clothing, a wide brimmed hat, and sunglasses.

Sunbeds or sunlamps

Sunbeds and lamps should not be used. They can be more dangerous than natural sunlight because they use a concentrated source of UV radiation. ⚠ It is illegal for people <18yrs to use a sunbed or be in an area that is allocated for sunbed users.

Sunscreen

Should be applied around 15min before going into the sun and reapplied every 2hrs. Take extra care to protect babies and children. Buy sunscreen suitable for skin type and which blocks both UVA and UVB radiation.

Sunscreens with a SPF of 15+ filters out 93% of UVB. ⚠ Sunscreens should not be used to ↑ time in the sun. No sunscreen has 100% protection. Choice of sunscreen should include:

• With a minimum SPF of 15—the higher, the better
• A star rating of >4, which indicates that it provides protection against UVA as well as UVB
• Water-resistant, to prevent being washed or sweated off
• With a valid 'use by' date. Most sunscreens have a shelf life of 2–3yrs. Expensive sunscreens are not more effective than cheaper ones.

Solar UV index

Indicates the strength of UV. It is shown in weather reports as a number in a triangle. The level of danger depends on skin type (i.e. fair burns, fair tans, brown, and black). UV index 10 means ↑ levels of UV, and advice for people of all skin types is to try to stay in the shade. Daily UV ratings are on UK Meteorological Office website.

Signs of skin cancer

Advise people to know what their skin normally looks like by looking regularly in a full-length mirror. ⚠ The following abnormalities and changes should be referred to the GP for further investigation:

Changes of non-melanoma skin cancer

Occurs mainly in older people, often on head, neck, and/or hands
• A new growth or sore that does not heal within 4wks
• A spot or sore that continues to itch, hurt, crust, scab, or bleed
• Persistent skin ulcers that are not explained by other causes

Signs of abnormality of malignant melanoma
• Moles which are asymmetrical or have blurred or jagged edges
• Moles that have changed colour, or with multiple colours in them
• Moles which are new, growing, or bigger than other moles
• Moles which are raised and/or have an uneven surface
• Moles which are bleeding, oozing, crusting, itchy, or painful

Further information

Cancer Research UK (*SunSmart*). Available at: ℘ https://www.cancerresearchuk.org/about-cancer/causes-of-cancer/sun-uv-and-cancer
UK Meteorological Office (*UV information*). Available at: ℘ https://www.metoffice.gov.uk/public/weather

Bowel cancer screening

Colorectal cancer is common in ♂ and ♀ (⊙ Colorectal cancer p. 715). About 1 in 20 people will get it in their lifetime.

Every 2 years, a home testing kit is offered to everyone in England aged 60–74 years. The test is called a faecal immunochemical test (FIT). The test kit includes a small plastic bottle with a stick attached inside the lid. The person uses the stick to collect the sample, which is then sealed in the bottle. The sample is returned to a laboratory in a pre-paid envelope. Results are returned within 2 weeks. There are two possible results: no further tests needed at this time, or further tests needed. Further tests involve an appointment with a specialist screening practitioner to assess whether the person is fit to undergo a colonoscopy. The colonoscopy will take place at an NHS bowel cancer screening centre. The procedure can detect both cancer and polyps. Polyps may be removed during the procedure and tested to ascertain whether they are cancerous. If polyps are found to be cancerous, or other signs of cancer are detected, the person will be referred to a bowel cancer specialist. If someone is not suitable for colonoscopy, they may be offered a computerized tomography (CT) colonography.

Further information

Bowel Cancer UK (*Bowel cancer screening*). Available at: ℛ https://www.bowelcanceruk.org.uk/about-bowel-cancer/screening/

PHE (*NHS bowel screening programme*). Available at: ℛ https://www.gov.uk/topic/population-screening-programmes/bowel

Breast cancer awareness and screening

Breast cancer (➔ Breast cancer p. 774) is the most common cancer to affect ♀ in the UK, with about one in eight affected in their lifetime. Early detection of changes is encouraged through 'breast awareness'. 2° prevention is by breast screening by mammography and clinical breast examination (➔ UK screening programme p. 362).

Breast awareness

Rationale for the promotion of breast awareness: ~90% of breast cancers detected by ♀ themselves or their partners; and early detection → better survival and ↓ requirement for mastectomy.

Teaching breast awareness

The most effective methods of promoting breast awareness are: provision of verbal and written information; demonstration and return demonstration on the ♀'s own breast; and feedback to the ♀ regarding her own ability. ♀ should practise breast awareness from the age of 18yrs onwards as part of overall bodily awareness.

Know what is normal for you

Check breasts during activities (e.g. bathing) to become aware of the normal state of the breasts. Breasts are sensitive to the presence of oestrogen and progesterone—in pre-menopausal ♀ and ♀ taking HRT, normal breasts feel different at different times of the month. Post-menopausal women's breasts may become softer and ↓ lumpy (➔ Menopause p. 364).

Look at your breasts and feel them

- Look: stand in front of the mirror, undressed to the waist, and raise arms above head and drop them to sides. Then place hands on hips and clench chest muscles.
- Look at the outline and rise and fall of each breast.
- Feel with the fingertips—breast is pear-shaped and extends into armpit, richly supplied by lymph nodes, so ensure whole breast and surrounding area is felt, including armpit, nipple, clavicle, and sternum.

Know what changes to look for

- Appearance change in the outline or shape of the breast, especially those caused by arm movements or lifting the breasts
- Skin puckering or dimpling of the skin
- Nipple change: direction, rash, position, shape, discharge, bleeding
- Lumps or thickening in breast or armpit, or seems different than the other breast
- Pain or discomfort, especially if new and persistent

⚠ Report any changes to the GP without delay.

Mammography screening

Mammography is part of the UK screening programme offered every 3yrs for ♀ aged 50–70yrs. ♀ aged >70yrs can make own appointment. It detects 75% of breast cancers in ♀ aged >50yrs (60% of which are impalpable). ♀ have a good prognosis in 70–80% of cancers detected by screening.

Screening more regularly does not improve outcomes and ↑ exposure to radiation. Many ♀ find having a mammogram uncomfortable and sometimes painful, but it is only for a few seconds.

Related topics
⮕ Breast problems p. 772

Further information
Breast cancer care (*Routine breast screening*). Available at: ℬ https://www.breastcancercare.org.uk/information-support/have-i-got-breast-cancer/referral-to-a-breast-clinic/routine-breast-screening

PHE (*NHS breast screening programme*). Available at: ℬ https://www.gov.uk/topic/population-screening-programmes/breast

Cervical cancer screening

In 2015, there were approximately 3,126 new diagnoses of cervical cancer and 854 deaths[22] (◑ UK health profile p. 2; ◑ Gynaecological cancers p. 776). This equates to 2% of all ♀ cancers. Incidence of cervical cancer is ↑ in women aged 25–29yrs; often related to lack of screening (◑ Cancer prevention p. 372).

Almost all cases of cervical cancer are caused by the human papilloma virus (HPV). Other risk factors for cervical cancer include smoking.[23] Survival rates for cervical cancer at 10yrs are around 63%.[22]

The UK has a robust national cervical screening programme[24] (◑ UK screening programmes p. 362). Cervical screening involves taking samples of cells from the cervix and examining these to detect cell abnormalities which, if left, can → cervical intraepithelial neoplasia (CIN) and, if untreated, cervical cancer (◑ Cervical sample taking p. 384).

Cervical screening programme

Cervical screening is an additional service in the General Medical Services contract (◑ General practice p. 18) and has specified points in the QOF (◑ Quality and Outcomes Framework p. 74).

Invitation to screening

Local call and recall agency invites ♀ for screening to GP practice. Some LAs offer opportunistic screening via contraceptive and sexual health clinics. In the UK, ♀ aged 25–64yrs:
• 3yrly between 25–49yrs
• 5yrly 50–64yrs

At >65yrs only those ♀ who have never been screened, have not been screened since age 50yrs, or have had recent abnormal tests are eligible. ♀ >65yrs who have had three consecutive negative smears are taken out of the call–recall system.

There is evidence (◑ Evidence-based healthcare p. 72) that screening women <25yrs will do more harm than good: one in six samples taken in women <25yrs will be abnormal, but in many cases these abnormalities will resolve without treatment.[23]

Transmen (people who have changed gender from ♀ to ♂) who have had a total hysterectomy do not need to have cervical screening tests. Transmen who still have a cervix are entitled to have cervical screening as outlined.

Cervical cell sampling

Cervical samples taken by liquid-based cytology. The test includes HPV triage and HPV test of cure. Practitioners who perform cervical screening should ensure they are appropriately trained.[22]

Results

Patients must receive results within 14 days. 90% have normal result and are recalled in 3–5yrs depending on age. For types of results and actions see Table 8.3. Abnormal results referred for colposcopy (i.e. examination with a low-powered light microscope). May also include biopsies or treatment (usually large loop excision of the transformation zone) with local anaesthetic.

Cytology/HPV	Wait/CWT pathway	NHSCSP standard
Three consecutive inadequate samples	18-wk pathway, upgraded to 62 days if cancer subsequently suspected	Offered an appointment with a colposcopist within 6wks
Borderline change/HR-HPV positive	18-wk pathway, upgraded to 62 days if cancer subsequently suspected	Offered an appointment with a colposcopist within 6wks
Low-grade/HR-HPV positive	18-wk pathway, upgraded to 62 days if cancer subsequently suspected	Offered an appointment with a colposcopist within 6wks
High-grade (moderate)	62-day pathway/2-wk urgent GP referral; (move to 18-wk pathway if cancer excluded)	Offered an appointment with a colposcopist within 2wks of referral
High-grade (severe)	62-day pathway/2-wk urgent GP referral; (move to 18-wk pathway if cancer excluded)	Offered an appointment with a colposcopist within 2wks of referral
? invasive squamous carcinoma	62-day pathway (move to 18-wk pathway if cancer excluded)	Offered an appointment with a colposcopist within 2wks of referral
? invasive glandular neoplasia	62-day pathway (move to 18-wk pathway if cancer excluded)	Offered an appointment with a colposcopist within 2wks of referral
Cells of endocervical origin—referral inside NHSCSP		
Cells of other origin—referral outside NHSCSP		Offered an appointment with a gynaecologist within 2 wks of referral
Abnormal cervix (outside the NHSCSP)	62-day pathway (move to 18-wk pathway if cancer excluded)	Offered an appointment with a gynaecologist within 2wks of referral
Symptomatic (outside the NHSCSP)	62-day pathway (move to 18-wk pathway if cancer excluded)	Offered an appointment with a gynaecologist within 2wks of referral

HPV: human papillomavirus; CWT: cancer waiting times; NHSCSP: NHS cervical screening programme; HR-HPV: high-risk HPV

PHE (2016) Summary of referral/waiting time standards. Available at: https://www.bsccp.org.uk/assets/file/uploads/resources/NHSCSP_20_Colposcopy_and_Programme_Management_(3rd_Edition)_(2).pdf. Reproduced under Open Government Licence for public sector information (http://www.nationalarchives.gov.uk/doc/open-government-licence/version/3/)

Quality assurance
The NHS cervical screening programme has a regional system of quality assurance. Every 3yrs, a regional team reviews the performance of the local cervical screening programmes against national quality standards.

HPV testing

HPV testing introduced in England in 2012. There are two tests:

HPV triage
- Offered to all ♀ with either borderline changes or mild dyskaryosis.
- If oncogenic HPV is detected, the ♀ referred immediately to colposcopy.
- If oncogenic HPV is not detected, ♀ returns to normal recall at 3 or 5yrs and need for ongoing surveillance will be removed.

HPV test of cure
- Offered to all ♀ who have been treated for CIN and who have either a normal or low-grade abnormality 6mths post treatment.
- If oncogenic HPV is not detected, ♀ is returned to normal recall—3yrs for all age groups. Removes approximately 80% of treated ♀ from the current 10-yr surveillance programme.
- If oncogenic HPV is detected, the ♀ remains under care of colposcopy service.

⚠ Women with glandular abnormalities (CGIN) do not come under this new protocol.

References

22. PHE (2016) *Cervical screening education and training*. Available at: https://www.gov.uk/guidance/cervical-screening-education-and-training
23. Cancer Research UK (2018) *Cancer statistics*. Available at: www.cancerresearchuk.org/cancerstats
24. PHE (2016) *NHS cervical screening programme: colposcopy and programme management*. Available at: https://www.bsccp.org.uk/assets/file/uploads/resources/NHSCSP_20_Colposcopy_and_Programme_Management_(3rd_Edition)_(2).pdf

Further information

Jo's Cervical Cancer Trust (Cervical screening for people with a learning disability). Available at: ᐰhttps://www.jostrust.org.uk/about-cervical-cancer/cervical-screening/cervical-screening-learning-disability
NICE Excellence (*Cervical screening*). Available ᐰ https://cks.nice.org.uk/cervical-screening

Cervical sample taking

Liquid-based cytology (LBC) is used for taking cervical samples in the UK (➔ Cervical cancer screening p. 380). The sample is obtained using a Cervex-Brush® and immediately placed into a vial of preservative liquid. There are two types of LBC used in the UK: ThinPrep® and SurePath™.

Timing

The sample can be taken at any time during the month except when the ♀ is menstruating. If it is unlikely that a ♀ will return for screening after menstruating, still take the sample, although this is less than ideal. Mid-cycle remains the optimum time, but is not essential. Appointment times should be available outside normal working hours to encourage attendance.

Patient comfort and understanding

Aim to minimize embarrassment, anxiety, and discomfort. A sensitive approach is required to ensure ♀ continue in the programme.
- Ensure understanding of purpose of screening.
- Explain the procedure before and during test.
- Obtain informed consent (➔ Consent p. 82), for sample and for HPV test.
- Offer opportunity to empty bladder before.
- Offer a chaperone (➔ Chaperone p. 84).
- Ensure privacy and use modesty paper sheet while on couch.
- Offer tissues and hand-washing after procedure.
- Offer an opportunity to ask questions.

Protection against infection

Vaginal speculae used to access the cervix must be either single-use items or sterilized via a central sterile supplies department. Brushes and vials for the test must be kept in a clean environment.

Taking a history and forms

A history should be taken using the request form as a template. Accurate and complete details are essential including:
- Screening history
- Any contraceptive method (➔ Contraception: general p. 400) and HRT (➔ Menopause p. 364)
- Any abnormal bleeding, dyspareunia, or discharge symptoms (consider whether referral to other service such as gynaecology is required)

Forms can be:
- National, e.g. HMR101 (England)
- Open Exeter form, pre-populated with the ♀ details and history
- An electronic requesting method used for all types of samples

Sample taking

The sample must be taken from the squamocolumnar junction (SCJ). This is usually around the cervical os. It is essential to obtain squamous cells and desirable to obtain some endocervical cells from the SCJ.

- Clean a trolley and lay out the equipment needed using a non-touch technique. Remove the lid of the specimen container ready to receive the Cervex-Brush®.
- Use an appropriately sized speculum to keep vaginal walls apart and visualize cervical os.
- Do not use any lubrication if possible; it may affect analysis of sample. If needed, avoid lubrication touching the tip of the speculum.
- Ensuring a light source is present, insert the speculum sideways and gently rotate until the handles are vertical. Gently squeeze the handles to view the cervix. Always check the ♀ is comfortable and stop is she asks you to.
- If cervix is posterior, ♀ may need to tilt pelvis by clenching fists under her sacrum. A Winterton speculum may be helpful when cervix is very posterior. Coughing can also help bring cervix into view.
- Insert Cervex-Brush® into endocervical canal, ensuring the tip is in the cervical os and the bristles are splayed out against the cervix. Rotate the brush 360° five times in a clockwise direction. Firm pressure is needed to obtain sufficient cells.
- If an ectropian/ectopy/eversion is present, take care to sample SCJ fully. If a wide ectropian is present, two Cervex-Brushes® may be needed.
- If intrauterine device /intrauterine system in situ, the five 360° sweeps start and end at thread position, gently moving thread aside (➲ Contraception: Intrauterine devices and systems p. 414).
- Remove the brush head with one hand and place sample in vial immediately, with bristles pointing down: with ThinPrep®, agitate the Cervex-Brush® in vial to release cells; with SurePath™, place thumb against brush pad and release brush head into vial.
- Label the vial.
- Agitate the bottle but do not shake.
- Record clinical observations of the cervix (e.g. contact bleeding, polyps) on the request form.
- Vial sealed in bag with request form and sent to the laboratory.
- Take additional bacterial and viral swabs only if indicated clinically.

Further information

NICE (*Cervical screening*). Available ✒ https://cks.nice.org.uk/cervical-screening
PHE (*NHS cervical screening programme: colposcopy and programme management*). Available at: ✒ https://www.bsccp.org.uk/assets/file/uploads/resources/NHSCSP_20_Colposcopy_and_Programme_Management_(3rd_Edition)_(2).pdf

Testicular self-examination

The aim of testicular self-examination (TSE) is the early detection of any changes from normal that may indicate testicular cancer. TSE is method of 2° prevention (➲ Cancer prevention p. 372). The majority of testicular cancers are first detected by ♂ themselves. Testicular cancer detected early responds extremely well to treatment, with a cure rate of 97%. Most of the testicular cancer deaths in UK occur in ♂ aged 30–50yrs.[25]

Known risk factors for testicular cancer

- Age 20–49yrs
- More common in white ♂
- Previous testicular cancer
- Risk ↑ in ♂ with cryptorchidism (undescended testis; risk ↓ if testicle repositioned by age 10yrs (➲ Congenital impairments p. 262)), inguinal hernia, subfertility

Guidelines

Barriers to TSE are embarrassment, ignorance, and lack of confidence. The easiest time for men to self-examine is after a bath or a shower, when the scrotal skin is relaxed. To be performed once/month.

Know what is normal
- Hold scrotum in palms of hands, and feel testicles' size and weight (it is usual for one testicle to be larger than other, or for one to hang lower).
- Feel each testicle and gently roll it between thumb and finger. It should feel smooth. Soft, tender tube toward back of each testicle is normal (i.e. epididymis).

Know what changes to look for
- Lump or swelling in part of testicle (most are not cancer)
- Lump may be small and hard (pea-sized), although it may be much larger
- A dull ache in the testicle and/or lower abdomen (there may be no pain)
- A heavy feeling in the scrotum

⚠ Report any changes without delay to GP (➲ General practice p. 18).

Reference

25. Cancer Research UK (2018) *About testicular cancer.* Available at: https://www.cancerresearchuk. org/about-cancer/testicular-cancer/about

New patient health check

Such a check provides the general practice (➔ General practice p. 18) with the opportunity to get to know the new patient, whilst ensuring their medical information is correct and up to date. The aim is to understand the new patient's health needs, ↓ the incidence of preventable conditions, encourage good health in the practice population, and record any relevant QOF indicators (➔ Quality and Outcomes Framework p. 74). Usually conducted by the practice nurse (➔ General practice nursing p. 40).

Practices should offer a routine NHS health check to all patients aged 40–75yrs every 5yrs. It is good practice for all patients >75yrs who have not been seen in the last year to be offered a routine heath check.

Suggested elements of the new patient health check

- Review current and past illnesses and operations.
- Identify family history of illnesses.
- Check and record current medications (➔ Principles of medication reviews p. 142).
- Check allergy status (➔ Allergies p. 694).
- Check screening tests are up to date (➔ UK screening programmes p. 362).
- Check immunization status (➔ Targeted adult immunization p. 392).
- Check and record smoking status and offer smoking-cessation advice (➔ Smoking cessation p. 356).
- Measure weight and height for BMI (➔ Adult body mass index chart p. 346), and waist circumference.
- Review alcohol units (➔ Alcohol p. 360).
- Undertake urinalysis for proteinuria, glycosuria, and haematuria.
- Measure BP (➔ Hypertension p. 628).
- Offer healthy lifestyle advice.
- Arrange appointments with appropriate healthcare professional if additional intervention necessary.

Abdominal aortic aneurysm screening

Aneurysms are weaknesses causing bulges in blood vessels. Abdominal aortic aneurysms (AAAs) cause ~6,000 deaths/yr in England and Wales (→ UK health profile p. 2). Those most at risk are ♂ >65yrs who smoke, have ↑ BP (→ Hypertension p. 628), or with close family history of AAA. All ♂ aged 65yrs are invited in the year of their birthday for screening (those older can contact the local programme for an appointment) (→ UK screening programmes p. 362). Invitation leaflets explain the reasons, procedure, and possible outcomes. The screening is by abdominal ultrasound (takes ~10min) and results are given at the time and in writing.

Possible results of screening

- Normal: no AAA detected. No further invitations
- Small aneurysm: aorta is wider than normal, and repeat invitations for regular checks will be issued
- Large aneurysm found: aorta much wider than normal (only 1 in 100 ♂). Referral to specialist service for further tests and possible treatment, usually surgery.

Further information

Circulation Foundation (*Abdominal aortic aneurysm*). Available at: ℳ http://www.circulationfoundation.org.uk/help-advice/abdominal-aortic-aneurysm

PHE (*Abdominal aortic aneurysm screening programme overview*). Available at: ℳ https://www.gov.uk/guidance/abdominal-aortic-aneurysm-screening-programme-overview

Immunization administration

The UK national immunization programme is detailed in the 'Green Book'[26] and updated online to reflect real-time policy decisions and recommendations of the Joint Committee on Vaccination and Immunization. The purpose of vaccination is to protect the individual, who in turn is less likely to be a source of infection to others. High percentages of vaccinated individuals provide 'population' or 'herd' immunity, which benefits those who cannot be vaccinated.

Key aspects of immunization provision

Information about the benefits and risks of each vaccination can be provided so that informed consent (❸ Consent p. 82) can be given. One individual (and a deputy) in each clinic or surgery is responsible for ordering, receipt, and proper storage of vaccines (❸ Storage, transportation, and disposal of medicines p. 148) including:

- No more than 2–4wks supply of vaccines to be stored and used by expiry date.
- Refrigerate immediately in specialized vaccine fridge.
- Store at 2–8°C as monitored and recorded at least once each working day.
- As vaccines are prescription-only medicines, the fridge should lock or be in lockable room.
- Cold chain must be preserved in transportation, with storage at manufacturer's recommended temperature to point of administration.
- Transporting vaccines to other clinics, care homes (❸ Care homes p. 32), etc. should only be in validated cool boxes with maximum/ minimum thermometers.
- All individuals advising and administrating vaccines should be trained and updated in immunization, and in recognizing and treating anaphylaxis (❸ Anaphylaxis p. 810).
- Anaphylaxis packs with adrenaline (epinephrine) and protocols must be immediately available at the time of vaccine administration.

Administration of vaccines

- Ensure suitability and no contraindications to individual vaccines.
- Ensure informed consent (❸ Consent p. 82).
- Ensure the patient or carer is aware of possible adverse reactions and how to treat them.
- Most vaccines given intramuscular (IM) except Bacillus–Calmette-Guerin (BCG) (given via intradermal route) and cholera vaccine (given orally) (❸ Injection techniques p. 576).
- Deltoid area of the upper arm or anterolateral aspect of the thigh are the preferred sites for IM and subcutaneous immunization.
- A 23-gauge (blue) 2.5cm-long needle is recommended for IM administration of most vaccines.
- If two or more injections are administered at same time, they should be given at separate sites, preferably in different limbs.

- Patient should be given a record of vaccination (➔ Client- and patient-held records p. 90).
- The nursing/medical records should include: the date of administration; vaccine and product name, batch number, and expiry date; dose administered and the site(s) used; name and signature of vaccinator (➔ Record keeping p. 86).

Related topics

➔ Childhood immunization schedules (UK) p. 166; ➔ Childhood immunization p. 164; ➔ Targeted adult immunization p. 392; ➔ Travel vaccinations p. 399

Reference

26. Public Heath England (PHE) (2014) *Immunization against infectious disease: 'The Green Book'.* Available at: https://www.gov.uk/government/collections/immunisation-against-infectious-disease-the-green-book#the-green-book

Further information

e-Learning for Health (*Immunization*). Available at: ℘ https://www.e-lfh.org.uk/programmes/immunisation/

PHE (*National minimum standards and core curriculum for immunization training of healthcare support workers*). Available at: ℘ https://www.gov.uk/government/publications/immunisation-training-of-healthcare-support-workers-national-minimum-standards-and-core-curriculum

Targeted adult immunization

Five doses of diphtheria, tetanus, and polio vaccines in childhood
(➔ Childhood immunization schedule (UK) p. 166) ensure long-term protection through adulthood. Those with <five doses should be offered the
rest. Those with unclear history should be offered all five. Adults at greater
risk are offered targeted immunization.

⚠ The 'Green Book'[27] is essential reading for immunizations.

Seasonal flu vaccine

The vaccine is prepared each year to WHO recommendations on likely
virus strains. Immunization in September–early November gives 70–80%
protection and lasts 1yr. Available to those not covered by NHS for a fee
in high-street pharmacies. NHS provides free immunization for those 'at
risk'. General practice (➔ General practice p. 18) identifies patients and
invites them to attend. The district nursing service (➔ District Nursing
p. 50) generally vaccinates the housebound. It is an enhanced service under
non-general medical services contract. Annual guidance should be checked,
but in general at-risk groups include:

• All patients 65yrs and over
• Pregnant women (in all trimesters) (➔ Pregnancy p. 424)
• Patients aged 6mths and over in a clinical risk group(s): chronic lung
  disease (not all patients (see Green Book)); heart disease; diabetes, liver
  disease; kidney disease; neurological disease; immunosuppressed (e.g.
  chemotherapy (consider also household members)); morbid obesity
  (BMI ≥40 kg/m²) (➔ Chronic obstructive pulmonary disease p. 614;
  ➔ Asthma in adults p. 608; ➔ Asthma in children p. 306; ➔ Coronary
  heart disease p. 624; ➔ Principles of diabetes management p. 664;
  ➔ Endocrine problems p. 304; ➔ Problems of the liver, gallbladder, and
  pancreas p. 718; ➔ Renal problems p. 754; ➔ Parkinson's disease p. 674;
  ➔ Motor neurone disease p. 672; ➔ Overweight and obesity p. 348;
  ➔ Principles of working with someone with compromised immunity
  p. 466)
• In addition, programmes usually include: care home residents (➔ Care
  homes p. 32), frontline health and social care workers, carers (➔ Carers
  p. 458), and those in contact with poultry (for H1N1)

Meningitis ACWY vaccine

Recommended for adults at risk of meningococcal disease: adults <25yrs,
if no prior immunization (single vaccination); and those with asplenia or
splenic dysfunction. See Green Book for boosters.

Pneumococcal vaccine

Recommended for adults where infection is more common or serious:

• All patients 65yrs and over
• Patients in clinical risk groups: asplenia or splenic dysfunction; chronic
  respiratory disease (not all patients (see Green Book)); heart disease;
  renal disease; liver disease; diabetes; immunosuppression; individuals
  with cochlear implants; individuals with potential for cerebrospinal
  fluid leaks

Shingles vaccine

Recommended for adults aged 70–79yrs.

Hepatitis A vaccine

Recommended for: patients with severe liver disease of whatever cause; haemophiliacs receiving plasma-derived clotting factors (⚠ Need SC injection); men who have sex with men (MSM); injecting drug users (➔ Substance use p. 476); and adults at occupational risk. Also consider for those with chronic Hepatitis B or C, or milder liver disease. See Green Book for boosters.

Hepatitis B vaccine

Recommended for: injecting drug users and their sexual partners and children; MSM; commercial sex workers; individuals receiving regular blood or blood products, and their carers; chronic liver disease; adopters and fosterers of children from countries with ↑ prevalence of Hepatitis B; chronic renal failure; prisoners; people with learning difficulties (➔ People with learning disabilities p. 456) in residential accommodation; workers at occupational risk; and travellers to ↑ risk areas (➔ Travel healthcare p. 394). See Green Book for doses and boosters.

BCG vaccine

Recommended for:
- Previously unvaccinated tuberculin-negative contacts of pulmonary TB (➔ Tuberculosis p. 728)
- Unvaccinated tuberculin-negative individuals <35yrs in occupational groups likely to have contact with person(s) with TB: healthcare and laboratory workers who may be exposed to TB; veterinary and abattoir workers; prison staff; workers in hostels for homeless (➔ Homeless people p. 446), and refugees and asylum seekers (➔ Asylum seekers and refugees p. 444)

Reference

27. PHE (2014) *Immunization against infectious diseases (The Green Book)*. Available at: ℛ https://www.gov.uk/government/collections/immunisation-against-infectious-disease-the-green-book

Travel healthcare

Every year, UK residents make >50 million journeys aboard. 1° care services provide a key role in travel health. Patients should consult their general practice (➔ General practice p. 18) 8wks before travel.

Pre-travel

Key elements of assessment depend on planned travel details (e.g. country, travel mode, length of stay):

- Assessment of fitness to travel to include general health (most serious illnesses abroad are due to pre-existing disease, not tropical disease) and medical history relevant to vaccination (e.g. contraception, pregnancy, mental health)
- Requirements for vaccination based on current vaccination status and current NHS advice on need for vaccination according to area of travel (➔ Travel vaccinations p. 399)
- Need for malaria prophylaxis (➔ Malaria prevention p. 398)
- Need for health promotion advice (➔ Travel health promotion p. 396)

The travel healthcare plan will include health promotion advice, vaccinations as required, and anti-malarial prophylaxis as required. Advice should be provided on medicines for people on long-term medication, including adequate prescribed medicine to cover trip and restrictions on taking medicines in other countries.

Post-travel care

Consider the presence of imported diseases, as well as usual UK health problems, in travellers consulting for up to 1yr (particularly in first 3mths) on return. Assessment should include details of dates, place, animal contact, swimming in inland waters, sexual contact, previous vaccinations, and health of others in travel party. If complaining of fever, suspect imported disease, including malaria (as first priority), typhoid, and paratyphoid. Investigations include full blood screen, including thick and thin films for malaria. If complaining of diarrhoea, suspect imported disease such as giardiasis, amoebic dysentery, and cholera. Investigations include microscopy, culture, and sensitivity of fresh stool sample.

Further information

National Travel Health Network and Centre (*Medicines and travel*). Available at: ℬ https://travelhealthpro.org.uk/factsheet/43/medicines-and-travel

NICE (*Travel immunizations*). Available at: ℬ https://cks.nice.org.uk/immunizations-travel

ONS (*Travel trends*). Available at: ℬ https://www.ons.gov.uk/peoplepopulationandcommunity/leisureandtourism/articles/traveltrends/2017

Travel health promotion

On the journey

On arrival

Travel health promotion

This may form part of a pre-travel assessment or be offered opportunistically during other consultations (➔ Travel healthcare p. 394). The emphasis is on prevention for a wide range of issues tailored according to travel plans, age, type of activity, length of stay, etc.

On the journey

Deep vein thrombosis prevention advice

For any travel involving sitting for long periods: avoid alcohol (➔ Alcohol p. 360), drink ↑ water, perform foot and leg exercises, and use of anti-embolytic stockings if severe risk (e.g. blood disorders) (➔ Varicose veins, thrombophlebitis, and deep vein thrombosis p. 656).

Combined oral contraception

Remind ♀ using combined oral contraception and travelling across time zones to keep track of the hours, not day of the week, for the next pill (➔ Combined hormonal contraceptive methods p. 402).

On arrival

Accidents and injuries

Main cause of death in travellers aged <40yrs, often alcohol-related. Advise on using same level of preventative measures as in UK (e.g. crash helmets with mopeds, not diving into shallow water). Emphasize need for first aid kit and adequate travel insurance.

Safe sex

Supply condoms if appropriate (➔ Sexual health: general issues p. 760; ➔ Sexually transmitted infections p. 764).

Blood-borne infections

Use of sterile medical kit (obtainable from chemists, outdoor retailers, on-line travel equipment shops). Avoidance of blood transfusion.

Avoid insect bites

The use of insect repellents; cover up, especially between dusk and dawn. Travellers to areas at risk of tick-borne encephalitis to wear long trousers tucked into socks and to spray clothes with insect repellent. ➔ Malaria prevention p. 398.

Avoid animal bites

Rabies occurs in animals in Europe and North America, as well as less-developed countries. Advise not to touch any wild or seemingly tame animals. Wound management is essential after any potential exposure. WHO guidance advises washing wound with soap and running water for 15min, then apply povidone iodine or alcohol to help kill rabies virus, and seek medical help immediately.

Other issues

- Sun protection (➔ Skin cancer prevention p. 374)
- Danger of altitude sickness if travel to altitudes >2500m
- No-go areas because of risk of violence

Food and drink

- Traveller's diarrhoea common in travellers (◆ Food-borne disease p. 730). Remind people of basic hygiene (e.g. hand cleaning after toilet).
- Avoid foods kept warm or likely to be touched by flies.
- Advise on oral rehydration (e.g. 1tsp sugar, pinch salt to 250mL boiled or bottled water, or use commercially available preparation).
- Anti-motility medicines, available OTC in UK for adults and some older children (patient to be advised by pharmacist)
- Antibiotics could be considered for those with serious pre-existing medical conditions.
- In areas with ↑ risk of cholera, typhoid, Hepatitis A (◆ Viral hepatitis p. 724), advise people to avoid tap water, salads, seafood, and ice cubes, to drink bottled or boiled water, and to peel fruit.

Travel health insurance

- Required for foreign travel in case of needing access to health services. Always inform company of any pre-existing medical problems.
- In Europe, a European Health Insurance Card provides evidence of eligibility for health services under reciprocal agreements (check post Brexit). Advise to check it is still in date before travel.

Related topics

◆ Malaria prevention p. 398; ◆ Travel vaccinations p. 399

Further information

Foreign and Commonwealth Office (*Passports, travel, and living abroad*). Available at: ℘ https://www.gov.uk/browse/abroad/travel-abroad

National Travel Health Network and Centre (*Malaria*). Available at: ℘ https://travelhealthpro.org.uk/search?s=malaria&ge_srch

NHS Business Authority (*European Health Insurance Card registration*). Available at: ℘ https://www.ehic.org.uk/Internet/startApplication.do

NHS Scotland (*Fit for travel*). Available at: ℘ https://www.fitfortravel.nhs.uk/home

TRAVAX (About TRAVAX: NHS website providing up-to-date information for UK healthcare professionals who advise the public about avoiding illness and staying healthy when travelling abroad). Available at: ℘ https://www.travax.nhs.uk/about-travax

Malaria prevention

Malaria is a parasitic disease spread by the bites of infected mosquitoes. Over 1,500 cases are imported to the UK each year. Over 70% are the potentially fatal Plasmodium falciparum strain, in which death can sometimes occur within 24hrs of developing symptoms of the disease. Malaria prevention advice centres on four essential principles:

- A: Awareness of risk (❍ Travel healthcare p. 394)
- B: Bite prevention (❍ Travel health promotion p. 396)
- C: Chemoprophylaxis
- D: Prompt diagnosis and treatment

Antimalarial prophylaxis is required according to the area of travel, as per recommendations from an authoritative source. Patients visiting countries with endemic malaria where they have previously lived should be warned that any earlier immunity is likely to be lost, and that children born in the UK have no immunity. Travel to malarial areas should be avoided in pregnancy (❍ Pregnancy p. 424). Breastfed infants require antimalarials (❍ Breastfeeding p. 182).

Antimalarial medication

Antimalarial medications are <100% effective against malaria, but if appropriately chosen, still give very good protection. Choice of antimalarials depends on:

- Presence of chloroquine-resistant malaria in the travel area
- Patient's medical history
- Specific advice for children and pregnant women
- Tablets being taken in accordance with instructions (❍ Medicine concordance and adherence p. 132)

Malaria prophylaxis is not prescribed from NHS, so requires a private prescription. Some are available OTC.

Antimalarial precautions to avoid being bitten

- Cover arms and legs with appropriate clothing from dusk to dawn.
- Use effective anti-mosquito repellent (including children over 2mths of age and pregnant women): most effective ones contain DEET (Diethyltoluamide) (up to 50% content). Reapply regularly.
- Sleep with windows closed, use a permethrin-impregnated mosquito net, spray room with knockdown spray, burn a mosquito coil overnight. Air conditioning is an effective deterrent.

Further information

National Travel Health Network and Centre (*Malaria*). Available at: ℘ https://travelhealthpro.org.uk/search?s=malaria&ge_srch

PHE (*Guidelines for malaria prevention in travellers from the UK: 2017*). Available at: ℘ https://www.gov.uk/government/publications/malaria-prevention-guidelines-for-travellers-from-the-uk

Travel vaccinations

All travellers should be up to date with routinely recommended vaccinations according to the national schedule. Vaccines available for the following diseases: cholera; typhoid; Hepatitis A; Hepatitis B; tetanus, diphtheria, polio; meningitis ACW135Y; rabies; Japanese B encephalitis; yellow fever; and tick-borne encephalitis.

Children

Routine child immunization (➡ Childhood immunizations p. 164; ➡ Childhood immunization schedule (UK) p. 166) given earlier if travelling to ↑ risk areas for prolonged stay or travel may delay the routine programme.

Live vaccines

There are special considerations for pregnant women (➡ Pregnancy p. 424), people with a suppressed immune response, and people treated with chemotherapy or radiotherapy (➡ Principles of working with someone with compromised immunity p. 466). If two live vaccines are required, they should be given simultaneously at different sites or 4wks apart.

Immunization advice by country

⚠ Authoritative up-to-date information on requirements for area and countries of travel should be consulted.

Prescribing and administration of vaccines

Prescribing and administration of vaccine should follow legal and good practice guidelines, as well as relevant protective procedures against bloodborne viruses (➡ Occupational exposure to blood-borne viruses p. 102) and sharps injuries ➡ Sharps injuries p. 108. Only travel vaccines available under the NHS can be administered under patient-group direction in NHS setting. Vaccines administered privately in NHS GP setting must be administered under a patient-specific direction or by prescription prior to administration.

Payment and availability of vaccines

Travel vaccination can be supplied at commercial travel clinics and in general practice. Protection against the diseases cholera, Hepatitis A, polio, and typhoid (and any combination vaccine containing any of these diseases) is free of charge to NHS patients in an NHS GP surgery. Other vaccines can be charged for privately. Yellow fever vaccination and the international certificate of vaccination or prophylaxis (required for entry to some countries) are available only at designated centres.

Further information

NICE (Immunizations— travel). Available at: ⌕ https://cks.nice.org.uk/immunizations-travel

Contraception: general

Fertility control is important for the health of ♀, families, and societies. Contraceptive services are available in NHS clinics, some sexual health clinics, young people's clinics, general practice (➔ General practice p. 18), and not-for-profit organizations (e.g. Marie Stopes and Brook Advisory Service (under 25yrs)). Contraception is free if provided in NHS clinics, prescribed in general practices, or commissioned by a CCG. Barrier methods (➔ Barrier contraceptive methods p. 416), fertility monitoring, and the emergency contraception can be bought OTC (➔ Emergency contraception p. 420). Choice of contraceptive method informed by:

- Patient preference and accurate knowledge of methods, effectiveness, benefits, and risks (Table 8.4)
- Patient age, medical history, immediate family medical history, gynaecological history
- Past contraceptive history and experience

Consultations as a health promotion opportunity

- Smoking cessation (➔ Smoking cessation p. 356)
- Weight management (➔ Nutrition and healthy eating p. 342) and exercise (➔ Exercise p. 354)
- Safer sex practices (➔ Sexual health: general issues p. 760), sexually transmitted infections (➔ Sexually transmitted infections p. 764) assessment, and screening (➔ UK screening programmes p. 362)
- Menopausal symptom management and prevention (➔ Menopause p. 364)

Table 8.4 Effectiveness of different contraceptives

>99% effective	Contraceptive implant
	Intrauterine system
	Intrauterine device
	Female sterilization
	Male sterilization or vasectomy
>99% effective but <95% effective with typical use	Contraceptive injection
	Combined pill
	Progestogen-only pill
	Contraceptive patch
	Vaginal ring
99% effective if used correctly	Symptothermal methods; natural family planning
98% effective if used correctly	Male condom
95% effective if used correctly	Female condom
92–96% effective if used correctly	Diaphragm or cap with spermicide

- Emergency contraception provision
- Self-examination and mammography programme for >50yrs (➔ Breast cancer awareness and screening p. 378)
- Cervical cancer screening (➔ Cervical cancer screening p. 380)
- Preconceptual care (➔ Preconceptual care p. 422)
- Osteoporosis prevention

Under 16s and contraception

Fraser Guidelines (a House of Lords ruling) should be applied when assessing anyone <16yrs. This states that a health professional is able to provide contraception, and sexual and reproductive health advice and treatment, without parental knowledge or consent (➔ Consent p. 82) provided:

- The young person understands health professional's advice.
- The health professional cannot persuade the young person to inform his/her parents or allow health professional/doctor to inform parents that s/he is seeking contraceptive advice.
- The young person is very likely to begin or continue having intercourse with or without contraceptive treatment.
- Unless he/she receives contraceptive advice or treatment, the young person's physical and/or mental health (➔ Child and adolescent mental health p. 246) are likely to suffer.
- The young person's best interests require health professional to give contraceptive advice, treatment, or both without parental consent.

Menopausal women and contraception

- ♀ <50yrs, contraception required 2yrs after last period
- ♀ >50yrs, contraception required 1yr after last period

Related topics

➔ Contraception: intrauterine devices and systems p. 414; ➔ Combined hormonal contraceptive methods contraceptive methods p. 402; ➔ Contraception: progestogen-only methods p. 410; ➔ Natural family planning and sterilization p. 418; ➔ Sexual health consultations p. 762; ➔ Incorrect use of combined hormonal contraception p. 406; ➔ Emergency contraception p. 420

Further information

Brook (Ask Brook). Available at: ℳ https://www.brook.org.uk/our-services/ask-brook-a-question-24-7
Faculty of Sexual and Reproductive Healthcare (UK medical eligibility criteria for contraceptive use). Available at: ℳ https://www.fsrh.org/ukmec/
Faculty of Sexual and Reproductive Healthcare (Standards and guidance). Available at: ℳ https://www.fsrh.org/standards-and-guidance/
Family Planning Association (About us). Available at: ℳ https://www.fpa.org.uk/about-us
Guillebaud, J. & MacGregor, A. (2017) Contraception: your questions answered (7th edn). Amsterdam: Elsevier

Combined hormonal contraceptive methods

Combined oral contraceptive pill

The combined oral contraceptive (COC) pill is an oral drug containing synthetic oestrogen and progestogen. It prevents pregnancy by suppressing ovulation, thickening cervical mucus, and thinning the endometrium. One pill taken for 21 days, at same time each day, then 7 days pill-free is standard use (see Table 8.5 for tailored regimen). 24-hr window to take the next pill before ↓ efficacy (➔ Incorrect use of combined hormonal contraception p. 406).

Advantages

These include ↓ bleeding (➔ Menstrual problems p. 778); ↓ dysmenorrhoea; ↓ premenstrual symptoms; protection against uterine and ovarian cancer (➔ Gynaecological cancers p. 776); ↓ ovarian cysts (➔ Problems of the ovaries and uterus p. 780); and ↓ pelvic inflammatory disease. Advantages of tailored regimens include more choice for the woman, avoiding accidentally prolonging pill-free intervals, avoiding bleeding, and reducing unwanted side effects.

Risks

Venous and arterial thrombosis (resulting in myocardial infarction (MI), cardiovascular accident (CVA), pulmonary embolism (PE), deep vein thrombosis (DVT) (➔ Varicose veins, thrombophlebitis, and deep vein thrombosis p. 656; ➔ Coronary heart disease p. 624)), and breast cancer (although risk returns to normal within 10yrs) (➔ Breast cancer p. 774).

Table 8.5 Standard and tailored regimens for use of combined hormonal contraception

Type of regimen	Period of combined hormonal contraceptive use	Hormone-free interval
Standard use	21days (21 active pills, or 1 ring, or 3 patches)	7days
Tailored use		
Shortened hormone-free interval	21days (21 active pills, or 1 ring, or 3 patches)	4days
Extended use (tricycling)	9weeks (3 x 21 active pills, or 3 rings, or 9 patches used consecutively)	4or 7 days
Flexible extended use	Continuous use (≥21 days) of active pills, patches, or rings until breakthrough bleeding occurs for 3–4 days	4days
Continuous use	Continuous use of active pills, patches, or rings	None

Reproduced from Faculty of Sexual and Reproductive Health (FSRH) (2019) *Combined hormonal contraception*. Available at: https://www.fsrh.org/standards-and-guidance/documents/combined-hormonal-contraception/. By permission of FSRH.

Absolute contraindications

Absolute contraindications are listed in Box 8.3. The use of the COC pill in such situations could cause death.

Relative contraindications

Caution should be used when prescribing the COC pill to patients with: sickle cell disease (→ Sickle cell disorders p. 308), severe depression (→ People with anxiety and depression p. 478), systemic lupus erythematosus (→ Bone and connective tissue disorders p. 738), Crohn's (→ Inflammatory bowel disease p. 712), splenectomy, diseases with high-density lipoprotein, diabetes (→ Diabetes: overview p. 660), diseases with drug treatments that interact (e.g. epilepsy (→ Seizures and epilepsy p. 740) and tuberculosis (→ Tuberculosis p. 728)), BMI >30kg/m² (→ Overweight and obesity p. 348), multiple risk factors for CVD.

Choice of COC

- First choice is low in progestogen and low in oestrogen, second-generation pill (e.g. Levest®, Microgynon 30®)
- COC with gestodene and desogestrel (e.g. Femodene®, Femodene ED®, Femodette®, Marvelon®, Mercilon®, Minulet®, Triadene®, and Tri-Minulet®), known as third-generation pills, associated with a slight ↑ venous thromboembolism risk than second-generation pills.

Starting routines

For immediate efficacy (otherwise additional contraception required for 7 days), are one of the following:

- Day 1–5 menstruation
- Day 21 post-partum and not lactating
- Same day as miscarriage/termination of pregnancy (→ Termination of pregnancy p. 788)
- Instant switch to higher-dose COC
- Switch to a lower dose COC after 7-day break

Box 8.3 Absolute contraindications for combined oral contraceptive pill

- Smokers >35yrs
- BMI >35kg/m² (→ Adult body mass index chart p. 346)
- Unexplained vaginal bleeding
- Focal migraines (→ Migraine p. 744)
- Pregnancy (→ Pregnancy p. 424), breastfeeding (→ Breastfeeding p. 182)
- First-degree relative with arterial or venous disease diagnosed <45yrs
- Oestrogen-dependent neoplasm
- Active liver disease, heart disease, lipid disorders, conditions affected by sex steroids (→ Problems of the liver, gallbladder, and pancreas p. 718)
- Past venous thrombolytic embolism, arterial thrombosis, cardiovascular accident, transient ischaemic attack, atrial fibrillation (→ Atrial fibrillation p. 641) 4wks before and 2wks after major or leg surgery

Advice on starting COC
- Seek medical attention if chest pain; pain and swelling in calf; shortness of breath; ↑ headaches, or with speech or visual disturbances; jaundice; severe stomach pain; BP >160mmHg systolic, 100mmHg diastolic (➔ Hypertension p. 628)
- Situations of ↓ effectiveness. Additional contraception (e.g. condoms) required if: severe vomiting and/or diarrhoea >24hrs; taking interacting drugs (e.g. enzyme-inducing drugs, such as anticonvulsants, antitubercule, St John's wort herbal preparation). Need to change to another method of contraception whilst taking them and for 4wks after stopping enzyme-inducing drugs.
- Missed pill rules (➔ Incorrect use of combined hormonal contraception p. 406)
- How to obtain emergency contraception if required (➔ Emergency contraception p. 420)
- Follow-up 3mths after starting or changing COC (earlier if problems) and then 6mths (or 1yr according to local protocols) (➔ Principles of medication reviews p. 142)

At each consultation and review, check the following:
- Age, BP, weight and BMI, smoking habits, change in health or family health status
- Any minor side effects
- Date and any problems with last menstrual period (➔ Menstrual problems p. 778)
- Problems with missed pills or missed pill rules
- Any questions or concerns
- Medications and allergies (➔ Allergies p. 694)

Minor short-term side effects
- Breakthrough bleeding: not unusual in first months, but check pill routine/missed pills/diarrhoea and vomiting/drug interactions/disease of cervix. Screen for sexually transmitted infections (➔ Sexually transmitted infections p. 764). If persistent, may need higher-dose pill.
- Nausea, bloating, weight gain, breast tenderness (➔ Breast problems p. 772), loss of libido (➔ Sexual problems p. 768), and depression: may need change of pill.

Contraceptive patch

A transdermal patch, releasing oestrogen and progestogen, stuck on skin for 21 days, then patch-free for 7 days, is standard use (see Table 8.5 for tailored use). As for COC for advantages, risks, contraindications, starting regimens, follow-up, and minor short-term effects. If patch falls off, see guidance on detachment (➔ Incorrect use of combined hormonal contraception p. 406).

NuvaRing®

The vaginal ring releases oestrogen and progestogen, and stays in situ for 21 days, then ring-free for 7 days (see Table 8.5 for tailored use). As for COC for advantages, risks, contraindications, starting regimens, follow-up, and minor short-term effects. If ring falls out, see guidance on unscheduled ring removal (→ Incorrect use of combined hormonal contraception p. 406).

Related topics

→ Smoking cessation p. 356; → Contraception: general p. 400

Further information

Brook (*Ask Brook*). Available at: ℘ https://www.brook.org.uk/our-services/ask-brook-a-question-24-7

Faculty of Sexual and Reproductive Healthcare (*Standards and guidance*). Available at: ℘ https://www.fsrh.org/standards-and-guidance/

Family Planning Association (*Your guide to the combined pill*). Available at: ℘ https://www.fpa.org.uk/sites/default/files/the-combined-pill-your-guide.pdf

Guillebaud, J. & MacGregor, A. (2017) Contraception: your questions answered (7th edn). Amsterdam: Elsevier

Incorrect use of combined hormonal contraceptive methods

Incorrect use of the COC pill, the combined vaginal ring, and the combined transdermal patch can lead to pregnancy. Figs.8.2–8.4 set out the actions to be taken when pills are restarted late or are missed, rings are restarted late or are removed at an unscheduled time, and patches are restarted late or detached at an unscheduled time.[28]

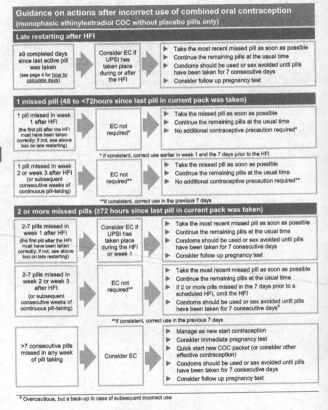

Fig. 8.2 Guidance on incorrect use of combined oral contraception.
Reproduced with the permission of the FSRH (2020). Available at: https://www.fsrh.org/documents/fsrh-ceu-guidance-recommended-actions-after-incorrect-use-of/fsrh-guidance-recommended-actions-after-incorrect-use-of-chc-march-2020.pdf.

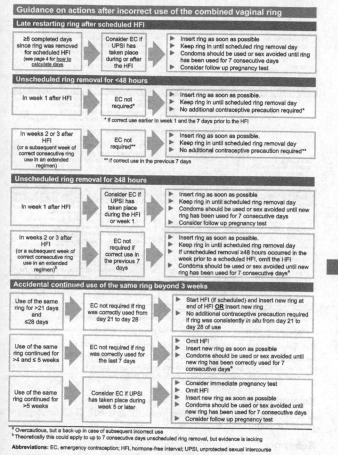

Fig. 8.3 Guidance on incorrect use of the combined vaginal ring (Nuvaring®).

Reproduced with the permission of the FSRH (2020). Available at: https://www.fsrh.org/documents/fsrh-ceu-guidance-recommended-actions-after-incorrect-use-of/fsrh-guidance-recommended-actions-after-incorrect-use-of-chc-march-2020.pdf

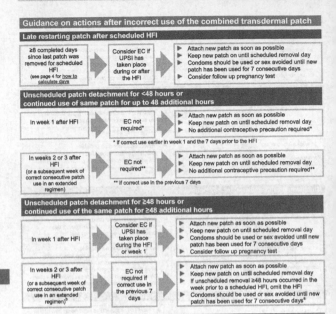

Fig. 8.4 Guidance on incorrect use of the combined transdermal patch.

Reproduced with the permission of the FSRH (2020). Available at: https://www.fsrh.org/documents/fsrh-ceu-guidance-recommended-actions-after-incorrect-use-of/fsrh-guidance-recommended-actions-after-incorrect-use-of-chc-march-2020.pdf

Related topics

➔ Combined hormonal contraceptive methods p. 402; ➔ Contraception: general p. 400

Reference

28. Faculty of Sexual and Reproductive Healthcare (FSRH) (2020) FSRH CEU guidance: recommended actions after incorrect use of combined hormonal contraception (e.g. late or missed pills, ring and patch). Available at: ℬ https://www.fsrh.org/documents/fsrh-ceu-guidance-recommended-actions-after-incorrect-use-of/

Contraception: progestogen-only methods

Progestogen-only contraceptive pill

The progestogen-only contraceptive pill (POP) is an oral method. It is sometimes known as the mini-pill. Prevents pregnancy by thickening cervical mucus, in some cycles suppressing ovulation, making endometrium unreceptive, and reducing fallopian tube function.

Advantages

Alternative to combined oral contraceptive (COC) pill when oestrogens are contraindicated (● Combined hormonal contraceptive methods p. 402). It may ↓ dysmenorrhoea and premenstrual symptoms (● Menstrual problems p. 778). It can be taken prior to surgery.

Initial consultation

Opportunity for health promotion, discussion of POP method, benefits, and side effects (particularly alteration of menstrual pattern).

Risks

↑ ovarian cysts (● Problems of the ovaries and uterus p. 780). If becomes pregnant, ↑ risk of ectopic (● Pregnancy p. 424); small ↑ risk breast cancer (but returns to normal within 10yrs) (● Breast cancer p. 774).

Contraindications

Pregnancy, past or present ischaemic heart disease, severe lipid abnormalities, liver disease or liver cancer, recent trophoblastic disease, current breast cancer concurrent enzyme-inducing drugs (e.g. anti-epileptics) (● Seizures and epilepsy p. 740; ● Problems of the liver, gallbladder, and pancreas p. 718).

Choice of POP

Desogestrel pill, as this inhibits ovulation and has ↑ efficacy compared with other POPs. Also has larger window to take the pill—12-hr compared with 3-hr with other POPs.

Starting POP

- Day 1–5 of menstruation: offers immediate protection. Additional contraceptive measures for 2 days if started later (● Barrier contraceptive methods p. 416).
- Changing from a COC: week 1 of CHC use additional precautions for 48hrs. Immediate protection if POP initiated week 2–3 of CHC or day 1–7 of pill-free interval.
- Post-partum: up to day 21, otherwise additional contraceptive measures for the first 2 days.

Taking the pill

Daily pill with no pill-free breaks, taken at the same time each day within 12hr for Desogestrel pill and 3hr for all other POPs.

Missed pills

If a pill is later than 12hr for Desogestrel pill and later than 3hr for all other POPs, continue taking POP at usual time and use additional precautions for 2 days. Ensure ♀ knows about emergency contraception (➔ Emergency contraception p. 420).

- Severe diarrhoea or vomiting within 2hr of taking pill: continue taking POP but assume pills 'missed' and additional precautions for 2 days.
- Enzyme-inducing drugs such as rifampicin and griseofulvin: reduce efficacy; need to use additional precautions or different method required whilst taking these and for 4wks after stopping them.

Review

3mths after starting POP, earlier if problems, then 6mthly or yearly according to local protocols (➔ Principles of medication reviews p. 142). Check age, BP (➔ Hypertension p. 628), weight, change in health or family health status, minor side effects, problems with menstruation or missed pills, any questions.

Side effects

- Menstrual irregularities: duration, volume, and flow may alter. May experience inter-menstrual episodes or amenorrhoea. This is the commonest reason for stopping method. Sexually transmitted infections (➔ Sexually transmitted infections p. 764) need to be excluded, and pregnancy test if amenorrhoea. Consider changing type of progestogen (i.e. to a different POP).
- Others: breast discomfort (➔ Breast problems p. 772), bloating, depression (➔ People with anxiety and depression p. 478), weight changes, nausea, skin problems (e.g. acne (➔ Acne vulgaris p. 300) or chloasma), changes in libido (➔ Sexual problems p. 768). Consider changing progestogen (i.e. to a different POP).

Progestogen injectables

Progestogen injectables have a main preventative action through suppression of ovulation.

Advantages

As for POP; lasts 8–12wks.

Disadvantages

Irregular bleeding, amenorrhoea, fertility may take up to 1yr to return (➔ Problems with fertility p. 784), may ↑ weight, may ↓ mood, cannot be withdrawn. Long-term use has a possible link to ↓ oestrogen levels and requires medical reassessment and review of risk factors for osteoporosis after 2yrs' use.

Contraindications

As for POP.

Initial consultation

As for POP.

Preparations

Preparations include Depo-Provera®, Sayana Press, and Noristerat®. Different preparations have different routes of administration and last for different periods of time. Some are licensed for long-term use and others for short-term use.

Starting injectables

Contraceptive effect immediate if first injection is given:
- Within 5 days of onset of menstruation
- <5 days post-partum if not breastfeeding or 6wks if breastfeeding (● Breastfeeding p. 182)
- 1–5 days after miscarriage or termination of pregnancy (● Termination of pregnancy p. 788)

Otherwise, advise ♀ to use additional contraception for 7 days after the first injection.

Repeat injections

Ensure timely repeat injections to prevent pregnancy (follow guidelines for each preparation). If repeat injection delayed, always exclude pregnancy before repeat injection (● Pregnancy p. 424).

Progestogen subdermal implants

For example, Nexplanon®. Small (40mm), thin rod inserted and removed by specially trained doctor or nurse into upper arm. Lasts for 3yrs with no check-ups required.

Action

As for injectables. Contraindications and side effects as for POP. Effect rapidly reversible.

Related topics

● Contraception: general p. 400

Further information

Faculty of Sexual and Reproductive Healthcare (*Standards and guidance*). Available at: ✍ https://www.fsrh.org/standards-and-guidance/

Contraception: intrauterine devices and systems

Intrauterine devices

Intrauterine devices (IUDs) are inserted via the cervical canal into the uterus. It is a small plastic device, often incorporating copper, with threads hanging into the vagina and tucked around the cervix. IUDs prevent pregnancy by impeding sperm transport, altering gametes, and blocking fertilization.

Disadvantages

Heavier and more painful periods (→ Menstrual problems p. 778), ↑ risk of ectopic if pregnant (→ Pregnancy p. 424), ↑ risk of pelvic inflammatory disease, rare risk of perforation of the uterus during insertion, risk of expulsion.

Advantages

Effective immediately, not reliant on user for efficacy, safe, and easily removable.

Contraindications

Previous ectopic pregnancy, abnormalities of uterus (→ Problems of the ovaries and uterus p. 780), allergy to copper (→ Allergies p. 694), at risk of sexually transmitted infections (STI) (e.g. multiple partners or short-term partners) (→ Sexually transmitted infections p. 764). History of fibroids and endometriosis, dysmenorrhoea, menorrhagia need careful individual assessment.

Pre-insertion

- Health promotion
- Counsel on advantages/disadvantages, particularly menstrual impact
- Sexually transmitted infection screening
- Ensure effective method of contraception until insertion, or abstinence from day 1 of period in that cycle. If changing IUD, no sex for 7 days before in case new IUD cannot be inserted and sperm survive.
- Information about insertion procedure, and likelihood of cramping pains that day

Insertion

- Performed by specially trained doctors and nurses
- Optimum time for insertion: end of main menstrual flow to days 14–28 of cycle; up to 48hrs post-partum, otherwise at or after 4wks
- Administration of oral analgesia (e.g. Mefenamic acid) prior to insertion to ↓ pain post-insertion

⚠ Emergency equipment should be available in case of vasovagal attack or anaphylaxis (→ Anaphalaxis p. 810). Insertions usually performed with two professionals for reassurance and in case of emergency.

Post-insertion

- ♀ encouraged to rest, then get up slowly
- Advise on feeling threads monthly and to return if cannot
- Advise on medical attention if pelvic pain and/or vaginal discharge
- Give patient a record of date of insertion and type of IUD (→ Client- and patient-held records p. 90)

Review and follow-up

Advise to return for review if any problems; no routine follow-up required. Ask about periods, pelvic pain, vaginal discharge, discomfort to partner, frequency of thread checks. Threads should be checked visually (through speculum) and also felt, as well as cervix moved gently side to side to detect partial expulsion of device.

Lifespan of device

Dependent on brand

Removal

• Any time if considering pregnancy
• 7 days after alternative method of contraception established
• 1yr after menopause (➔ Menopause p. 364)

Intrauterine systems

Intrauterine systems (IUSs) (Mirena®, Levosert®, and Jaydess®) have a slow-release progestogen (levonorgestrel) reservoir around the vertical stem.

Advantages

As IUDs, plus ↓ heavy periods, ↓ dysmenorrhoea, and suitable for women with history of pelvic inflammatory disease.

Disadvantages

Associated with irregular bleeding; may be constant spotting over first few months, although this settles down. Amenorrhoea after first few months is possible. More expensive than IUDs, so it is important ♀ fully understands disadvantages. Risk of expulsion and possible ↑ risk of ectopic pregnancy.

Pre-insertion, insertion, post-insertion, and removal

As IUDs

Related topics

➔ Contraception: general p. 400

Further information

Faculty of Family Planning and Reproductive Health (*Intrauterine contraception*). Available at: ℘ https://webcache.googleusercontent.com/search?q=cache:6LkD4bBXub0J:https://www.fsrh.org/standards-and-guidance/documents/ceuguidanceintrauterinecontraception/ceuguidanceintrauterinecontraception.pdf+&cd=1&hl=en&ct=clnk&gl=uk

Faculty of Sexual and Reproductive Healthcare (*Standards and guidance*). Available at: ℘ https://www.fsrh.org/standards-and-guidance/

Family Planning Association (FPA) (*Your guide to the IUD*). Available at: ℘ https://www.fpa.org.uk/sites/default/files/intrauterine-device-iud-your-guide.pdf

FPA (*Your guide to the IUS*). Available at: ℘ https://www.fpa.org.uk/sites/default/files/ius-your-guide.pdf

NICE (*Long-acting reversible contraception [CG30]*). Available at: ℘ https://www.nice.org.uk/guidance/cg30

Barrier contraceptive methods

Male condoms

♂ condom is a single-use sheath. It is applied to the erect penis before contact with vulva. The closed end is squeezed to expel air before unrolling down the length of the penis. After ejaculation, the penis is withdrawn, holding condom firmly in place.

Advantages and disadvantages

Protection against sexually transmitted infections (➔ Sexually transmitted infections p. 764), no systemic effects, easily available (➔ Contraception: general p. 400). Perceived as an interruption to sex, loss of sensitivity. Plain-ended and thin condoms ↑ sensitivity. Allergy problems. Hypoallergenic brands available if allergic to latex (➔ Allergies p. 694). Contraindicated in people with erectile problems (➔ Sexual problems p. 768).

⚠ Should only be used with water-based lubricants (e.g. KY jelly®). Oil-based products (e.g. baby oil, Vaseline®) damage latex and ↓ effectiveness.

Female condoms

♀ condom is a lubricated polyurethane tube with inner and outer ring, inserted into vagina. Inner ring aids insertion. Outer ring at open end, sits flat against vulva. Femidom® is the only female condom licensed in UK.

Advantages and disadvantages

Advantages as for ♂ condom. It can be used with oil-based products. Can be perceived as noisy during sex.

Vaginal diaphragms and caps

A diaphragm is a silicone rubber dome used with spermicide and inserted into vagina to cover the cervix (Fig. 8.5).

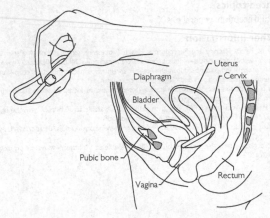

Fig. 8.5 Inserting a diaphragm.

Reproduced from Szarewski, A. & Guillebaud, J. (2000) Contraception. Oxford: Oxford University Press. By permission of Oxford University Press.

Advantages and disadvantages

Non-systemic, can be used during menstruation. Requires motivation, may be perceived as messy. Contraindicated in people with poor vaginal tone or prolapse (→ Vaginal and vulval problems p. 786), allergy to rubber or spermicide, recurrent UTIs (→ Urinary tract infections p. 756), past history of toxic shock syndrome.

Type of diaphragm and fitting

A coiled spring diaphragm or arcing spring diaphragm which is suitable for ♀ with posterior cervix. Sizes available from 60mm to 90mm. Femcap sizes 22mm, 26mm, and 30mm. Fitting must be performed by a doctor or nurse trained to fit diaphragms. The ♀ then practises in the clinic room: insertion, checking the diaphragm covers the cervix, and removal. Then ♀ has a trial period for >1wk in which she uses the diaphragm while using another form of contraception. Any problems of insertion, fit, removal, and comfort are addressed at a follow-up appointment, and size and fit checked before prescribing the diaphragm for contraceptive use.

Advice on correct use and follow-up

- Diaphragm used with 2cm strips of spermicide on both sides.
  Spermicide effective for 3hrs. If intercourse takes place 3hrs later, more spermicide is needed.
- Insert diaphragm before intercourse and leave in place 6hrs afterwards but no longer than 24–48hrs, depending on the brand.
- After use, wash diaphragm in warm soapy water, dry, and store in box.

⚠ Caps can be damaged by some oil-based products (e.g. Vaseline®, baby oil) and vaginal medications (e.g. Nystan® cream).

Advise to return for check of fit if problems or after pregnancy (→ Sexual problems p. 768). New diaphragm prescribed annually, or if develops hole, or after treatment of a vaginal infection.

Spermicides

Used in combination with barrier methods and are not protective on their own.

Further information

Brook (*Ask Brook*). Available at: ℘ https://www.brook.org.uk/our-services/ask-brook-a-question-24-7
Faculty of Sexual and Reproductive Healthcare (*Standards and guidance*). Available at: ℘ https://www.fsrh.org/standards-and-guidance/
Guillebaud, J. & MacGregor, A. (2017) *Contraception: your questions answered* (7th edn). Amsterdam: Elsevier

Natural family planning and sterilization

Natural family planning involves fertility awareness through observation of changes that indicate ovulation (usually 12–16 days before menstruation). From this information, the couple will either decide to abstain or use additional contraception (→ Contraception: general p. 400) or have sex for a pregnancy (→ Pregnancy p. 424).

Methods of estimating ovulation

A hand-held computerized system

Used for testing early morning urine for hormone changes. Commercial system (Persona®) available to buy, plus additional urine dip sticks. Not suitable if menstrual cycle <23 days or >35 days, menopausal (→ Menopause p. 364), breastfeeding (→ Breastfeeding p. 182), has kidney (→ Renal problems p. 754) or liver disease (→ Problems of liver, gallbladder, and pancreas p. 718), or using hormonal treatment.

Temperature

Taken orally in morning, prior to drinking or getting up (ovulation thermometer available on FP10). Charted from first day of period. ↑ 0.2–0.4°C indicates progesterone release from corpus luteum. Once temperature has ↑ and been maintained for 3 days, then intercourse can be unprotected until next period.

Mucus texture (Billing's method)

Texture of vaginal secretions is felt between finger and thumb daily (more frequently at first). Prior to ovulation, mucus becomes profuse, clear, stretchy (looks like raw egg white). 4 days after peak, mucus changes to thick, sticky, and opaque. Advise no unprotected intercourse from day the mucus becomes more profuse until 3 days after it becomes sticky.

Temperature and mucus texture often used in combination as a double-check method.

Sterilization

Sterilization is a surgical, permanent procedure preventing egg and sperm meeting. It is used by people who are certain they do not want children or more children. In the UK, about 45% couples >40yrs rely on sterilization of one partner. Referral is to specialist services (NHS or private) after initial counselling.

Counselling and information process

Very important, particularly with those <25yrs, without children, pregnant women, those in reaction to a loss of relationship, or those who may be at risk of coercion by their partner (→ Domestic violence p. 450). Prior sanction by a high court judge sought in all cases where there is doubt over an individual's mental capacity (→ Mental capacity p. 470; → Sexual health and adults with learning disability p. 770) to consent (→ Consent p. 82). Key information should include:

- Sterilization should be thought of as permanent (reversal is <50% successful)
- Post-procedure pregnancy rate: 1:200 ♀ (plus ↑ ectopic risk); 1:2000 ♂

- Procedures: ♀ laparoscopic tubal occlusion with clips or rings, usually done under general anaesthetic as a day case; ♂ vasectomy, usually done under local anaesthetic as a day case
- Risk of operative complications
- Need for contraception before and after operation: ♀, other contraception until first post-procedure menstruation; ♂, other contraception until two consecutive (but 2–4wks apart) semen analyses (>8wks post-vasectomy) show sperm-free

Further information

Faculty of Sexual and Reproductive Healthcare (*Standards and guidance*). Available at: ℜ https://www.fsrh.org/standards-and-guidance/

Family Planning Association (*About us*). Available at: ℜ https://www.fpa.org.uk/about-us

Guillebaud, J. & MacGregor, A. (2017) *Contraception: your questions answered* (7th edn). Amsterdam: Elsevier

NICE (*Contraception—sterilization*). Available at: ℜ https://cks.nice.org.uk/contraception-sterilization

Emergency contraception

Three time-limited forms of emergency contraception (EC) are available to prevent pregnancy (→ Pregnancy p. 424) post unprotected sexual intercourse (UPSI):

- Levonorgestrel tablets
- Ulipristal acetate tablets
- Insertion of copper IUD (→ Contraception: intrauterine devices and systems p. 414)

Choice depends on time from earliest UPSI in that cycle, and medical, contraceptive, and menstrual history.

Levonorgestrel (Levonelle®)

May be used <72hrs after UPSI. Given as a single oral dose. Most effective closest to UPSI in time. Acts to prevent ovulation or by blocking implantation of egg. If pregnant, ↑ risk of ectopic. If given from 27 to 120hrs after UPSI, as unlicensed use.

Contraindications
Porphyria

Cautions
Efficacy reduced with liver disease (→ Problems of liver, gallbladder, and pancreas p. 718), enzyme-inducing drugs (may need a higher dose), severe malabsorption syndromes, active trophoblastic disease.

Side effects
Nausea and vomiting, menstrual irregularities (→ Menstrual problems p. 778), breast tenderness (→ Breast problems p. 772).

Advice
- Take tablet immediately
- Not 100% effective and if pregnant may ↑ risk of ectopic pregnancy
- If vomit within 2hrs of taking, return for replacement dose
- Levonorgestrel deals with UPSI in last 72hrs, not future
- To seek medical attention if lower abdominal pain
- To reconsult if period unusual or >5 days late
- Advise sexually transmitted infection (→ Sexually transmitted infections p. 764) screening in 14 days, if appropriate

Discuss future contraceptive needs
Suitable hormonal contraception may be started immediately after Levonorgestrel EC with extra precautions for 7 days for combined hormonal contraception (CHC), injectables, and implants (→ Combined hormonal contraceptive methods p. 402), 2 days for the progesterone-only pill (POP) (→ Contraception: progesterone-only methods p. 410), and pregnancy test in 3wks. Alternatively, wait for next normal period. An intrauterine system may not be fitted until the next normal period, to exclude pregnancy.

Ulipristal acetate (EllaOne®)

This may be used up to 120hrs after UPSI. Given as a single oral dose.

Contraindications

Hepatic impairment, breastfeeding (➜ Breastfeeding p. 182), severe asthma (➜ Asthma in adults p. 608).

Cautions

EllaOne® ↓ the efficacy of combined and progestogen-only methods. With enzyme-inducing drugs, advice is to give Levonelle® (see above) or, if suitable, fit IUD.

Side effects

Nausea and vomiting, menstrual irregularities, breast tenderness, and headaches.

Advice

- Take tablet immediately
- Not 100% effective and if pregnant may ↑ risk of ectopic pregnancy
- If vomit within 3hrs of taking tablet, return for replacement dose
- To seek medical attention if lower abdominal pain
- To reconsult if period unusual or >5 days late
- Advise sexually transmitted infection screening in 14 days, if appropriate

Discuss future contraceptive needs

If starting oral hormonal contraception, should start on day 1 of next normal period or commence 120hr after EllaOne®, with extra precautions for 7 days for CHC, injectables, and implants, and for 2 days for the POP, and pregnancy test in 3wks. An IUS may be fitted at next normal period.

Insertion of copper IUD

Acts as a post-coital method by preventing implantation and may also block fertilization (100% effective). May be inserted up to 5 days after single occasion of UPSI or, if several occasions in that cycle, up to 5 days after the earliest calculated date of ovulation (usually 12–16 days before next menstrual period). At insertion, chlamydia results will not be available; therefore, prophylactic antibiotics may be given.

Related topics

➜ Victims of crime p. 452

Further information

Brook Advisory Service (*Emergency contraception (including the morning after pill)*). Available at: ℬ https://www.brook.org.uk/your-life/emergency-contraception

Faculty of Sexual and Reproductive Healthcare (*Emergency contraception*). Available at: ℬ https://www.fsrh.org/news/fsrh-launches-new-emergency-contraception-guideline/

Preconceptual care

Preconceptual care and advice can be offered as part of other consultations, including those for contraception (→ Contraception: general p. 400), cervical screening checks (→ Cervical cancer screening p. 380), etc. It may be given opportunistically or as part of a planned consultation. The aims are to ↓ problems in pregnancy (→ Pregnancy p. 424) and ↑ chances of conceiving in an optimum state of health.

Key areas to discuss

Rubella

Rubella infection in early pregnancy results in ↑ risk of fetal abnormalities, including deafness and blindness. Rubella status should be checked. If not immune, should be immunized with the measles, mumps, and rubella (MMR) vaccination (exclude pregnancy beforehand) and advised to avoid pregnancy for 1mth (→ Targeted adult immunization p. 392).

Screening

♀ should be encouraged to ensure any screening is up to date (e.g. cervical cancer screening) or undertaken if at risk (e.g. sexually transmitted infections (→ Sexually transmitted infections p. 764), and HIV (→ Human immunodeficiency virus p. 462)).

Genetic screening and counselling

Genetic screening and counselling are aimed at detecting carriers (→ Genetic problems p. 270), identifying levels of risk, and couples having informed choices about pregnancy. It may be required if: personal or family history of genetic abnormality; a previous pregnancy, baby with genetic abnormality; or an ethnic background in which ↑ risk of carrier status. Ethnic backgrounds with ↑ risk of carrier status include: Northern European descent for cystic fibrosis (→ Cystic fibrosis p. 318); African descent for sickle cell disease (→ Sickle cell disorders p. 308); Southeast Asian, African, West Indian, and Mediterranean descent for alpha thalasseamia (→ Thalasseamia p. 312); Mediterranean, Asian, Middle Eastern, Hispanic, and West Indian descent for beta thalassemia; and Ashkenazi Jewish, French Canadian, and Cajan descent for Tay sachs.

Diet

Encourage healthy diet and BMI (→ Adult body mass index chart p. 346) in normal range plus: folate-rich foods (e.g. breakfast cereals, leafy green foods) prior to pregnancy and in the first 12wks; avoid high levels of vitamin A (do not eat liver, liver products, or take supplements containing vitamin A); and do not eat shark, marlin, or swordfish and limit tuna consumption to 140g cooked and 170g raw per week (due to ↑ levels of mercury which can damage baby's developing nervous systems). Folic acid supplements are recommended in preconceptual period and through the first trimester of pregnancy (→ Neural tube defects p. 274).

Avoid food poisoning

Maintain good hand and food preparation hygiene (→ Home food safety and hygiene p. 352). ↓ risk of a bacterial infection called listeriosis, which can lead to miscarriage, stillbirth, or severe illness in newborns, by avoiding unpasteurized milk and any products made from it. Avoid soft ripened cheeses such as camembert, brie, goat's and sheep's cheeses and mould-ripened (blue-veined) cheeses, and any type of pâté. Ensure ready meals are heated until piping hot throughout, and pre-prepared salads are thoroughly washed. Prevent salmonella by avoiding uncooked meat, especially poultry. Only eat eggs with red lion logo stamped on their shells. ➋ Food-borne disease p. 730.

Smoking and alcohol

Encourage cessation in both partners because it can affect ovulation and sperm count, quality, and mortality (➋ Smoking cessation p. 356). In pregnancy, tobacco smoking increases the risk of miscarriage, growth retardation, pre-term birth (➋ Pre-term infants p. 176), cleft lip and palate (➋ Cleft lip and palate p. 259), placental abruption, stillbirth, and sudden infant death (➋ Sudden infant death syndrome p. 278). If pregnancy is planned or suspected, the safest approach is not to drink any alcohol because no safe consumption limit is known (➋ Alcohol p. 360). Drinking in pregnancy can cause long-term harm to the baby. The more alcohol consumed, the greater the risk of fetal alcohol syndrome. This can cause ↓ growth, facial malformations, and potential long-term learning and behavioural needs (➋ Behavioural disorders in children p. 326).

Toxoplasmosis

This is a parasitic infection causing fetal brain damage and blindness. Avoid raw meat, contact with cat faeces, sheep and goat's milk.

Fertility awareness

If sexual intercourse occurs within a day or so of ovulation, pregnancy is most likely to occur. This is usually about 14 days after the first day of the last period.

Pre-existing medical conditions and OTC medicines

Should consult their GP for review and advice, particularly on suitability of medication in pregnancy (➋ Prescribing for special groups p. 138). Few OTC medicines have been established as safe in pregnancy, so avoid whilst trying to conceive.

Previous problems in pregnancies

Should consult their GP for advice and early referral to specialist.

Pregnancy

Pregnancy is a continuous process of growth and development from the time of conception to the birth of the baby. The early signs and symptoms include missed period (or very light spotting), sickness and/or nausea, breast tenderness and enlargement, tiredness, frequency of urine, and constipation. OTC urine dipstick pregnancy tests can detect hormone human chorionic gonadotrophin on first day period is missed (see instructions on different brands).

Estimated delivery date

Duration of pregnancy is measured from the first day of the last menstrual period, not from the day of conception. So 4wks pregnant is 2wks after conception. The average duration is 40wks, and full term is 37–42wks. The estimated date of delivery is confirmed by ultrasound scan. Scans preformed in the first 12wks of pregnancy are generally accurate to within 3–5 days.

First trimester

During first 12wks of pregnancy, baby develops from an early embryo into fetus, with all organs and systems in place. Placental circulation also becomes established. If a ♀ is going to experience a miscarriage, it is more likely to happen in first trimester, most likely due to developmental problems with either fetus or placenta, or genetic defects. Antenatal screening for fetal abnormality takes place towards the end of the first trimester (➲ Antenatal care and screening p. 426).

Second trimester

From 12–28wks, ♀ experiences a growing sense of well-being as early symptoms, like nausea, diminish. Baby continues to grow and develop, with nervous system maturing progressively, so fetal movements become more pronounced. The baby can experience sensations like warmth and can taste amniotic fluid swallowed. Some even develop hiccups from time to time. A baby born late in this trimester would require respiratory and nutritional support to survive (➲ Pre-term infants p. 176).

Third trimester

From 28wks to birth is a time of continued growth and maturation. Baby doubles in weight between 34 and 40wks. Every week spent in mother's uterus is significant in respect of maturity of respiratory and digestive system. Full term is from 37 completed weeks. Fat stores develop subcutaneously to protect from hypothermia and hypoglycaemia in neonatal period.

Further information

National Childbirth Trust (*Pregnancy*). Available at: ℘ https://www.nct.org.uk/pregnancy

Antenatal education and preparation for parenthood

Antenatal education can take place during any encounter a pregnant ♀ may have with a health professional (e.g. during antenatal visits to a midwife) (➍ Pregnancy p. 424).

Parent education classes

♀ are also invited to locally held, free NHS parent education classes. Some localities offer a range of different preparations to suit local needs (e.g. aqua-natal classes that take place in a swimming pool under the direction of a midwife or other specially trained instructor). In many areas, health visitors (➍ Health visiting p. 46) work with midwives to provide community antenatal classes. Other organizations (e.g. National Childbirth Trust) also offer parent education, but will charge a fee to attend (see ✎ https:// www.nct.org.uk/pregnancy).

The aim of antenatal education is to build confidence to enable parents to take control over their labour and the birth of their child (➍ Group health promotion p. 336). Antenatal classes provide a place to discuss fears and worries, and exchange views with other parents-to-be. Parents attending classes find meeting new friends who will be going through the same experiences beneficial, particularly if first-time parents (➍ Support for parenting p. 172). Objectives: obtain balanced, realistic information so they know what to expect; learn skills that will help them to cope during labour; learn about emotional and social aspects of birth and parenthood; and learn about life after birth and caring for their new baby. Content of classes:

• Development and growth of the baby
• What parents might expect during pregnancy
• Common screening tests/blood tests
• Healthy eating for pregnancy
• Going into hospital to give birth and what to take
• Recognizing when labour has started and when to seek advice
• Coping skills for labour
• What will happen if help is needed to give birth (assisted birth)
• Common types of pain relief available during labour
• Breastfeeding (➍ Breastfeeding p. 182) and caring for new baby
• Life at home with new baby/how partners can help
• Common problems in the postnatal period

Some sessions might include practising labour-coping skills, such as relaxation and breathing techniques.

Antenatal care and screening

Pregnancy (➔ Pregnancy p. 424) is a time of tremendous physical, psychological, social, and emotional change. Professional care and advice at an early stage of pregnancy allows identification and management of any initial problems. Midwife or GP (➔ General practice p. 18) can be the first point of contact. Antenatal care is then carried out by midwives, GPs, and obstetricians depending on need and risks of developing problems during the pregnancy. Antenatal care can be given in mother's home, GP surgery, community clinic, or hospital. Care is best delivered by same midwife or team for continuity of care. Mothers hold their own pregnancy record so that continuity is maintained (➔ Client- and patient-held records p. 90). The aim of antenatal appointments is to check on the mother's and baby's progress, and provide information, explanations about care, and health promotion advice. The pattern varies according to need.

Antenatal care appointments

All women should have appointments and screening (Fig. 8.6).

First appointment before 12 weeks
Full assessment is undertaken. This may be a lengthy appointment. Routine blood tests include: full blood count (FBC), blood group and Rhesus factor, Venereal Disease Research Laboratory test, rubella antibodies. Recommended but optional blood tests include HIV (➔ Human immunodeficiency virus p. 462) and Hepatitis B (➔ Viral hepatitis p. 724).

Around 14 weeks
Perform ultrasound for dating/fetal anomaly/nuchal fold measurement and serum Down's risk screening (➔ Genetic problems p. 270).

16 weeks
Review results of scan and screening tests. If a congenital abnormality is detected, the ♀ and her family will need to choose whether or not to continue with pregnancy (➔ Congenital impairments p. 262). Genetic counselling available for all ♀ in this situation.

18–20 weeks
If mother requests a fetal anomaly scan.

28 weeks
To offer prophylactic anti-D to ♀ who are Rhesus negative (second dose at 34wks) and obtain FBC to monitor mother's haemoglobin level.

34 and 36 weeks
Presentation of baby checked.

38 weeks
To monitor mother and baby.

+38 weeks
All ♀ not delivered by 41wks will receive a further visit to arrange induction of labour. Nulliparous ♀ have another three appointments, to a total of 12 visits.

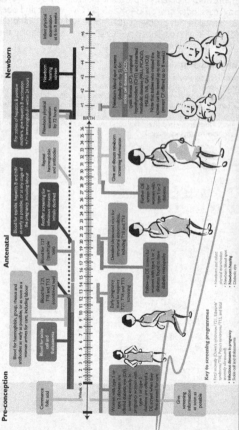

Fig. 8.6 Antenatal and newborn screening timeline: optimum times for testing.

PHE (2019) *NHS population screening: education and training.* Available at: © https://assets.publishing.service.gov.uk/government/uploads/system/uploads/attachment_data/file/768805/ANNB_Timeline_v8.4.pdf. Reproduced under the Open Government License for public sector information (℗ https://www.nationalarchives.gov.uk/doc/open-government-licence/version/3/).

Monitoring

- BP and urinalysis for proteinuria at each visit
- Measurement of symphysis fundal height at each visit from 25wks
- Pregnant ♀ are also offered the opportunity to disclose domestic violence (◗ Domestic violence p. 450)
- If, at any time, a complication arises, the ♀ should be referred to obstetrician for advice (◗ Common problems in pregnancy p. 432)

Women whose pregnancies are assessed as medium or high risk

Extra antenatal visits if long-term condition (e.g. diabetes (◗ Diabetes: overview p. 660)), previous problems in pregnancies, age >40yrs or <18yrs, BMI (◗ Adult body mass index chart p. 346) >35 (◗ Overweight and obesity p. 348) or <18, mental health problems (◗ People with anxiety and depression p. 478; ◗ People with psychosis p. 486; ◗ People with bipolar affective disorder p. 482), or problematic social circumstances.

Further information

National Childbirth Trust (*Antenatal care*). Available at: ℘ https://www.nct.org.uk/about-us/professional/research/pregnancy-birth-and-postnatal-care/antenatal-care

NHS Scotland (*Ready steady baby*). Available at: ℘ http://www.readysteadybaby.org.uk

NICE (*Antenatal care for uncomplicated pregnancies [CG62]*). Available at: ℘ http://guidance.nice.org.uk/CG62

Public Health Agency Northern Ireland (*Pregnancy book*). Available at: ℘ http://www.publichealth.hscni.net/publications/pregnancy-book-0

Maternity rights and benefits

Pregnant ♀ and new mothers in employment are protected by a number of regulations specific to their welfare and well-being while at work, and protected against discrimination on the basis of pregnancy (➋ Pregnancy p. 424). Employers of pregnant ♀ must:

- Carry out a risk assessment (➋ Health and safety at work p. 92) and if aspects of job pose a risk to the health of ♀, adjust working conditions/hours or offer another job
- Provide a rest area, preferably smoke-free
- After returning to work, provide a private room for breastfeeding mothers to express and store their milk (➋ Breastfeeding p. 182)

Pregnant ♀ in employment have a right to:

- Paid time off to attend antenatal care (➋ Antenatal care and screening p. 426)
- Normal sick pay rights for pregnancy-related illness
- Accrual of contracted holiday entitlement while on maternity leave
- A right to return to the same job

Maternity leave

All employed ♀ are entitled to 26wks ordinary maternity leave and 26wks additional maternity leave, irrespective of whether they are entitled to maternity benefits.

Key regulations

- They must inform the employer, preferably in writing with a medical certificate (MATB1), by the end of the 15th week before baby is due, when they wish to commence maternity leave. MATB1 is signed by midwife or GP (➋ General practice p. 18) to verify pregnancy and expected delivery date (EDD) at 20wks before EDD.
- Maternity leave can start any time after 11wks before EDD.
- Maternity leave starts automatically if a ♀ is sick with a pregnancy-related illness during the 4wks before EDD.
- A ♀ may not return to work within 2wks of birth (4wks if they work in a factory).
- Maternity leave rights remain if baby is stillborn after 24wks or born earlier than EDD.

Maternity benefits

Statutory maternity pay (SMP)

- A weekly payment made by employers to employees or former employees if they meet the qualifying conditions: employed for 26wks continuously by the 15th week before the EDD; earning at least an average of £107/week before tax
- An entitlement whether or not they intend to return to work for that employer
- Paid for a maximum of 39wks, can start 11wks before EDD
- First 6wks of SMP are 90% of weekly earnings; then 33wks of £145.18 or 90% of earnings, whichever is less

Maternity allowance

- Available to some employed and self-employed ♀ who do not qualify for statutory maternity pay, but meet criteria on weeks of continuous employment, paying National Insurance (NI), and earning on average £30/week
- Paid by Department of Work and Pensions and claimed on form MA1 from Jobcentre Plus
- Pays 39wks at £145.18 or 90% of weekly earnings, whichever is less
- Reduces amount received from other state benefits

Paternity leave and pay

Fathers are entitled to statutory paternity leave of 1–2wks at time of birth if they have been employed continuously for 26wks at the 15th week before EDD. They have to inform employer in writing. A self-certification form (SC3) is required (available at ℰ https://www.gov.uk/government/collections/statutory-pay-forms). This leave is paid if they are earning enough to pay NI, otherwise the father may be able to claim income support.

Sure Start maternity grants

Available to parents on ↓ incomes receiving Jobseeker's Allowance, Income Support, Pension Credit, Child Tax Credit at a rate higher than family element, or Working Tax Credit where a disabled worker is included in the assessment. This grant is only available if there are no other children under 16yrs of age in the family, or it is a multiple birth. A payment of £500, which does not have to be paid back. Claimed on SF100 Sure Start form from local Jobcentre Plus office, or Social Security office.

Other benefits

Pregnant ♀ and up to 12mths after birth are entitled to:

- Free prescriptions on production of exemption card (MATEX) from prescription pricing authority on completion of form FW8 (obtainable from GP or midwife) (➔ Help with costs of medicines p. 134)
- Free NHS dentistry
- Healthy Start tokens for milk, fruit, or vegetables if receiving low income benefits, from 10wks of pregnancy, by claiming on form (available at ℰ www.healthystart.nhs.uk) countersigned by health visitor (➔ Health visiting p. 46) or midwife

Further information

Citizens Advice (*Maternity leave—what you're entitled to and how to get it*). Available at: ℰ https://www.citizensadvice.org.uk/work/rights-at-work/parental-rights/maternity-leave-what-youre-entitled-to-and-how-to-get-it/

HM Government (*Pregnancy and birth*). Available at: ℰ www.gov.uk/browse/childcare-parenting/pregnancy-birth

Common problems in pregnancy

During pregnancy, a ♀ may experience a range of problems for which she can be given timely advice, making these easier to manage and improving her well-being (➲ Pregnancy p. 424). Problems include nausea, constipation, indigestion, varicosities, backache, and frequency of micturition. These so-called minor disorders of pregnancy are a series of commonly experienced symptoms related to effects of pregnancy hormones and consequences of enlargement of the uterus as the fetus grows.

Nausea

- Nausea and vomiting are common, with about 50% of pregnant ♀ suffering anything from mild nausea on awakening, to nausea throughout day with some vomiting, during first half of pregnancy.
- For many ♀ symptoms subside after 12th–14th week of pregnancy, coinciding with ability of placenta to take over support of growing embryo.
- Advice includes maintaining good fluid intake, eating little and often throughout the day, and avoiding caffeine and spicy/fatty foods.
- Doctor should be consulted if a ♀ is vomiting more than four times a day, if she is losing weight, or fluids are not being kept down.

Indigestion

- Caused when progesterone relaxes smooth muscle in cardiac sphincter, leading to reflux of acid into oesophagus
- Taking fluids separately to mealtimes, and sleeping with >two pillows so chest is raised slightly higher than abdomen can ease the symptoms

Constipation

- Caused by progesterone relaxing the smooth muscle in bowels
- The ♀ can be advised to take extra fluids, increase amount of fruit and vegetables consumed, and that exercise such as walking may help

Varicosities

- They are caused when weight of growing uterus creates back pressure in veins of lower body, overcoming normal flow of blood
- Accompanied by smooth muscle relaxation in vessel walls due to influence of progesterone
- Can occur in legs, vulva, or anal canal (haemorrhoids) (➲ Anal conditions p. 706)
- Support tights and close-fitting supportive underwear will minimize leg and vulval varicose veins. If legs are aching, resting with them elevated will ease symptoms.

Backache

- Complaint is common, both during and after pregnancy
- Ligaments supporting lower spine and pelvis become softer and stretch more readily during pregnancy. Poor posture exacerbates this, leading to backache.
- Advice includes not standing or sitting for long periods. Pay attention to posture, particularly if ♀ uses keyboard or computer at work. Using a chair with good lumbar support at work and at home, and regular gentle exercise such as walking, can all be beneficial.

Frequency of micturition

- Usually apparent during early pregnancy when uterus is still a pelvic organ, and later in pregnancy when fetal head enters maternal pelvis
- Both situations create pressure on bladder, reducing amount of space available; hence, the need to pass urine more often
- This does not normally inconvenience ♀, but she should be asked about other symptoms, such as burning, stinging, or discomfort during micturition to rule out UTI (➲ Urinary tract infection p. 756)

Further information

National Childbirth Trust (*Antenatal care*). Available at: ℛ https://www.nct.org.uk/about-us/professional/research/pregnancy-birth-and-postnatal-care/antenatal-care

NHS Scotland (*Ready steady baby*). Available at: ℛ http://www.readysteadybaby.org.uk

NICE (*Antenatal care for uncomplicated pregnancies [CG62]*). Available at: ℛ http://guidance.nice.org.uk/CG62

Public Health Agency Northern Ireland (*Pregnancy book*). Available at: ℛ http://www.publichealth.hscni.net/publications/pregnancy-book-0

Birth options and labour

For most mothers to be, planning the birth of the baby is an exciting prospect. Previous experience can, however, make this a daunting prospect. The midwife usually discusses options with the mother and her family once a risk assessment (including medical history, pregnancy, and previous complications) is completed, as it may limit the ♀ choices.

Place

A mother may give birth at home, in a birth centre, in a midwife-led unit, or in a hospital consultant-led unit. Healthy, ↓ risk mothers whose pregnancies are progressing normally can deliver with their midwife at home or in a midwife-led setting. Arrangements may change if complications occur in pregnancy and mother is referred to a consultant obstetrician. A mother may prefer a particular type of care (e.g. epidural pain relief) which requires she is cared for in hospital.

Care in labour

During labour, the mother will be cared for on a one-to-one basis by a midwife, if she is low risk. Mothers with high-risk pregnancies are cared for by a midwife, working alongside the consultant obstetrician. In a hospital setting, an obstetrician, anaesthetist, paediatrician, and operating department staff are also available if required. It is very rare that mothers being cared for at home will require any assistance other than that of the midwife; however, the midwife can request assistance from any other clinician as necessary. A decision to transfer into hospital is made if there is any deviation from normal during the labour or birth.

Pain relief

Usually, a discussion about such choices will have taken place during pregnancy and any preferences included in the birth plan. During labour in any setting, a mother also has choices about how she will be cared for. She may wish to be upright and mobile, and give birth in a standing, kneeling, squatting, all fours, or seated position. A range of pain relief is available including epidural analgesia (not during home deliveries), opiates, nitrous oxide, and O_2. A range of complementary therapies may be available if the mother wishes to use these.

During pregnancy the uterus contracts painlessly and passively to assist circulation of blood to the uterine muscles and placenta. These are called Braxton Hicks contractions. At the end of pregnancy, hormone changes result in the uterus becoming more sensitive to oxytocin, and so these formerly passive contractions become more active.

The process of labour

Initiation of labour

The cervix has to become softer and thinner to allow it to dilate during labour. In a first-time mother, these changes start to occur from 36wks' gestation. Prostaglandins are responsible for these changes, and some mothers might experience a blood-stained mucous discharge as the cervix alters. This is because the protective plug sealing the cervix is disturbed as the cervix alters its shape and size.

First stage

- Effacement of the cervix: i.e. cervix gradually becomes shorter (3cm long to almost flat) as early labour contractions pull cervical tissues up into lower part of uterus. These contractions can stop and start again several times before labour establishes.
- Cervix then gradually dilates until completely open in response to contractions and pressure from baby's head.
- Meanwhile, membranes containing amniotic fluid in front of baby's head start to bulge through opening cervix. This 'bag' of water does not normally break until cervix is fully open
- First stage of labour can last anything up to 12–18hrs.

Second stage

- Characterized by contractions becoming more expulsive in nature, creating an almost uncontrollable urge to push as descending baby's head is pressed against rectum.
- Mother will push during contractions and gradually this stretches perineum allowing baby's head to be born. The next contraction delivers baby's body.
- Second stage of labour can last from 30min to 1hr or more, depending on type of analgesia used. Use of epidural analgesia lengthens this stage as mother does not experience bearing-down sensations.

Third stage

Uterus continues to contract until placenta and membranes delivered. Most ♀ are offered an injection of oxytocin/ergometrine (Syntometrine) to prevent excessive bleeding during this stage, which lasts 5–15min.

Related topics

➔ Complicated labour p. 436; ➔ Pregnancy p. 424

Further information

NHS Scotland (*Ready steady baby*). Available at: ℘ http://www.readysteadybaby.org.uk
Public Health Agency Northern Ireland (*Pregnancy book*). Available at: ℘ http://www.publichealth.
hscni.net/publications/pregnancy-book-0
Royal College of Midwifes (*Clinical practice and guidance*). Available at: ℘ https://www.rcm.org.uk/
clinical-practice-and-guidelines

Complicated labour

Induction of labour

Labour may be induced with the mother's consent if she is 10–14 days overdue, or earlier if there are any concerns about maternal or fetal well-being at any other point during late pregnancy (➲ Birth options and labour p. 434). Induction methods aim to mimic normal labour so synthetic prostaglandin gel or pessaries are used to soften cervix, followed by IV oxytocin, which causes regular contractions to become established. Process of labour then continues as normal. Because contractions are artificially induced, they may be more painful, especially if rupture of membranes is also performed.

Caesarean section

This operation is performed with the mother's consent (➲ Consent p. 82) if it is anticipated that a vaginal birth poses unacceptable risks to the mother and/or the baby. This can be planned in advance if a problem is identified before labour or be carried out in an emergency should a problem develop unexpectedly either during pregnancy or during labour. Key points:

- Common for this operation to be performed under epidural anaesthetic as this leads to ↓ post-operative complications.
- Caesarean section on demand is discouraged as it is statistically more likely for a woman to die as a result of a Caesarean than a vaginal birth.
- Postnatal recovery can be delayed due to giving birth by Caesarean section.
- Complications such as infection (➲ Wound infection p. 526), urinary problems, haemorrhage, and thromboembolic disorders are managed by administering prophylactic antibiotics and low molecular weight heparin.
- Before surgery, an indwelling urinary catheter is inserted to prevent urinary complications.
- Analgesia is usually required for a number of days/weeks after birth. The mother stays in hospital approx. 48hrs afterwards.
- Caesarean section can sometimes lead to delay in lactation, so extra support is required by breastfeeding mothers (➲ Breastfeeding p. 182).
- There are also some risks to baby of being delivered by this method. These include difficulties establishing respiration, transient tachyapnoea of newborn, which requires admission to special care baby unit, (if delivered <39wks' gestation), and scalpel cuts to head, face, or neck area.

Forceps/ventouse

These instruments are used in 12% of births when either the mother or baby become tired or distressed, or the second stage of labour is considered too slow. Having an epidural ↑ the risk of needing an instrumental delivery. After use of ventouse, oedema on baby's head can take up to 2wks to resolve (➲ New babies p. 178).

Episiotomy

This is a cut made by the midwife or doctor into the perineum under local or epidural anaesthetic. Its purpose is to enlarge the vaginal opening and assist birth. It can be performed if the baby is in distress and needs to be born quickly, or during an instrumental delivery to protect the vaginal wall, or to assist a slow birth. 12% of births are aided by episiotomy. An episiotomy is repaired with dissolvable stitches (as are tears). It heals in about 2wks. Mothers are advised by midwife on perineal hygiene, pain relief, and other remedies (e.g. ice packs, warm baths) that may ease discomfort.

Further information

NICE (*Caesarean section [CG132]*). Available at: ℜ www.nice.org.uk/cg132

Royal College of Midwives (*Clinical practice and guidance*). Available at: ℜ https://www.rcm.org.uk/clinical-practice-and-guidelines

Royal College of Obstetricians and Gynaecologists (*Assisted vaginal birth—ventouse or forceps*). Available at: ℜ https://www.rcog.org.uk/en/patients/patient-leaflets/assisted-vaginal-birth-ventouse-or-forceps/

Postnatal care

The postnatal period is the time when the mother recovers from the birth, her reproductive and other organs regain their normal function, and lactation is established if she is breastfeeding (**➲** Breastfeeding p. 182). She adjusts to motherhood and becomes confident in the care of her baby, receiving advice and support initially from the midwife and, subsequently, from the health visitor (HV) (**➲** Health visiting p. 46). The midwife visits according to the needs of the mother and baby up to 28 days (although may be involved up to 6wks—there is variation according to national and local frameworks), visiting frequently in the first 10 days. The midwife liaises with the HV and in most instances the HV will visit around day 14.

Most of the physical changes take place in the first 6wks after the birth. Social, psychological, and emotional adjustment can take considerably longer and even up to a year after the birth. The rate at which a woman recovers will depend on several factors: her health during pregnancy (**➲** Pregnancy p. 424); the length of labour; whether birth was complicated or uncomplicated (**➲** Complicated labour p. 436); whether baby is healthy and makes normal progress; whether there were any problems in immediate postnatal period; and level of support she receives as she recovers.

Maternal health

At first postnatal contact, the mother will be offered information on the physiological process of recovery after birth and common health problems. The midwife will advise the mother about the signs and symptoms of potentially life-threatening conditions, and to contact a healthcare professional immediately if any of the following occur: sudden and profuse loss of blood or persistent increased blood loss; signs and symptoms of infection; headache in first 72hrs, accompanied by visual disturbances, vomiting, or feeling faint; signs and symptoms of thromboembolism (**➲** Varicose veins, thrombophlebitis, and deep vein thrombosis p. 656); and if the mother has not passed urine within 6hrs of birth.

During the first week after birth, the mother is given guidance and advice on the following: tiredness, a normal consequence of new parenthood; perineal hygiene or care of Caesarian wound; involuntary leakage of small amounts of urine (**➲** Urinary incontinence p. 504); haemorrhoids, common in postnatal period (**➲** Anal conditions p. 706); importance of appropriate diet and fluid intake (**➲** Nutrition and healthy eating p. 342); contact details for expert contraceptive advice (**➲** Contraception: general p. 400); that intercourse may be uncomfortable at first and contraception should be used to prevent further pregnancies; and normal patterns of emotional changes. The mother is advised to contact a midwife, GP, or HV if: any changes in mood outside of normal pattern; itching or bleeding around anus; or faecal urgency or frank faecal incontinence.

Between 2 and 6wks, the mother is advised to contact a midwife, GP, or HV if: still bleeding after 6wks; sex still painful; or severe, long-lasting backache is preventing normal daily activities. Midwife and HV remain alert to signs of domestic violence during this period (**➲** Domestic violence p. 450).

Infant feeding

Infant feeding information and advice is given during the first week. The midwife will support each mother in her feeding method of choice and knows to contact midwife or GP urgently if signs of mastitis (flu-like symptoms, red and painful breasts) (➲ Breastfeeding p. 182; ➲ Bottle feeding p. 186; ➲ Breast problems p. 772).

Infant health

At each postnatal contact, the parents are offered information and advice to help them to assess their baby's general condition, identify warning signs to look for if their baby is unwell (➲ The sick baby and child p. 276), and how to contact a healthcare professional or emergency service if required.

The midwife will assess the physical well-being of the baby during each postnatal contact, as well as advising the parents on:

- Parenting and attachment, social capabilities of baby
- Neonatal screening: obtaining neonatal blood spot screen (➲ Child screening tests p. 160; ➲ UK screening programmes p. 362)
- Health promotion and well-baby care: including skin, thrush infection, nappy rash, constipation, diarrhoea, colic, fever, jaundice, vitamin K, and care of umbilicus before and after cord separation (➲ Baby hygiene and skin care p. 194)
- Relevant safety issues and safety equipment (➲ Accident prevention p. 168; ➲ Promoting baby development safely 0–1 years p. 202), and reinforcing the recommendations about sudden infant death (➲ Sudden infant death syndrome p. 278)

Midwife will be alert to risk factors, and signs of child abuse and children in need (➲ Safeguarding children p. 248; ➲ Identifying the child in need of protection p. 250). Either the midwife or HV will give the parents a parent-held child health record (➲ Client- and patient-held records p. 90) and NHS-produced child health promotion information, according to local protocols.

Related topics

➲ New birth visits p. 174

Postnatal depression

Definition and onset

A depressive illness that occurs during the first 12mths following childbirth and lasts for several weeks/months, with a second peak at 6–8mths post-partum. Often more long-lasting and debilitating than depression at other times (➲ People with anxiety and depression p. 478). It occurs in 10–15% of women. It is distinguishable from postnatal 'blues' (i.e. brief low mood felt at some point by many women in first 2wks postnatally) by greater severity and longer duration. It is also distinguishable from more severe post-partum psychosis (symptoms include loss of contact with reality, hallucinations, severe thought disturbance) (➲ People with psychosis p. 486), which only occurs in 2 in 2000 births, and requires immediate medical assessment and treatment.

Causes

Unknown, probably no single reason. In some cases, may be a result of hormonal changes. Stress of looking after a young baby, and having sleep disrupted may also help to bring on illness in susceptible people.

Risk factors

* Previous history of depression
* Stressful life events: especially during pregnancy (negative life events, previous miscarriage/stillbirth)
* Family and marital difficulties: poor marital relationship, conflict between woman and parents (➲ Domestic violence p. 450)
* Inadequate levels of social support
* Personality factors and attitudes: perfectionism, low self-esteem, negative maternal attitudes towards child rearing
* Mood during pregnancy
* Family history of depression
* Infant temperament and mother–infant difficulties
* Early experiences: poor relationship with own mother, history of sexual abuse
* Unrealistic expectations of motherhood

Symptoms

Variable, but persist most of the time and include low mood, tearfulness/crying, anxiety/panic attacks, self-blame/guilt, undue health worries, lethargy/tiredness, irritability, ↓ appetite, inadequacy, emotionally labile, loss of interest in activities.

Assessment and management

* Assessment should be through simple, brief self-report on symptoms of depression, at a minimum, on antenatal booking (➲ Antenatal care and screening p. 426) and postnatally at 4–6wks and 3–4mths (➲ Postnatal care p. 438).
* Edinburgh Postnatal Depression Scale is not a screening tool and is not ratified by the UK National Screening Committee. However, clinical guidance[29] suggests it can aid in assessment of mood when used by

trained professionals. Local protocols apply in management and referral to GP (→ General practice p. 18) and mental health services of women identified at different levels of risk.

- 1° prevention: focuses on raising awareness antenatally, provision of extra support, and prevention of social isolation, e.g. through Sure Start (→ Social support p. 28; → Support for parenting p. 172). Additional 'listening visits' may be offered by health visitors (HVs) (→ Health visiting p. 46) to women identified as 'at risk' of depression (→ Talking therapies p. 472).
- Management of women diagnosed with postnatal depression is as for any depression. It may include 'listening visits' by HVs, non-directive counselling, dynamic psychotherapy, cognitive behavioural therapy, and antidepressants. Occasionally, hospital admission to a mother and baby unit is necessary.
- ♀ diagnosed with puerperal psychosis are managed in the same way as any psychotic illness and may be admitted to mother and baby unit.

Potential long-term effects

- May predispose for future postnatal depression
- May have a negative influence on the mother–infant relationship and future child development
- May have a negative effect on partner/marital relationship

Reference

29. NICE (2014) *Antenatal and postnatal mental health: clinical management and service guidance [CG162]*. Available at: https://www.nice.org.uk/guidance/cg192

Further information

Association for Postnatal Illness (*About us*). Available at: ℒ www.apni.org

Health Care Improvement Scotland and Scottish Intercollegiate Guidelines Network (*Management of perinatal mood disorders*). Available at: ℒ www.sign.ac.uk/assets/sign127_update.pdf

National Childbirth Trust (*Postnatal depression and support services*). Available at: ℒ https://www.nct.org.uk/local-activities-meets-ups/region-east-england/branch-herts-north/branch-health-information-herts-north/postnatal-depression-support-and-services

NICE (*Antenatal and postnatal mental health: clinical management and service guidance [CG192]*). Available at: ℒ www.nice.org.uk/CG192

Service users
with extra needs

Asylum seekers and refugees 444
Homeless people 446
Gypsies and travellers 448
Domestic violence 450
Victims of crime 452
Adults at risk from harm and abuse 454
People with learning disabilities 456
Carers 458
Human immunodeficiency virus (HIV) 462
Principles of working with someone with compromised
    immunity 466
Principles of working with someone with an infectious
    disease 467
Transition of young people to adult services 468
Mental capacity 470
Talking therapies 472
People with eating disorders 474
Substance use 476
People with anxiety and depression 478
People with bipolar affective disorder 482
People with psychosis 486
Post-traumatic stress disorder 490
Female genital mutilation 492
Suicidal intent and deliberate self-harm 494
People with dementia 498
Armed forces veterans 502

Asylum seekers and refugees

The UK is a signatory to the 1951 United Nations (UN) Convention relating to the Status of Refugees.[1]

Refugee

A person who has a 'well-founded fear of being persecuted for reasons of race, religion, nationality, membership of a particular social group or political opinion, is outside the country of his nationality and is unable or, owing to such fear, is unwilling to avail himself of the protection of that country; or who, not having a nationality and being outside the country of his former habitual residence as a result of such events, is unable or, owing to such fear, is unwilling to return to it'.[1] In the UK, a person is recognized as refugee only when application for asylum has been accepted by the Home Office (HO).

Asylum seeker

Those in the application process to be granted refugee status are referred to as 'asylum seekers'. In the UK, they need to lodge an asylum claim with the HO and wait for a decision on the claim.

People seeking asylum

People make their application at an asylum screening unit in South London. Asylum seekers are not allowed to work and have to comply with restrictions and stay in contact with their case worker. Those without personal means of support and classed as destitute (homeless (➲ Homeless people p. 446) or without means to buy food) may qualify for free housing (➲ Homes and housing p. 26) and financial help. Accommodation is provided on a no-choice basis outside of London and the South-East. People making an application have the right to NHS care (➲ NHS Entitlements p. 10) and education for children. Refused asylum seekers are expected to arrange to leave the UK. If a person does not leave the UK after their claim has been refused, the UK Border Agency may arrange an enforced return. Secure detention centres are used to accommodate people and children when there are strong grounds for believing that an asylum seeker is likely to abscond or refuse to co-operate with authorities, for identity/security verification, and in connection with significant unfounded or abusive claims.

People recognized as refugees

People recognized as refugees by the UK Border Agency are given a residence permit for 5yrs in the first instance, at which point their case will be reviewed again and they may have to return to their own country or be given indefinite leave to remain. Those not recognized as refugees, within the terms of the Refugee Convention, but who can demonstrate a need for international protection, may be granted humanitarian protection or discretionary leave.

Health issues

Refugees and asylum seekers are a vulnerable group with significant and complex health needs (⊙ Children with complex health needs and disabilities p. 238). They often originate from ↓ income countries with an ↑ prevalence of infectious diseases (⊙ Infectious diseases in childhood p. 290; ⊙ Infectious disease notifications p. 104; ⊙ Principles of working with someone with an infectious disease p. 467) such as Hepatitis B (⊙ Viral hepatitis p. 724), tuberculosis (TB) (⊙ Tuberculosis p. 728), and human immunodeficiency virus (HIV) (⊙ Human immunodeficiency virus p. 462). Poor hygiene conditions during flight from conflict and inadequate vaccine coverage aggravate health issues. This group has ↑ sexual and reproductive health needs (⊙ Sexual health: general issues p. 760) with ↑ levels of sexual and gender-based violence (⊙ Domestic violence p. 450; ⊙ Victims of crime p. 452) and limited access to contraception (⊙ Contraception: general p. 400). Refugees and asylum seekers also suffer from non-communicable diseases such as hypertension (⊙ Hypertension p. 628), musculoskeletal (MSK) disease (⊙ Common musculoskeletal problems p. 734), chronic respiratory disease (⊙ Chronic obstructive pulmonary disease p. 614; ⊙ Asthma in children p. 306; ⊙ Asthma in adults p. 608), and diabetes (⊙ Diabetes: overview p. 660; ⊙ Principles of diabetes management p. 664), which may not have been managed as they fled their countries.[2]

Mental health is also a concern. Violence experienced in countries of origin may include war, sexual abuse, and torture leading to psychological and physical trauma (⊙ Post-traumatic stress disorder p. 490; ⊙ People with anxiety and depression p. 478). This is exacerbated by loss of social networks, changing roles, and the stress of trying to integrate into a new country. A significant proportion suffer post-traumatic stress disorder.

Refugees and asylum seekers are not homogeneous. Health needs have to be assessed individually. While all refugees and asylum seekers have experienced loss, they also demonstrate resilience and courage in facing enormous challenges.

Related topics

⊙ Adults and children with additional communication needs p. 122; ⊙ Female genital mutilation p. 492; ⊙ Anti-discriminatory healthcare p. 81; ⊙ Child and adolescent mental health p. 246

References

1. United Nations High Commissioner for Refugees (2010) *Convention and protocol relating to the status of refugees.* Available at: http://www.unhcr.org/protection/basic/3b66c2aa10/convention-protocol-relating-status-refugees.html
2. Robertshaw, L., Dhesi, S., & Jones, L. (2017) Challenges and facilitators for health professionals providing primary healthcare for refugees and asylum seekers in high-income countries: a systematic review and thematic synthesis of qualitative research. *BMJ Open*, 7(8). Available at: https://bmjopen.bmj.com/content/7/8/e015981

Homeless people

Types of homelessness include rough sleeping, living in temporary accommodation, and sofa surfing between friends and family. To be legally defined as homeless, someone must either lack a secure place in which they are entitled to live or are not reasonably able to stay. Local authorities (LAs) (● Social services p. 30) have a legal duty to provide advice to all those who meet the criteria and a duty to provide emergency accommodation to those with a priority need such as dependent children (● Children and young people in need p. 158) and pregnancy (● Pregnancy p. 424).

Causes of homelessness

Complex, interrelated, and different for different age groups: mental health needs; family breakdown; abuse (● Safeguarding children p. 248; ● Adults at risk from harm and abuse p. 454) or violence in the home (● Victims of crime p. 452); alcohol (● Alcohol p. 360), drug and substance misuse (● Substance use p. 476); debt and unemployment; lack of affordable housing (● Homes and housing p. 26); and leaving armed forces (● Armed forces veterans p. 502), prison, or residential care (e.g. looked-after children (● Looked-after children p. 254).

Health needs

In addition to health needs that have contributed to homelessness, people are vulnerable to a wide range of health problems: mental health problems, including depression (● People with anxiety and depression p. 478); drug misuse; TB (● Tuberculosis p. 728); respiratory problems (● Chronic obstructive pulmonary disease p. 614; ● Asthma in adults p. 608; ● Asthma in children p. 306); hepatitis (● Viral hepatitis p. 724); skin problems (● Eczema/dermatitis p. 684; ● Fungal infections p. 686), including leg ulceration (● Leg ulcer assessment p. 536); and malnutrition (● Malnutrition p. 350). Homeless people are 40 times less likely to register with a GP (● General practice p. 18) than members of the general population. The average life expectancy of homeless people is 47yrs (● UK health profile p. 2).

Access to healthcare

Health organizations and LAs have local plans for improving access to healthcare for families in temporary accommodation and homeless people (● Health needs assessment p. 15). It is important to ensure close liaison between mental health service providers, charitable providers, and 1° healthcare. In urban areas, where there are ↑ numbers of homeless, more likely to be specialist providers/teams and GPs offering enhanced services.

Help with housing

Local Citizens Advice Bureaus and Housing Action Centres are key resources for advice and help on housing issues. Shelter also provides access to expert housing advisers and an urgent helpline (● 0808 8004444).

Emergency accommodation
- Night shelters: often found in public buildings (e.g. churches)
- Hostels: provide a few nights' to a few months' accommodation, requires payment, and may need to book ahead. Some have entry criteria (e.g. age, no substance abuse, and religious)
- Nightstop: for single homeless aged 16–25yrs for one night only, provided by people with spare rooms
- Foyers: for young people, provide accommodation up to 9mths, support to acquire new skills, and long-term housing

Support and advice for other forms of accommodation
For example, bed and breakfast (subject to eligibility), housing association, council housing, and private rental can be accessed through local council, homeless outreach teams (charitable or council-based), and main homeless charities (e.g. Shelter, Crisis).

Related topics
→ Asylum seekers and refugees p. 444; → Anti-discriminatory healthcare p. 81; → Child and adolescent mental health p. 246

Further information
Crisis (*Ending homelessness*). Available at: https://www.crisis.org.uk/ending-homelessness/
Nightstop (*Preventing homelessness through community hosting*). Available at: www.depaulnightstopuk.org/
Shelter (*Homelessness*). Available at: https://england.shelter.org.uk/housing_advice/homelessness

Gypsies and travellers

Definition

- Romany gypsies and Irish travellers
- New travellers
- Scottish travellers
- European Roma
- Show people (fairground workers and circus people)
- Bargees (occupational boat dwellers)

Discrimination and marginalization

Romany gypsies and Irish travellers are a recognized minority ethnic group who have the full protection of the Equality Act 2010. They are one of most marginalized ethnic minorities in the UK and subject to widespread prejudice (➔ Anti-discriminatory healthcare p. 81).

Accommodation

Trailers (caravans) on privately-owned or rented sites, or on unauthorized encampments (➔ Homes and housing p. 26). Cultural importance of close proximity to extended family for support (➔ Carers p. 458) and well-being. Around half the population live in houses. House dwelling is associated with long-term illness, poorer health state, and anxiety (➔ People with anxiety and depression p. 478).

Health

Gypsies and travellers have significantly worse health than the general population: ↑ respiratory problems (➔ Chronic obstructive pulmonary disease p. 614; ➔ Asthma in adults p. 608; ➔ Asthma in children p. 306); ↑ suicide (➔ Suicidal intent and deliberate self-harm p. 494), anxiety, and depression; and excess prevalence of stillbirths, neonatal deaths (➔ Sudden infant death syndrome p. 278), and premature death of older offspring. Possibly the highest maternal death rate among all minority ethnic groups. ↓ life expectancy and ↑ mortality rates for all causes compared to general population (➔ UK health profile p. 2).

Access to services

Reluctance of GPs (➔ General practice p. 18) to register travellers or visit sites. Mismatch of expectations between travellers and health staff (➔ Patient and public experience p. 75). Attitudinal barriers (➔ Professional conduct p. 80). Cultural inappropriateness of service delivery. Lack of readily available health records for continuity of care (➔ Continuity of care p. 598). ↓ literacy levels and poor knowledge of services amongst travellers.

Good practice guidance

Never make assumptions about cultural practices. Use client-held health records (➔ Client- and patient-held records p. 90). Involve specialist health workers for gypsies and travellers. Maximize opportunistic health promotion (➔ Models and approaches to health promotion p. 334; ➔ Group health promotion p. 336).

At an organizational level: involve gypsies and travellers in cultural competence training (➔ Continuing professional development p. 53); use specialist health workers in partnership with gypsy and traveller communities and agencies to address wider determinants of health through community development and capacity development (➔ Health needs assessment p. 15; ➔ Community approaches to health p. 338); and include in NHS ethnic monitoring to address 'invisibility' in public health practice.

Related topics

➔ Child and adolescent mental health p. 246

Further information

Friends, Families and Travellers (*Working towards equality*). Available at: ℅ www.gypsy-traveller.org

National Federation of Gypsy Liaison Groups (*Resources*). Available at: ℅ http://www.nationalgyps ytravellerfederation.org/resources.html

Queen's Nursing Institute (*Outreach nurse for the gypsy and traveller commu-nity in Leeds*). Available at: ℅ https://www.qni.org.uk/2019/02/08/an-outreach-nurse-for-the-gypsy-and-traveller-community-in-leeds/

Domestic violence

Definition

Domestic violence (DV) is any incident or pattern of incidents of controlling, coercive, or threatening behaviour, violence, or abuse between those aged ≥16yrs who are or have been intimate partners or family members, regardless of gender or sexuality. This can encompass, but is not limited to, the following types of abuse: psychological, physical, sexual, financial, and emotional. Controlling behaviour comprises a range of acts designed to make a person subordinate and/or dependent by: isolating them from sources of support; exploiting their resources and capacities for personal gain; depriving them of the means needed for independence, resistance, and escape; and regulating their everyday behaviour. Coercive behaviour is an act or a pattern of acts of assault, threats, humiliation, and intimidation or other abuse that is used to harm, punish, or frighten their victim (➤ Victims of crime p. 452).

Key facts

- Affects ~one in four ♀
- One in seven ♂ will experience DV
- Two ♀ murdered every week by partners or ex-partners
- ♀ suffer ~35 assaults before contacting police
- Often starts or ↑ during and after pregnancy (➤ Pregnancy p. 424)
- ~52% of reported ♀ rapes committed by current or former partner
- In 50% cases where mother abused, children also abused (➤ Safeguarding children p. 248; ➤ Identifying the child in need of protection p. 250)
- Accounts for ~one in ten homelessness applications (➤ Homeless people p. 446)
- One in four lesbian, gay, bisexual, and transgender people have experienced DV
- Disabled ♀ are two times more likely to experience DV than non-disabled ♀
- DV in teen relationships is a serious issue (➤ Working with teenagers p. 232; ➤ Sex and relationship education p. 236)
- There is an impact not just on the health of the person experiencing DV, but also on children. Both are likely to have long-term emotional and mental consequences (➤ People with anxiety and depression p. 478; ➤ Post-traumatic stress disorder p. 490; ➤ Behavioural disorders in children p. 326; ➤ Emotional problems in children p. 330). ♀ stay in abusive relationships for many reasons, including self-blame, shame, loss of confidence, fear of losing children, financial dependency, and fear that no one will believe them.

Potential indicators of domestic violence

- Multiple injuries at various stages of healing (➤ Sprains, strains, and fractures p. 824; ➤ Burns and scalds p. 816)
- Explanations vague or inconsistent with injuries
- Partner insists on being present at all appointments
- Person experiencing DV appears depressed or overly anxious
- Person experiencing DV fails to attend appointments

⚠ ♀ are at particular risk during pregnancy and following separation from a violent partner (➤ Working with parents p. 170).

Key principles for health professionals

Create a supportive environment that allows the person to talk (→ Principles of good communication in patient assessment p. 120). Ask ♀ (only if alone) direct questions about DV. Have information available on local agencies that can help, in a format the person can easily conceal. Always keep the safety of both the person experiencing DV and that of any children in mind. Know how to refer people to local support agencies if that is what they want. Never try to mediate between partners. Ensure own and colleagues' safety (→ Health and safety at work p. 92; → Lone working p. 94).

Routine enquiry

Ask all ♀, but particularly pregnant ♀, about DV as part of usual care. Routine enquiry includes being clear on the limits of confidentiality.

On disclosure of domestic violence

Reassure and support. Give 24-hr National DV freephone helpline number (☎ 0808 2000 247). Provide local specialist DV services contact details (e.g. women's refuge, police DV unit). Undertake a risk assessment with the person experiencing DV to determine extent of danger (→ Clinical risk management p. 78). ↑ risk includes children present, pregnancy, previous violence, alcohol (→ Alcohol p. 360) and/or drug misuse (→ Substance use p. 476), weapons present, stalking, separation, suicide threat (→ Suicidal intent and deliberate self-harm p. 494). Document fully in records (that cannot be accessed by perpetrator) all observations, actions, and events (→ Record keeping p. 86).

⚠ If immediate risk (e.g. partner acting aggressively in the same building) call police. ⚠ If there are children in the household, follow local child protection procedures. ⚠ If ↑ risk, seek senior clinician/manager support to follow multi-agency guidelines.

Help person experiencing DV think through need for a safety plan if still living with perpetrator (e.g. think about escape routes, call ☎ 999 if violence starts, keep money and keys easy to grab) and if now living separately (e.g. change locks, think about escape routes).

Legislation in the UK may be changing. The Domestic Abuse Bill (2019–2021) was debated at second reading on 28 April 2020 and has now been sent to a Public Bill Committee.

Related topics

→ Child protection processes p. 252; → Child and adolescent mental health p. 246

Further information

Department of Health (Health visiting and school nursing programmes. Supporting implementation of the new service model no.5: domestic violence and abuse). Available at: ℰ https://assets.publishing.service.gov.uk/government/uploads/system/uploads/attachment_data/file/211018/9576-TSO-Health_Visiting_Domestic_Violence_A3_Posters_WEB.pdf

Refuge for Women and Children (Get help). Available at: ℰ https://www.refuge.org.uk/get-help-now/

Women's Aid (Resource for children). Available at: ℰ www.thehideout.org.uk

Victims of crime

Over recent decades, overall reported crime has ↓ in the UK. However, this hides geographical variation and variation in different types of crime, including an ↑ in offences involving knives in metropolitan areas.[3] Most people do not experience crime, but some groups experience greater risk:[4] mixed, Asian, and Black ethnic groups; younger people; long-term unemployed; and people with severe mental health problems (◑ People with psychosis p. 486; ◑ People with bipolar affective disorder p. 482).

Impact of crime of communities

Communities are adversely affected by ↑ levels of crime. Residents may become withdrawn and less likely to participate in community activities. Property prices are affected and home insurance premiums ↑. New businesses may avoid the area and existing businesses may close down due to repeated theft, vandalism, etc.

Impact of crime on individuals

Being a victim of crime has a range of short- and long-term effects: emotional and psychological problems (◑ People with anxiety and depression p. 478; ◑ Post-traumatic stress disorder p. 490; ◑ Emotional problems in children p. 330); physical health problems; financial problems; and relationship problems. Crime does not affect everyone in the same way. The impact is influenced not solely by the seriousness of the incident but a range of factors. The physical impact of crime is most obviously associated with violent crime and abuse; however, victims of burglary also report deterioration in their general physical health.[5]

Reporting crime

Reporting the crime to the police → the person who committed the crime being brought to justice, which could help ↓ further crimes and protect others. A police crime number will be provided, which is needed to apply for financial assistance, make an insurance claim for damaged or stolen property, and claim criminal injuries compensation. To report a crime to the police:

- Emergencies: ☎ 999 and ask for the police
- Non-emergency situations: ☎ 101 and ask for the police. Some crimes can also be reported online. Local police forces have their own online crime-reporting websites.
- Anonymously: ☎ 0800 555111 or complete an form at ⌨ www. crimestoppers-uk.org

Support for victims of crime

Victim Support is a national charity that provides free and confidential support for people affected by crime and traumatic events, regardless of whether these were reported to the police:

- Victim Support (England and Wales): ☎ 08 08 16 89 111 or visit ⌨ https://www.victimsupport.org.uk/help-and-support/get-help
- Victim Support Scotland: ☎ 0345 603 9213 or visit ⌨ https://www. victimsupportsco.org.uk/contact-us/

- Victim Support Northern Ireland: ☎ 02890 243133 (Belfast) or 02871 370086 (Foyle) or visit ✆ http://www.victimsupportni.com/about-us/contact-us/

The support services provided are tailored to the needs of each person and include; information and advice; immediate and long-term emotional and practical help; advocacy; restorative justice; personal safety services; and help navigating the criminal justice system.

Related topics

➔ Adults at risk from harm and abuse p. 454; ➔ Domestic violence p. 450; ➔ Safeguarding children p. 248; ➔ Child and adolescent mental health p. 246

References

3. ONS (2018) *Crime in England and Wales: year ending March 2018.* Available at: https://www.ons.gov.uk/peoplepopulationandcommunity/crimeandjustice/bulletins/crimeinenglandandwales/yearendingmarch2018
4. Home Office (2018) *Victims of crime.* Available at: https://www.ethnicity-facts-figures.service.gov.uk/crime-justice-and-the-law/crime-and-reoffending/victims-of-crime/latest
5. Victim Support (2017) *Understanding victims of crime: the impact of the crime and support needs.* Available at: https://www.victimsupport.org.uk/sites/default/files/VS_Understanding%20victims%20of%20crime_web.pdf

Adults at risk from harm and abuse

Safeguarding adults at risk from harm and abuse is everyone's responsibility (◆ Professional accountability p. 83. In England, the Care Act 2014 sets out a clear legal framework for how health and social care (◆ Social services p. 30) organizations should protect adults who are at risk of harm and abuse. Similar legislation exists in Scotland (Adult Support and Protection (Scotland) Act 2007) and Wales (Social Services and Well-Being (Wales) Act 2014).

Definition of an adult at risk

Someone aged ≥18yrs who has needs for care and support (whether or not the LA is meeting any of those needs) and is experiencing, or at risk of, abuse or neglect, and as a result of those care and support needs is unable to protect themselves from either the risk of, or the experience of, abuse or neglect. Types of abuse are summarized in Box 9.1. Abuse may constitute a single act or repeated acts, be intentional or non-intentional, involve one type of abuse or a combination of types, and involve one or more person at risk. Perpetrators may include family members, carers (◆ Carers p. 458), neighbours, professionals, or strangers.

> ### Box 9.1 Types of abuse
> - Physical abuse
> - Domestic violence or abuse
> - Sexual abuse
> - Psychological or emotional abuse
> - Financial or material abuse
> - Modern slavery
> - Discriminatory abuse
> - Organizational or institutional abuse
> - Neglect or acts of omission (including self-neglect)

Acting on a suspicion or disclosure of abuse

Follow local multi-agency procedures and share concerns with your line manager or the adult safeguarding lead in your organization (◆ Quality governance p. 68). Action should be underpinned by the following six principles:
- Empowerment: encourage adults to make their own decisions
- Prevention: strategies to promote resilience and self-determination
- Proportionate: a proportionate and least intrusive response balanced with the level of risk
- Protection: adults are offered ways to protect themselves, and there is a co-ordinated response to adult safeguarding
- Partnership: local solutions through services working together (◆ Teamwork p. 58)
- Accountable: accountability and transparency in delivering a safeguarding response

Action in response to a suspicion or disclosure

Your responsibilities include:[6]

- Assessing the situation, i.e. are emergency services required?
- Ensuring the safety and well-being of the individual
- Establishing what the individual's views and wishes are
- Maintaining any evidence
- Following local procedures for reporting incidents/risks (➔ Clinical risk management p. 78)
- Remaining calm and trying not to show any shock or disbelief
- Listening carefully and demonstrating understanding (➔ Principles of good communication in patient assessment p. 120; ➔ Adults and children with additional communication needs p. 122)
- Informing the person that you are required to share information (➔ Confidentiality p. 89; ➔ Consent p. 82)
- Making a written record (➔ Record keeping p. 86)

Information sharing

The LA has statutory responsibility for adult safeguarding. Consent to sharing information with the LA should be sought from the adult at risk. If they deny permission, consider:[7] exploring the reasons for objection; explaining why you think it is important to share the information; stating who you intend sharing the information with; explaining the benefits to them or others of sharing information; discussing the consequences of not sharing information; and reassuring them that they are not alone and support is available.

If the adult at risk continues to refuse permission, in general, their wishes should be respected. However, such a decision may be overridden in some circumstances, including when:[8] they lack mental capacity (➔ Mental capacity p. 470), other people are at risk (➔ Safeguarding children p. 248), sharing information could prevent a serious crime, a serious crime has been committed, and staff are implicated (➔ Professional conduct p. 80). Discuss exceptions with the adult safeguarding lead.

Related topics

➔ Domestic violence p. 450; ➔ Whistleblowing p. 85; ➔ Victims of crime p. 452

References

6. NHS England (2017) *Safeguarding adults: a guide for healthcare staff*. Available at: ℘ https://www.england.nhs.uk/wp-content/uploads/2017/02/adult-pocket-guide.pdf

7. Association of Directors of Social Services (2016) *London multi-agency adult safeguarding policy and procedures*. Available at: ℘ http://londonadass.org.uk/wp-content/uploads/2015/02/Pan-London-Updated-August-2016.pdf

8. Social Care Institute for Excellence (2014) *What if the person does not want to share their information?* Available at: ℘ https://www.scie.org.uk/care-act-2014/safeguarding-adults/sharing-information/does-not-want-to-share.asp

People with learning disabilities

Learning disability (LD) is ↓ intellectual ability and ↑ difficulty with everyday activities. All types of LD are lifelong. People with profound and multiple LDs require significant help, while those with mild/moderate LDs will often be able to live independently with support. Government policies emphasize: rights, independence, choice, and inclusion (➔ Anti-discriminatory healthcare p. 81).

Health profile

Children and adults with LDs have significantly worse health in comparison to the general population (➔ UK health profile p. 2), in particular, respiratory problems (➔ Chronic obstructive pulmonary disease p. 614; ➔ Asthma in adults p. 608; ➔ Asthma in children p. 306), diabetes (➔ Diabetes: overview p. 660), gastrointestinal problems (➔ Dyspepsia, gastro-oesophageal reflux disease, and peptic ulceration p. 708) (including gastrointestinal cancers), heart disease (➔ Coronary heart disease p. 624), epilepsy (➔ Seizures and epilepsy p. 740; ➔ Febrile convulsions and epilepsy p. 280), depression (➔ People with anxiety and depression p. 478), schizophrenia (➔ People with psychosis p. 486), hypothyroidism (➔ Thyroid p. 702), and sensory impairments (➔ Blindness and partial sight p. 748; ➔ Deafness in children p. 268; ➔ Deafness p. 696; ➔ Speech and language acquisition p. 218). Mortality rates are ↑ for all causes compared with the general population. Mental health and well-being may be challenged by bullying, victimization, stigmatization, and alienation in society.

Access to health services

There is an inverse relationship between ↑ level of health needs and ↓ use of health services. Contributory factors: attitudinal barriers (➔ Professional conduct p. 80); communication difficulties (➔ Adults and children with additional communication needs p. 122); diagnostic overshadowing (i.e. the disability masks the illness); lack of accessible information; and confusion about law regarding consent (➔ Consent p. 82).

Good practice points

Never make assumptions. Speak clearly and not too fast (➔ Principles of good communication in patient assessment p. 120). Avoid medical jargon, use simple everyday language. Use photographs and objects to accompany information. Use concrete terms. Try to avoid negative words such as 'don't'. Use key events in the person's life (e.g. birthdays) to help recall. Use open-ended questions. Use active language (e.g. Jane will give you a blood test). Use health action plans or personal hand-held records (➔ Client- and patient-held records p. 90). Use Makaton or British sign language when required. Talk to the person, not their carer.

Specialist support for children and young people

May be located at children's centres. Some areas may have specialist staff working in mainstream services such as Child and Adolescent Mental Health Services (CAMHS). Children and young people with LDs are often at risk of harm and abuse (➔ Safeguarding children p. 248). Local child protection guidance should be available (➲ Identifying the child in need of protection p. 250; ➲ Child protection processes p. 252). Transition from adolescence to adulthood is a vital transitional point, and it is crucial that services work in partnership with the young person to ensure that they are actively involved in the choices and decisions about their future (➲ Transition of young people to adult services p. 468).

Specialist support services for adults

Many adults will access care through single access points via LD teams. These teams co-ordinate health and social care (➲ Teamwork p. 58; ➲ Social support p. 28; ➲ Social services p. 30. Team members may include LD nurses, social workers, physiotherapists, occupational therapists, psychologists, speech and language therapists, and psychiatrists. Many LD teams will have an open referral system. These services can help with housing (➲ Homes and housing p. 26), benefits, personal independence payments (PIP), occupation, education, leisure, bereavement (➲ Coping with bereavement p. 574), respite care, family support, relationships, health access, communication, mobility, etc. People with LDs are often at risk of harm and abuse (➲ Adults at risk from harm and abuse p. 454). Local adult protection guidance should be available. Adults with LDs are living longer and require service supports to be robust, as they often do not have close family support. Palliative care needs (➲ Services for the dying patient p. 552) may be overlooked.

Behaviour that is seen as challenging

This is a term used to describe a wide range of behaviours that some people with LDs may use to communicate an unmet need. These behaviours may be self-injurious, risky to other people, or socially inappropriate. Physical complaints should always be considered as a cause of change in behaviour, and a mental health assessment should be carried out, as the behaviour may be due to an unmet emotional need. These behaviours should be considered a form of communication.

Related topics

➲ Sexual health and adults with a learning disability p. 770; ➲ Mental capacity p. 470; ➲ Children with complex health needs and disabilities p. 238; ➲ Child and adolescent mental health p. 246

Further information

NICE (Mental health problems in people with learning disabilities: prevention, assessment and management). Available at: ℛ www.nice.org.uk/guidance/ng54

Scottish Consortium for Learning Disability (The keys to life). Available at: ℛ https://www.scld.org.uk/the-keys-to-life/

Carers

Anyone who provides unpaid care for a friend or family member who due to illness, disability, a mental health problem, or an addiction (◆ Substance use p. 476) cannot cope without their support (e.g. child looking after parent with alcohol problem (◆ Alcohol p. 360), older person looking after spouse with dementia (◆ People with dementia p. 498)). ♀ more likely to be carers. Other groups with ↑ propensity to care include:

- Bangladeshi, Pakistani, and Indian groups: due to socioeconomic factors (e.g. intergenerational households), cultural factors, and differing levels of health and employment
- Older people: due to socioeconomic factors (e.g. ↓ intergenerational households and geographical dispersal of children) and ↑ levels of ill health and disability amongst older dependents

Care activities and impact of caring

Include a range of activities including: keeping an eye on and keeping company; laundry services and providing transport; shopping, housework and paperwork; and personal care and medication management. Caring can be a positive experience, but it can also negatively impact on many aspects of life.

Financial

Combining work and caring responsibilities is often difficult due to problems with co-ordination of care and inflexibility in employment. Detrimental to pension, e.g. people who have breaks in pension contribution due to time out of work to care. Additional expenditure, e.g. care-related costs such as travel.

Health and well-being

- Tiredness (due to interrupted sleep)
- Physical strain associated with moving and handling (◆ Patient moving and handling p. 96)
- Anxiety and depression (◆ People with anxiety and depression p. 478)
- ↑ susceptibility to illness
- Deterioration of existing health conditions
- Neglecting own health

Socializing and learning

Caring can be isolating as it can be difficult to leave the house. It may be hard to sustain friendships or develop new ones, or to maintain interests and activities previously enjoyed. Young carers can experience educational difficulties due to missing school because of caring responsibilities.

What carers want

- To keep a normal home routine
- To be spoken to about their needs
- Help with well-being and mental health
- Information about carer breaks and respite
- Help identifying, anticipating, and preventing crises

- Help accessing support to manage care alongside paid employment/ childcare responsibilities
- Professionals to recognize ↑ frailty (● Frailty p. 678) amongst older carers and the likelihood of spouses undertaking mutual caring roles
- Support young carers with their transition to adult carers (● Transition of young people to adult services p. 468)

Legislation

The Care Act 2014 strengthened the rights and recognition of adult carers in England, giving them specific rights to personal budgets, direct payments, information and advice, assessment, and support to maintain their health and well-being. Young carers in England have a right to an assessment under the Children and Families Act 2014. Similar legislation exists in Scotland (The Carer (Scotland) Act 2016) and Wales (Social Services and Well-being (Wales) Act 2014).

Support carers to identify themselves

Self-identification can be difficult as many see their relationship with the person they care for as being that of a child, sibling, neighbour, or partner. Identification by health professionals especially important. GP practices (● General practice p. 18) should register carers to ensure they get appointments at convenient times, and are offered free annual health checks and flu vaccinations (● Targeted adult immunization p. 392).

Recognize carers in individual care planning

Carers have expert knowledge about the person they care for and their contribution can improve outcomes. To facilitate participation: carers and the essential role they play are identified at first contact; staff are 'carer aware' and trained in carer engagement strategies (● Patient and public experience p. 75); policy and practice protocols relating to confidentiality (● Confidentiality p. 89) and sharing information are in place; defined post(s) responsible for carers are in place; a carer introduction to the service and staff is available; and a range of carer support services is available.

Adult carer assessment

Can request a statutory carer's assessment. Responsibility of LA (● Social services p. 30). Takes place face-to-face or over the telephone. Includes review of how caring role affects: health and well-being, relationships and family, housing and living environment, work and finances, and hobbies and interests. Should establish feelings and choices about caring, and planning for emergencies.

Young carer assessment

LA has a duty to assess on the appearance of need without a request being made. Assessment must look at: whether or not the young carer wishes to continue caring; whether it is appropriate for them to continue caring; and any education, training, work, or recreational activities the young carer participates in or wishes to partake in (● Identifying the child in need of protection p. 250; ● Child protection processes p. 252; ● Child and adolescent mental health p. 246).

Types of carer support available

After the carer's assessment, the LA will write to the carer about whether they have eligible care and support needs. If the LA decides the carer is eligible, help might include: money to pay for things that make caring easier; respite care and short breaks; referral to local support groups; support to attend medical appointments; support if the carer needs to go into hospital; training (e.g. moving and handling); help with housework or gardening; buying a laptop, so they can keep in touch with family; and membership of a gym, so they can look after their own health (⊃ Exercise p. 354).

Benefits

Carers may be eligible for a range of benefits including: Carer's Allowance, Carer's Credit, Carer's Premium, and Pension Credit.

Further information

Carers' Trust (*The triangle of care: carers included*). Available at: ℰ https://professionals.carers.org/sites/default/files/thetriangleofcare_guidetobestpracticeinmentalhealthcare_england_0.pdf

Queen's Nursing Institute (*Free online resources to support district nurses, general practice nurses and school nurses who work with carers*). Available at: ℰ https://www.qni.org.uk/nursing-in-the-community/supporting-carers/

Human immunodeficiency virus (HIV)

HIV is a retrovirus that infects immune system cells, particularly the CD4 (T-helper cells), and over a number of years the CD4 cells (T-helper cells) malfunction and die to a point where they jeopardize immunity (➲ Principles of working with someone with compromised immunity p. 466). There are two main types of HIV: HIV1 which is highly virulent; and HIV2 found mainly in West Africa. In the UK ~13% of those infected with HIV are unaware of their infection.[9] ↑ prevalence in ♂ who have sex with ♂ (MSM), and Black African ♂ and ♀.

Transmission

Through body fluids including semen, vaginal fluids, menstrual fluids, breast milk, amniotic fluid, pleural effusions, cerebrospinal fluid, and blood. Injecting drug users are also at ↑ risk. Transmission vertically from mother to baby and through infected blood products is possible but rare in the UK. HIV cannot be transmitted by social interactions such as shaking hands and kissing.

Prevention

- Safer sex practices (e.g. use ♀ and ♂ condoms with lubricant) (➲ Barrier contraceptive methods p. 416)
- Stop IV drug abuse and ↓ needle sharing (➲ Substance use p. 476)
- All donated blood screened for HIV
- Risk ↓ of mother to child transmission by antiretroviral treatment given antenatally (➲ Pregnancy p. 424; ➲ Antenatal care and screening p. 426), during delivery, and to the baby for 6wks. Also, elective Caesarian delivery and not breastfeeding (➲ Breastfeeding p. 182).

Post-exposure prophylaxis (PEP)

For occupational exposure or following sexual assault (➲ Sexual health: general issues p. 760). A combination of antiretroviral medicines started as soon as possible after exposure and taken for 4wks. Available through genitourinary medicine clinics, emergency departments, and some GPs.

Pre-exposure prophylaxis (PrEP)

HIV prevention strategy that uses antiretroviral drugs to protect HIV-negative people from HIV infection. Made available to 10,000 people in England as part of the IMPACT trial since 2017. ⚠: PrEP is not a vaccine and only provides protection from HIV as long as taken as prescribed (➲ Medicine concordance and adherence p. 132).

Diagnosis and stages of HIV progression

Four main types of HIV diagnosis test: blood test, point-of-care test, home sampling kit, and home testing kit. The blood test is the most accurate and can normally give reliable results 1mth after infection. Stages of HIV progression are summarized in Table 9.1.

HIV in children

HIV disease in children has a different progression to adults, should be treated differently, and be under a paediatric HIV clinical network. Pregnant ♀ with possible or confirmed HIV should have access to diagnostic tests and interventions as early as possible or provided as early as possible after birth.

- All ♀ with HIV must have a birth plan for prevention of transmission, and elective Caesarian should be considered.
- All children at risk of HIV infection should have an HIV test.
- Children and young people with HIV should be referred urgently to a specialist paediatric HIV service (appointment within 2wks).
- Children with HIV should have the HIV infection monitored and access a range of multidisciplinary services.
- Children living with HIV should be prescribed antiretroviral therapy (ART) by a qualified clinician and receive individualized support to achieve adherence.
- Talking to children diagnosed with HIV about condition needs to take place over time, as appropriate for age and level of understanding.

Table 9.1 Stages of HIV progression

Stage	Symptoms
Seroconversion illness	Also known as 1° HIV infection, usually short illness after infection (can also go unnoticed) and when the person is ↑ infectious
Asymptomatic HIV	Once seroconversion is over, there are limited or no symptoms and this can last for several years. The virus is active and replicating.
Symptomatic HIV	The immune system is weakened and the person is more at risk of infections. Longstanding HIV infections can lead to constitutional symptoms (such as fever, weight loss, sweats), respiratory conditions, neurological and visual conditions, cancers, skin conditions, oral conditions, gastrointestinal conditions, genital conditions, and haematological conditions.
Late-stage HIV	Serious damage made to immune system, and opportunistic infections leading to acquired immune deficiency syndrome (AIDS)-defining illnesses (e.g. cancer, TB, and pneumonia).

Monitoring HIV infection

Usually done in specialist clinics using the CD4 lymphocyte cell count and viral load. The CD4 count reflects the degree to which immunocompromised, and the viral load reflects rates of viral replication. The CD4 cell count of a person who does not have HIV can be 500–1500. People living with HIV who have a CD4 count >500 are usually in good health. Those with a CD4 cell count <200 are at ↑ risk of serious illnesses.

Management with antiretroviral medicines

Antiretroviral medicines limit HIV replication. Several combinations can be prescribed. Side effects are common and some are serious. Adherence to treatment is key as the HIV virus replicates. Several blood tests are indicated to identify drug resistance. Highly active antiretroviral therapy (HAART) for children was introduced in 1997 and d mortality rates considerably. Once babies are diagnosed with HIV, HAART and pneumocystis carinii pneumonia (PCP) prophylaxis started.

Living with HIV

Specialist teams and services available to help address a wide range of psychological, emotional, social, as well as physical needs arising from the infection, treatments, and progression of the disease. 1° care services work in partnership, as with any LTC (➔ Teamwork p. 58). Also have health promotion role, encouraging: safe sex practices (even when both partners have HIV diagnosis, as they are at risk of acquiring drug-resistant strain); cancer screening (as ↑ at risk of malignancies) (➔ UK screening programmes p. 362); immunization (including annual influenza immunization, and Hepatitis A immunisation for MSM) (➔ Targeted adult immunization p. 392); and good antenatal and postnatal care (➔ Postnatal care p. 438). Monitor mental health, as people living with HIV are at ↑ risk of mental health problems due to stigma, isolation, and discrimination (➔ People with anxiety and depression p. 478). Adolescents and young people living with HIV should have an individualized care plan to transition them to adult services over time (➔ Transition of young people to adult services p. 468).

Related topics

➔ Sexual health consultations p. 762; ➔ Child and adolescent mental health p. 246

Reference

9. UK Government (2016) *HIV in the UK*. Available at: https://assets.publishing.service.gov.uk/government/uploads/system/uploads/attachment_data/file/602942/HIV_in_the_UK_report.pdf

Further information

Children's HIV Association (*Professionals*). Available at: ℘ "https://www.chiva.org.uk/professionals/" https://www.chiva.org.uk/professionals/
Nam Aidsmap (*The basics*). Available at: ℘ http://www.aidsmap.com/thebasics
NICE (*HIV infection and AIDS*). Available at: ℘ https://cks.nice.org.uk
Young People with HIV (including infants born to mothers with HIV). Available at: ℘ https://www.chiva.org.uk

Principles of working with someone with compromised immunity

Healthy people fight infections through the immune system, mainly the lymphatic system. This can be compromised by age (➔ Frailty p. 678), infection, burns (➔ Burns and scalds p. 816), neoplasms, metabolic disorders (➔ Diabetes: overview p. 660; ➔ Principles of diabetes management p. 664), irradiation, foreign bodies, cytotoxic drugs, and steroids. Most people with compromised immunity live independently. Care is related to the severity and type of symptoms. Many of the associated disorders (e.g. rheumatoid arthritis (➔ Rheumatoid arthritis p. 602) and HIV (➔ Human immunodeficiency virus p. 462)) have support groups and organizations providing information (➔ Expert patients and self-management programmes p. 340).

Principles of care for people with immunodeficiency disorders

Lack of awareness about antibody defects → considerable ↓ diagnosis. Be alert to patients with multiple infections per year (ear, sinus, chest, skin (➔ Bacterial skin infections p. 680; ➔ Viral skin infections p. 690)), failure of an infant to gain weight (➔ Growth 0–2 years p. 190), or when family history of immune deficiency. Aim to prevent infections and complications and to enable a normal working capability and life expectancy. Involve the multidisciplinary team (➔ Teamwork p. 58). Educate patient in self-care and disease management and encourage smoking cessation (➔ Smoking cessation p. 356).

Prevention of infection

⚠ Adhere to principles of infection prevention and control.
- Patients exposed to specific infections (e.g. rheumatic fever, TB (➔ Tuberculosis p. 728), meningitis) should receive prophylactic antibiotics
- Prophylactic treatment of patients with HIV and pneumocystis and granulocytopenia for prevention of bacterial infections
- Immunization against influenza, meningococcal, and pneumococcal infections (➔ Targeted adult immunization p. 392)
- Hepatitis B immunization given to people who regularly receive blood products

Related topics

➔ Oral chemotherapy in the home p. 546; ➔ Principles of working with someone with an infectious disease p. 467

Further information

International Patient Organization for Primary Immunodeficiencies (*What are primary immunodeficiencies?*). Available at: ℛ https://ipopi.org/pids/what-are-pids/

Principles of working with someone with an infectious disease

Infectious or communicable diseases are illnesses caused by micro-organisms not normally present in the body: bacteria (e.g. Streptococcus aureus, salmonellosis, meningococcal meningitis); viruses (e.g. influenza, hepatitis, chickenpox); protozoa (e.g. malaria, toxoplasmosis); and infestation (e.g. head lice). Transmission may be by ingestion, inhalation, inoculation (through a cut, skin abrasion, or needle stick injury), and direct contact.

NICE suggest standard principles for common infectious diseases:

- Hand hygiene (→ Hand hygiene p. 98)
- Personal protective equipment as per national and local guidelines (→ Personal protective equipment p. 100)
- Safe disposal of sharps (→ Managing healthcare waste p. 106)
- Food hygiene (→ Home food safety and hygiene p. 352)
- Personal hygiene
- Appropriate disposal of clinical waste (→ Managing healthcare waste p. 106)

Related topics

→ Principles of working with someone with compromised immunity p. 466; → Sexually transmitted diseases p. 764; → Vomiting and diarrhoea in children p. 287; → Viral hepatitis p. 724; → Human immunodeficiency virus p. 462; → Pandemic influenza p. 726; → Infectious disease notifications p. 104; → Pneumonia p. 750; → Infectious diseases in childhood p. 290; → Methicillin-resistant Staphylococcus aureus (MRSA) p. 722; → Tuberculosis p. 728; → Antimicrobial stewardship p. 146; → Fungal infections p. 686

Further information

NICE (Infectious diseases prevention and control). Available at: ℘ https://www.nice.org.uk/guidance/health-protection/communicable-diseases/infectious-disease-prevention-and-control
PHE (*Primary care guidance*). Available at: ℘ www.hpa.org.uk/Topics/InfectiousDiseases/InfectionsAZ/PrimaryCareGuidance

Transition of young people to adult services

The journey from adolescence into adulthood can be especially challenging for young people with a disability, LTC, or mental health problem. Adult and child services are different in expectations, style, and culture.[10]

Transition can impact on health outcomes and health behaviours (e.g. a young person with diabetes may experience a change in glycaemic control and difficulty accessing and maintaining healthcare (➔ Endocrine problems p. 304; ➔ Diabetes: overview p. 660; ➔ Principles of diabetes management p. 664)). The components of practice that promote continuity in this period include:[11]

- Start planning transition by school year 9 (aged 13–14yrs).
- Annually review transition planning for each young person.
- Allocate each young person a named worker to co-ordinate care and support before, during, and after transfer.
- Ensure young people meet a practitioner from each of the adult services they will move to before they transition.
- Contact young people who do not attend their first meeting or appointment with adult services and give them further opportunities to engage.

⚠ The point of transfer to adult services should not be based on a rigid age threshold but should take place at a time of relative stability for the young person.[11]

Related topics

➔ Children with complex health needs and disabilities p. 238; ➔ Continuity of care p. 598; ➔ People with learning disabilities p. 456; ➔ School nursing p. 42; ➔ Working in schools p. 44; ➔ Child and adolescent mental health p. 246

References

10. Royal College of Nursing (2013) *Lost in transition: moving young people between child and adult health services*. Available at: https://www.rcn.org.uk/professional-development/publications/pub-003227
11. NICE (2016) *Transition from children's to adults' services (QS140)*. Available at: https://www.nice.org.uk/guidance/qs140

Further information

Queen's Nursing Institute (2017) *Transition from children's to adult community services: e-learning resource*. Available at: ♪ https://www.qni.org.uk/child_to_adult/index.php

Mental capacity

Always encourage and empower people to share decisions about their treatment and care. Whilst people have the right to make what others might regard as an unwise decision, there are occasions when a person's refusal to consent (➔ Consent p. 82) to treatment will raise concerns about their decision-making ability. The assessment of capacity to consent to treatment and care is a fundamental component of shared nurse–patient decision making.

Mental Capacity Act (MCA) 2005

Legislation designed to protect and empower people who may lack the mental capacity to make their own decisions about care and treatment. Applies to people ≥16yrs in England and Wales. Similar legislation exists in Scotland (Adults with Incapacity Act 2000). In Northern Ireland, decision making is governed by the common law. Key principles: begin by assuming that people have capacity; people must be helped to make decisions; unwise decisions do not necessarily mean lack of capacity; decisions must be taken in the person's best interests; and decisions must be as least restrictive of freedom as possible.

Assessment

Accurate and timely assessment is important to ensure those who suffer a loss of autonomy are identified and appropriately supported (➔ Principles of good communication in patient assessment p. 120). The person most closely involved in the decision being made is responsible for carrying out the assessment of capacity. The MCA sets out a two-stage test.

Stage 1 (Diagnostic test)
Is there an impairment of, or disturbance in, the functioning of the person's mind or brain? If so, progress to Stage 2.

Stage 2 (Functional test)
Is that impairment or disturbance sufficient that the person lacks the capacity to make a particular decision? A person lacks capacity to make a particular decision if they cannot either: understand information relevant to the decision; **or** remember the information long enough to make a decision; **or** use that information as part of the decision-making process; **or** communicate their decision by talking, using sign language, etc.

If the person is found to lack capacity, then a best-interests decision may be made on their behalf.

Best-interests decisions

Checklist to consider when deciding best interests: encourage participation; identify all relevant circumstances; find out the person's views; avoid discrimination (➔ Anti-discriminatory healthcare p. 81); and assess whether the person might regain capacity. Always consult with others (➔ Teamwork p. 58), in particular close relatives and friends (➔ Carers p. 458), any attorney appointed under a lasting power of attorney or enduring power of attorney, and any deputy appointed by the Court of Protection to make decisions for the person. Find the least restrictive option. ⚠ In certain cases, the restrictions applied may amount to 'deprivation of liberty'. Where this might happen, the care provider has to apply to their LA who will assess whether the deprivation of liberty is in the best interests of the person concerned.

Advance statements and advance decisions

Advance statements are written statements setting out person's preferences, wishes, beliefs, and values regarding their future. Not legally binding,
but may guide decisions in a person's best interests if they have lost mental
capacity. Advance decisions are legally binding decisions that allow someone
≥18yrs, while still capable, to refuse specified medical treatment for a time
in the future when they may lack capacity to consent to refusal of that
treatment.

Lasting power of attorney (LPA)

Can be made at any time when the person making it has the mental capacity
to do so. A person can grant a LPA to another person or people to enable
them to make decisions about their health and welfare, or decisions about
property and financial affairs. There will be a separate legal document in
respect of each of these, appointing one or more attorneys. LPAs must be
registered with the Office of the Public Guardian.

Court of Protection

Oversees the MCA and deals with all issues, including financial and serious healthcare matters, concerning people who lack the mental capacity to
make their own decisions. It is involved in disputes when there is disagree-
ment about what's in the person's best interests, or when the views of the
attorneys in relation to property and welfare conflict. Also hears important
cases, such as whether the NHS should withdraw treatment. They can appoint 'deputies' who can also take decisions on health and welfare, as well
as in financial matters. They will come into action when the court needs to
delegate an ongoing series of decisions, rather than one decision.

Independent mental capacity advocate

Established by the MCA to support people who do not have mental capacity, who have not given a LPA to anyone, who do not have a court-
appointed deputy, and who may not have friends or family to speak on their
behalf. Role to ensure people have their views and wishes heard.

Related topics

➲ Care homes p. 32; ➲ People with dementia p. 498; ➲ Adults at risk
from harm and abuse p. 454; ➲ People with learning disabilities p. 456;
➲ People with psychosis p. 486; ➲ Suicidal intent and deliberate self-harm
p. 494

Further information

Department for Constitutional Affairs (*Mental Capacity Act 2005: code of practice*). Available at: ℘
    https://assets.publishing.service.gov.uk/government/uploads/system/uploads/attachment_
    data/file/497253/Mental-capacity-act-code-of-practice.pdf

NICE (*Decision-making and mental capacity [NG108]*). Available at: ℘ https://www.nice.org.uk/
    guidance/NG108

Office of the Public Guardian (*Making decisions: a guide for people who work in health and social care*).
    Available at: ℘ https://assets.publishing.service.gov.uk/government/uploads/system/uploads/
    attachment_data/file/348440/OPG603-Health-care-workers-MCA-decisions.pdf

Talking therapies

Talking therapies may also be called counselling, psychological therapies, or psychotherapies. They involve talking to a suitably trained person to help explore thoughts and feelings that may be impacting negatively on a person. Talking therapies are now recommended as a first-line approach for many mental health conditions from anxiety and depression (⊃ People with anxiety and depression p. 478) to people at risk of developing psychosis (⊃ People with psychosis p. 486). In the NHS, therapies may be provided by counsellors, psychologists, psychiatrists, psychotherapists, nurses, or social workers. There may be variation in local availability (⊃ Commissioning of services p. 12). Anyone seeking a private therapist should ensure they belong to a recognized professional body such as the British Association for Counselling and Psychotherapy (⊃ Professional accountability p. 83).

Counselling

Counselling can help with many problems including bereavement (⊃ Coping with bereavement p. 574), relationship problems, minor anxiety, and depression. A key element is active and reflective listening to encourage people to think about their own difficulties and feelings, and to try to find ways to address them. It does not involve giving advice. Usually short-term (e.g. six sessions of 45–50min). Counsellors may be available in general practice (⊃ General practice p. 18), local mental health services, or sometimes 1° care nurses may be involved in offering brief intervention counselling or active listening sessions (⊃ Postnatal depression p. 440). Also available through the local voluntary sector (e.g. Relate (relationship counselling)).

Cognitive behavioural therapy (CBT)

Aims to help people explore how their thoughts affect their feelings and behaviour. It aims to change behaviour and associated feelings by understanding and changing the thought processes underlying them. The person can then develop more effective coping skills. CBT has been shown to be effective for a variety of mental health problems, including depression, anxiety, panic attacks (⊃ Post-traumatic stress disorder p. 490), phobias (⊃ People with anxiety and depression p. 478), obsessive compulsive disorder, and eating disorders (⊃ People with eating disorders p. 474). It can be helpful for some people with psychoses, as part of treatment. It is a structured approach, with goals for treatment and activities to complete between sessions.

Psychoanalytical and psychodynamic therapies

Helps the person to know themselves better, even at an unconscious level. The therapist listens to the person's experiences, and explores connections between present feelings, actions, and past events. This type of therapy often continues for >1yr. It can help people with long-term or recurring problems get to the root of their difficulties. Some evidence that it can help depression and some eating disorders. Psychoanalysis and psychodynamic therapy does not suit everyone and requires significant time and emotional commitment.

Solution-focused therapy (SFT)

Widely used approach that focuses on solutions rather than problems. Uses techniques such as asking the person to imagine their perfect future and then exploring steps to reach it. It is a strengths-focused approach which looks at what the person can do rather than what they cannot.

Risks of talking therapies

Work for some, but not all people. People may not relate to their therapist or dislike them for unconscious reasons, which can stall the therapeutic process. There are examples of therapists undertaking misguided interventions which can have a negative impact on a vulnerable person (➲ Adults at risk from harm and abuse p. 454).

Further information

British Association for Counselling and Psychotherapy (*Thinking about therapy*). Available at: ℅ https://www.bacp.co.uk/about-therapy/we-can-help//

MIND (*Types of talking therapies*). Available at: ℅ https://www.mind.org.uk/information-support/drugs-and-treatments/talking-therapy-and-counselling/types-of-talking-therapy/

NICE (*Generalized anxiety disorder and panic disorder in adults: management [CG113]*). Available at: ℅ www.nice.org.uk/guidance/cg113

NICE (*Common mental health disorders: identification and pathways to care [CG123]*). Available at: ℅ http://publications.nice.org.uk/common-mental-health-disorders-cg123

NICE (*Psychosis and schizophrenia in adults: prevention and management [CG178]*). Available at: ℅ www.nice.org.uk/guidance/CG178/resources

People with eating disorders

Anorexia nervosa

Anorexia nervosa is a condition where there is a marked distortion of body image, ↓ weight, and weight-loss behaviours. Presentation: children with poor growth (➔ Growth and nutrition 5–11 years p. 222; ➔ Growth and nutrition 12–18 years p. 234); low body weight (15% below expected BMI) (➔ Adult body mass index chart p. 346; self-induced weight loss including vomiting, purging, ↑ exercise [➔ Exercise p. 354), use of appetite suppressants; and body image distortion (including imposed ↓ weight threshold).

Causes include a family history of eating disorders. Physical or sexual abuse can be risk factors (➔ Safeguarding children p. 248). Psychodynamic factors may also play a part including: family relationships (may be rigid, overprotective, weak parental boundaries, lack of conflict resolution), individual (disturbed body image due to dietary problems in early life, parental preoccupation with food, lack of sense of identity), and analytical (regression to childhood, fixation on the oral stage, avoidance of problems in adolescence).

Health-related complications
Patients who are pregnant (➔ Pregnancy p. 424) or who have diabetes (➔ Diabetes: overview p. 660; ➔ Principles of diabetes management p. 664) are at particular risk. Everyone involved in their care should be aware of the eating disorder. See Box 9.2.

> **Box 9.2 Complications of anorexia nervosa**
>
> - Impaired memory
> - Irritability
> - Poor decision-making ability
> - Anxiety and depression (➔ People with anxiety and depression p. 478)
> - Fatigue, fainting, and dizziness
> - Sensitivity to the cold
> - Reduced immunity
> - Amenorrhoea (➔ Menstrual problems p. 778)
> - Hair loss and dry skin
> - Loss of muscle mass
> - Reduced libido (➔ Sexual problems p. 768)
> - Compromised cardiac function
> - Anaemia (➔ Anaemia in adults p. 652)
> - Calluses on finger joints
> - Eroded tooth enamel (➔ Dental health in older children p. 226)
> - Hypotension, bradycardia (➔ Abnormal cardiac rhythms p. 640)
> - Atrophy of the breasts
> - Swollen tender abdomen
> - Loss of sensation in extremities
> - Brittle nails

Screening questions
- Do you worry excessively about your weight?
- Do you think you have an eating problem?

Treatment
People with anorexia are referred to specialist eating disorder clinics, where available. Often treated as an outpatient, with a combined approach including: pharmacological (antidepressants and appetite stimulants), psychological (family therapy and individual therapy, including CBT (→ Talking therapies p. 472)), and educational (nutritional and self-help manuals).

Hospital admission required if there are serious medical problems. Compulsory admission when feeding is regarded as treatment (→ Consent p. 82). Ethical issues around a person's right to die and their right to refuse treatment (→ Euthanasia, assisted suicide, and assisted dying p. 572). Poor prognostic factors include: chronic illness, late-age onset, bulimic features (see following), anxiety when eating with others, excessive weight loss, poor childhood social adjustment, poor parental relationships, male.

Bulimia nervosa

Recurrent episodes of binge eating in excess of normally accepted amounts of food. Behaviours to prevent ↑ in weight include vomiting and use of laxatives, diuretics, and appetite suppressants.

Management
Evidence-based self-help programmes (→ Expert patients and self-management programmes p. 340). Refer to GP for assessment of mental health. Refer as appropriate to eating disorders clinic. Refer as appropriate for CBT for binge eating disorder. Where there is laxative abuse, advice to gradually reduce intake. Family members, including siblings, should normally be included in treatment of children and adolescents with eating disorders. Interventions may include sharing information, advice on behavioural management, and facilitating communication.

Related topics

→ Nutrition and healthy eating p. 342; → Assessment of children, young people, and families p. 156; → Child and adolescent mental health p. 246; → Malnutrition p. 350; → Puberty and adolescence p. 228; → Working with teenagers p. 232

Further information

BEAT Eating Disorders (*Types of eating disorder*). Available at: ℘ https://www.beateatingdisorders.org.uk/types

NICE (*Eating disorders: recognition and treatment [NG69]*). Available at: ℘ http://publications.nice.org.uk/eating-disorders-cg9/implementation-in-the-nhs

Substance use

Substance use refers to the use of any substance (e.g. alcohol (❯ Alcohol p. 360), street drugs) or misuse of prescribed drugs (❯ Prescribing p. 136). Many people use drugs 'recreationally' and experience minimal harms. Their drug use tends to ↓ as they grow older and have ↑ life responsibilities. Some people may be more prone to developing a substance use disorder or addiction due to:

- Genetic factors which ↑ a predisposition to addiction
- Personality traits such as impulsivity or ↑ sensation seeking
- Psychosocial factors such as ineffective parenting and poverty
- Early age of first use

See Table 9.2

Substances tend to have three main effects (some share these effects): stimulant (↑ energy, euphoria, dilated pupils, ↑ libido, reduced appetite, ↓ sleep); depressant (sedation, feelings of calm and relaxation); or hallucinogenic (induction of hallucinatory experiences in any of the five senses).

Dependence syndrome

Describes the features of substance dependence:

- Primacy of drug-seeking behaviour
- Narrowing the drug-taking repertoire
- ↑ tolerance to the effects of drug
- Loss of control of consumption
- Signs of withdrawal on attempted abstinence
- Drug taking to avoid withdrawal symptoms
- Continued drug use despite negative consequences
- Rapid reinstatement of previous pattern of drug use after abstinence

Aims of care

- ↓ or modify drug-using behaviour
- ↓ risk of other health problems (e.g. infections, depression)
- ↓ social consequences of substance use (e.g. homelessness (❯ Homeless people p. 446)

Care and management

Multidisciplinary team (❯ Teamwork p. 58) endeavour involving community substance use teams. Will include: education (harm reduction, safer routes of administration, risk of overdose, hepatitis immunization for injecting drug users and close contacts (❯ Viral hepatitis p. 724; ❯ Targeted adult immunization p. 392, needle exchange); treatment of dependence (provided as part of 1° healthcare team, involving community pharmacist and specialist services); and family and carer (❯ Carers p. 458) support (including liaison with voluntary agencies and support groups). Talking therapies (❯ Talking therapies p. 472) and alternative therapies, such as acupuncture, may also be offered (❯ Complementary and alternative therapies p. 838).

Table 9.2 Features of substance abuse

Acute intoxication	Pattern of reversible physical and mental abnormalities caused by direct effect of substance (e.g. disinhibition, ataxia, euphoria, visual, and sensory distortion)
Risky use	Where person is at ↑ risk of harming their physical or mental health. Not dependent on how much taken, but on situations and associated behaviours (e.g. cannabis use while driving)
Harmful use	Continuation of substance misuse despite damage to mental health, social, occupational, or familial wellbeing. Damage is denied or minimized
Dependence	Includes both physical and psychological dependence
Withdrawal	Where abstinence leads to features of withdrawal. Different substances have different symptoms. Clinically significant withdrawals are recognized in alcohol, opiates, benzodiazepines, amphetamines, and cocaine
Complicated withdrawal	Development of seizures, delirium, or psychotic features (● Seizures and epilepsy p. 740; ● People with psychosis p. 486)
Substance-induced psychotic disorder	Hallucinations and/or delusions occurring as a direct result of substance neurotoxicity (● Poisoning and overdoses p. 822)
Cognitive impairment syndromes	Reversible cognitive deficits occur during intoxication, persist in chronic misuse → dementia (● People with dementia p. 498). Occurs in alcohol, volatile chemicals, benzodiazepines, and possibly cannabis
Residual disorders	Continuing symptoms exist despite discontinuing substance
Exacerbation of pre-existing conditions	Some mental health problems can be made worse through the use of substances. There is a known worsening of positive psychotic symptoms for some people when cannabis is used. Depression can be made worse by alcohol use (● People with anxiety and depression p. 478). Antidepressants can be made ineffective by alcohol. Cannabis does not affect most psychotropic medications.

Related topics

● Child and adolescent mental health p. 246

Further information

Adfam (*Supporting families of drug abusers*). Available at: ℜ www.adfam.org.uk
Talk to FRANK (*Drugs A to Z*). Available at: ℜ https://www.talktofrank.com/drugs-a-z

People with anxiety and depression

Depression and anxiety are the most common mental health conditions seen in 1° care. Causes and risk factors include: biological and genetic factors; stress vulnerability models; past history of anxiety or depression; long-term health problems; history of traumatic events; and history of drug or alcohol misuse (➔ Substance use p. 476; ➔ Alcohol p. 360).

Anxiety

Anxiety is a type of fear usually associated with the thought of a threat or something going wrong in the future or something happening now. Types of anxiety include: generalized anxiety disorder; social anxiety or social phobia; phobias; health anxiety; obsessive compulsive disorder; and panic disorder. Signs and symptoms may include any of those in Box 9.3, and usually a combination, but different for everyone.

> **Box 9.3 Signs and symptoms of anxiety**
> - Muscle tension
> - Butterflies in the stomach
> - Intrusive thoughts
> - Confusion
> - Hot or cold sweats
> - Dizziness or wobbly legs
> - ↑ heart rate (➔ Abnormal cardiac rhythms p. 640)
> - Hyperventilation
> - Sweaty palms
> - Shaking, especially hands
> - Tingling sensations on head and in fingers and toes

People who experience long-term anxiety can develop a number of health issues including: sleep problems, fluctuations in energy due to the prolonged or intense panic experiences, gastric ulcers (➔ Dyspepsia, gastro-oesophageal reflux disease, and peptic ulceration p. 708), changes in metabolism, nausea, irritable bowel syndrome (➔ Irritable bowel syndrome p. 710), and constipation (➔ Constipation and encopresis p. 286; ➔ Constipation in adults p. 512).

Screening tools include:
- Screening for Childhood Anxiety-Related Disorders (SCARED)
- (Adults) Patient Health Questionnaire Scale (PHQ-9)

Anxiety management

Mild anxiety is usually managed in 1° care.
- Sleep hygiene
- Avoid caffeinated drinks
- Reduce alcohol intake
- Mindfulness and other relaxation techniques
- ↑ exercise can be useful (➔ Exercise p. 354)

- Self-help literature/online CBT (➔ Talking therapies p. 472)
- Referral to mental health workers in GP surgery
- Referral to Increased Access to Psychological Therapies (IAPT)

⚠ If there are associated risk-taking behaviours, including thoughts, plans, or intent to harm self or others (➔ Suicidal intent and deliberate self-harm p. 494), refer to GP in first instance or ☎ 999 if the risk is immediate.

For moderate or severe anxiety, follow the NICE pathway and refer to 2° care services.[12] If the risk is indicated as ↑, refer to local crisis team for assessment, support, and guidance. ⚠ If risk is immediate, ☎ 999.

Depression

Can occur to anyone. May occur as a one-off episode or develop into a LTC. Defined as a mood disorder that causes a persistent feeling of sadness and loss of interest. It affects how you feel, think, and behave and can lead to a variety of cognitive, emotional, and physical problems. Signs and symptoms may include any of those in Box 9.4, and usually a combination, but different for everyone. If anyone reports experiencing four or more for most of the day, nearly every day, for >14 days, refer to IAPT or mental health worker at GP surgery.

Box 9.4 Signs and symptoms of depression

- Anhedonia (inability to feel pleasure in normally pleasurable activities)
- Avolition
- Negative/catastrophic thinking
- Sense of hopelessness
- Lethargy
- ↓ self-esteem/self-confidence
- Feeling like a burden to others
- Feelings of guilt/shame
- Tearfulness
- Sleep disturbance/trouble getting to sleep
- Early morning wakening
- Ruminating on events
- Changes to appetite
- Change in personality
- ↓ libido (➔ Sexual problems p. 768)
- Physical or psychosomatic presentations of aches and pains
- Preoccupation with mortality/morbidity
- Thoughts of deliberate self-harm or actual self-harm
- Intention to harm self /suicide
- Some people experience psychotic ideations

Screening tools include:
- (Adults) Patient Health Questionnaire Scale (PHQ-9). Available in different languages
- Becks Depression Inventory. Developed for service users over 13yrs ago

Always ask service users about risk of self-harm or suicidal thoughts. You will not put the idea into someone's mind and it is important to open this conversation for an accurate risk assessment.

The NICE guidelines[13] advise a stepped approach to treatment:
- Mild depression: managed at 1° care level
- Moderate depression: may require specialist support from mental health services. Talking therapies will be considered first, and then medication
- Severe depression: refer to specialty mental health team

⚠ If there is a risk of deliberate self-harm or suicidal thoughts, refer to specialist mental health services. You can also accompany the service user to A&E, who will have a mental health liaison team to assess and support. Inpatient treatment may be indicated. If the risk is immediate, ✆ 999 ambulance for assistance.

Related topics
⮞ Postnatal depression p. 440; ⮞ Post-traumatic stress disorder p. 490; ⮞ Child and adolescent mental health p. 246; ⮞ Depression and spiritual distress in palliative care p. 564

References
12. NICE (2014) *Anxiety disorders [QS53]*. Available at https://www.nice.org.uk/guidance/qs53/chapter/Quality-statement-3-Pharmacological-treatment
13. NICE (2018) *Depression in adults: recognition and management. Clinical guidelines [CG90]*. Available at: https://www.nice.org.uk/guidance/cg90

People with bipolar affective disorder

Bipolar affective disorder is a relapsing and remitting mood disorder. Characterized by episodes of both elated mood or euphoria (mania) and depression (➲ People with anxiety and depression p. 478). Previously called manic depression. Age of onset is ~15–19 years.[14] People with bipolar affective disorder are at ↑ risk of harm by accident and deliberate self-harm (➲ Suicidal intent and deliberate self-harm p. 494). Associated with a lifetime risk of suicide 15 times greater than in the general population[15] (➲ UK health profile p. 2). Multifactorial triggers including brain structure and functioning, and genetics and family history (either parent or sibling). Those at risk will not always develop the condition as it is also dependent on variables including stressors and social factors.

Mania and depression

Depression symptoms are listed in Box 9.4. Mania is characterized by prolonged and intense periods of euphoria and can include psychotic features (see Table 9.3). Hypomania is characterized by a less severe episode of euphoria.

Table 9.3 Signs and symptoms of mania

Increased energy	• Overactivity • Pressured speech • Flight of ideas • Racing thoughts • ↓ need for sleep • Restlessness • Agitation
Increased self-esteem	• Grandiosity • ↓ social inhibitions • Over-familiarity • Facetiousness • Reduced attention span • Tangential thinking and speech
Risk-taking behaviour	• Preoccupation with impractical schemes • Spending recklessly • ↑ libido and ↓ ability to consider consequences of unsafe sexual encounters
Other manifestations	• Excitement • Irritability • Aggressiveness • Suspiciousness • Disruption to daily routines and activities • Lack of insight into mental state • Catatonic or manic stupor can occur

Types

Biploar I is defined by manic episodes that last >7 days, or by manic symptoms that are so severe that the person needs immediate hospital care. Usually, depressive episodes occur as well, typically lasting >2wks. Episodes of depression with mixed features (having depression and manic symptoms at the same time) also possible. Bipolar II is defined by a pattern of depressive episodes and hypomanic episodes, but not the full-blown manic episodes just described. Cyclothymic disorder is defined by numerous periods of hypomanic symptoms, as well as numerous periods of depressive symptoms lasting for >2yrs (1yr in children and adolescents). However, the symptoms do not meet the diagnostic requirements for a hypomanic episode and a depressive episode. Other specified and unspecified bipolar and related disorders are defined by bipolar disorder symptoms that do not match the three categories listed here.

Prognosis

Prognosis is highly individual but shorter duration of elevated mood, lack of psychotic features, later onset, and ↑ degree of insight (including engagement with treatment, psychological and pharmacological) is linked to improved outcomes. Prognosis is less good when the person has any substance misuse issues, less support networks, lack of engagement with treatment, and/or prolonged and repeated episodes of depression occur between the manic episodes.

The life course of the disorder varies. A person can experience a one-off manic/hypomanic episode and repeated periods or prolonged depressive episodes, or repeated episodes of elevated mood and few depressive periods. There are sometimes years between episodes.

Some people experience a rapid cycling of mood from ↑ to ↓, and this can occur within a very short space of time (e.g. hours). This can be very distressing for the person and their family. It is associated with ↑ risk of harm from accident, to both self and potentially others. If treated, hypomania can be short-lived, for days rather than weeks.

Diagnosis

Bipolar disorder may not be diagnosed accurately and can be attributed to unipolar depression. If a person presents with depressive symptoms, ask about previous overactivity or euphoria lasting >4 days. Upon suspicion of bipolar disorder, refer to 2° mental health services for assessment and diagnosis.

Supporting the person with bipolar disorder

Some people will require support from specialist mental health services for shorter or longer periods. Other people will be managed in 1° care only. When working with people diagnosed with bipolar disorder who have a care co-ordinator in 2° care: develop an ongoing relationship with the person and their carers (→ Carers p. 458); support the person to carry out care plans developed in 2° care and achieve their recovery goals, as part of the Care Programme Approach (including triggers, early warning signs, crisis plans); share any risk assessments with 2° care and vice versa (→ Clinical risk management p. 78; → Teamwork p. 58; → Continuity of care p. 598); and review treatment and care, including medication, at least annually and more if there are concerns (→ Principles of medication reviews p. 142).

If bipolar disorder is managed solely in 1° care, re-refer to 2° care if any one of the following applies: there is a poor or partial response to treatment; the person's functioning declines significantly; treatment adherence is poor (➔ Medicine concordance and adherence p. 132); intolerable or medically important side effects from medication (➔ Medicine optimization p. 128); comorbid alcohol (➔ Alcohol p. 360) or drug misuse (➔ Substance use p. 476) is suspected; or a woman with bipolar disorder is pregnant (➔ Pregnancy p. 424) or planning a pregnancy (➔ Preconceptual care p. 422).

⚠ Refer people urgently for a specialist mental health assessment if mania or severe depression is suspected, or they are a risk to themselves or others, or deterioration of health. This may require the CRISIS team or attendance at A&E to be seen by the mental health liaison team. Where there is a serious ↓ in mental state, it may be necessary for the person to be in hospital as an informal patient. When there are immediate risks to self, others, or health, an assessment under the Mental Health Act (1983, amended 2007) may → formal detention in hospital (➔ Consent p. 82).

Monitoring physical health

Weight gain (➔ Overweight and obesity p. 348; ➔ Adult body mass index chart p. 346), metabolic syndrome, smoking (➔ Smoking cessation p. 356), and diabetes (➔ Diabetes: overview p. 660; ➔ Principles of diabetes management p. 664) contribute to cardiovascular disease (➔ Angina p. 626; ➔ Hypertension p. 628; ➔ Coronary heart disease p. 624) and death in people with bipolar affective disorder. Monitor the physical health of people with bipolar affective disorder at least annually. A copy of the results should be sent to the care co-ordinator and psychiatrist if the person has 2° care support.

Related topics

➔ Children and adolescent mental health p. 246

References

14. Smith, D.J., et al. (2013) Prevalence and characteristics of probable major depression and bipolar disorder within UK Biobank: cross-sectional study of 172,751 Participants. *Plos*, 8 (11), e75362. DOI:10.1371/journal.pone.0075362

15. Hayes, J.F., Miles, J., Walters, K., King, M., & Osborn, D.P. (2015) A systematic review and meta-analysis of premature mortality in bipolar affective disorder. *Acta Psychiatr Scand*, 131(6), 417–25

People with psychosis

Psychotic disorders are characterized by changes in perception, thinking, and experience of reality. For the person and their family (→ Carers p. 458), these changes can be ↑ distressing. There is ↑ risk in inner city and deprived areas. More ♂ are given the diagnosis than ♀. Black and minority ethnic groups are proportionally more highly represented. Age of peak onset ~15–17yrs, though can occur earlier. People can recover from psychosis. Early recognition and support can positively influence prognosis. A diagnosis of schizophrenia, bipolar disorder, or psychotic depression is a likely final diagnosis.

The stress-vulnerability model is often used to describe how a psychosis can develop. People all have some vulnerability to psychosis. Whether the person develops psychosis depends on the levels and severity of stress. A single, highly stressful event could → psychosis for someone or a gradual ↑ in stress over time. This is an individual response, as we all have differing levels of stress that we can tolerate before becoming unwell. Types of stress which can trigger psychosis include work pressures (→ People with anxiety and depression p. 478), relationship difficulties, exams, unemployment, bereavement (→ Coping with bereavement p. 574), physical illness, and sleep deprivation. There are also inherited predispositions, difficult early childhood experiences (→ Safeguarding children p. 248), and life circumstances, including giving birth (→ Complicated labour p. 436).

Psychosis can manifest in many ways and be unique to the individual. It can occur as a sudden onset or, more usually, gradually over time. Positive symptoms refer to additional or new experiences, and negative symptoms to the loss of others (see Table 9.4).

Anyone presenting with a suspected first episode of psychosis should be referred to the locality Early Intervention Service (EIS), who will assess the person, usually over an 8-wk period. A care plan is developed, including crisis planning and early warning signs of relapse. If the person meets the threshold, the EIS team will support that person for 3yrs. A differential diagnosis may be given, and diagnostic uncertainty underpins the work. Comorbidities of depression, anxiety, or substance misuse (→ Substance use p. 476) are common. The stigma associated with certain diagnoses requires sensitivity and education.

Post-partum psychosis

Post-partum psychosis (puerperal psychosis) is a mental health emergency (→ Postnatal care p. 438). Rapid-onset psychosis, usually within 2wks of giving birth (but can be later). Risk of neglect or harm to self or baby (→ Identifying the child in need of protection p. 250). ↑ risk if previous diagnosis or severe mental illness, or family history.

Treatment and management of psychosis

Treatment interventions include talking therapies (→ Talking therapies p. 472), and most people will also be offered medication. Ongoing psychological education and relapse prevention interventions are important.

1° care may be the only services involved with the person and will monitor at least 6mthly as per QOF (→ Quality and outcomes framework

Table 9.4 Symptoms of psychosis

Positive symptoms (within the first 3mths)	Negative symptoms (within the first 3mths)	First-rank symptoms (usually indicative of schizophrenia*)
• Hallucinations: abnormal perceptions of the senses—visual and auditory are most common, although olfactory, gustatory, and tactile regularly occur • Delusions: a false belief that no-one else shares; can be very frightening • Persecutory ideas: feeling victimized for actions, beliefs, or personality characteristics.	• Flattened mood • Depression • ↓ problem solving • ↓ sleep • ↓ cognition • ↓ insight • ↓ motivation • ↓ social awareness	• Auditory hallucinations: can be others arguing about you or talking about you (third-person hallucinations); a running commentary is suggestive of schizophrenia • Thought withdrawal, insertion, and interruption • Thought broadcasting • Somatic hallucinations • Delusional perception—a usual event is given an alternative meaning • Feelings or actions experienced as made or influenced by external agents

* Schizophrenia is used to describe a prolonged episode or a series of discrete episodes of psychosis.

p. 74). 2° care may be involved after the 3yrs of EIS support, with transfer to a longer-term team to support. At times of acute crisis, a crisis team referral may be needed to provide additional support to the person and their family/carers (➲ Teamwork p. 58).

People benefit, at different stages, from mental health supported activities or socially inclusive mainstream projects. MIND and Rethink mental health charities have local Hearing Voices groups (➲ Expert patients and self-management programmes p. 340). Carers will require an assessment of need.

⚠ At times of immediate risk to self or others, or deterioration of health, the person may require inpatient admission. If informal admission is declined, assessment under the auspices of the Mental Health Act (1983, amended 2007) may → formal inpatient treatment (➲ Consent p. 82).

Risk of suicide

⚠ The lifetime risk of death by suicide is estimated at 5.6% for people with schizophrenia and other psychotic disorders[16] (➲ Suicidal intent and deliberate self-harm p. 494). Regular and comprehensive risk assessment is vital (➲ Clinical risk management p. 78). Collateral information from carers can be very important to note.

Related topics

➜ Child and adolescent mental health p. 246

Reference

16. Nordentoft, M., Madsen, T., & Fedyszyn, I. (2015) Suicidal behaviour and mortality in first-episode psychosis. *Journal of Nervous and Mental Disease*, 203(5), 387–92

Further information

MIND (*Understanding psychosis*). Available at: ℘ https://www.mind.org.uk/media/4862926/understanding-psychosis_2016.pdf

Rethink (*Psychosis–what?*). Available at: ℘ https://www.rethink.org/diagnosis-treatment/conditions/psychosis/what

The Hearing Voices Network (*Hearing Voices groups*). Available at: ℘ https://www.hearing-voices.org/hearing-voices-groups/

Post-traumatic stress disorder

Post-traumatic stress disorder (PTSD) is a syndrome that develops following exposure to an extremely threatening or horrific event or series of events.[17] Such events might include:

- Violent crime (⊋ Victims of crime p. 452), including sexual abuse and domestic violence (⊋ Domestic violence p. 450)
- War, torture, and terrorism (⊋ Asylum seekers and refugees p. 444; ⊋ Armed forces veterans p. 502)
- Natural or man-made disasters or accidents
- Diagnosis of a life-threatening illness or long-term condition (LTC)
- Traumatic childbirth (⊋ Complicated labour p. 436)

Not everyone will develop PTSD who experienced the same events, and the symptoms may sometimes take years to develop. It is usual for the symptoms to be severe and last >4wks before consideration of a diagnosis of PSTD.

Those at risk of PTSD include not only those who are directly affected by a horrific event, but also witnesses, perpetrators, and those who help PTSD sufferers. People at ↑ risk include those who have experienced repeated trauma, have existing or previous depression or anxiety (⊋ People with anxiety and depression p. 478), are managing other stressors at the same time, or lack informal and/or professional support.

Characteristics

The characteristics of PTSD are summarized in Table 9.5 These experiences must occur over several weeks and significantly impair social functioning, including relationships, interactions with family/friends, or educational or occupational ability, or impact negatively upon the person.

Complex PTSD may develop following exposure to an event or series of events of an extremely threatening or horrific nature, most commonly prolonged or repetitive events from which escape is difficult (e.g. torture, prolonged domestic violence, repeated childhood sexual abuse (⊋ Safeguarding children p. 248)). It is characterized by the symptoms of PTSD together with severe and ongoing mood dysregulation, ↓ self-image (often with guilty feelings), and difficulty sustaining relationships.

Table 9.5 Characteristics of post-traumatic stress disorder (PTSD)

Re-experiencing traumatic events	Avoidance of thinking about the event	Perception of threat increased
Intrusive memories, nightmares, or flashbacks; these can occur without stimuli and cause intense emotional distress, disorientation, and agitation	The area where it occurred, people who were associated with it, smells or other sensory remembrances	Including hypervigilance and ↑ startle response; can also manifest as suspicion towards others' actions and motives

Treatment and management

For PTSD sufferers presenting in 1° care, GPs should take responsibility for the initial assessment and co-ordination of care. This includes the determination of the need for emergency medical or psychiatric assessment. Trauma-focused psychological therapies are recommended, though only when the sufferer considers it safe to proceed (➔ Talking therapies p. 472). The therapy is specialized and requires training. Limited evidence for pharmacological intervention. People who experience PTSD may develop other mental health issues such as severe anxiety, phobia, depression, dissociative disorder, or suicidal feelings (➔ Suicidal intent and deliberate self-harm p. 494). Service users may use alcohol and drugs to try to manage symptoms. In the long term, people with PTSD may develop physical illnesses such as heart disease (➔ Coronary heart disease p. 624), hypertension (➔ Hypertension p. 628), and obesity (➔ Overweight and obesity p. 348).

Related topics

➔ Child and adolescent mental health p. 246

Reference

17. International Classification of Disease (ICD-11) *Mortality and morbidity statistics*. Available at: https://icd.who.int/browse11/l-m/en#/http://id.who.int/icd/entity/2070699808

Further information

MIND (*Post-traumatic stress disorder*). Available at: ℘ https://www.mind.org.uk/information-support/types-of-mental-health-problems/post-traumatic-stress-disorder-ptsd/treatments-for-ptsd/#.W6uHtGhKg2w
NICE (*Post-traumatic stress disorder [NG116]*). Available at: ℘ https://www.nice.org.uk/guidance/ng116

Female genital mutilation

Female genital mutilation (FGM) is the ritual cutting or removal of some or all of the external ♀ genitalia. The practice is found in Africa, Asia, and the Middle East, and in communities from countries where FGM is common. Typically carried out by a traditional circumciser using a blade, FGM is conducted from days after birth to puberty (⊃ Puberty and adolescence p. 228) and beyond. ⚠ FGM has no health benefits.

Classification

WHO has identified four types of FGM.[18] All are associated with health risks (see Box 9.5).

- Type 1: Often referred to as clitoridectomy, this is the partial or total removal of the clitoris (a small, sensitive, and erectile part of the female genitals), and in very rare cases, only the prepuce (the fold of skin surrounding the clitoris).
- Type 2: Often referred to as excision, this is the partial or total removal of the clitoris and the labia minora (the inner folds of the vulva), with or without excision of the labia majora (the outer folds of skin of the vulva).
- Type 3: Often referred to as infibulation, this is the narrowing of the vaginal opening through the creation of a covering seal. The seal is formed by cutting and repositioning the labia minora, or labia majora, and sometimes through stitching, with or without removal of the clitoris (clitoridectomy).
- Type 4: This includes all other harmful procedures to the female genitalia for non-medical purposes, e.g. pricking, piercing, incising, scraping, and cauterizing the genital area.

UK legislation

Legislation includes the Female Genital Mutilation Act 2003 in England, Wales, and Northern Ireland, and the Prohibition of Female Genital Mutilation (Scotland) Act 2005. It is illegal to carry out FGM in the UK. It is also a criminal offence for UK nationals or permanent UK residents to perform FGM overseas or take their child abroad to have FGM.

Mandatory reporting

In England and Wales, health and social care professionals and teachers have a mandatory duty to report to the police if they are informed by a ♀ <18yrs that they have undergone FGM, or if they observe physical signs which appear to show an act of FGM has been carried out on a ♀ <18yrs. FGM is a safeguarding issue (⊃ Safeguarding children p. 248; ⊃ Identifying the child in need of protection p. 250; ⊃ Child protection processes p. 252; ⊃ Adults at risk from harm and abuse p. 454).

Box 9.5 Health risks of female genital mutilation (FGM)

Immediate complications
- Severe pain
- Haemorrhage
- Shock
- Infections
- Urination problems (➲ Urinary incontinence p. 504)
- Impaired wound healing (➲ Wound infection p. 526)
- Death
- Psychological trauma (➲ Post-traumatic stress disorder p. 490)

Long-term complications
- Pain
- Chronic genital infections
- UTIs (➲ Urinary tract infection p. 756)
- Menstrual problems (➲ Menstrual problems p. 778)
- Scar tissue and keloids
- Sexual problems (➲ Sexual problems p. 768)
- Obstetric problems (➲ Complicated labour p. 436)

Reference

18. WHO (*Female genital mutilation*). Available at: https://www.who.int/news-room/fact-sheets/detail/female-genital mutilation

Further information

NSPCC (*Female genital mutilation*). Available at: ✍ https://learning.nspcc.org.uk/child-abuse-and-neglect/fgm/#heading-top

Suicidal intent and deliberate self-harm

Suicidal intent is the intention to die by suicide. Suicidal thoughts can be persistent or fleeting and may escalate over time. They can include negative thoughts about oneself and the world, overwhelming wishes to die, that life is not worth living, and not seeing another way out.

Suicidal ideation and deliberate self-harm are not always related. Suicide is the action of taking one's life intentionally. Deliberate self-harm is to injure or poison oneself with the intention of causing harm. Some who harm themselves have no plans to die, just as some who take their own life have no history of self-harming. However, people who self-harm are at ↑ risk of suicide, whether by intention or accident, especially with those who repeatedly harm or use violent or dangerous methods.

Deliberate self-harm

Children and young people

NICE guidance starts from aged 8yrs.[19] It is not always clear why a child or adolescent starts harming themselves. It can be a one-off event or → repeated or compulsive behaviours.

Self-harm cycle

Self-harming results in a chemical being released to which the brain can become addicted. The person may feel immediate relief of pressure, but this relief is short-lived. It can → feelings of remorse or shame and ↑ the pressures and stressors felt by the person (➲ People with anxiety and depression p. 478). This in turn may cause the person to harm again. Early recognition is important. Triggers for children include being bullied, under too much pressure to do well at school/work, and being emotionally abused (➲ Working with teenagers p. 232; ➲ Puberty and adolescence p. 228). These experiences can → feelings that the person is unsure how to manage including: ↓ self-esteem and ↓ confidence; loneliness; sadness; anger; numbness; and lack of control over their lives. Signs of self-harm are summarized in Box 9.6.

⚠ There could be other causes of the physical signs of self-harm, including the possibility these marks were left by others (➲ Safeguarding children p. 248; ➲ Identifying the child in need of protection p. 250; ➲ Adults at risk from harm and abuse p. 454).

Suicide

High-risk groups include: prior suicide attempt/s; depression and other major mental health disorders (➲ People with psychosis p. 486; ➲ People with bipolar affective disorder p. 482; ➲ Post-traumatic stress disorder p. 490); substance misuse (➲ Substance use p. 476); family history of a mental health problem or substance misuse or suicide; family violence (➲ Victims of crime p. 452), including physical or sexual abuse; having weapons or poisons readily available (➲ Poisoning and overdoses p. 822); feelings of hopelessness; impulsive or aggressive tendencies; cultural beliefs (e.g. belief that suicide is a noble resolution); local epidemics of suicide; and isolation, a feeling of being cut off from other people.

Box 9.6 Signs of self-harm

- Bruising
- Cuts
- Hair missing (from pulling)
- Burns (⊕ Burns and scalds p. 816)
- Wearing long sleeves even in the hot weather
- Posting messages related to death/suicide on social media
- Depressed mood
- Anxious or nervous affect
- Social isolation
- Substance misuse (⊕ Substance use p. 476)
- Weight fluctuations (⊕ People with eating disorders p. 474)
- ↓ self-esteem or self-confidence
- Change in routines/activities/friendship groups
- Secretiveness

Barriers to accessing mental health treatment
- Loss (relational, social, work, or financial)
- Being in prison
- Exposure to others' suicidal behaviour (e.g. peer or media figure)
  Physical ill health, especially if a LTC or in pain
- Unwillingness to seek help because of the stigma attached

Protective factors
- Effective clinical care for mental, physical, and substance misuse
- Easy access to a variety of clinical interventions
- Family and community support (connectedness)
- Support from ongoing medical and mental healthcare relationships Skills in problem solving and conflict resolution
- Cultural beliefs that discourage suicide
- Support to develop resilience

Support and management for self-harm/suicide attempts

For some, 1° care management may be indicated. However, if the risk taking is severe, repeated and/or leads to significant harm, referral to 2° care should occur for children and some adults. This may be local Child and Adolescent Mental Health Services (CAMHS) (⊕ Child and adolescent mental health p. 246). If this risk is unmanaged, the person does not feel safe, or if the assessment outcomes are unclear, A&E is needed. If self-poisoning has occurred, A&E will always be indicated.

Questions to consider (⊕ Clinical risk management p. 78):
- Is the risk imminent?
- Does the person continue to wish to die?
- Have they left a note or equivalent?
- Did they use a violent/lethal method/large quantity of tablets?
- Did they expect not to be found in time?
- Are the means still available (tablets, weapons, or poisons)?
- Did they use readily available means or is there evidence of preplanning?

- Do they have a history of self-harm/ suicidal attempts?
- Do they have any specialized support?
- Are they engaged with that support currently?
- Are they alone or is there someone to support them at home (➲ Carer p. 458)?

People may be referred to CAMHS or community mental health teams (CMHTs) for longer-term support, including talking therapies (➲ Talking therapies p. 472; ➲ Teamwork p. 58). For children, GP counsellors and school supports are available (➲ Working in schools p. 44); NSPCC, Childline, and other non-statutory organizations can be perceived as more acceptable to the young person. ⚠ Peer support groups can be useful to some, but beware of potential to escalate behaviour (➲ Expert patients and self-management programmes p. 340).

Related topics

➲ School nursing p. 42; ➲ Postnatal depression p. 440; ➲ Depression and spiritual distress in palliative care p. 564; ➲ Child protection processes p. 252

Reference

19. NICE (2011) *Guidance: self-harm in over 8s: long-term management [CG133]*. Available at: https://www.nice.org.uk/guidance/cg133/resources

Further information

Campaign Against Living Miserably (*Support after suicide*). Available at: ♫ https://www.thecalmzone.net/help/get-help/support-after-suicide/

Childline (*Coping with suicidal thoughts and feelings*). Available at: ♫ https://www.childline.org.uk/info-advice/your-feelings/mental-health/coping-suicidal-feelings/

Papyrus (*Prevention of young suicide*). Available at: ♫ https://papyrus-uk.org/

Rethink Mental Health (*Suicidal thoughts*). Available at: ♫ https://www.rethink.org/diagnosis-treatment/symptoms/suicidal-thoughts

Samaritans (*Contact us now*). Available at: ♫ https://www.samaritans.org/how-we-can-help-you/contact-us

Silver Line Helpline for Older People (*Our helpline*). Available at: ♫ https://www.thesilverline.org.uk/what-we-do/our-helpline/

People with dementia

Progressive neurodegenerative condition affecting 5–7% of people ≥65yrs. Incidence ↑ with advancing age (⊋ Frailty p. 678). Prevalence ↑ in people with learning disabilities (⊋ People with learning disabilities p. 456). Defined as an acquired significant cognitive impairment in a minimum of one of the following: learning and memory; social cognition; language; executive function; complex attention; and perceptual motor function. The deficit must → an impairment of activities of daily living (ADL) and involve a continuous cognitive decline from a previous ↑ level of functioning. Common types of dementia include: Alzheimer's disease; vascular dementia; dementia with Lewy Bodies; frontotemporal dementia; and Parkinson's disease (⊋ Parkinson's disease p. 674) dementia. People may suffer from dual pathologies (mixed dementia).

Signs and symptoms of dementia

- Cognitive changes (amnesia, aphasia, apraxia, and agnosia)
- Attention and concentration changes (dysexecutive syndrome and changes in thinking, judgement, and mental capacity)
- Psychological symptoms (psychotic symptoms and mood disturbances)
- Behavioural changes (apathy, agitation, and aggression, purposeful walking, abnormal vocalization, and sexually inappropriate behaviour)
- Biological symptoms (sleep disturbances and changes in eating habits and appetite)

Diagnosis

Timely diagnosis provides people with knowledge about what is happening to them, gives them access to treatment and support services, and allows them to plan their future (⊋ Mental capacity p. 470). Barriers to diagnosis include patient and family (⊋ Carers p. 458) fear, and professional attitudes due to the perception that, in the absence of a cure, there is no point, and if the patient is content, there is no point intervening.

Initial assessment should include:[20] history taking from the patient (and family); physical examination; appropriate blood and urine tests to exclude reversible causes; and cognitive testing using a validated brief structured instrument (⊋ Standardized assessment tools p. 118). Refer person to specialist dementia diagnostic service (e.g. memory clinic) if reversible causes of cognitive decline or impairment have been investigated and dementia still suspected.

Prognosis

Average survival after diagnosis is ~7yrs. Markers of poor short-term survival include: aspiration, UTIs (⊋ Urinary tract infection p. 756), sepsis (⊋ Sepsis p. 826), pressure ulcers (⊋ Pressure ulcer prevention p. 520), and weight loss (⊋ Malnutrition p. 350).[21] ⚠ Dementia is a terminal illness and needs to be perceived as such to ensure good-quality outcomes at end of life.

Pharmacological treatment

Plays a relatively small role in management; used to allow patients to maintain functional independence for as long as possible and then aid management of problem behaviours in advanced disease.

Role of nurse

Varies depending on the phase of dementia and area of practice.[22]

Learning that the condition is dementia

• Provide compassionate support following diagnosis.
• Advocate on behalf of the person/family/carers.
• Know how dementia might affect person/family/carers.
• Recognize the person as a unique individual and citizen.
• Know how the condition might affect any coexisting conditions.

Learning more about dementia, treatment, care, and support

• Provide information and advice about living well with diagnosis.
• Ensure people from Black and minority ethnic communities access services and support that meet their needs.
• Work in partnership with the person/family/carers to identify needs, preferences, and outcomes.
• Know about local services, community resources, and opportunities to enable people to get the support they need to live well.
• Support the person to overcome barriers and stigma.
• Consider Imaginative and creative treatment and care options.
• Ensure person/family/carers know who to contact in a crisis.

Getting the right help at the right time, preventing crises

• Work in partnership with the person/family/carers and colleagues to plan care, identify possible crisis situations, and establish strategies to pre-empt or manage crises (➔ Teamwork p. 58).
• Work in partnership with colleagues and voluntary sector organizations to identify a care co-ordinator to help the person/family/carers navigate services (➔ Continuity of care p. 598).
• Work with the person/family/carers to identify and articulate future needs, and support family with lasting power of attorney and advance care planning.
• Support the person to access psychological and other relevant therapies (➔ Talking therapies p. 472), including exercise (➔ Exercise p. 354), creative therapies, and meaningful activities relevant to the person's interests.
• Liaise with relevant services to ensure that they know about dementia, the person, plans, and possible crisis points.
• Understand the carer's needs and concerns; welcome and support the carer as a partner in care provision.
• Ensure that physical health and care needs are identified and met.

Getting help to stay at home or, if needed, move to a care home

- Work together with other relevant health, social care, and voluntary sector services to enable the person to remain at home and maintain their independence as long as possible.
- Where possible work to prevent admission to an acute hospital (→ Services to prevent unplanned hospital admission p. 22).
- Work to enable safe, timely discharge from hospital (→ Services to promote hospital discharge p. 23).
- Support the person/family/carers in decision making regarding alternatives to living at home (→ Care homes p. 32).
- Work with care home colleagues to ensure the person receives compassionate and safe care, and participates in stimulating activities.

Receiving care, compassion, and support at the end of life

Record a person's wishes and preferences for end-of-life care (→ Mental capacity p. 470). Understand potential difficulties in communicating pain (→ Pain assessment and management in palliative care p. 554) and distress (→ Depression and spiritual distress in palliative care p. 564), and work with multidisciplinary team (→ Teamwork p. 58) to ensure effective pain relief. Ensure good communication between palliative care, 1° care, and other relevant colleagues and family/carers. Support the family/carers through the last days of life and signpost them to relevant services and bereavement support (→ Coping with bereavement p. 574).

References

20. NICE (2018) *Dementia: assessment, management and support for people living with dementia and their carers.* Available at: https://www.nice.org.uk/guidance/ng97
21. Widera, E. & Bernacki, R. (2015) Dementia. In: Cherny, N., Fallon, M., Kassa, S., Portenoy, R., & Currow, D. (eds) *Oxford Textbook of Palliative Medicine* (5th edn). Oxford: Oxford University Press
22. Department of Health (2016) *Making a difference in dementia: nursing vision and strategy* (refreshed edn). Available at: https://www.gov.uk/government/publications/dementia-nursing-vision-and-strategy

Armed forces veterans

A veteran is someone who has served in HM Armed Forces for at least one day. For serving personnel, 1° healthcare is provided by the Ministry of Defence. On leaving the forces, healthcare is the responsibility of the NHS. According to the Armed Forces Covenant, those injured in service should be cared for in a way that reflects the nation's moral obligation to them.[23] Thus, veterans are entitled to receive priority NHS care (including hospital, 1°, or community care) for any condition related to their service.

Veterans' trauma network

Veterans may have complex healthcare needs related to their war injuries. NHS England established a network of ten veterans' trauma centres: Plymouth, Oxford, London (three centres), Birmingham, Nottingham, Leeds, Liverpool, and Middlesbrough. Within these centres are health professionals with an understanding of Armed Forces culture. To refer to the network, the veteran's GP can email england. veterantraumanetwork@nhs.net.

Mental health

Poor mental health can affect veterans and their families. If someone is worried about their mental health, they should speak to their GP or contact the Combat Stress 24-hr helpline. Combat Stress is the UK's leading military charity specializing in mental health. ☎ 0800 138 1619, text 07537 404 719, or email helpline@combatstress.org.uk. Within the NHS in England, expert help is available from: NHS Veterans' Mental Health Transition, Intervention, and Liaison Service (TILS), and NHS Veterans' Mental Health Complex Treatment Service (CTS). Veterans can self-refer or ask their GP to refer them.

Related topics

➔ People with anxiety and depression p. 478; Post-traumatic stress disorder p. 490; ➔ Alcohol p. 360; ➔ Substance use p. 476; ➔ Suicidal intent and deliberate self-harm p. 494

Reference

23. Ministry of Defence (2011) *The Armed Forces Covenant*. Available at: https://assets.publishing. service.gov.uk/government/uploads/system/uploads/attachment_data/file/49469/the_ armed_forces_covenant.pdf

Further information

NHS (*Mental health care for veterans*). Available at: ♫ https://assets.nhs.uk/prod/documents/673_ NHS_Veterans_Mental_Health_leaflet_S23_Online_for_web.pdf

Adult care provision

Urinary incontinence 504
Indwelling urinary catheter care 508
Constipation in adults 512
Faecal incontinence 514
Stoma care 516
Spinal cord injury 518
Pressure ulcer prevention 520
Wound assessment 522
Post-operative wound care 524
Wound infection 526
Wound debridement 528
Malignant fungating wounds 530
Wound dressings 532
Leg ulcer assessment 536
Venous leg ulcers 540
Compression therapy for venous leg ulcers 542
Oral chemotherapy in the home 546
Lymphoedema 548
Palliative care in the home 550
Services for the dying patient 552
Pain assessment and management in palliative care 554

Nausea and vomiting in palliative care 558
Breathlessness in palliative care 560
Fatigue in palliative care 562
Depression and spiritual distress in palliative care 564
Palliative care emergencies 566
Caring for patients in the dying phase 568
Syringe drivers 570
Euthanasia, assisted suicide, and assisted dying 572
Coping with bereavement 574
Injection techniques 576
Venepuncture 580
Care of central venous catheters 582
Recording a 12-lead electrocardiogram 584
Tracheostomy care 586
Ear care 590
Enteral tube feeding 594

Urinary incontinence

Types of urinary incontinence

Stress incontinence

Leakage of urine when doing anything that causes abdominal pressure to be stronger than urethral sphincter mechanisms (e.g. coughing, laughing, lifting, and jogging). Incompetent urethral sphincter can be related to childbirth (➔ Complicated labour p. 436; ➔ Birth options and labour p. 434), surgery, pelvic floor weakness, obesity (➔ Overweight and obesity p. 348), hormone deficiency, chronic constipation (➔ Constipation in adults p. 512), and ageing (➔ Frailty p. 678). Rare in ♂ except post-prostatectomy (➔ Prostrate problems p. 758). Amount of leakage usually small but can be ↑ if bladder very full.

Urge incontinence

Caused by sudden involuntary contraction of bladder muscle and associated with a strong desire to urinate and inability to delay voiding long enough to get to the toilet. Person may experience nocturia. Part of a group of symptoms called overactive bladder syndrome, where bladder muscle is ↑ active than usual. Can occur with multiple sclerosis (➔ Multiple sclerosis p. 670), Parkinson's disease (➔ Parkinson's disease p. 674), poor fluid intake, and urinary tract infections (UTIs) (➔ Urinary tract infection p. 756). Symptoms antagonized by caffeinated and fizzy drinks, and alcohol (➔ Alcohol p. 360). Smoking and obesity also contributory factors. Usually only a small amount of urine at a time.

Mixed incontinence

Combination of the symptoms of stress and urge incontinence.

Overflow incontinence

Frequent leakage without the urge to void or the inability to urinate normal volumes. Often caused by a blockage or obstruction of the bladder (e.g. enlarged prostate, bladder stones, and constipation). Can also occur due to multiple sclerosis and Parkinson's disease. The amount of urine that exceeds the bladder's capacity leaks out, but the bladder remains full.

Total incontinence

Complete absence of control, with either continuous leakage or periodic uncontrolled emptying of the bladder's contents.

Assessment

History of symptoms

Explore: when problem first started; whether anything provokes leakage or makes it worse; completion of 3–7 days' diary detailing fluid intake (type and volume) and leakage/emptying episodes (frequency and volume); associated symptoms (e.g. pain and haematuria); and impact on lifestyle (incontinence-specific quality-of-life scales available).

Past medical/surgical history

Explore: underlying conditions that cause polyuria, nocturia, increased abdominal pressure, or central nervous system disturbances (e.g. cardiac failure (➔ Heart failure p. 636), chronic renal failure (➔ Renal problems

p. 754), diabetes (**⊃** Diabetes: overview p. 660), chronic obstructive pulmonary disease (COPD) (**⊃** Chronic obstructive pulmonary disease p. 614), neurological disease (including stroke and multiple sclerosis), cognitive impairment (**⊃** People with dementia p. 498), and depression (**⊃** People with anxiety and depression p. 478). Also: abdominal surgery; pregnancy and childbirth (number, mode of delivery, and birthweight); constipation; menopausal status (**⊃** Menopause p. 364); and weight and BMI (**⊃** Adult body mass index chart p. 346).

Drug history

Some medications can disrupt normal process of storing and passing urine or ↑ amount produced (e.g. diuretics, opioids, angiotensin converting enzyme (ACE) inhibitors, antidepressants, and sedatives).

Social history

Establish smoking status (**⊃** Smoking cessation p. 356) and alcohol intake. Consider functional incontinence due to poor access to toilet (**⊃** Homes and housing p. 26).

Abdominal examination

Taken by appropriately trained professional to exclude urinary retention and pelvic masses (**⊃** Gynaecological cancers p. 776; **⊃** Colorectal cancer p. 715). Also perineal examination including external genitalia, vaginal or rectal examination, and pelvic floor contraction. Offer chaperone (**⊃** Chaperones p. 84).

Urinalysis and additional investigations

Always perform urinalysis as part of initial assessment. Refer patients with voiding symptoms, complicated urinary incontinence, or recurrent UTIs for post-voiding residual volume with ultrasonography. Refer patients with complicated urinary incontinence for urodynamics—a series of tests to evaluate how well bladder, sphincters, and urethra are storing and releasing urine.

Urgent referral

Patients with the following symptoms should be referred for urgent review: haematuria, pain, recurrent UTIs, previous pelvic radiotherapy, associated faecal incontinence (**⊃** Faecal incontinence p. 514), or suspected neurological disease. In ♀, urgent referral for: Grade 3 or symptomatic prolapse, previous surgery for urinary incontinence, pelvic pass, or suspicion of fistula. In ♂, urgent referral for: abnormal rectal examination, findings suspicious of voiding dysfunction.

Management

Simple medical interventions

- Treat UTI
- Optimize management of underlying disease (e.g. heart failure (**⊃** Heart failure p. 636)) (**⊃** Medication optimization p. 128)
- Explore adjustment of medication impacting on urinary symptoms
- Relieve constipation

Lifestyle interventions

- ↓ caffeine, fizzy drinks, and alcohol
- Advising modification of ↑ or ↓ fluid intake

- Weight management (→ Nutrition and healthy eating p. 342; → Exercise p. 354)
- Smoking cessation
- Timed or promoted voiding in people with cognitive impairment

Bladder training
Indicated in people with urge or mixed incontinence (Box 10.1).

Pelvic floor muscle training
Indicated in people with stress or urinary mixed incontinence (Box 10.2). Also offer to ♂ undergoing radical prostatectomy to speed recovery from incontinence.

Box 10.1 Bladder training

Aim to establish a normal pattern of bladder emptying (between 6–8 times a day) by ↑ length of time of holding urine, so bladder is trained to fill and stay relaxed. Based on frequency of passing urine, set a target that lengthens the time before going to the toilet to pass urine and ↑ the volume passed. For example:
- Week 1: each time you feel the urge, wait and hold for 5mins
- Week 2: wait and hold for 10mins
- Week 3: wait and hold for 15mins
- Week 4: wait and hold for 20mins
- Week 5: wait and hold for 25mins
- Week 6: wait and hold for 30mins

The urge feeling is the first sign that your bladder is filling up, but it will subside. Strategies that can help control the initial urge to pass urine include:
- Sitting on a hard seat or tightly rolled towel to put pressure on pelvic floor muscles
- Five quick squeezes of the pelvic floor muscles

When going to the toilet, do not rush. Sit down on the seat, do not hover over it, and do not push or strain to empty.

Box 10.2 Pelvic floor exercises

Exercise 1
- Tighten muscles around anus, vagina, and urethra and lift up as if trying to stop passing urine and wind at the same time.
- Hold for as long as possible. Build up to a maximum of 10secs, then rest for 4secs, and repeat to a maximum of ten contractions.

Exercise 2
- Practise quick steady contractions, drawing in the pelvic floor muscles and holding for 1sec before releasing muscles.
- Aim for strong muscle tightening with each contraction, up to maximum of ten times.

Do one set of slow contractions (Exercise 1) followed by one set of quick contractions (Exercise 2) six times a day.

Containment products

Containment products include continence pads (including shaped pads, all-in-ones, and pull-ups) and devices (e.g. handheld urinals, urinary sheaths). Most people can achieve a successful resolution without containment products. For others, the appropriate product gives confidence and an improved quality of life. Following assessment, patients may be able to get products free, but it depends on their local NHS organization. Indwelling urinary catheters (➔ Indwelling urinary catheter care p. 508) rarely used to manage urinary incontinence due to risk of catheter-related infection. Intermittent self-catheterization might be useful in some patients (e.g. patients with neuropathic bladder conditions).

Medication

Patients with urge incontinence may be offered antimuscarinics, but review after 4wks (➔ Principles of medication reviews p. 142) and caution in older people (➔ Prescribing for special groups p. 138). Use of desmopression may be considered in patients with urge incontinence, specifically for nocturia. Post-menopausal ♀ with vulvovaginal atrophy may benefit from vaginal oestogren therapy. If treatments not successful or unsuitable, surgery or other procedures may be recommended.

Access to public toilets

Radar key gives independent access to over 9,000 toilets in the UK. Purchased from disability charities. Smartphone toilet finder apps also available.

Related topics
➔ Gynaecological cancers p. 776

Further information

European Association of Urology (*Guidelines on urinary incontinence*). Available at: ℘ https://www.guidelines.co.uk/urology/eau-urinary-incontinence-guideline/452979.article

NICE (*Urinary incontinence in women: management*). Available at: ℘ https://www.nice.org.uk/guidance/cg171/chapter/1-Recommendations

Royal College of Nursing (*Continence resource*). Available at: ℘ https://www.rcn.org.uk/clinical-topics/continence

Indwelling urinary catheter care

Urinary catheters are a last resort. Clinical indicators include:[1] chronic urinary retention, draining residual urine volumes, bypassing an obstruction, facilitating continence (➋ Urinary incontinence p. 504), and maintaining skin integrity. The main risk is catheter-associated UTIs (➋ Urinary tract infections p. 756); therefore, indwelling catheters may not be the best option for some patients (e.g. patients with an artificial heart valve or a heart defect, patients who are immunosuppressed (➋ Principles of working with someone with compromised immunity p. 466), and patients with one kidney). Other potential problems include allergic reaction (➋ Allergies p. 694; ➋ Anaphylaxis p. 810) to the material used in the catheter, injury to the urethra when the catheter is inserted, and bladder stones. Indwelling catheters might not be suitable for some people with dementia due to non-comprehension and their trying to remove them (➋ People with dementia p. 498).

Long-term urethral catheters

Expected to stay in place >28 days. Inserted into bladder and held in place with a water-filled balloon.

Catheter length and diameter, and balloon size

The adult ♀ urethra is 3–4cm long and the adult ♂ urethra is 18–22cm. Adult catheters come in different lengths: ♀ length (20–26cm) and standard length (40–45cm): ♀ length catheters are used for ♀ who are ambulant and of normal weight; and standard-length catheters are used for ♂ in all situations and for ♀ who are bedbound, immobile, or obese (➋ Overweight and obesity p. 348) with large thighs. Always choose the smallest size (gauge) to maintain adequate drainage. The Charrière (ch) denotes the measurement of the external diameter of the catheter: 12ch or 14ch or 16ch for long-term use in ♂; and 12ch or 14ch for long-term use in ♀. Balloon size refers to the amount of water needed to inflate the balloon. Large balloons (30ml) are only used post urological surgery or when the bladder neck is damaged; otherwise, a 10ml balloon should be used in adults. Over or under inflation of the balloon can cause pain, bladder spasm, bypassing, mucosal trauma, and catheter expulsion.

Long-term catheter material

• All silicone
• Silicone-elastomer-coated latex ⚠ Not suitable for people with an allergy to latex
• Hydrogel-coated latex ⚠ Not suitable for people with an allergy to latex
• Hydrogel-coated silicone
• Silver-alloy-coated catheters

Suprapubic catheters

Inserted into the bladder through the abdominal wall; performed in hospital under local or light general anaesthetic. Used when urethral catheterization is not possible or contraindicated (e.g. vulva carcinoma (➋ Gynaecological cancers p. 776). May ↓ risk of urethral trauma associated with long-term urethral catheters. Benefits include ↑ comfort and freedom to remain sexually active. Potential complications include infection and over granulation at cystostomy site (➔ Wound infection p. 526; ➔ Wound assessment p. 522).

Catheter length and diameter, and balloon size
• Standard length
• 16ch or 18ch
• Balloon size as per long-term urethral catheters

Catheter material
Ensure the catheter type is licensed for suprapubic use. All silicone may be contraindicated due to cuffing on balloon deflation and trauma on removal.

Changing urethral and suprapubic catheters

Long-term catheters have a maximum time *in situ* of ~12wks (see local and manufacturer guidelines). When encrustation is a problem, estimate lifespan by monitoring and recording blockage patterns. Blockages should be responded to promptly. ⚠ For patients with spinal cord injury at or above thoracic spine 6 (T6) (➔ Spinal cord injury p. 518), change catheter immediately to avoid autonomic dysreflexia.

Considerations when changing catheters
• Knowledge, education, and competency of person performing procedure
• First suprapubic change should be performed by urology team
• Local policy regarding catheterization of a ♀ patient by a ♂ nurse
• Local policy regarding circumstances nurses can undertake ♀ catheterizations (e.g. may be prohibited if patient has a history of pelvic trauma or bleeding on cathetherization)
• Consider using a chaperone (➔ Chaperone p. 84)
• Should always be performed using an aseptic, no-touch technique
• Only use antibiotic prophylaxis when changing catheters in patients with a history of catheter associated UTIs or those at risk of endocarditis.[2]

Drainage and support systems

Type depends on individual assessment. Intermittent drainage using a catheter valve may promote independence and ↓ risk of encrustation. Not suitable for patients with ↓ dexterity, confusion, a small bladder capacity, ↓ bladder sensation, renal impairment (➔ Renal problems p. 754) or ureteric reflux, or an overactive bladder. Should be changed every 5–7 days. Continuous drainage systems:
• Closed systems: where catheter and drainage bag remain connected for 5–7 days and drained using an outlet tap in the bag
• Link systems: where catheter and leg bag remain connected for 5–7 days, and for night-time drainage, a bed bag is linked to the outlet tap of the leg bag and is then discarded on a daily basis

Catheter self-management

Patients should be advised:

- Wash hands before and after touching the catheter/drainage system (carers to wash hands and wear non-sterile gloves)
- Fluid intake 1.5–2L per day
- Avoid constipation (➔ Constipation in adults p. 512)
- Avoid kinking the tubing and keep drainage bag below bladder
- Keep a closed system of drainage
- Cleanse meatus twice daily with a gentle soap and water
- ♂ should apply a condom to secure catheter during sex.

Catheter-associated UTI

Diagnosis will involve assessing clinical signs and symptoms: fever, new onset or worsening confusion, malaise/lethargy, back pain, pelvic pain, and acute haematuria. Obtain urine sample from sampling port. Depending on the severity of symptoms, consider waiting until results are available before prescribing.[3] Consider removing or changing the catheter before treating the infection. ⚠ Be alert to potential for sepsis (➔ Sepsis p. 826). Reassess if symptoms worsen or do not improve in 48hrs. Refer if infections are recurrent.

Record keeping

Documentation to include: choice of catheter length, diameter, balloon size, material, date due to be changed, date changed (and reason for change if related to blockage), and choice of drainage and support systems (➔ Record keeping p. 86). Patient should be provided records of the same (➔ Client- and patient-held records p. 90).

References

1. Royal College of Nursing (RCN) (2012) *Catheter care: RCN guidance for nurses.* Available at: https://www.rcn.org.uk/professional-development/publications/pub-003237
2. NICE (2012) *Healthcare associated infections: prevention and control in primary care and community care (CG139).* Available at: https://www.nice.org.uk/guidance/cg139
3. NICE (2018) *Urinary tract infection (catheter associated): antimicrobial prescribing— draft for consultation.* Available at: https://www.nice.org.uk/guidance/indevelopment/gid-apg10005

Constipation in adults

The diagnostic criteria for constipation includes two or more of the following: straining during ≥25% of defecations; lumpy or hard stools ≥25% of defecations; sensation of incomplete evacuation ≥25% of defecations; sensation of anorectal obstruction/blockage ≥25% of defecations; manual manoeuvres to facilitate ≥25% of defecations; and < three spontaneous bowel movements per week.[4] Constipation can be acute or chronic. Chronic constipation occurs when symptoms are present for ≥12wks in the preceding 6mths. Functional constipation is chronic constipation without a known cause. 2° constipation is constipation caused by a drug or underlying medical condition.

Assessment

History of the presenting problem

Explore: onset (duration of problem, whether constipation is a long-term problem, and usual habit); character (abdominal pain, back passage pain, flatus, distension, and appearance of the stool (see Bristol Stool Chart)); associated symptoms (nausea or vomiting, rectal bleeding, urinary retention, overflow diarrhoea (➔ Faecal incontinence p. 514), fever, and loss of appetite/ weight); and relieving factors (self-help measures).

Past medical history

Explore: spinal cord injury (particularly patients with spinal cord injury at risk of autonomic dysreflexia) (➔ Spinal cord injury p. 518); carcinoma of the bowel (➔ Colorectal cancer p. 715); diverticular disease (➔ Appendicitis, diverticulitis, hernias, and intestinal obstruction p. 716); haemorrhoids (➔ Anal conditions p. 706); diabetes (➔ Diabetes: overview p. 660); hypothyroidism (➔ Thyroid p. 702); irritable bowel syndrome (➔ Irritable bowel syndrome p. 710); irritable bowel disease; abdominal surgery; anaemia (➔ Anaemia in adults p. 652); and any recent surgery or inflammation which may have caused paralytic ileus.

Drug history

Explore use of opioids, atropine, and antidepressants.

Social history

Explore: alcohol intake (➔ Alcohol p. 360); use of recreational drugs (➔ Substance use p. 476); dietary and fluid intake; stress (➔ People with anxiety and depression p. 478); and access to toilet facilities (➔ Homes and housing p. 26).

Family history

History of malignancy

Physical examination

Including consideration of general appearance, digital rectal examination, and inspection, auscultation, palpation, and percussion of abdomen. Offer chaperone (➔ Chaperone p. 84).

Differential diagnoses

Organic obstruction (e.g. carcinoma and hernias); painful anal conditions (e.g. haemorrhoids and rectal prolapse); adynamic bowel (e.g. hypothyroidism and spinal cord injury); drugs (e.g. opioids and anticholinergics);

habit and diet (e.g. dehydration and low-fibre diet); and psychiatric problems (e.g. depression and anorexia (⊃ People with eating disorders p. 474)).

⚠ New onset constipation, especially in people aged >50yrs, or accompanying symptoms such as anaemia, abdominal pain, weight loss, or blood in the stool, should be urgently investigated due to the risk of malignancy.

⚠ Symptoms of intestinal obstruction vary depending on level of blockage, including vomiting with or without nausea, abdominal distension and generalized discomfort, colic may be a feature, and altered bowel sounds. Intestinal obstruction is a medical emergency. In end-of-life care, patient wishes will inform treatment.

Self-management

Healthy diet (including whole grains, fruits high in sorbitol, and vegetables) (⊃ Nutrition and healthy eating p. 342); an adequate fluid intake (1.5L per day); ↑ activity levels (⊃ Exercise p. 354); and helpful toileting regimens (e.g. responding immediately to sensation of needing to defecate).

Pharmacological management

Pharmacological management will be guided by a variety of factors including whether the working diagnosis is short-duration constipation, opioid-induced constipation, faecal impaction, or chronic constipation. Types of laxative are classified by their mechanism of action and include bulk-forming laxatives, stimulant laxatives, osmotic laxatives, and faecal softeners.

Bulk-forming laxatives retain fluid in the stool and ↑ stool weight and consistency. Examples include ispaghula husk and methylcellulose. Onset of action is up to 72hrs. It is important to advise the patient to drink plenty of fluids for these laxatives to be effective. ⚠ Lack of water → bloating and bowel obstruction.

Stimulant laxatives stimulate the submucosal plexus and deeper myenteric plexus, which ↑ motility and intestinal secretions. Examples include senna and bisacodyl. Often causes abdominal cramps and should be avoided in intestinal obstruction. Onset of action ~6–12hrs.

Osmotic laxatives ↑ the amount of water in the large bowel, either by drawing fluid into the bowel (e.g. lactulose) or by retaining the fluid they were administered with (e.g. macrogols). ⚠ Laxatives that draw fluid into the bowel have dehydrating effects. Onset of action ~24–72hrs for lactulose and ~24–48hrs for macrogols.

Faecal softeners allow passage of water into the stool mass by ↓ the surface tension of the stool mass. Examples include docusate sodium (either as an oral preparation or rectal suppository) and glycerol suppositories. ⚠ Avoid rectal preparations in patients with haemorrhoids and anal fissure. Onset of action ~24–48hrs for oral preparations and ~20mins for rectal suppositories.

Reference

4. Drossman, D.A., Chang, L.C., Kellow, W.J., Tack, J., & Whitehead, W.E. (2016) *Rome IV functional gastrointestinal disorders: disorders of gut–brain interaction* (4th edn). Raleigh, NC: The Rome Foundation.

Further information

NICE (*Constipation*). Available at: ℘ https://cks.nice.org.uk/constipation#!topicsummary
Scottish Palliative Care Guidelines (*Bowel obstruction*). Available at: ℘ http://www.palliativecareguidelines.scot.nhs.uk/guidelines/symptom-control/bowel-obstruction.aspx

Faecal incontinence

Faecal incontinence (FI) is a common problem in 1° care. It involves involuntary loss of faeces (liquid or solid) from the bowel. Severity varies from infrequent seepage to complete loss of rectal contents. It is a socially embarrassing and disabling condition.

Assessment

In some patients, cause will be multifactorial. Subjective assessment will always include a drug history and the following topics.

History of presenting problem

Explore: onset (duration, whether a long-term problem, and usual habit); character (frequency, urgency, passive soiling, and appearance of stool (see Bristol Stool Chart); associated symptoms (abdominal pain and bloating, flatus, rectal bleeding (⊃ Colorectal cancer p. 715), urinary incontinence (⊃ Urinary incontinence p. 504), fever, loss of appetite/weight); relieving factors (self-help measures); and effects of symptoms on psychological and social functioning.

Past medical history

Explore: surgical damage to anal sphincter (e.g. haemorrhoidectomy); anal sphincter trauma (e.g. during childbirth with third/fourth degree vaginal tears) (⊃ Anal conditions p. 706; ⊃ Complicated labour p. 436)); and neurological disorders affecting sensory or motor function (e.g. spinal cord injury (⊃ Spinal cord injury p. 518), multiple sclerosis (⊃ Multiple sclerosis p. 670), and spina bifida).

Social history

Explore dietary and fluid intake (especially fibre and caffeine) (⊃ Nutrition and healthy eating p. 342), and ease of toilet access. Rule out overflow diarrhoea related to constipation (⊃ Constipation in adults p. 512).

Physical examination

Physical examination may be performed including consideration of general appearance, digital rectal examination, and inspection, auscultation, palpation, and percussion of abdomen. Offer chaperone (⊃ Chaperone p. 84). Consider risk of cross infection, skin excoriation, incontinence-associated dermatitis (⊃ Eczema/dermatitis p. 684), pressure ulceration (⊃ Pressure ulcer prevention p. 520), and wound contamination (⊃ Wound infection p. 526).

Management

⚠ Immediate referral if red flag symptoms for colorectal cancer present: rectal bleeding, unintentional weight loss, anaemia, unexplained change in bowel habit. Management varies according to underlying disorder and impact of problem on patient's quality of life.[5]

Conservative treatment

- Pelvic floor muscle training
- Biofeedback
- Use of constipating agents and laxatives

- Dietary modification
- Use of pads (including shaped pads, all-in-ones, and pull-ups. Following assessment, patient may be able to get products provided for free, but it depends on their local NHS organization.)
- Use of anal plugs

Surgical treatment
- Sphincter repair
- Neo-sphincter formation
- Formation of colostomy or stoma (➔ Stoma care p. 516)

Other treatments
Sacral nerve simulation

Faecal management systems
May be indicated for short-term use (<29 days) in patients who have liquid to semi-liquid stools, have little or no bowel control, and who are bedbound.[6] Contraindicated with the following conditions: sensitivities or allergies (➔ Allergies p. 694; ➔ Anaphylaxis p. 810) to the materials used in the faecal management system, history of rectal or anal surgery, severe rectal or anal stricture or stenosis, rectal mucosal impairment, rectal/anal tumour, severe haemorrhoids, faecal impaction, and spinal cord injury at thoracic spine 6 (T6) or above.

Access to public toilets
Radar key gives independent access to over 9,000 accessible toilets in the UK. Purchased from various disability charities. Smartphone toilet finder apps also available.

References

5. Omar, M. & Alexander, C. (2013) *Cochrane database of systematic reviews: drug treatment for faecal incontinence in adults.* Available at: https://www.cochranelibrary.com/cdsr/doi/10.1002/14651858.CD002116.pub2/full

6. Evans, J., Price, J., Yates, A., & Young, T. (2010) *All Wales guidelines for faecal management systems: guidelines for best practice.* Available at: http://www.welshwoundnetwork.org/files/6313/8555/6979/all_wales-faecal_systems.pdf

Further information

National Institute for Care and Health Excellence (*Faecal incontinence in adults [CG49]*). Available at: M https://www.nice.org.uk/guidance/cg49

Stoma care

Colostomies and ileostomies

Colostomies and ileostomies are surgically created openings of the bowel and the abdominal wall used in the management of bowel cancer (➔ Colorectal cancer p. 715), inflammatory bowel disease (➔ Inflammatory bowel disease p. 712), following major trauma, and sometimes in functional bowel disorders (➔ Constipation in adults p. 512; ➔ Faecal incontinence p. 514). They can be either permanent or temporary.

Colostomy

Most common type of stoma. Formed from large bowel (colon). Located in the left iliac fossa. Bowel movements are usually solid as faeces has travelled through colon undergoing water absorption. Stoma will be flush to the skin.

Ileostomy

Second most common type of stoma. Formed of small bowel (ileum). Located in right iliac fossa. Bowel movements are liquid and light in colour. Enzymes in faeces are toxic to the skin. Therefore, the stoma has a spout protruding above skin level to allow faeces to drain without touching the skin.

Stoma appliances and accessories

Prior to use, stoma nurse will have undertaken a full assessment of the patient. Two key appliances are the flange and bag. The flange is the adhesive part, which is made from material similar to hydrocolloid dressings, which acts as a skin-protective barrier, and additional security is provided by the adhesive. If the stoma is irregular in shape, it is appropriate to use a cut-to-fit flange. Care should be taken when cutting the flange: too large an opening may cause skin to become excoriated; and too small an opening may constrict the stoma (⚠ in severe cases, ischaemia can occur). Mouldable flanges are available and instead of being cut to shape are moulded into shape. Bags may be closed, drainable, or taped.

Appliances come as one-piece or two-piece systems. In the one-piece system, the flange and the bag are joined together. In the two-part system, the flange is separate from the bag and joined together using clips or adhesive. With the two-part system, the flange can be left in place for up to 4 days and the bag changed as required.

Convex appliances are available, which may be useful for a flush or retracted stoma or a leaking appliance. These may be held in place with small elastic belt. ⚠ Convex appliances may result in peristomal skin damage.

Colostomy bags are usually changed when a third to half full of faeces. Patients with a colostomy can use a plug or similar device to 'hold back' faeces so they are released at a convenient time. Colostomies can also be irrigated, which can allow the patient to wear a stoma cap rather than a bag. A patient with an ileostomy will require a drainable one-piece or two-piece system to be emptied four to six times a day.

Accessories include adhesive paste, adhesive remover spray, adhesive remover wipe, protective cream, protective stoma powder, protective spray, protective wipe, retention strip, seal/washer, and strip paste. Prescriptions can be taken to the chemist or sent to a specialist supplier, who will deliver the products (➔ Prescribing p. 136). In England, prescription charges do not apply for appliances or accessories for a permanent ileostomy or colostomy (but charges do apply for temporary stomas).

Urostomies

Surgically created to divert urine from the kidneys and ureters to the abdominal wall, bypassing the bladder. Treatment in bladder cancer, neurogenic bladder disease, birth defects, and chronic inflammation of the bladder. A urostomy is permanent. Located in the right iliac fossa. An isolated part of the small bowel (ileum) is brought onto the surface of the abdomen and the other end sealed. The ureters are detached from the bladder and reattached to the isolated section of intestine. This forms the ileal conduit. Stoma has a spout protruding above skin level.

Stoma appliances and accessories

Prior to use, the stoma nurse will have undertaken a full assessment of the patient. Appliances come as drainable one-piece or two-piece systems. The tap or bung at the bottom of the bag can be attached to a night drainage bag to allow additional drainage overnight. With the two-part system, the flange can be left in place for several days (4 days maximum) and the bag changed as required. Accessories available as per above. Prescriptions can be taken to the chemist or sent to a specialist supplier, who will deliver the products. In England, prescription charges do not apply for appliances and accessories for a urostomy.

Supporting patients at home

Monitor for complications associated with ileostomies, colostomies, and urostomies, including parastomal hernia, stoma blockage, skin problems, stomal fistula, stoma retraction, stoma prolapse, stomal stricture, leakage, stomal ischaemia. Additional complications with ileostomies and colostomies include rectal discharge and bowel obstruction (➔ Appendicitis, diverticulitis, hernias, and intestinal obstruction p. 716). Additional complications with ileostomies include dehydration and vitamin B12 deficiency.

The stoma care nurse should provide ongoing support to patients following discharge from hospital. They should be contacted by patients or community nurses for further advice. Self-help groups also available (e.g. Colostomy UK ♫ http://www.colostomyuk.org/support-groups/, Internal Pouch Support Group ♫ http://www.iasupport.org/, and the Urostomy Association ♫ https://urostomyassociation.org.uk/support/) (➔ Expert patients and self-management programmes p. 340).

Further information

PrescQIPP (Bulletin 105: stoma). Available at: M https://www.prescqipp.info/our-resources/bulletins/bulletin-105-stoma/

Spinal cord injury

Spinal cord injury (SCI) damage can be caused by trauma or as a result of infection or disease. Damage → temporary or permanent disability. Extent of paralysis depends on level of injury. The higher the damage, the more movement and sensation will be lost (Table 10.1).

Injuries are either complete or incomplete. In the former, there is complete loss of sensation and muscle control below the level of injury. In the latter, some areas remain sufficiently intact to retain some function.

There are ~12 SCI centres in the UK and Ireland. It is expected that all patients with actual or potential SCI are referred to a specialist centre. Services include:[7]

- Initial admission (addressing all aspects of a patient's life as part of rehabilitation and reintegration/resettlement planning process)
- Community liaison (providing comprehensive community liaison services—a useful resource for specialist guidance once patient has left hospital, for both patients and healthcare professionals)
- Outpatient (reviewing patients and providing management advice on planned regular basis or as requested, and providing referrals to specialist physiotherapists, occupational therapists, nurses, and psychologists)
- Readmission (further assessment and/or treatment of a particular problem or planned specialist additional rehabilitation).

Neurogenic bladder

All patients with SCI will have a neurogenic bladder. Depending on the level of lesion and the type of neurogenic bladder, symptoms include incontinence (➔ Urinary incontinence p. 504), overactive bladder, and urinary retention. Management approaches will be initiated by a specialist and may include intermittent catheterization, indwelling urinary catheters, or suprapubic catheters (➔ Indwelling urinary catheter care p. 508). Pharmacological management may be indicated. UTIs (➔ Urinary tract infections p. 756) are a frequent complication of neurogenic bladder. Symptoms may be atypical and include fever, nausea, headache, and ↑ spasticity. ⚠ Noxious stimulation of the bladder, including bladder distension, is a common cause of autonomic dysreflexia.

Neurogenic bowel

All patients with SCI will have a neurogenic bowel. Depending on the level of lesion and the type of neurogenic bowel, symptoms include ↑

Table 10.1 Level of injury and associated impairment

Level of injury	Associated impairment
Cervical (C1–C8)	Impairs function from the neck down, including swallowing, speech, and movement of the arms and hands (in addition to the loss of function in the thoracic, lumber, and sacral regions).
Thoracic (T1–T12)	Causes difficulties with breathing and digestion (in addition to loss of function in the lumbar and sacral regions).
Lumbar (L1–L5)	Impairs movement of the legs and feet (in addition to loss of function in the sacral region).
Sacral (S1–S5)	Impairs bladder and bowel control and sexual function.

colonic transit time, paralysis of the external anal sphincter, constipation (⊃ Constipation in adults p. 512), difficulty with evacuation, incontinence (⊃ Faecal incontinence p. 514), and faecal impaction. Management aims to promote regular and thorough bowel emptying, and maintain continence. Management approaches will be initiated by a specialist. Interventions dependent on the type of neurogenic bowel and may include dietary advice, rectal stimulants, oral laxatives, abdominal massage, digital rectal removal of faeces, and transanal irrigation. ⚠ Constipation is a common cause of autonomic dysreflexia.

Respiratory complications

Patients with a SCI above L1 will have some form of lung dysfunction. Impairment will be more severe in high cervical injuries and involve diminished inspiratory capacity and reduced cough effectiveness. Respiratory complications include atelectasis, pneumonia (⊃ Pneumonia p. 750), and respiratory failure. Management approaches will depend on the level of injury and include positioning and postural changes, breathing techniques, seasonal influenza and pneumococcal vaccination (⊃ Targeted adult immunization p. 392), suctioning, pharmacological interventions, and smoking cessation (⊃ Smoking cessation p. 356).

Autonomic dysreflexia

Patients with SCI at or above T6 are at risk of autonomic dysreflexia (AD). Caused by spinal reflex mechanisms initiated by a noxious stimulus entering the spinal cord below the level of injury, such as bladder distension, constipation, pressure ulcers (⊃ Pressure ulcer prevention p. 520), ingrown toenails, mensuration, and anal fissures (⊃ Anal conditions p. 706). → potentially life-threatening hypertension (⊃ Hypertension p. 628). Signs and symptoms include: pounding headache, flushed appearance of the skin above the level of lesion, profuse seating above the level of the lesion, tightness in the chest, nasal congestion, and hypertension. Patients with SCI at or above T6 should have a baseline BP available so that an increase above what is normal can be detected. ⚠ AD is a medical emergency due to risk of intracranial haemorrhage.

Treatment

Treatment is to sit the patient upright and drop the feet, loosen restrictive clothing, remove noxious stimulant as soon as possible, and monitor BP closely. Administer medication prescribed for AD. One of the most commonly used hypotensive agents is nifedipine (either sublingually (SL) or using the bite-and-swallow technique, according to local guidelines). Alternative treatments include SL or topical nitrates. Men with SCI will sometimes use phosphodiesterase type 5 (PDE5) inhibitors (e.g. sildenafil (Viagra)) for sexual dysfunction; ⚠ use of nitrates is contraindicated in this situation. Transfer patient to hospital if the cause of AD cannot be identified or the hypertension cannot be controlled.

Pressure ulceration

SCI is a risk factor for pressure ulcer development.

Reference

7. Royal National Orthopaedic Hospital NHS Trust (undated) *Medical management advice*. Available at: https://www.rnoh.nhs.uk/our-services/spinal-cord-injury-centre/medical-management-advice

Pressure ulcer prevention

Localized injuries to the skin or underlying tissue, caused by pressure, or pressure in combination with strain between the skeleton and a support surface. According to the International Pressure Ulcer (PU) Classification System:[8]

- Stage I: Non-blanchable erythema
- Stage II: Partial-thickness skin loss
- Stage III: Full-thickness skin loss
- Stage IV: Full-thickness tissue loss
- Unstageable: Depth unknown
- Suspected deep tissue injury: Depth unknown

Risk assessment

Patient risk factors include immobility, poor general skin status, a history of previous ulceration, and ineffective tissue perfusion. All patients receiving healthcare should be assessed for their risk of developing a PU using a validated scale (e.g. Waterlow, Braden) (→ Standardized assessment tools p. 118). Reassess risk if there is a change in the patient's condition or circumstances (e.g. falls (→ Falls prevention p. 368), infection), or more frequently as per local policy. Risk assessment will help determine if someone is at: risk, ↑ risk, or very ↑ risk.

Skin inspection should be offered to all at risk. Should include: heels; sacrum; ischial tuberosities; shoulders; back of head; toes; parts of body affected by anti-embolic stockings, equipment, and clothing; and parts of the body where pressure, friction, and shear is exerted. Patients should also be encouraged to inspect their own skin using a mirror. Check for: skin integrity; colour changes or discolouration; and variations in heat, firmness, and moisture. All risk assessments and skin inspections should be documented (→ Record keeping p. 86).

Prevention interventions

Timely, tailored information to patients and their family or carers (→ Carers p. 458). In collaboration with the patient, develop and document an individualized care plan guided by the acronym SSKIN:[9]

- Support surface: Pressure redistributing overlays, mattresses, and cushions (including high-specification foam mattresses and active support surfaces). Also consider offloading at risk heels. (→ Assistive technology and home adaptations p. 834)
- Skin inspection: See 'Risk assessment' section
- Keep moving: Repositioning according to patient risk factors and support surface provided. Teach patients to do pressure relief lifts. Use the 30° tilted side-lying position if the patient can tolerate and their condition allows.
- Incontinence/continence management: Develop and implement a continence management plan, ensuring skin is promptly cleaned after incontinence. Consider use of barrier preparations.
- Nutrition and hydration: Assess nutritional status using a validated tool (e.g. Malnutrition Universal Screening Tool) (→ Malnutrition p. 350), provide advice regarding nutrition and hydration, and refer to dietician as needed (→ Nutrition and healthy eating p. 342).

Safeguarding adults

Whilst some community-acquired PUs are unavoidable, they are largely considered avoidable and should be reported according to local clinical risk management policies (➲ Clinical risk management p. 78). Also follow guidelines on reporting as an adult safeguarding concern[10] (➲ Adults at risk from harm and abuse p. 454).

References

8. National Pressure Ulcer Advisory Panel, European Pressure Ulcer Advisory Panel, and Pan Pacific Pressure Injury Alliance (2014) *Prevention and treatment of pressure ulcers: quick reference guide*. Available at: https://www.npuap.org/wp-content/uploads/2014/08/Updated-10-16-14-Quick-Reference-Guide-DIGITAL-NPUAP-EPUAP-PPPIA-16Oct2014.pdf

9. Healthcare Improvement Scotland (2011) *SSKIN care bundle*. Available at: http://www.healthcareimprovementscotland.org/programmes/patient_safety/tissue_viability/sskin_bundle.aspx

10. Department of Health and Social Care (2018) *Safeguarding adults protocol: pressure ulcers and the interface with a safeguarding enquiry*. Available at: https://assets.publishing.service.gov.uk/government/uploads/system/uploads/attachment_data/file/675192/CSW_ulcer_protocol_guidance.pdf

Further information

NICE (*Pressure ulcers: prevention and management [CG179]*). Available at: ℘ https://www.nice.org.uk/guidance/cg179

Wound assessment

Defined as information obtained using observation, questioning, physical examination, and clinical investigations in order to formulate a management plan[11]. Assessment should be of the patient and the wound. Holistic assessment will include consideration of factors impacting on healing: comorbidities, medications, systemic or local infections, reduced oxygenation and tissue perfusion, age, pain, poor nutrition and hydration (➲ Malnutrition p. 350), smoking, alcohol intake (➲ Alcohol p. 360), and obesity (➲ Overweight and obesity p. 348).

Frequency of assessment

Initial or baseline assessments should be performed when wound is first identified. Follow-up assessments provide comparison data to determine response to treatment. Serial assessments should be performed at least weekly, with dressing changes (➲ Wound dressings p. 532), whenever a change occurs in the wound, or more frequently according to local policy.[12]

Framework for assessment

Only cleanse wound if debris present on wound bed. Triangle of wound assessment advocates an assessment of three areas:[13]

Wound bed

Identify location and take measurements of size (length, width or area, and depth). Ensure consistency in measurement—usually a single-use measuring guide. In relation to depth, consider tissue involvement (e.g. epidermis, dermis, subcutaneous tissue, tendon, muscle, fascia, bone). Record appearance (➲ Record keeping p. 86):

- *Tissue types* (e.g. necrotic, sloughy, granulating, epithelializing) and % of tissue type visible in wound bed
- *Exudate level* (e.g. dry, low, medium, high) and type (e.g. thin/watery, thick, cloudy, purulent (yellow/brown/green), pink/red). No standard method for assessing exudate levels; what is normal varies depending on wound type, size, and stage of healing.
- *Signs and symptoms of local infection* (increased pain or new onset; erythema; oedema, local warmth; increased exudate; delayed healing, bleeding/friable granulation tissue; malodour; and pocketing) (➲ Wound infection p. 526)
- *Signs and symptoms of spreading/systemic* (as above plus: increased erythema; pyrexia; abscess/pus; wound breakdown; cellulitis; general malaise; raised white blood cells; and lymphangitis)

Wound edge

Assess edges to identify impediments to migration of epithelial cells across wound bed: maceration; dehydration; undermining; and rolled edges.

Periwound skin

Assess skin within 4cm of the wound edge and under dressing for signs of: poor exudate management, infection, dressing-related injury, etc.; maceration (can easily become infected with bacteria or fungi); excoriation; dry skin; hyperkeratosis; callus; and eczema (➲ Eczema/dermatitis p. 684).

Wound photography

Digital photographs provide an objective visual representation to accompany written record. Follow local guidelines relating to equipment, patient confidentiality (→ Confidentiality p. 89), and data protection.

Additional investigations

Some wound types will require additional investigations, e.g. patients with a leg ulcer will require an ankle-brachial pressure index measurement (→ Leg ulcer assessment p. 536). Microbiological tests and wound biopsy may be indicated in some circumstances.

Record keeping

Documentation essential to review previous status and facilitate multidisciplinary team approach (→ Teamwork p. 58) and continuity of care (→ Continuity of care p. 598). Formal standardized assessment charts and documents may be provided in some areas (→ Standardized assessment tools p. 118).

Related topics

→ Post-operative wound care p. 524; → Malignant fungating wounds p. 530; → Sepsis p. 826

References

11. Nix, D. (2012) Skin and wound inspection and assessment. In: Bryant R. & Nix, D. (eds) *Acute and chronic wounds*. Missouri, USA: Elsevier Mosby
12. Doughty, D. & McNichol, L. (2015) Wound, Ostomy and Continence Nurses Society® core curriculum: wound management. Philadelphia, USA: Wolters Kluwer
13. Dowsett, C., Protz, K., Drouard, M., & Harding, K. (2015) *Triangle of wound assessment made easy.* Available at: http://www.woundsinternational.com/media/other-resources/_/1189/files/twa-made-easy_web.pdf

Post-operative wound care

The aims of post-operative wound care are to promote healing, minimize complications, and produce the best cosmetic result possible.

Complications

- Infection (⊃ Wound infection p. 526)
- Dehiscence
- Pain
- Haematoma
- Sinus and/or fistula formation

Wound closure

Surgical wounds can be closed by 1° or 2° intention. 1° intention is where the edges are brought together with stitches, staples, glue, or adhesive skin tapes. 2° intention is where the wound edges cannot be brought together (e.g. cavities following surgery to treat an anal abscess (⊃ Anal conditions p. 706)) and requires a granulation tissue matrix to be built to fill the wound. Occasionally, wounds are closed by 3° intention, where the wound is left open initially due to poor circulation or infection and surgically closed at a later date.

Changing dressings and wound cleansing

Removal of a dressing reduces the temperature of the wound and may disrupt healing; therefore, dressing changes should be kept to a minimum. In general, it is recommended that surgical wounds are undisturbed for the first 48hrs.[14,15] In order to protect the patient from healthcare-acquired infections, aseptic technique should be used during dressing changes (⊃ Wound dressings p. 532).

Sterile saline should be used for wound cleansing up to 48hrs after surgery. Thereafter, the patient is usually able to shower.[15] Freshly drawn tap water can be used for wound cleansing after 48hrs if the surgical wound has separated or has been surgically opened to drain pus.[15]

A light absorbent dressing pad may be required in wounds healing by 1° intention until haemostasis is achieved and the wound is sealed by a fibrin scab. Thereafter, a film dressing may be applied and left in place until the wound closure material is removed. Film dressings should not be used with adhesive skin-closure materials.

NICE recommend the use of interactive dressings to manage surgical wounds healing by 2° intention.[15] Interactive wound dressings include hydrocolloid dressings, foam dressings, alginate dressings, hydrofibre dressings, hydroactive dressings, and hydrogel dressings. Further advice can be sought from tissue viability nurse specialist.

Removal of surgical staples

Should be timed to ↓ the risk of permanent scarring but not so soon as to cause the wound to reopen. Usually removed after 7–10 days. The surgeon will determine the timing of removal according to the site of the wound (e.g. staples may remain *in situ* longer in ↑ tension areas). Prior to removing staples, the patient should be encouraged to shower and the wound should be assessed to identify signs of infection and determine whether removal is appropriate. If the wound looks inflamed or if any exudate is present, seek advice, as it may be necessary to remove some but not all staples to allow the exudate to drain. An aseptic dressing technique should be used when performing the procedure. Establish the number of staples *in situ* (see discharge letter) and check that they are visible. Always use a staple remover and slide the lower part under the centre of the staple. Squeeze the handles together until the staple is automatically released. Remove alternate staples. If the wound begins to gape, removal should be stopped and advice sought. If wound remains intact, remove remaining staples.

References

14. Health Protection Scotland (2015) *Preventing surgical site infections.* Available at: https://www.hps.scot.nhs.uk/haiic/ic/resourcedetail.aspx?id=663
15. NICE (2008) *Surgical site infections: prevention and treatment (last updated February 2017).* Available at: https://www.nice.org.uk/guidance/cg74/chapter/1-Guidance

Wound infection

↑ risk of morbidity and mortality (➔ Sepsis p. 826). Can occur in any wound and should be prevented, detected (➔ Wound assessment p. 522), and effectively managed.

Wound infection continuum

Wound healing not usually impaired by the presence of bacteria alone. Factors determining impact include: number, virulence, mix, and host resistance. The wound infection continuum outlines the ↑ in number and virulence of micro-organisms, together with the response they invoke within the host.[16]

Contamination

Existence of non-proliferating microbes within a wound at a level that does not evoke a host response.

Colonization

Existence of microbial organisms that undergo limited proliferation within a wound without evoking a host reaction.

Local infection

Bacterial or other microbes penetrate deeper into the wound tissue. The amount of proliferation provokes a host response. Local infection is contained in a single location, system, or structure. Signs and symptoms: covert (hypergranulation; bleeding, friable granulation; epithelial bridging and pocketing in granulation tissue; wound breakdown and enlargement; delayed wound healing beyond expectations; new or increasing pain; and increasing malodour); and overt (erythema; local warmth; swelling; purulent discharge; delayed wound healing beyond expectations; new or increasing pain; and increasing malodour).

Spreading infection

Invasion of the surrounding tissue by infective organisms. Signs and symptoms extend beyond the wound border: induration with or without erythema; lymphangitis; crepitus; wound breakdown/dehiscence with or without satellite lesions; malaise/lethargy or non-specific general deterioration; and inflammation/swelling of lymph glands.

Systemic infection

Infection from the wound affects the whole body. Signs and symptoms: severe sepsis; septic shock; organ failure; and death.

⚠ Patients who are immunocompromised may not show typical signs of infection (➔ Principles of working with someone with compromised immunity p. 466).

Investigations

Clinical assessment and judgement can be supplemented by investigations including wound cultures, bloods, and imaging. Aim of investigations:[15]

- Identify specific pathogen strains
- Establish microbes are sensitive to antibiotic type
- Identify possible complications (such as osteomyelitis)
- Inform management strategies

Wound cultures should be collected only if indicated:[15]
- Acute wounds with classic signs and symptoms of infection
- Chronic wounds with signs of spreading or systemic infection
- Infected wounds that have failed to respond to antimicrobial intervention, or are deteriorating despite appropriate antimicrobial treatment
- In compliance with local protocols for the surveillance of drug-resistant microbial species
- Wounds where the presence of certain species would contraindicate a surgical procedure

Management of wound infection

⚠ Patients with spreading infection or systemic infection require systemic antibiotics. Seek appropriate medical help immediately. Management strategies also include[1] optimising individual host response (e.g. improving nutritional status (⊃ Nutrition and healthy eating p. 342), pain management, and the management of comorbidities), reducing wound microbial load (e.g. managing wound exudate and optimising the wound bed), promoting environmental and general measures (e.g. ensuring a clean environment and appropriate cleansing technique), and regular reassessment.

Reference

16. International Wound Infection Institute (2016) *Wound infection in clinical practice: principles of best practice*. Available at: http://www.woundinfection-institute.com/wp-content/uploads/2017/03/IWII-Wound-infection-in-clinical-practice.pdf

Wound debridement

Removal of damaged and necrotic tissue, extraneous debris, and bacteria from wound to encourage formulation of healthy granulation tissue. Devitalized material and debris can: mask or mimic signs of infection (→ Wound infection p. 526); serve as a source of nutrients for bacteria; block delivery of topical preparations; prolong inflammation; inhibit growth of new tissue; hinder wound assessment (→ Wound assessment p. 522); and ↑ exudate and odour.

Types of debridement

- Surgical
- Sharp
- Larval therapy
- Mechanical
- Autolytic
- Hydrosurgical
- Ultrasonic

Risk management

Comprehensive assessment of both wound and patient necessary to inform decision to debride, speed of debridement, and what method to use. Principal concern is patient safety (→ Clinical risk management p. 78).

Each type of debridement has advantages and disadvantages. Practitioner must have appropriate skills, knowledge of anatomy, and certainty of diagnosis. Multidisciplinary team decision making necessary in some situations (→ Teamwork p. 58).

⚠ Debridement in some locations entails ↑ risk: face, hands, feet, and genitalia; ischaemic limbs; wounds associated with malignancy (→ Malignant fungating wounds p. 530) or congenital malformations; and wounds in close proximity to blood vessels, nerves, and tendons. Caution should also be exercised in patients with clotting disorders (→ Patients on anticoagulant therapy p. 642), possible implants and/or dialysis fistulas, and inflammatory conditions (e.g. Pyoderma gangrenosum).

Surgical debridement

Excision or wider resection of necrotic tissue, including removal of healthy tissue from wound margins. Undertaken in a surgical environment by a surgeon, podiatrist, or specialist practitioner with appropriate training. Anaesthesia usually required.

Sharp debridement

Removal of dead or devitalized tissue using scalpel, scissors, and forceps. Performed in the home or clinic. More than one session may be required. Does not remove healthy tissue. Used in conjunction with autolytic debridement. Undertaken by a doctor with surgical skills, a podiatrist, or a skilled practitioner with specialist training.

Larval therapy

Larvae of green bottle fly to remove necrotic and devitalized tissue. Larvae born in sterile conditions and available on prescription, usually in a mesh bag. When applied to wound, stay in place for 48–72hrs. Need to be applied by competent practitioners with specialist training.

Mechanical debridement

Necrotic and devitalized tissue removed by application of a certain amount of force. ⚠ Traditional wet-to-dry treatment no longer recommended due to risk of additional tissue damage and patient discomfort. New methods include use of a monofilament soft pad, which can be used by competent practitioners in the patient home or clinic.

Autolytic debridement

Commonest method of debridement. Harnesses body's own enzymes and moisture to rehydrate, soften, and liquefy hard dead tissue and slough. Use of occlusive and semi-occlusive dressings helps to achieve moisture balance (◆ Wound dressings p. 532). Slow process, often requiring multiple treatments. Used by competent practitioners in the patient home or clinic.

Further information

Wounds UK (*Effective debridement in a changing NHS: a UK consensus*). Available at: ℛ https:// lohmann-rauscher.co.uk/downloads/clinical-evidence/Effective_debridemen.pdf

Malignant fungating wounds

Defined as infiltration of the tumour or the metastasis into the skin, and can involve the afferent blood and lymph vessels.[17] Unless controlled through intervention (such as chemotherapy, radiotherapy, or hormone therapy), wound will grow, and the goal is palliation not healing. Common sites: breast, head, and neck area (➔ Breast cancer p. 774).

Fungating wounds have a significant psychosocial impact, including: body image alteration, denial, depression (➔ People with anxiety and depression p. 478), embarrassment, shame, revulsion, social isolation, problems with sexual expression (➔ Sexual problems p. 768), and fear.[18] Physical symptoms include: haemorrhage/bleeding (➔ External bleeding p. 814; ➔ Palliative care emergencies p. 566), odour, pain, pruritus, and exudate.

Assessment

Key points for clinical practice include:[17]

Patient assessment

- Holistic assessment
- Impact of the wound on psychosocial functions
- Comorbidities
- Functional limitations from wound location and symptoms

Wound assessment

- ➔ Wound assessment p. 522
- Clinical assessment
- Consideration of symptoms of HOPES (haemorrhage, odour, pain, exudate, and superficial infection)
- Swab cultures if showing signs of spreading infection (➔ Wound infection p. 526)

Management

Key strategies for the management of wounds include:[17]

Cleansing

- Reduces odour by removing necrotic tissue and ↓ bacterial load
- Gently irrigate with normal saline as required

Odour control

- Wound cleansing as already outlined
- Metronidazole (orally or topically) can be helpful
- Use of activated charcoal and antimicrobial dressings (➔ Wound dressings p. 532)
- Careful disposal of soiled dressings (➔ Managing healthcare waste p. 106)
- Provision of environmental agents (e.g. room deodorizers and aromatherapy oils). ⚠: Some products may cause nausea or breathing difficulties.

Local bacterial colonization

- Wound cleansing as already outlined
- Autolytic or enzymatic debridement of sloughy tissue if required
- Use of antimicrobial agents
- Oral or intravenous antibiotics if signs of spreading infection are present

Exudate
- Use of supra-absorbent dressings
- Dressings may require changing twice/day
- Protect surrounding skin using a suitable barrier preparation

⚠: If there is high fluid output from the wound, patients will have ↑ protein and hydration requirements (➲ Nutrition and healthy eating p. 342).

Pain
- Assess to determine type of pain
- Specialist advice may be required (➲ Teamwork p. 58)
- Low-dose topical opioids may help reduce wound pain
- Reduce pain at dressing changes: administer analgesia prior to dressing changes, remove dressing carefully, and use non-adherent wound contact dressings

Bleeding
- Non-adherent dressings and moist products that do not dry out
- If bleeding occurs, apply direct pressure for 10–15mins
- Local ice packs can assist in controlling bleeding
- Haemostatic dressings or pressure dressings may be required

⚠: If there is a risk of a fatal arterial bleed, this risk should be discussed with the patient and family members. Pain control and sedation should be available, and dark-coloured towels provided.

Pruritus
Some evidence for the use of transcutaneous electrical nerve stimulation. Provision of cotton garments and bed linen. Refrigerated hydrogel sheet dressings.

References

17. European Oncology Nursing Society (2015) *Recommendations for the care of patients with malignant wounds*. Available at: https://www.cancernurse.eu/documents/EONSMalignantFungatingWounds.pdf
18. O'Brien, C. (2012) Malignant wounds: managing odour. *Canadian Family Physician*, 58(3), 272–4

Wound dressings

Phases of wound healing

Wound healing is a complex process. It is generally described in four distinct but often overlapping phases: inflammatory phase (lasts 0–3 days), destructive phase (lasts 1–6 days), proliferation phase (lasts 3–24 days), and maturation (lasts 21 days–2yrs). As a wound moves through these phases, different types of dressings will be required (➔ Wound assessment p. 522).

Maintaining a moist healing environment

Exudate provides a moist environment and promotes healing, but excessive exudate can cause maceration of the wound and surrounding healthy tissue. The ideal dressing for moist wound healing needs to ensure that the wound remains:[19]

- Moist with exudate, but not macerated
- Free of clinical infection (➔ Wound infection p. 526) and excessive slough
- Free of toxic chemicals, particles, or fibre
- At the optimum temperature for healing
- Undisturbed by the need for frequent dressing changes
- At the optimum pH value.

⚠ There are certain circumstances where moist wound healing is not appropriate. For example, necrotic toes should not be rehydrated as the tissue may become a focus for infection. In such cases, specialist tissue viability and vascular assessment is essential (➔ Teamwork p. 58).

Factors determining dressing selection

Dressing selection should be guided by an assessment of the wound and the patient. In relation to the wound, consideration should be given to the type of wound, the location of the wound, the type of wound closure (➔ Postoperative wound care p. 524), the phase of wound healing, the level of exudate, and the presence of infection. In relation to the patient, consideration should be given to allergies and sensitivities (➔ Allergies p. 694; ➔ Anaphylaxis p. 810), comorbidities (e.g. diabetes (➔ Diabetes: overview p. 660)), pain and discomfort, and patient preference.

There have been few clinical trials able to establish a clear advantage for any particular product; therefore, cost is an important consideration (➔ Evidence-based healthcare p. 72). Many organizations will have a wound-dressing formulary, providing practitioners with guidance and a selection of products which are preferred for use in that organization, based on effectiveness, suitability, acceptability, and cost effectiveness. Practitioners are encouraged to use a product included in the formulary in most cases and only use a non-formulary product when there is a good clinical reason (➔ Professional accountability p. 83).

Moisture-retentive dressings

Understanding the indications for these dressings and how to apply them is an important skill. Moisture-retentive dressings include films, hydrogels, hydrocolloids, foams, alginates, and hydrofibres.[20]

Film

- Properties: transparent self-adhesive sheets of polyurethane; gas- and water-permeable; impermeable to fluid and bacteria; flexible and conformable; allow visualization of the wound.
- Wound types: low exudating wounds; shallow wounds (e.g. superficial lacerations, burns, and donor sites); retention dressings (e.g. cannulas); may be used as a 2° dressing over alginates or hydrogels.
- Instructions for use: wear time ~3 days.
- Cautions and contraindications: not suitable for moderately or ↑ exudating wounds; risk of trauma on removal.

Hydrogels

- Properties: cross-linked starch polymers comprised of up to 96% water; available as sheets and gels; ability to rehydrate and maintain moist environment.
- Wound types: dry, sloughy, and necrotic wounds.
- Instructions for use: wear time ~1–3 days; 2° non-absorbent dressing is required.
- Cautions and contraindications: avoid on infected wounds; do not use on necrotic toes; may → maceration and excoriation of the peri-wound area.

Hydrocolloid

- Properties: cross-linked polymer matrices with integrated adhesives and starches; available as sheets, pastes, and powders; upon contact with the wound exudates, absorb exudates and form gels; ability to rehydrate and maintain a moist environment.
- Wound types: abrasions; superficial pressure ulcers; shallow leg ulcers.
- Instructions for use: sheet form is self-adhesive, waterproof, and does not require a 2° dressing; wear time ~3–5 day (some >7 days); warm with hand to ↑ pliability and adhesion; requires 1.5–2cm border/margin to ensure adhesion.
- Cautions and contraindications: avoid in infected wounds; do not use on necrotic toes; avoid on highly exudating wounds; gel formed by these products can be mistaken for infection.

Foam

- Properties: comprised of polyurethane or silicone centre and semi-occlusive outer layer; outer layer is permeable to water vapour and serves to protect against bacterial penetration and leakage; polyurethane or silicone centre provides absorptive quality; cushioning provides ↑ comfort.
- Wound types: light to highly exudating wounds.
- Instructions for use: may be adhesive or non-adhesive; non-adhesive forms will require 2° dressing (do not use occlusive 2° dressing); wear time ~1–7 days.
- Cautions and contraindications: absorptive capacity will be compromised under compression bandaging; saturated dressings may → maceration and excoriation of the peri-wound area; avoid using on very dry, sloughy, or necrotic wounds.

Alginate
- Properties: comprised of seaweed or kelp-based polysaccharides; calcium ions within the dressing exchange with the sodium ions in the wound exudate to form a highly absorbent alginate gel; calcium released from the dressing have haemostatic properties that can promote clotting.
- Wound types: medium to ↑ exudating wounds.
- Instructions for use: available as a sheet or rope; sheet may be adhesive or non-adhesive; non-adhesive will require a 2° dressing; rope useful in sinus or cavity wounds; wear time ~1–3 days; remove alginate dressing by soaking with saline or water.
- Cautions and contraindications; avoid in ↑ bleeding wounds; caution in fungating tumours with friable tissue; avoid in dry or necrotic wounds; risk of adherence, pain, and damage on removal.

Hydrofibre
- Properties: ↑ absorbent sodium carboxymethylcellulose; when hydrofibres absorb wound exudate, they transform into gels; ability to maintain a moist environment; more absorbent than alginates.
- Wound types: medium to highly exudating wounds.
- Instructions for use: available as a sheet or rope; sheet may be adhesive or non-adhesive; non-adhesive will require a 2° dressing; rope useful in sinus or cavity wounds; maximum wear time 1wk; change daily for infected wounds.
- Cautions and contraindications: pack only 80% of cavity as dressing expands when converted to gel form.

Antimicrobial dressings

These may be categorized as specialist products by some organizations, which should only be prescribed on the recommendation of a tissue viability nurse specialist (➔ Antimicrobial stewardship p. 146).

Silver
Considered a broad-spectrum antimicrobial that can be used in superficially infected wounds. Silver particulates can be impregnated into hydrogels, alginates, foams, and hydrofibres. Avoid in acute wounds and third-degree burns (➔ Burns and scalds p. 816). Limited evidence to support in patients with venous leg ulcers (➔ Venous leg ulcers p. 540). ⚠ Do not use in patients with a sensitivity to silver.

Iodine
Considered a broad-spectrum antimicrobial. Available as a sheet or a gel. Iodine is absorbed systemically. Do not use in children, during pregnancy (➔ Pregnancy p. 424) or lactation (➔ Breastfeeding p. 182), or in patients with an iodine allergy, thyroid disease (➔ Thyroid p. 702), impaired renal function (➔ Renal problems p. 754), or on lithium therapy (➔ Prescribing for special groups p. 138). Do not apply to large wounds or use over a prolonged period.

Medical-grade honey

Medical-grade Manuka honey from New Zealand and Australia is thought to have peroxide and non-peroxide antibacterial activity. Do not use in venous leg ulcers or heavily bleeding wounds. Do not use in patients with a known sensitivity to honey, bee products, or bee stings. Monitor blood glucose levels of patients with diabetes during use (➲ Principles of diabetes management p. 664). Non-medical honey can contaminate wound: only use medical-grade honey.

References

19. NICE (no date) *Wound management products and elasticated garments*. Available at: https://bnf.nice.org.uk/wound-management/

20. Broussard, K. & Gloeckner Powers, J. (2013) Wound dressings: selecting the most appropriate type. *American Journal of Clinical Dermatology*, 14, 449–59

Further information

Nurse Prescribers' Advisory Group (2018) Nurse prescribers' formulary for community practitioners (September 2017–19). London: Pharmaceutical Press

Wounds International (*Best pPractice*). Available at: ℘ https://www.woundsinternational.com/resources/all/0/date/desc/cont_type/45

Leg ulcer assessment

Prevalence of leg ulcers equates to 1.5% of adult population and ↑ with age. Healing rates range from 45–80% at 24wks for all ulcer types. Ulceration is characterized by alternating phases of ulceration, healing, and recurrence (➲ Wound assessment p. 522). 75% of all leg ulcers are venous in origin (➲ Venous leg ulcers p. 540) and 25% are arterial, mixed aetiology, or neuropathic. Many patients have never had the aetiology of their ulcer correctly diagnosed. Ulcer aetiology determines the management strategy. Assessment and treatment should be commenced as soon as possible.

General assessment

Patient-related factors
Explore: medical and surgical history; medication; family history (FH); nutrition and hydration status (➲ Malnutrition p. 350); presenting symptoms (including pain); mobility; previous ulceration (including treatment and healing outcomes); and knowledge and understanding of leg ulceration.

Psychosocial-related factors
Explore: lifestyle (physical activity (➲ Exercise p. 354) and smoking (➲ Smoking cessation p. 356)); occupation; impact of ulceration on quality of life and sleeping; social activity and care network; expectations of treatment; and weight/BMI (➲ Adult body mass index chart p. 346).

Leg assessment

Limb-related factors
Consider: limb size and shape; presence and distribution of oedema (➲ Lymphoedema p. 548); mobility and/or ankle movement; and colour and condition of the skin (➲ Eczema/dermatitis p. 684).

Vascular-related factors
Undertake doppler ultrasound and consider: vascular history; limb temperature; erythema, pallor and/or cyanosis; signs of arterial insufficiency; and signs of venous insufficiency.

Wound/skin assessment

Record: location; size (length, width, area, and depth); tissue (non-viable or deficient); infection or inflammation (➲ Wound infection p. 526); moisture imbalance; edge of wound; and surrounding skin.

Doppler ultrasound

Compares blood flow in the arm with blood flow in the lower limb to calculate the ankle-brachial pressure index (ABPI). ↑ accuracy of ulcer assessment by excluding concomitant arterial disease and defining a safe level of compression bandaging. All patients should have their ABPI calculated prior to treatment (Table 10.2). For arterial ulcers, the ABPI reading provides an indication of severity of arterial disease.

Table 10.2 Significance of ankle-brachial pressure index (ABPI) readings

ABPI reading	Significance of reading
0.8–1.3	Normal arterial blood flow; safe to compress
>1.3	Consider calcification. Consider referral to vascular centre or tissue viability services
0.5–0.8	Mixed disease. Refer to vascular centre, tissue viability team. Reduced compression: follow specialist advice
<0.5	Severe arterial disease. Urgent vascular referral. No compression

Additional investigations

A variety of additional investigations may be indicated, including: urinalysis; bloods, including full blood count and erythrocyte sedimentation rate (ESR); wound swabs for culture and sensitivity testing; and patch testing.

Significance of assessment findings for diagnosis

All elements of the assessment will inform diagnosis. Table 10.3 compares clinical signs and symptoms of venous and arterial leg ulceration. ⚠ Regular reassessment is needed to determine effectiveness of treatment and changes in vascular status.

Referral criteria

If ABPI is <0.5, an urgent referral should be made to a vascular centre. Referral to specialist service (e.g. tissue viability service) (➔ Teamwork p. 58) when:
• ABPI outside 0.8–1.3 range
• Area ≥100cm²
• Present for more than 6mths

Table 10.3 Comparison of clinical signs and symptoms of venous and arterial leg ulceration

	Venous ulceration	Arterial ulceration
Previous medical history	Previous leg fracture, deep vein thrombosis, skin staining, eczema, family history of leg ulcers, varicose veins	History of stroke, heart disease, peripheral arterial disease, hypertension, diabetes
Site/position	Often between the ankle and knee (gaiter area)	Usually on the foot, between the toes, or close to the medial malleolus
Appearance	Large, shallow wounds producing copious exudate	Often small, deep wounds producing less exudate
Surrounding skin condition	Characteristic pigmentation—lipodermatosclerosis, atrophy blanche. Contact dermatitis and eczema common	Hairless, shiny skin. Skin colour ranges from white to dusky pink and purple. Dusky pink feet turn pale when raised above heart.
Pain/discomfort	Aching/heaviness of legs, localized ulcer pain	Severe rest pain, constant ulcer pain, often worse at night

- Cardiac failure (➔ Heart failure p. 636)
- Current infection/history of infections
- Non-adherence to treatment regimen
- Wound has failed to ↓ in size by 20–30% at 4–6wks
- Fixed ankle or ↓ range of movement
- Foot malformation
- Poor pain control
- Contact dermatitis (➔ Eczema/dermatitis p. 684)
- Uncertain aetiology of ulceration
- Symptoms of arterial disease even if ABPI within normal range
- Mixed aetiology ulcers
- Neuropathic ulcers

Reassessment

- Assess patient at every dressing change
- Formally reassess wound at least every 4wks
- Measure wound size at least every 4wks
- ABPI readings should be reassessed every 3, 6, or 12mths depending on initial and ongoing assessments.

Record keeping

Documentation (➔ Record keeping p. 86) essential to review previous status and facilitate multidisciplinary team approach and continuity of care (➔ Continuity of care p. 598). Formal standardized assessment charts and documents may be provided in some areas (➔ Standardized assessment tools p. 118).

Related topics

➔ Compression therapy for venous ulcers p. 542

Further information

NICE (*Leg ulcers—venous*). Available at: ℘ https://cks.nice.org.uk/leg-ulcer-venous#!topicsummary
Wounds UK (*Holistic management of venous leg ulceration*). Available at: ℘ https://lohmann-rauscher.co.uk/downloads/VLU_BPS_Web.pdf

Venous leg ulcers

One of the most common types of chronic wound. Patients frequently experience wound leakage, offensive odour, wound pain, and lack of sleep. This can ↑ dependence on carers (➲ Carers p. 458), ↓ quality of life, and affect self-esteem (➲ People with anxiety and depression p. 478).

Key terms

- Venous leg ulcer: a break in the skin of the lower leg present for over 2wks, caused by disease in the venous system
- Lipodermatosclerosis: characteristic skin changes in lower extremities including fat necrosis, skin staining, fibrosis of skin, and subcutaneous tissues that become hard and 'woody'
- Atrophe blanche: refers to the presence of white satellite scars in the ankle area, commonly seen in venous stasis due to occlusion of dermal vessels causing tissue death.

Risk factors

- Deep vein thrombosis (➲ Varicose veins, thrombophlebitis, and deep vein thrombosis p. 656)
- ↑ age
- Vein trauma/surgery
- ↓ mobility
- Pregnancy (➲ Pregnancy p. 424)
- Phlebitis
- Reduced mobility
- Congenital valve defect (➲ Congenital heart defects p. 260)
- Obesity (➲ Overweight and obesity p. 348)
- Smoking (➲ Smoking cessation p. 356)
- Intravenous drug use (➲ Substance use p. 476)

Clinical signs of venous hypertension

Signs of venous hypertension are initially mild and become more pronounced overtime: ankle and lower limb oedema (dependent); ankle flare (distended venous medial aspect of ankle); varicose veins; abnormal leg shape—'inverted champagne bottle'; lipodermatosclerosis; atrophie blanche; and varicose eczema (➲ Eczema/dermatitis p. 684).

Complications

- Recurrent infection (➲ Wound infection p. 526)
- Lymphoedema: Refer to specialist services (➲ Lymphoedema p. 548)
- Malignant changes (rare): Refer for biopsy
- Contact dermatitis: Refer for patch testing

Management

Compression therapy is the cornerstone of treatment, which aims to ↓ venous hypertension and improve venous ulcer healing (➲ Compression therapy for venous ulcers p. 542).

Exudate

Can produce ↑ levels of exudate which ↓ healing. Select dressings that will absorb excess exudate, but still maintain a moist wound environment to avoid dressing adhesion and trauma (❂ Wound dressings p. 532). Super absorbent dressings can be used under compression. Skin barrier preparations can be an effective method of ↓ damage and excoriation.

Debridement

Infection or uncontrolled oedema are the commonest causes of slough accumulation on the ulcer surface, and require removal. Refer to specialist services for sharp debridement (❂ Wound debridement p. 528).

Pain

Pain is common and often underestimated how much it contributes to sleep disturbance, anxiety, depression, and poor compliance with treatment. Important to assess and manage.

Skincare

Remove hyperkeratosis scales with cleansing. Treat eczema as required. Establish an ongoing emollient-based skincare regime. Encourage self-care; support in skin hygiene and self-care issues.

Prevention of recurrence

Once healed, follow-up care is essential as recurrence rates are ↑. Appropriate skincare, exercise (❂ Exercise p. 354), leg elevation, and avoidance of prolonged standing should be emphasized, together with the permanent use of fitted compression stockings to minimize recurrence. Provide smoking cessation and weight management advice (❂ Nutrition and healthy eating p. 342) and support.

Useful dressing types

Refer to local prescribing formularies for product choice and guidance:
- Clean ulcers with freshly drawn tap water or normal saline solution
- Solution soaks of polyexamethylene biguanide (PHNB) may be helpful for biofilm and bacteria reduction
- Simple non-adherent dressings
- Alginate dressings for exudate management
- Wound gel for debridement
- Absorbent pads 2° to 1° dressing
- Topical antimicrobials if signs of biofilm or infection present
- ⚠ Use for 2wks, then review
- Skin barrier preparations may minimize skin excoriation/maceration

Treatment

Compression therapy should be first-line treatment.

Further information

NICE (Leg ulcers—venous). Available at: ℛ https://cks.nice.org.uk/leg-ulcer-venous#!topicsummary
SIGN (Management of chronic venous leg ulcers). Available at: ℛ https://www.sign.ac.uk/assets/sign120.pdf
Wounds UK (Holistic management of venous leg ulceration). Available at: ℛ https://lohmann-rauscher.co.uk/downloads/VLU_BPS_Web.pdf

Compression therapy for venous leg ulcers

Compression should be first-line treatment to optimize healing, ↓ pressure in superficial venous system, encourage venous return and tissue perfusion, minimize oedema, and improve lymphatic drainage for venous leg ulcers (➲ Venous leg ulcers p. 540). Compression should be started as early as possible. Full compression systems should be the aim for full therapeutic compression. It is vital to involve the patient in all stages of care, especially decision making around treatment.

Contraindications

- Arterial disease (ABPI less than 0.5)
- Coexisting vascular conditions
- Patients with narrow ankles/calves
- Patients with ↓ sensation
- Uncontrolled heart failure (➲ Heart failure p. 636)

⚠ Extreme caution should be exercised for patients with venous leg ulcers and diabetes (➲ Diabetes: overview p. 660) or rheumatoid arthritis (➲ Rheumatoid arthritis p. 602).

Different compression systems available

Compression hosiery kits

- Do not require a high level of skill to apply
- Deliver consistent compression levels
- Deliver compression to the foot
- No limits to footwear/clothing
- Facilitate self-care
- Not suitable for unusual limb sizes and shapes
- Not suitable for rapidly ↓ limb sizes
- Exudates need to be contained using dressings

Compression wraps

- Compression value adjustable
- Allow for adjustment as limb volume ↓
- Deliver compression to the foot
- No limits to footwear/clothing
- Facilitate self-care
- Not indicated if ulcer highly exuding
- Some systems do not compress the foot

Compression bandages

- Allow good anatomical fit
- Suitable for most limb sizes and shapes
- ↑ stiffness systems produce greatest improvements in venous blood flow
- Compression value dependent on application technique
- Some systems do not compress the foot
- Limits to footwear/clothing
- Do not facilitate self-care

Bandage types

Elastic (highly extendable) bandages
Contain highly elastic materials and apply more constant pressure with little change in pressure on movement.

Inelastic (short-stretch) bandages
Contain inelastic materials providing a rigid structure. The pressure ↑ when the calf muscle expands against the rigid cuff during activity, causing pressure to be forced into the tissues. Generates ↑ working pressures on movement and ↓ resting pressure.

Bandage application

⚠ Should only be performed by practitioners trained in compression therapy. In a venous ulcer with a reading of >0.8, standard compression should be applied which exerts a sub-bandage pressure of ~40mmHg at the ankle. The ↑ pressure should be exerted at the ankle, gradually falling to 50% at the knee. ↓ levels of compression may also be safely used in patients with mild arterial disease (ABPI 0.5–0.8) following specialist advice. Table 10.4 outlines a range of regimens that may be used.

Bandage tension and pressure on the limb
The more the bandage is stretched on application, the ↑ in sub-bandage pressure. Generally, elasticated bandages are applied with 50% extension. The aim is to apply the bandage with constant extension. Inelastic bandages are commonly applied at 100% stretch.

Limb circumference and pressure on the limb
For effective graduation, ankle circumference should measure ~50% of the calf circumference. A bandage applied with constant tension and 50% overlap will exert ↑ pressure at the ankle than the calf. Bony prominences are prone to ↑ pressure. Apply padding to protect the skin and to ↑ the size of small ankles. To determine the bandage regimen, remeasure ankle circumference weekly and refer to manufacturer's guidance on bandage application according to ankle circumference. Distorted limb shapes and skin folds should be protected and shaped using padding.

Table 10.4 Compression regimes related to arterial status

ABPI	Compression regimen	Comments
>0.8–1.3	Full compression	Bandage pressure ~40mmHg. Use local policies for product choice. Caution in patients with concurrent conditions, e.g. diabetes and heart failure.
0.5–0.8	Reduced compression	Bandage pressure ~20–25mmHg. Refer to specialist teams for advice. Use local guidance for product choice.
<0.5	No compression	Patients should be referred for urgent vascular opinion.

Bandage layers and pressure on the limb

The more layers applied, the ↑ sub-bandage pressure gained. When applying a spiral application using 50% overlap, two layers are being applied. Conversely, a figure-of-eight application applies four layers.

Practical application

- Measure ankle circumference.
- Cover ulcer with 1° dressing.
- Apply wool bandage layer to shape the leg, and remeasure ankle. Apply bandage from base of toes to knee (refer to manufacturer's instructions).
- Oedema management should be considered when choosing bandage type system; inelastic systems are most suitable for large amounts of oedema and limb distortion (➔ Lymphoedema p. 548).
- Avoid double turns of the bandage which doubles the pressure exerted in a single turn.
- Do not apply additional layers of bandage under the knee in an attempt to use up bandage surplus.
- Ask patient to inform staff if bandage feels uncomfortable and remove if necessary.

Prevention of recurrence after healing

Compression hosiery or wrap systems should be used in the maintenance phase. Studies have found that when using hosiery kits for ulcer treatment, it is more likely that hosiery will be worn for maintenance.[21] Refer to local policy and formulary for product choice. The maintenance system needs to be simple and practical to use on an ongoing daily basis. Promoting skincare, self-care, and exercise regimes will → more positive outcomes.

Related topics

➔ Wound dressings p. 532

Reference

21. Ashby, R., Gabe, R., Ali, S., et al. (2014) Clinical and cost-effectiveness of compression hosiery versus compression bandages in treatment of venous leg ulcers (Venous Leg Ulcer Study IV, VenUS IV): a randomised controlled trial. *Lancet*, 383(9920), 871–9

Further information

NICE (*Leg ulcers—venous*). Available at: ⅁ https://cks.nice.org.uk/leg-ulcer-venous#!topicsummary
SIGN (*Management of chronic venous leg ulcers*). Available at: ⅁ https://www.sign.ac.uk/assets/sign120.pdf
Wounds UK (*Holistic management of venous leg ulceration*). Available at: ⅁ https://lohmann-rauscher.co.uk/downloads/VLU_BPS_Web.pdf
Wounds UK (*Compression hosiery*). Available at: ⅁ http://legsmatter.org/wp-content/uploads/2018/02/content_11547.pdf

Oral chemotherapy in the home

↑ in oral chemotherapy for the treatment of cancer offers benefits in terms of allowing care closer to home and improved cost effectiveness. Despite these benefits, it has been associated with ↑ number of errors and adverse events (→ Clinical risk management p. 78). In 1° care, sources of error include medication non-adherence (→ Medicine concordance and adherence p. 132) and delayed reporting of medication side effects.

Patient non-adherence to oral chemotherapy

Despite the gravity of a cancer diagnosis and expectations that patients will be ↑ motivated to take their medication, adherence levels are 50–70%.[22] Oral chemotherapy doses are set to ensure sustained and mild plasma concentrations over time. Patient non-adherence to oral chemotherapy can result in: treatment resistance, ↑ toxicity, disease progression, and death.

Importance of side effects

Patients experience the same side effects as they would with intravenous chemotherapies (e.g. diarrhoea, constipation (→ Constipation in adults p. 512), nausea, fatigue, skin changes, and loss of appetite). ⚠ Presence of side effects can be a sign of serious problems. Delays in reporting can → treatment delays, ↑ hospitalization, ↓ quality of life, and fatality.[23]

Oncology emergencies
- Neutropenic sepsis (→ Sepsis p. 826)
- Severe nausea and vomiting
- Severe mucositis (→ Mouth and throat problems p. 698)
- Tumour lysis syndrome
- Severe diarrhoea
- Hypersensitivity/anaphylactic reactions (→ Anaphylaxis p. 810)

Symptom-reporting tool

National Chemotherapy Board provide an example traffic-light symptom-reporting tool:[22]

RED
☏ 999 immediately in the following circumstances:
- Chest pain
- Difficulty breathing

Call hospital immediately in the following circumstances:
- Generally unwell
- Shivery episodes or flu-like symptoms
- Temperature >37.5°C or <36°C
- Being sick (vomiting)
- Diarrhoea (>four loose bowel movements in 24hrs)
- Bleeding or unusual bruising
- Swollen or painful legs
- Sore mouth that stops the patient eating or drinking

AMBER

Call the hospital within 24hrs in the following circumstances:
- Sore mouth but the patient can still eat and drink
- Itchy or painful skin changes
- Sore, watery eyes
- ↑ in pain
- Nausea
- Diarrhoea (two to four loose bowel movements in 24hrs)

GREEN

Call the hospital within 48 hours in the following circumstances:
- Tiredness
- Skin changes that are not itchy or painful
- Mood changes
- Difficulty coping with the treatment
- Loss of appetite

Related topics

→ Palliative care emergencies p. 566

References

22. Hohneker, J., Shah-Mehta, S., & Brandt, P. (2011) Perspectives on adherence and persistence with oral medications for cancer treatment. *Journal of Oncology Practice*, 7(1), 65–7
23. National Chemotherapy Board (2016) *Good practice guideline: promoting early identification of systemic anti-cancer therapies side effects.* Available at: https://webcache.googleusercontent.com/search?q=cache:blFPZCbNmxsJ:https://www.rcplondon.ac.uk/file/4805/Jownload%3Ftoken%3DDWCtyB9a+&cd=1&hl=en&ct=clnk&gl=uk

Lymphoedema

A long-term problem caused by failure of lymphatic drainage, causing oedema, affecting one or more limbs and adjacent trunk.

Causes of chronic oedema

1° lymphoedema is due to an intrinsic genetic abnormality of the lymphatic system. More common is 2° lymphoedema due to damage to lymphatic system caused by: obstruction from malignancy (◑ Breast cancer p. 774); infection (e.g. cellulitis, lymphadenitis, tuberculosis (◑ Tuberculosis p. 728)); trauma (e.g. lymph node dissection, radiotherapy, and burns (◑ Burns and scalds p. 816)); venous disease; inflammation (e.g. rheumatoid arthritis (◑ Rheumatoid arthritis p. 602)); dermatitis (◑ Eczema/dermatitis p. 684); psoriasis (◑ Psoriasis p. 688); endocrine disease (e.g. pretibial myxedema); ↓ mobility and paralysis (◑ Spinal cord injury p. 518); and obesity (◑ Overweight and obesity p. 348).

Clinical features

Initially, the swelling may be intermittent and soft and easy to 'pit'. Overtime, the swelling becomes more permanent and subcutaneous tissues become firmer due to the deposition of fat and fibrosis.

Stemmer's sign describes the inability to pinch and lift a skinfold at the base of the second toe and is usually positive in lymphoedema of the legs when it has been present for some time.

In chronic lymphoedema, skin changes such as abnormal thickening (hyperkeratosis), benign skin growths (papillomatosis), and clear or haemorrhagic papules (lymphangiectasia) are seen as the condition progresses.

Cellulitis

A serious complication of lymphoedema, characterized by pain, warmth, swelling, and erythema (◑ Bacterial skin infections p. 680). Prompt treatment with antibiotics is needed as it can lead to further lymphatic damage and recurrent cellulitis. A decision whether hospital admission is indicated should be based on the level of systemic upset[24] (◑ Sepsis p. 826). If patients are managed at home, they need to be closely monitored by their GP (◑ General practice p. 18). Bed rest and elevation of the affected limb is essential.

Care and management

Aim to relieve pain and discomfort, prevent and reduce build-up of fluid, and prevent complications (e.g. cellulitis).

Skincare

Important to have good skincare to ↓ risk of infection. Moisturize skin everyday with non-perfumed cream/oil; clean and treat small cuts; wear gloves for housework and gardening to ↓ risk of cuts; use insect repellant to avoid bites, and use sun protection. Treat fungal infections (e.g. athlete's foot) (◑ Fungal infections p. 686).

External support/compression

Elastic compression garments (e.g. sleeves and stockings) will help prevent further swelling in the limb. Compression garments need to be specially fitted. Multi-layered lymphoedema bandaging may be indicated (e.g. deep skin folds, chronic skin changes, limb too large to fit hosiery, distortion in shape, fragile, damaged, or ulcerated skin). Lymphoedema specialist to advise on what approach to support/compression and on application of bandages.

Exercise and movement

To maximize lymph drainage without over-exertion. Gentle exercise (◆ Exercise p. 354) following advice from lymphoedema specialist. Should always wear compression garment when doing exercise. Stop exercise if skin becomes red.

Simple lymphatic drainage

Manual lymphatic drainage (MLD) is a specialized massage technique to promote drainage that should only be practiced by trained therapists. However, simple lymphatic drainage is a gentle fingertip massage technique based on principles of MLD. Patient will be taught how to perform this by lymphoedema specialist.

Psychosocial support

Focusing on depression, concordance with treatment, loneliness and isolation, and poor coping. Lymphoedema Support Network provides support and information to people with lymphoedema including a telephone support line ☎ 020 7351 4480 (Monday–Friday, 9.30am–4.30pm) (◆ Expert patients and self-management programmes p. 340).

Reference

24. British Lymphology Society and the Lymphoedema Support Network (2016) *Consensus document on the management of cellulitis in lymphoedema (revised cellulitis guidelines)*. Available at: https://www.lymphoedema.org/images/pdf/CellulitisConsensus.pdf

Further information

International Lymphoedema Framework (*Best practice for the management of lymphoedema*). Available at: ℘ https://www.lympho.org/wp-content/uploads/2016/03/Best_practice.pdf

Palliative care in the home

Most people would like to die at home, but only the minority do. Palliative care emphasizes the improvement of quality of life of patients with advanced illness and their families (➔ Carers p. 458) through: prevention and relief of distress; and early detection, assessment, and treatment of symptoms and other problems (e.g. physical, psychosocial, and spiritual problems).

General palliative care

Focuses on patients with ↓ to moderate palliative care needs, also those with complex needs supported by specialist palliative care services (➔ Services for the dying patient p. 552).

Specialist palliative care

Specialist palliative care services include hospice inpatient services, hospital services, and community services. Specialist palliative care is provided by practitioners for whom palliative care is their main role. Community specialist palliative care refers to teams of palliative care clinical nurse specialists with palliative medicine specialist support. They focus on patients with moderate to complex palliative care needs and their families. They can visit patients in their own homes as well as provide telephone advice. They also support GPs and 1° care nurses.

End-of-life care

Usually last year of life for patients with advanced, progressive, incurable illness. Aims to enable patients to live as well as possible until they die. Includes the identification of patients' and their families' supportive and palliative care needs in the last phase of life and into bereavement (➔ Coping with bereavement p. 574).

Dying phase

Management of patients from the time it is apparent the patient is in a progressive and sometimes rapid state of decline, i.e. last few hours/days of life (➔ Caring for patients in the dying phase p. 568). Important to make this stage as comfortable as possible for patients and their carers, with everyone working together confidently, honestly, and consistently (➔ Teamwork p. 58; ➔ Continuity of care p. 598).

Ambitions for palliative and end-of-life care

In England, the National Palliative and End-of-Life Care Partnership has set out six ambitions to improve palliative and end-of-life care:[25]

- Each person is seen as an individual
- Each person gets fair access to care
- Maximizing comfort and well-being
- Care is co-ordinated
- All staff are prepared to care
- Each community is prepared to help.

Gold Standard Framework (GSF)

The GSF is intended to enable a gold standard of care for all people in the last years of life, supporting them to live well until they die. It is a proactive model provided by generalist staff in all care settings. It emphasizes a whole-team approach and involves a number of key steps:

- Identify (proactive): patients considered to be in their last year of life should be recorded on a register (consider the question: would you be surprised if this patient died within the next 12mths?)
- Assess (person-centred): clinical and personal needs (e.g. advance care planning)
- Plan (systematic): anticipate needs (e.g. pre-emptive prescribing)

Following these steps should ensure the right person receives the right care in the right place at the right time.

Organizations can apply for the GSF Quality Accreditation Hallmark Award if they demonstrate: patients and their needs are identified; advance care planning discussions (➲ Mental capacity p. 470) have been offered; plans in place to enable patients to live well; plans in place to enable patients to die well, carers and families are supported; compassionate care; and a systematic approach to care.

Advance care planning

Process of discussion that intends to make clear a person's wishes. Includes advanced statements (preferred priorities for care), and advance decisions (including advance decision to refuse treatment) and 'Do not attempt cardiopulmonary resuscitation (CPR)' instruction (➲ Adult basic life support and automated external defibrillation p. 792). The latter is completed by the clinician responsible for the individual (e.g. GP), usually following discussion with the patient. If cardiac or respiratory arrest is an expected part of the dying process, and CPR will not be successful, making and recording the 'Do not attempt cardiopulmonary resuscitation' decision will help to ensure that the patient dies in a dignified manner and in their preferred place of care, by avoiding emergency admission from a community setting to hospital.

References

25. National Palliative and End-of-Life Care Partnership (2015) *Ambitions for palliative and end-of-life care: a national framework for local action 2015–2020*. Available at: http://endoflifecareambitions. org.uk/wp-content/uploads/2015/09/Ambitions-for-Palliative-and-End-of-Life-Care.pdf

Further information

GSF (*About us*). Available at: ℘ http://www.goldstandardsframework.org.uk/about-us

Services for the dying patient

1° healthcare team (GP (➲ General practice p. 18) and district nurse (DN) (➲ District nursing p. 50)) provide generalist palliative care (➲ Palliative care in the home p. 550). They establish ongoing relationships with patients, assessing needs, providing direct care, and liaising with specialists in palliative care, social care, and 2° services (➲ Teamwork p. 58). Other services include:

- Out-of-hours care: greater likelihood of maintaining a patient at home when there is 24-hr DN availability
- Specialist palliative care services: multidisciplinary specialist palliative care team, e.g. consultant, palliative care clinical nurse specialist, social worker, and allied health professionals (AHPs)
- Hospice services: inpatient care for complex and holistic symptom management and end-of-life care; outpatient hospice day centres and clinics (e.g. Breathlessness Clinic (➲ Breathlessness in palliative care p. 560)) and outreach/hospice-at-home teams
- Paid carers are commissioned through the NHS or social services. Other services that may be available include: night sitters, respite care, and carers' support groups
- Care homes and community hospitals: may provide respite and short-stay support, particularly for people who live alone. These facilities may have GSF accreditation
- Charities can help with respite care, extra nursing at home, financial support, and bereavement support (➲ Coping with bereavement p. 574).

Service provision is locally determined (➲ Commissioning of services p. 12). Poor recognition of palliative care needs for patients with non-malignant advanced illness and their carers leads to less support than for people with advanced cancer. Both patient groups can have a similar symptom burden and psychological and psychosocial issues.

Further information

e-Learning for Healthcare (*End-of-life care programme*). Available at: ℬ https://www.e-lfh.org.uk/programmes/end-of-life-care/

Pain assessment and management in palliative care

Pain is an unpleasant sensory and/or emotional experience linked to actual or potential tissue damage (e.g. muscle, nerve, bone). It is a subjective experience and can be influenced by psychological, social, and spiritual factors. It is always the patient who defines it and its severity. Pain can go unrecognized, especially in older people or those with cognitive impairment (◆ People with dementia p. 498).

Assessment

Open-ended questions to allow the patient to define the pain experience. Follow up with questions to locate and monitor the pain (SOCRATES):

- Site: Where is the pain? Is it in more than one site?
- Onset: When did the pain start? Was it sudden or gradual?
- Character: What is the pain like? Aching? Stabbing?
- Radiation: Does the pain radiate anywhere?
- Associations: Any other symptoms associated with the pain?
- Time course: What is the duration? Does the pain follow any pattern?
- Exacerbating/relieving factors: What triggers the pain and has this changed over time? Is it worse at different times of the day? What relieves the pain (e.g. analgesia, relaxation, distraction)?
- Severity: How bad is the pain? Use numerical rating scale 0–10 with 0 being 'no pain' and 10 being 'worst pain'

Observational assessment is essential for patients with cognitive impairment, e.g. facial expressions such as grimacing, body movements such as rocking and guarding, vocalizations such as moaning, and changes in mental state including increased tearfulness.

Pain assessment tools

Tools to initially assess pain and chart effectiveness of pain-reduction strategies and interventions (◆ Standardized assessment tools p. 118).

Body map

Record location(s) and characteristics; useful when there are multiple pain sites (◆ Record keeping p. 86).

Visual analogue scales

A line with 'no pain' and 'worst pain' at each extreme. Patient marks point on the line that reflects their pain severity. Variations on the analogue scales include verbal rating scales and numerical rating scales. A hand is useful if the patient has limited numeracy.

Pain questionnaires
- Brief Pain Inventory: measures location, intensity, and triggers
- McGill Pain Questionnaire: useful if nerve (neuropathic) pain (e.g. shooting pain) suspected
- For patients who cannot verbalize (e.g. patients with dementia or communication difficulties) consider the Abbey Pain Scale.

Causes of pain and pain management

Pain can be related directly to the tumour (such as compression/infiltration) or from cancer treatment (such as chemotherapy and radiotherapy). It can also be related to associated factors (e.g. constipation (⊃ Constipation in adults p. 512)), procedures (e.g. dressing changes (⊃ Wound dressings p. 532)), or comorbidities (e.g. arthritis).

Use of the pain relief ladder is helpful (Fig. 10.1). All types of pain can show some response to opioids. The cause of pain always needs to be established as the approach to management will be dependent on the pain type and cause (Table 10.5). Morphine is the gold standard opioid (second-line opioid is oxycodone). Seek advice when converting strong opioids. For complex pain management, consider referral to a specialist palliative care service. Monitor for opioid toxicity symptoms, including: myoclonus, pin-point pupils, hallucinations, or delirium. Reduce dose and seek specialist advice, and consider switching opioid.

In addition to pharmaceutical interventions, management options may include massage, repositioning, application of heat packs, and distraction therapy (e.g. playing music, reading a book out loud).

Related topics

⊃ Syringe drivers p. 570; ⊃ Complementary and alternative therapies p. 838; ⊃ Hyper- and hypocalcaemia p. 704

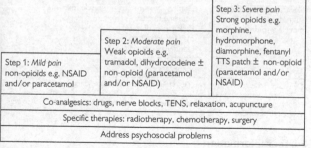

Fig. 10.1 WHO pain relief ladder.

Reproduced with permission from Watson, M. (2005) *Oxford Handbook of Palliative Care.* Oxford: Oxford University Press

Table 10.5 Types, causes, and management of pain

Type of pain	Possible causes	Management options
Bone pain: dull, aching, exacerbated by movement, tender over bone	Bone metastases, arthritis, consider if hypercalcaemia	NSAIDS, bisphosphonates, oncology/orthopaedic referral
Liver capsule pain: sharp, stabbing, right upper quadrant or right shoulder tip	Liver metastases, other liver disease	NSAIDS, dexamethasone
Raised intracranial pressure: headache worse in the morning, associated with vomiting	Brain tumour, brain metastases	Dexamethasone, neurological referral
Pancreatic pain: central abdominal pain, radiating through to the back	Pancreatic tumour, pancreatitis	Combination of opioid, NSAID, and neuropathic agents; intervention pain referral
Smooth muscle spasm: crampy, colicky, intermittent pains	Bowel/bladder/biliary: constipation, bowel obstruction, ureteric obstruction, bladder spasm	Treat constipation if present; review medication as prokinetic drugs may be the cause; use an anticholinergic
Oesophageal pain: intermittent chest pain, related to swallowing	Oesophageal tumour, candida infection	Treat candida infection; drugs to relieve smooth muscle spasm
Rectal and pelvic pain: tenesmus, pain worsened by bowel action, deep-seated pelvic pain	Pelvic and rectal tumours, constipation	If constipation excluded: NSAIDS, neuropathic agents, drugs to relieve smooth muscle spasm, local steroid, oncological referral, intervention pain referral
Skeletal muscle pain: ache, stiffness, worse in the morning, spasms	Debility, motor neurone disease, Parkinson's disease; may be difficult to identify if overlying long bone or spinal metastases	Muscle relaxants

© Wessex Palliative Care Physicians (2014) *Palliative care handbook* (8th edn). Available at:⅏ https://www.oakhavenhospice.co.uk/wp-content/uploads/2015/10/Palliative-Care-Handbook-8th-edition-2014-Wessex-Palliative-Physicians.pdf. Reproduced with permission from Wessex Palliative Care Physicians.

Further information

Marie Curie, Palliative Care Knowledge Zone (*Pain control at the end of life*). Available at: https://www.mariecurie.org.uk/professionals/palliative-care-knowledge-zone/symptom-control/pain-control

NICE (*Palliative care for adults: strong opioids [CG140]*). Available at: ⅏ http://www.nice.org.uk/cg140

Palliative Care Adult Network Guidelines ᴾᴸᵁˢ .. Available at: ⅏ http://book.pallcare.info/

Twycross, R., Wilcock, A., & Howard, P. (2017) *Palliative care formulary* (6th edn). Nottingham: Palliativedrugs.com

Nausea and vomiting in palliative care

Nausea and vomiting are common symptoms in advanced diseases; present in up to 70% of patients with advanced cancer and up to 50% of patients with non-malignant disease such as heart failure (➔ Heart failure p. 636), renal failure (➔ Renal problems p. 754), and COPD (➔ Chronic obstructive pulmonary disease p. 614). Severity can increase as disease progresses.

Care and management

Identify and treat the cause (Table 10.6). Consider impact on hydration, ADL, quality of life, and anxiety and depression (➔ People with anxiety and depression p. 478; ➔ Depression and spiritual distress in palliative care p. 564). Refer to local formularies and protocols for care. Consider diversion and relaxation techniques.

Related topics

➔ Syringe drivers p. 570; ➔ Complementary and alternative therapies p. 838; ➔ Hyper- and hypocalcaemia p. 704; ➔ Oral chemotherapy in the home p. 546; ➔ Renal problems p. 754; ➔ Principles of medication reviews p. 142; ➔ Constipation in adults p. 512; ➔ Teamwork p. 58; ➔ Appendicitis, diverticulitis, hernias, and intestinal obstruction p. 716

Table 10.6 Causes/risk factors for nausea and vomiting

Cause	Clinical feature	Drug therapy
Raised intracranial pressure	Worse in the morning, headache, drowsiness	Dexamethasone, cyclizine, levomepromazine
Cerebellar disease	Ataxia, past-pointing, dysarthria	As above
Anxiety	For example, pre-chemotherapy	Levomepromazine, benzodiazepines
Motion, positional	Worse on movement or travelling	Cyclizine, prochlorperazine, hyoscine hydrobromide
Drugs, endogenous toxins	May be apparent from drug history (coincides with starting a drug), renal failure, hypercalcaemia	Metoclopramide, haloperidol, levomepromazine
Chemotherapy and radiotherapy	Symptoms worse at time of treatment or in subsequent days or weeks	Consult oncology colleagues
Gastric stasis	Inability to eat a meal or fullness after small meal	Metoclopramide, domperidone, erythromycin
Gastric irritation	May be associated with epigastric discomfort, acid indigestion	Review medication, antacids, proton pump inhibitors, misoprostol if caused by NSAIDS
Intestinal stasis	Constipation, abdominal fullness, reduced bowel sounds	Metoclopramide
Intestinal obstruction	Dependent on level of blockage. Limited bowel movement or flatus, vomiting brings some relief, faeculent material in vomit, colic, abdominal distension, empty rectum, scanty or tinkling bowel sounds	Management will depend on: site of obstruction; whether complete or incomplete; bowel motility; and the patient's wishes and general condition. Will include consideration of reversible causes, non-drug measures, and drug therapies.
Constipation	Reduced frequency of passing stool	Better to anticipate and prevent constipation than to wait until treatment is urgent.
Indeterminate	No discerning features	Metoclopramide, levomepromazine, cyclizine, trial of others

© Wessex Palliative Care Physicians (2014) *Palliative care handbook* (8th edn). Available at: ℘ https://www.oakhavenhospice.co.uk/wp-content/uploads/2015/10/Palliative-Care-Handbook-8th-edition-2014-Wessex-Palliative-Physicians.pdf. Reproduced with permission from Wessex Palliative Care Physicians.

Further information

Twycross, R., Wilcock, A., & Howard, P. (2017) *Palliative care formulary* (6th edn). Nottingham: Palliativedrugs.com

Palliative Care Adult Network Guidelines ᴾᴸᵁˢ .. Available at: ℘ http://book.pallcare.info/

Breathlessness in palliative care

Breathlessness is when breathing feels uncomfortable and/or difficult. The emotional experience of breathlessness is inextricable from the sensation and biomedical causes. It is a significant symptom for patients with COPD (➜ Chronic obstructive pulmonary disease p. 614), heart failure (➜ Heart failure p. 636), and 1° lung cancer (➜ Lung cancer p. 751). It is also seen in patients with other cancers, with no evidence of lung or pleural involvement. Results in ↓ activity, social life, and self-esteem. Often characterized by: rapid respiration; nasal flaring and using accessory muscles to breath; feelings of panic and being unable to get enough breath; and fears of impending death. May be accompanied by cough, sputum, haemoptysis, fatigue (➜ Fatigue in palliative care p. 562), insomnia, pain (➜ Pain assessment and management in palliative care p. 554), loss of appetite, and anxiety and depression (➜ People with anxiety and depression p. 478; ➜ Depression and spiritual distress in palliative care p. 564).

Causes of breathlessness

- Heart failure and COPD
- 1° or 2° cancer: airway constriction/obstruction (always look for stridor), size and site of tumour, inflammation, involvement of pleura, pericardium, and vessels (e.g. superior vena cava obstruction)
- Indirect consequences of cancer: pulmonary embolism, pneumonia (➜ Pneumonia p. 750), pneumothorax, ascites, fatigue/weakness, and anaemia (➜ Anaemia in adults p. 652)
- Respiratory muscle weakness: motor neurone disease (➜ Motor neurone disease p. 672), cachexia-anorexia, and drug-induced (corticosteroids, benzodiazepines)
- Following cancer treatments: radiotherapy and surgery

Care and management

Breathlessness from responsive anaemia, pleural effusions, airway obstruction, ascites, and superior vena cava obstruction can improve with targeted interventional treatments. Involve multidisciplinary team in assessment (➜ Teamwork p. 58).

Non-pharmacological management

Careful assessment of what relieves or exacerbates symptoms. Exploration of what breathlessness means to patients about their disease and their feelings about the future. Simple measures to relieve breathlessness include keeping the room cool and improving air circulation.[26] Encourage exercise within the person's capabilities. Discuss adaptations to ADL and lifestyle expectations.

Relaxation and breathing techniques

Approaches include: pursed lip breathing to help relieve perception of breathlessness during exercise or when breathlessness triggers—people inhale through their nose for several seconds with their mouth open, then exhale slowly through pursed lips for 4–6secs; relaxing and dropping the shoulders to reduce the hunched posture associated with anxiety; sitting upright to ↑ peak ventilation and ↓ airway obstruction; and leaning forward with arms bracing a chair or knees with the upper body supported to improve ventilator capacity.

Pharmacological management

Pharmacological approaches include opioids, which alter the sensation of breathlessness and feelings of distress; however, caution should be exercised in older patients and patients with renal impairment. O_2 can provide symptomatic relief of acute breathlessness and panic; however, nasal cannula should be used to minimize oral dryness. If O_2 saturations are within normal range, reassure patient that O_2 is not required. Benzodiazepines may ease anxiety related to breathlessness. Other pharmacological interventions include antibiotics (for an infection), diuretics (for pulmonary oedema), high-dose steroids and corticosteroids (for inflammation), bronchodilators and anticholinergics (for bronchoconstriction), and nebulized saline (for viscous secretions).

Related topics

➲ Drugs commonly used in the treatment of respiratory conditions p. 620;
➲ Nebulizers p. 623

Reference

26. NICE (2016) *Clinical knowledge summaries: palliative care (dyspnoea)*. Available at: https://cks.nice.org.uk/palliative-care-dyspnoea#!scenario:1

Further information

Palliative Care Adult Network Guidelines ᴾᴸᵁˢ .. Available at: ℘ http://book.pallcare.info/
Scottish Palliative Care Guidelines (*Breathlessness*). Available at: ℘ http://www.palliativecareguidelines.scot.nhs.uk/guidelines/symptom-control/breathlessness.aspx
Twycross, R., Wilcock, A., & Howard, P. (2017) *Palliative care formulary* (6th edn). Nottingham: Palliativedrugs.com

Fatigue in palliative care

A common, distressing symptom in progressive chronic disease. It occurs on a continuum from tiredness to exhaustion and → a combination of physical, emotional, and cognitive difficulties. Severe fatigue is unrelated to activity levels and cannot be resolved by sleeping. Causes:[27]

- Anaemia (➲ Anaemia in adults p. 652)
- Cachexia (wasting syndrome) and nutritional deficiencies (➲ Malnutrition p. 350)
- Breathlessness (➲ Breathlessness in palliative care p. 560)
- Hypothyroidism (➲ Thyroid p. 702), hypogonadism, adrenal insufficiency (➲ Adrenal disorders p. 700)
- Metabolic disorders
- Reduced activity and deconditioning
- Pain (➲ Pain assessment and management in palliative care p. 554)
- Depression (➲ People with anxiety and depression p. 478; ➲ Depression and spiritual distress in palliative care p. 564)
- Chemotherapy, radiotherapy, and surgery
- Adverse effects of medications

Management of fatigue

- Treat potentially reversible factors as appropriate
- Physical activity: promotes ↑ functional capacity and mood (➲ Exercise p. 354)
- Diet: advise to eat when hungry, frequent small amounts
- Pacing of activities: prioritize and plan for activities
- Sleep: good sleep routine
- Psychosocial interventions, including: stress/anxiety management, relaxation/complementary therapy (➲ Complementary and alternative therapies p. 838), and counselling (➲ Talking therapies p. 472).

Only limited evidence to recommend pharmacological treatment[28,29] (➲ Evidence-based healthcare p. 72). Patients undergoing cancer treatment may be encouraged to keep a fatigue diary to keep a daily record of their energy levels and when they have treatment, to work out how treatment affects them.

References

27. Care Search Palliative Care Knowledge Network (2017) *Fatigue*. Available at: https://www.caresearch.com.au/caresearch/ClinicalPractice/Physical/Fatigue/tabid/235/Default.aspx
28. Scottish Palliative Care Guidelines (2015) *Weakness/fatigue*. Available at: http://www.palliativecareguidelines.scot.nhs.uk/guidelines/symptom-control/weakness-fatigue.aspx
29. Macmillan Cancer Support (2015) *A practical guide to living with and after cancer: coping with fatigue* (7th edn). Available at: https://be.macmillan.org.uk/Downloads/CancerInformation/ResourcesForHSCP/InformationResources/MAC11664Copingwithfatigue.pdf

Depression and spiritual distress in palliative care

Depression

Depression is common but often under-recognized in palliative care (● People with anxiety and depression p. 478). Time is precious for individuals with life-limiting illness and early detection is imperative. Risk factors include: poorly controlled physical symptoms, increasing disability, advanced disease at diagnosis, social isolation, coexisting life stresses, and personal or family history of depression. Signs and symptoms:

• Loss of interest in everyday activities
• Feelings of hopelessness, worthlessness, and guilt
• Suicidal thoughts and wish for an earlier death
• Reduced emotional reactivity

Distinguish appropriate sadness versus depressive disorder, and recognize that there is some overlap with somatic symptoms (e.g. ↓ appetite, fatigue, sleep disturbance). In appropriate sadness, people will still feel intimately connected to others, able to enjoy happy memories, feel a sense of self-worth, look forward to things, and retain a capacity for pleasure. Sadness is likely to come in waves rather than be unremitting.

Screening

The Patient Health Questionnaire (PHQ-9) can be used as a screening tool. The Brief Edinburgh Depression Scale is also suited to palliative care patients (● Standardized assessment tools p. 118).

Management of depression in advanced illness

Good palliative care with comprehensive assessment and optimal management of physical symptoms (e.g. pain and fatigue) and attention to psychological well-being (e.g. spiritual issues) and social wellbeing is important (e.g. resolving conflicts and maintaining social networks).

Care and management

Pharmacological management may include the prescription of antidepressants. Non-pharmacological management may include brief psychological therapy (e.g. cognitive behavioural therapy (● Talking therapies p. 472)).

Spiritual distress

Palliative care emphasizes care of the whole person. Spiritual needs are understood broadly and include all the existential concerns of an individual and their family and carers (● Carers p. 458). Spirituality can give meaning and purpose in life. It is how people make sense of their joys and difficulties. May not include a belief in a particular god but could include belief in a power greater than oneself. Spiritual care is important throughout the illness trajectory and into bereavement. Tools available to take a spiritual history include the HOPE mnemonic:[30]

• Sources of **h**ope, meaning, strength, peace, love, and connection
• **O**rganized religion
• **P**ersonal spirituality and **p**ractices
• **E**ffects on medical care and end-of-life issues

Reference

30. Anandarajah, G. & Hight, E. (2001) Spirituality and medical practice: using the HOPE questions as a practical tool for spiritual assessment. *American Family Physician*, 1(63), 81–9

Further information

European Palliative Care Research Collaborative (*Management of depression in palliative care*). Available at: ℗ https://www.kcl.ac.uk/nursing/departments/cicelysaunders/attachments/depression-guidlines/the-management-of-depression-in-palliative-care.pdf

NICE (*End-of-life care for adults*). Available at: ℗ https://www.nice.org.uk/guidance/qs13/chapter/Introduction-and-overview

Scottish Palliative Care Guidelines (*Depression*). Available at: ℗ http://www.palliativecareguidelines.scot.nhs.uk/guidelines/symptom-control/Depression.aspx

Palliative care emergencies

Some emergency conditions can be reversed if identified early and treated in hospital settings. However, some patients may decline treatment (➲ Consent p. 82; ➲ Mental capacity p. 470) and prefer to remain at home for end-of-life care. It is crucial to recognize such emergencies and respond quickly. If a patient chooses not to have active treatment, it is important that anticipatory medication for pain and other symptoms are prescribed.

Sepsis in the neutropenic patient

Patients can become neutropenic during or following chemotherapy. The patient can become septic and die if they are not treated quickly (➲ Sepsis p. 826).

Metastatic spinal cord compression (MSCC)

Bone metastases in the spinal column can progress to MSCC when tumours in the pedicles of the vertebrae directly invade the spinal canal and cause pressure on the spinal cord. Debilitation and paralysis will differ depending on where on the spine the compression occurs. Key symptoms include back pain (particularly a band-like pain around the abdomen), altered sensation/ weakness in the legs, and unexplained incontinence (➲ Urinary incontinence p. 504; ➲ Faecal incontinence p. 514) or constipation/urinary retention (➲ Constipation in adults p. 512). ⚠ Requires emergency imaging, followed by treatment with high dose steroids, radiotherapy, and occasionally surgery. Treatment is not always successful.

Superior vena cava (SVC) obstruction

Occurs when blood flow to the SVC is obstructed by external compression, thrombosis, or direct invasion of the SVC, particularly from lung tumours (➲ Lung cancer p. 751). Key symptoms include: breathlessness; engorged veins in the neck/chest; swelling with discolouration in the face, chest, and arm; headache/fullness if bending forwards; swelling around the eyes. If untreated, the patient can die within days. ⚠ Requires urgent referral for imaging. High doses of steroids and diuretics may alleviate symptoms.

Hypercalcaemia

Related to lytic bone lesions and the production of parathyroid hormone-related peptide (➲ Hyper- and hypocalcaemia p. 704). Common in patients with breast cancer (➲ Breast cancer p. 774), lung cancer, and multiple myeloma. Key symptoms include: drowsiness, confusion, nausea, vomiting, thirst, weakness, constipation, polyuria, and coma. Treatment consists of rehydration with fluids and an intravenous (IV) infusion of bisphosphonates. If treated, it can be reversed successfully, although it is likely to reoccur within 2–4wks. It is a poor prognostic sign.

Haemorrhage

In patients with malignant tumours (➲ Malignant fungating wounds p. 530), oesophageal, throat, and/or oral tumours, or varices, there is a possibility that there can be severe haemorrhage which can be fatal. Important to plan well in advance if a patient has an identified risk. The patient and their family should be informed about their risk and what may occur. In the event of a severe haemorrhage, stay with the patient and carer (➔ Carers p. 458). Sedation (given either IV or intramuscular) and morphine, if required, to reduce distress and pain. Provide dark towels to mask serious bleeding.

Further information

Marie Curie (*Recognising emergencies*). Available at: ℘ https://www.mariecurie.org.uk/professionals/palliative-care-knowledge-zone/symptom-control/recognising-emergencies

NICE (*Hypercalcaemia*). Available at: ℘ https://cks.nice.org.uk/hypercalcaemia#!topicsummary

Scottish Palliative Care Guidelines (*Superior vena cava obstruction*). Available at: ℘ http://www.palliativecareguidelines.scot.nhs.uk/guidelines/palliative-emergencies/Superior-Vena-Cava-Obstruction.aspx

Watson, M., Lucas, C., Hoy, A., & Wells, J. (2009) *Oxford Handbook of Palliative Care* (2nd edn). Oxford: Oxford University Press

Caring for patients in the dying phase

One chance to get it right

Five key priorities have been recommended nationally to ensure that patients and their carers (➋ Carers p. 458) receive the care that they need when they are dying[31] (➋ Services for the dying patient p. 552).

Recognize

The possibility that a person may die within the next few days or hours is recognized. When patients are approaching the dying phase, in the context of an advanced and life-limiting illness, they may display:

- ↑ weakness/bedbound
- Drowsy or ↓ cognition
- ↓ interest or ability to eat and drink
- Difficulty swallowing oral tablets

Following an unexpected deterioration or change in condition, a doctor should assess whether the condition is potentially reversible. If so, appropriate decisions about treatment need to be taken. If it is agreed that the person is imminently dying, goals for treatment and care must be communicated clearly to the patient, their carers, and professionals.

Communicate

Communicate sensitively, honestly, and openly. Information should be given clearly and at the right pace, with opportunities to repeat and revisit. Everyone should be aware the patient appears to be dying, but acknowledge that predicting prognosis can be difficult (➋ Continuity of care p. 598). All planned care and key conversations must be documented. Ensure 'Do not attempt cardiopulmonary resuscitation' status is clearly documented (➋ Adult basic life support and automated external defibrillation p. 792). Include information about how to summon urgent help if needed and what to do when the person dies.

Involve

Information about benefits, risks, and burdens of treatments should be given. Decision making should include the dying patient's views, which should be documented (➋ Record keeping p. 86). The extent someone wishes to be involved in such decisions will vary. If they no longer have capacity, best interests decisions must be made (➋ Mental capacity p. 470).

Support

Regularly assess the emotional and practical needs of carers. Acknowledge their expertise as carers. Check their own religious, spiritual, and cultural needs.

Plan and do

Assess the patient to ensure their needs inform an individual plan of care. The plan must include food and drink, and other practical aspects such as mouth care, bladder, bowel, and skincare. The dying patient must be supported to eat and drink as long as they are able, unless they are at risk of choking (➋ Adult choking p. 798). If they are able to make an informed decision, they can continue to do so, even if they are at risk of aspiration.

For patients unable to swallow, decisions about clinically assisted nutrition and hydration must comply with guidance from the General Medical Council.[32] The plan also needs to include symptom management and psychological, social, and spiritual support.

Managing symptoms in the dying phase

When a patient is dying, they lose their ability to swallow oral medications, and non-essential medications should be discontinued. Anticipatory prescribing is good practice. The subcutaneous (SC) route (➔ Injection techniques p. 576) is preferred for patient comfort. All patients should be prescribed medications for key symptoms as needed ('prn'): pain (➔ Pain assessment and management in palliative care p. 554); agitation, restlessness, and distress; respiratory tract infections; nausea and vomiting (➔ Nausea and vomiting in palliative care p. 558); and breathlessness (➔ Breathlessness in palliative care p. 560). Individual medications required will vary depending on the clinical history and local protocols. If the patient experiences frequent or continuous symptoms, and/or has been taking regular oral medications for pain or other symptoms, a syringe driver should be considered (➔ Syringe drivers p. 570).

References

31. Leadership Alliance for the Care of Dying People (2014) *One chance to get it right*. Available at: http://wales.pallcare.info/files/One_chance_to_get_it_right.pdf
32. General Medical Council (2010) *Treatment and care towards the end of life. good practice in decision making*. Available at: https://www.gmc-uk.org/ethical-guidance/ethical-guidance-for-doctors/treatment-and-care-towards-the-end-of life

Syringe drivers

Palliative care drugs are commonly administered by continuous SC infusion (◆ Injection techniques p. 576), using portable battery-powered syringe drivers delivering a measured volume of drugs at a predetermined rate. Provide an important alternative route when patients are in the deteriorating/dying phase and assessed as requiring continuous analgesic and/or continuous relief of other symptoms, and to prevent the need for regular injections when medication cannot be swallowed or absorbed (◆ Caring for patients in the dying phase p. 568). Indications:

- Intractable vomiting (◆ Nausea and vomiting in palliative care p. 558)
- Severe dysphagia
- Impaired consciousness
- Patient too weak to swallow oral drugs
- Poor alimentary absorption (rare)
- Intestinal obstruction
- Patient's preference

Advantages include: drug mixtures can be administered; infusion timing is accurate; mobility and independence is retained; and provides continuous pain relief (◆ Pain assessment and management in palliative care p. 554) and ↓ the need for breakthrough analgesia. A full explanation should be provided to the patient and family carer (◆ Carers p. 458) about what a syringe driver is, how it works, and why its use is indicated.

Types of syringe driver

⚠ Different syringe drivers deliver infusions in different ways. It is best to use one type of syringe driver, with standardized procedures across the health organization, to ↓ risk of dose error (◆ Clinical risk management p. 78). McKinley T34 Medical Syringe Drivers are commonly used in community settings. Always check manufacturer's instructions before use and date of last service. Training is essential before setting up and using a syringe driver. Always refer to local policy and standard operating procedure. ⚠ Always check for correct conversion ratios if converting from oral to SC route.

Further information

CME Medical Clinical (*T34 pump*). Available at: ℘ http://www.cmemedical.co.uk/training/clinical-training/clinical-elearning/

NICE (*Prescribing in palliative* care). Available at: ℘ https://bnf.nice.org.uk/guidance/prescribing-in-palliative-care.html

Scottish Palliative Care Guidelines (*Syringe pumps*). Available at: ℘ http://www.palliativecareguidelines.scot.nhs.uk/guidelines/end-of-life-care/syringe-pumps.aspx

Euthanasia, assisted suicide, and assisted dying

Euthanasia, assisted suicide, and assisted dying are controversial subjects engendering on one hand strong feelings about the right to desire and demand death and, on the other, strong feelings that life is so precious that we have a duty to preserve it at all costs.

Definitions are contentious and problematic. Nevertheless, euthanasia is generally defined as the act of deliberately ending a person's life to relieve suffering. It is important to recognize that where the 1° intention is to prevent suffering, it is not considered euthanasia (Box 10.3). Assisted suicide is the act of deliberately assisting or encouraging another person to kill themselves (➔ Suicidal intent and deliberate self-harm p. 494).

The law

Euthanasia is illegal in the UK. Assisted suicide is illegal in England, Wales, and Northern Ireland (including assisting someone to travel overseas to die). There is no legislation in Scotland concerning assisted suicide; however, someone who assists someone to end their lives is nevertheless likely to be prosecuted.

In the event someone asks for your assistance to die

The Royal College of Nursing (RCN) provides guidance for nurses on responding to a request to hasten death.[33] This emphasizes that conducting difficult conversations is central to the provision of ↑ quality end-of-life care. Patients and carers may raise the subject of euthanasia and/or assisted suicide. The nurse must work within the law to support the patient and those who are important to them.

If a patient directly requests assistance in hastening death:
- Check you have understood the patient.
- Do not use metaphors that can be confusing.
- Acknowledge the request and resist the inclination to ignore it.
- Tell the patient it is not possible to keep such a request private.
- Inform the patient of the legal position in the UK.
- Document all conversations (➔ Record keeping p. 86).

Issues to consider when a patient requests assistance in hastening death include whether: pain (➔ Pain assessment and management in palliative

---

Box 10.3 What euthanasia is *not*
- Withholding or withdrawing futile, burdensome treatment. This includes nutrition and hydration if the patient is dying and is unable to swallow.
- Giving opioids, or any other medications, to control symptoms including pain, fear, and overwhelming distress.
- Sedating a patient in the terminal stages if all other practical methods of controlling symptoms have failed.
- Issuing a 'Do not resuscitate' order.

Adapted from Watson, M., Lucas, C., Hoy, A., et al. (2009) *Oxford Handbook of Palliative Care* (2nd edn). Oxford: Oxford University Press

control p. 554) and symptom relief is effective; there is reversible clinical depression (➔ People with anxiety and depression p. 478; ➔ Depression and spiritual distress in palliative care p. 564); there is appropriate social support; and the patient has been given a voice in planning their future care.

⚠ If you are in any doubt about the safety and well-being of the patient and consider them to be an adult at risk, it is important to raise a safeguarding alert as per local policy (➔ Adults at risk from harm and abuse p. 454).

References

33. RCN (2016) *When someone asks for your assistance to die* (2nd edn). Available at: https://www. rcn.org.uk/professional-development/publications/pub-005822

Coping with bereavement

Grief is a normal reaction to bereavement. Traditional models see it as a process where an individual moves to 'recovery'. Not a linear process: individuals likely to oscillate between loss and restoration, memories of the dead person and getting on with life.

Normal manifestations of grief

Physical
- Hollowness in the stomach
- Tightness in the throat and chest
- Shortness of breath
- Sensitivity to noise
- Dry mouth
- Muscle weakness

Emotional
- Initial response often shock and numbness
- Feelings of anger, guilt, anxiety, disorganization, and helplessness
- Sadness most common manifestation (but might be delayed)
- Sense of relief and freedom can → feelings of guilt

Cognitive
- Sense of unreality and disbelief, even denial in early bereavement
- Short-term memory and concentration can be affected
- Not uncommon to have sense of the presence of the deceased

Behaviour
- Appetite and sleep disturbed
- Individual may withdraw socially
- May consider rapid changes in their life (e.g. new relationship and moving house) to avoid pain of loss, but not advisable

Health consequences of bereavement

- ↑ risk of mortality
- Alcohol abuse (➔ Alcohol p. 360)
- Depression (➔ People with anxiety and depression p. 478)
- Suicidal thoughts (➔ Suicidal intent and deliberate self-harm p. 494)
- ↓ immune response

Where there has been nursing involvement and relationship with the family/carers, appropriate for nurse to visit in the month after the death to see how the bereaved are coping, allowing them to express how they are feeling and to remember the deceased (➔ Talking therapies p. 472). Signpost as necessary to bereavement mutual support groups (e.g. Widowed and Young Foundation (see ℘ https://www.widowedandyoung.org.uk/) and the Loss Foundation (see ℘ https://www.thelossfoundation.org/)) and bereavement counselling (e.g. Cruse Bereavement Care (see ℘ https://www.cruse.org.uk/)).

Bereaved children

Children understand what death is by 8yrs, and even by 2–3yrs will have some understanding. If possible, prepare children for death with the opportunity to ask questions. Excluding children to protect them can ↑ the pain and feelings of being isolated. Specialist help may be appropriate.

Complicated grief reactions

Grief does not usually need clinical intervention. However, grief can sometimes become a chronic debilitating condition called complicated grief. Symptoms include: intense yearning, longing, or emotional pain; frequently preoccupying thoughts and memories of the deceased; a feeling of disbelief or an inability to accept the loss; and difficulty imagining a meaningful future without the deceased.[34] If complicated grief is suspected, monitor carefully and consider referral for bereavement counselling, and possibility of clinical depression.

Reference

34. Shear, K. (2015) Complicated grief. *New England Journal of Medicine*, 372(2), 153–60

Injection techniques

Drugs are given via parenteral routes when they need to be absorbed quickly or when they would be altered by ingestion. Some drugs are re-leased over a long period of time and need a parenteral route that will absorb the drug more steadily. Key principles:

- Be familiar with medication and local policies/protocols.
- Do not prepare injectable medicines in advance of immediate use.
- Only administer injectable medicine you have prepared yourself or which has been prepared in your presence.
- Ensure anaphylactic shock kit is easily accessible (◆ Anaphylaxis p. 810).
- Assess patient anxiety and if reassurance needed (◆ People with anxiety and depression p. 478).
- Assess condition of proposed injection site and avoid sites if the skin is broken, oedematous, or scarred.
- Where frequent injections are given (e.g. insulin (◆ Principles of diabetes management p. 664), sites should be rotated to prevent damage (use of rotation charts may be considered).
- Use aseptic non-touch technique.
- Use needles with engineered sharps injury protection, if available. (◆ Sharps injuries p. 108).
- Ensure prompt disposal of sharps in sharps bin. (◆ Managing healthcare waste p. 106).
- Document procedure (drug name, dose given, site, batch, and expiry date) (◆ Record keeping p. 86).

Intramuscular (IM) injections

The effect of medicines given IM will be faster than those given via the SC route but slower than drugs given IV. Suitable for small volumes (e.g. <5ml in adults, <2ml in children, and <1ml in infants). Large volumes as-sociated with ↑ discomfort. May need to divide doses between sites to ensure comfort.

Adult sites

- Ventrogluteal (gluteus medius)
- Lateral aspects of the vastus lateralis
- Dorsogluteal (gluteus maximus) ⚠ ↑ risk due to proximity of large blood vessels and nerves. If the patient is obese, the injection may not reach the gluteus maximus.
- Deltoid ⚠ Only suitable for small volumes (<2ml)

Child sites

- Ventrogluteal: considered suitable for children >7mths
- Dorsogluteal ⚠ Not recommended for immunization (◆ Childhood immunizations p. 164) due to poor absorption and risk of sciatic nerve injury.
- Vastus lateralis: preferred site in infants and children <2yrs
- Rectus femoris: painful but suitable for self-administration
- Deltoid ⚠ Only suitable for small volumes (<1ml for children and <0.5ml for infants)

Preparation

- Perform hand hygiene and put on apron (➲ Hand hygiene p. 98;
  ➲ Personal protective equipment p. 100).
- Attach blunt needle to syringe.
- Loosen needle guard so that it will slip off easily.
- Tap the top of the ampoule to remove any liquid and snap off the top.
- Draw up liquid.
- Replace the needle guard using a non-touch technique.
- Expel air from syringe.
- See that a drop of liquid appears at the top of the syringe.
- Discard the blunt needle into a sharps container.
- For adults, attach a sterile 21G needle onto the syringe (needle length
  for infants and children will depend on weight and age).
- Explain procedure and gain patient consent (➲ Consent p. 82).
- Put on non-sterile gloves.
- Wash skin if visibly dirty.
- Use of alcohol and chlorhexidine-impregnated swabs according to local
  policy.
- Pick up syringe and allow needle cover to slip off.

Z-track technique

- Pull the skin sideways or downwards away from the injection site.
- Hold syringe like a pen and insert at 90° in a dart-like motion up to the
  hub of the needle to ensure the full length is used.
- Aspirate with dorsogluteal sites due to the presence of the gluteal
  artery, but unnecessary with other sites.
- Depress the plunger at a rate of 1ml/10secs.
- Wait a few seconds before smoothly withdrawing the needle from
  the skin.
- Discard needle and syringe.
- Release tension from the skin.
- Press firmly on the site with a swab if any bleeding occurs.

⚠ Do not massage the skin.

- Remove gloves and apron and wash hands.

Subcutaneous (SC) injections in adults

Used for slow, sustained absorption of medication in small volumes (≤2ml).

Sites

- Lateral aspects of upper arms
- Anterior aspects of the thighs
- Abdomen

Preparation

- Perform hand hygiene and put on apron.
- Explain procedure and gain patient consent.
- Put on non-sterile gloves.
- Wash skin if visibly dirty.

Procedure
- Pinch skin.
- Insert the needle at an angle of 80–90°.
- Inject the solution, maintaining the skin pinch.
- Wait a few seconds before withdrawing the needle.
- Release skin pinch.
- Discard needle (and syringe).
- Remove gloves and apron and wash hands.

Explore potential for self-administration.

Related topics

➔ Targeted adult immunization p. 392; ➔ Managing healthcare waste p. 106; ➔ Immunization administration p. 390

Further information

Forum for Injection Technique (*Diabetes care in the UK: the UK injection and infusion technique recommendations* (4th edn)). Available at: ℛ http://www.fit4diabetes.com/files/4514/7946/3482/FIT_UK_Recommendations_4th_Edition.pdf

Venepuncture

The introduction of a needle into a vein to obtain blood samples for haematological, biochemical, or bacteriological analysis. Common sites:

- Median cubital vein
- Cephalic vein
- Basilic vein
- Avoid using the dominant arm and arms affected by stroke. ⚠ Do not use arms where there is a fistula or vascular graft, oedematous (➔ Lymphoedema p. 548) or scarred areas, sites above an IV cannula, and, in mastectomy patients, the arm on the same side as the mastectomy.

Complications

- Pain
- Phlebitis
- Haematoma
- Arterial puncture
- Nerve injury
- Sharps injury (➔ Sharps injuries p. 108)

Training and ↑ competency essential to ↓ the risk of complications.

Preparation

- Assemble equipment.
- Perform hand hygiene and put on apron (➔ Hand hygiene p. 98; ➔ Personal protective equipment p. 100).
- Explain procedure and gain consent (➔ Consent p. 82).
- Check allergy status (e.g. to plasters) (➔ Allergies p. 694).
- Confirm patient has adhered to any requirements prior to sampling (e.g. when last ate before fasting samples, and time and dose of last medication before drug samples and hormone levels).
- Ensure patient sitting or lying comfortably.
- Apply tourniquet. ⚠ Apply pressure to impede venous not arterial flow (check pulse).
- Inspect the arm to identify a suitable vein.
- Release the tourniquet.
- Put on non-sterile gloves.
- Clean the skin thoroughly and allow to dry completely.
- Attach needle to the plastic holder.

Procedure using vacuum sampling system

- Replace tourniquet as before.
- With patient's arm in a downward position, apply traction to skin below the puncture site.
- Bevel side upwards, align needle with vein, and smoothly insert needle at a 15°angle.
- Hold needle and plastic holder securely.
- Attach the sampling tube by pushing it firmly onto the needle attachment in the plastic holder.
- Allow sampling tube(s) to automatically fill.

- When blood sampling nearly finished, release tourniquet.
- When blood sampling is complete, gently place a cotton wool ball over puncture site.
- Fully withdraw the needle.
- Discard needle and plastic holder in sharps bin (⊃ Managing healthcare waste p. 106).
- When needle is withdrawn, apply pressure over cotton wool ball (ask the patient to continue to apply pressure for 2–3mins).
- Apply a plaster to puncture site.
- Invert sample tubes to mix with additives. ⚠ Do not shake.
- Remove gloves and apron and wash hands.
- Label sample tubes.
- Ensure safe and timely transport of specimens in biohazard container.
- Discuss arrangements for patients and carers (⊃ Carers p. 458) to receive results.
- Document procedure (⊃ Record keeping p. 86).

Care of central venous catheters

Devices inserted into the central venous system, with the distal tip sitting within the superior or inferior vena cava or right atrium. Enables patients requiring long-term IV therapy (chemotherapy, total parental nutrition, blood products, fluids, medication, and blood sampling) to receive treatment without the multiple venepuncture. Three types of central venous catheter are encountered in 1° and community care:

- Tunnelled (e.g. Hickman, Groshong) for long-term use
- Peripherally inserted, for medium- or short-term use
- Totally implantable (e.g. portacath) for long-term use

Complications

- Bloodstream infections
- Air embolism
- Upper extremity deep vein thrombosis
- Occlusion
- Catheter dislodgement

Site care for tunnelled and peripherally inserted catheters

In hospital settings, the patient will be assessed at least daily for signs of possible thrombosis or thrombophlebitis. Similarly, the catheter insertion site will be examined at least daily for signs of infection, catheter dislodgement, or leakage. In 1° and community care, local guidelines should be followed relating to the frequency of assessment and examination. However, the dressing should be replaced weekly, and sooner if indicated.

Dressing the site

- Explain procedure and check allergy status (➲ Allergies p. 694).
- Perform hand hygiene (➲ Hand hygiene p. 98) and put on apron (➲ Personal protective equipment p. 100) and non-sterile gloves.
- Remove and discard the dressing (➲ Wound dressings p. 532).
- Inspect catheter, catheter site, and surrounding skin for complications.
- Apply sterile gloves.
- Clean site with 2% chlorohexidine in 70% alcohol for 30secs.
- Allow to air dry.
- Ensure catheter securely attached to the skin.
- Apply sterile, transparent, occlusive dressing.
- Encourage use of showers rather than baths, and avoid swimming.

Keeping the line clear

If line is not used regularly, aspirate and flush all lumens weekly. See local guidelines relating to flushing solutions.

- Explain procedure and check allergy status.
- Perform hand hygiene and put on apron.
- Draw up two 10ml syringes of sterile saline 0.9%.
- Apply non-sterile gloves.
- Remove and discard the dressing.
- Inspect catheter, catheter site, and surrounding skin for complications.
- Apply sterile gloves.
- If clamp present, ensure closed.

- If bung present, remove and discard, and clean the hub of the line with 2% chlorohexidine in 50% alcohol and allow to air dry.
- If using needle-free connector, this will need changing weekly. If using needle-free connector, change prior to flushing.
- Attach first 10ml saline syringe.
- If present, open clamp.
- Flush using push–pause technique and repeat with second syringe.

⚠ Never force the flush.

- If clamp present, line must be clamped as the last 1ml is being administered.
- If using a bung, attach a clean bung to the hub.
- Ensure catheter securely attached to the skin.
- Redress as per above.

When to refer to hospital

- Pyrexia
- Rigor after flushing
- Patient feeling generally unwell
- Inflammation and tenderness at exit site
- Catheter is sluggish or there is complete occlusion
- Pain or swelling when the catheter is used
- Fluid leaks from the exit site when catheter flushed
- Fluid leaks from external portion of catheter when flushed
- Increase in external length of peripherally inserted catheter
- Pain or swelling of arm, neck, or shoulder
- Palpitations
- Cardiopulmonary symptoms

Further information

London Cancer North and East (*Central line care guidelines*). Available at: ✆ http://www.londoncancer.org/media/80146/London-Cancer-Central-Line-Policy-v1.pdf

Recording a 12-lead electrocardiogram

The collection of electrical waveforms produced by the heart. Indications for recording a 12-lead electrocardiogram (ECG) include chest pain (➔ Angina p. 626), palpitations (➔ Abnormal cardiac rhythms p. 640), and history of syncope.

Procedure

- Ensure the room is warm and try to relax the patient.
- Position the patient in a semi-recumbent comfortable position.
- Prepare the skin if necessary.
- Ask patient to remain still and breathe normally during procedure.

Application of limb electrodes and leads

- Refer also to manufacturer's guidance, as colours can vary.
- Red: inner right wrist
- Yellow: inner left wrist
- Black: inner right leg, just above ankle
- Green: linner left leg, just above ankle

Apply the chest electrodes and leads

- Refer to Fig. 10.2.
- V1: 4th intercostal space, just to right of sternum
- V2: 4th intercostal space, just to left of sternum.
- V3: midway between V2 and V4

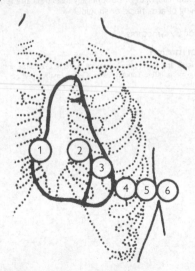

Fig. 10.2 Positioning of chest electrodes and leads.

Reproduced with permission from Longmore, M., Wilkinson, I., Davidson, E., et al. (2004) Oxford Handbook of Clinical Medicine (6th edn). Oxford: Oxford University Press

- V4: 5th intercostal space, mid-clavicular line
- V5: on anterior axillary line, on same horizontal line as V4
- V6: mid-axillary line, on same horizontal line as V4 and V5

After recording the ECG

- Print out ECG following manufacturer's recommendations.
- Check the quality of the trace and repeat as necessary.
- Correctly label ECG (e.g. patient's name, date of birth, date and time of recording, ECG serial number), including any relevant information (e.g. if patient was pain free or complaining of chest pain during recording)

Accuracy, quality, and standardization

- Accuracy: ensure all the electrodes and leads are correctly applied.
- Quality: minimize interference (e.g. patient movement and electrical interference) as this can produce a 'fuzzy' trace.
- Standardization: standard calibration (1mV = 10mm), standard paper speed (25mm/sec), and standard patient position.

Tracheostomy care

A tracheostomy is an artificial opening in the trachea below the level of the larynx, into which a tube is inserted. Performed to secure and maintain a safe airway. Reasons include progressive neurological conditions and carcinoma causing upper airway obstruction. Patients with advanced cancer of the larynx may require a laryngectomy, which entails removal of the larynx, where the lower trachea is diverted to create a permanent opening, which disconnects the lungs from the mouth. Tracheostomy tube includes:

- Outer tube
- Inner tube (important for patients with a lot of secretionscan be cleaned and removed if a mucus plug forms, so the outer tube serves as the airway)
- Flange
- +/− a cuff
- +/− a subglottic port

Held in place with a tracheostomy tube holder (cotton and/or Velcro).

Complications

- Accidental decannulation or displacement
- Tracheal damage
- Pneumonia (➔ Pneumonia p. 750)
- Occlusion
- Communication problems (➔ Adults and children with additional communication needs p. 122)

Safe discharge

Key members of the 1° and 2° care team (➔ Teamwork p. 58) include: tracheostomy specialist practitioner, speech and language therapist, dietician, physiotherapist, occupational therapist, nursing team, and GP (➔ General practice p. 18). Patients and carers (➔ Carers p. 458) must be taught tube management and action to be taken in an emergency. Additional activities prior to discharge include:

- Arranging community support and follow-up
- Sharing important contact details
- Provision of a tracheostomy alert card
- Provision of equipment for first 7 days (or as per local policy)
- Informing ambulance service that the patient is a neck breather (➔ Adult basic life support and automated external defibrillation p. 792)
- Setting up emergency SMS (short message service) text service to ambulance and police
- Informing utility provider that the patient is a priority for restoration of electricity in the event of a power cut

Discharge information to community services to include:

- Rationale for tracheostomy
- Presence or absence of larynx
- Requirement for supplementary O_2
- Type and size of tube
- Type and characteristics of secretions
- Cough effort

- Ability to swallow
- Frequency of suctioning and cleaning of inner cannula
- Condition of stoma site and requirement for dressing
- Availability of spare and emergency equipment
- Type of humidification device
- Routine observations
- Oral health assessment
- Tube and any humidification device care
- Patient's communication methods
- Advice in emergency

Healthcare professionals caring for patients with tracheostomies should have completed tracheostomy competencies.

Living with a tracheostomy

Tracheostomy passport

Every patient should carry written documentation detailing: type of tracheostomy in place; when the tracheostomy needs changing; current information regarding swallowing, eating, drinking, and communication; and previous issues there may have been with the tracheostomy's management.[36] Tubes may need to be changed electively (following multidisciplinary discussion and performed by a tracheostomy specialist practitioner) or require replacement under emergency conditions due to tube blockage, accidental decannulation, or displacement.

Speech

Ability to speak is dependent on whether larynx is present and whether a cuffed or uncuffed tube is used. If larynx is functioning and patient has an uncuffed tube, they may be able to speak using a speaking valve or by covering their tube with a finger and forcing air through vocal cords.

Humidification

Must be provided to keep secretions thin and avoid mucus plugs. Device dependent on needs of patient. They include heat moisture exchangers (e.g. Swedish nose and Thermovent) and stoma filters or bibs. Saline nebulization may be required. Ensure adequate hydration. Mobilization helps improve clearance of secretions. Chest physiotherapy may be indicated.

Suctioning

Some patients able to project mucus by forced expirations, but many require suctioning. Tracheal damage may be caused by suctioning: managed by using appropriately sized tracheal suction catheter, appropriate suction pressures, and only suctioning within the tracheostomy tube. Depth of tube can be determined by measuring a spare tube of the same type and size. Use premeasured suction catheters where available. Follow sterile nontouch technique and standard infection control precautions (including goggles). Use lowest effective pressure (do not exceed 120mmHg), with each suction lasting 5–10 secs. Do not apply suction to catheter when inserting tube. Assess patient for respiratory distress.

Stoma care
- Frequency of cleaning stoma is dependent on individual patient requirements.
- Use sterile non-touch technique and follow standard infection control precautions (including goggles).
- Use two-person procedure due to risk of accidental decannulation (i.e. one person holds the tube in place whilst the other removes tracheostomy holder and soiled dressing etc.).
- Observe for trauma, infection (➙ Wound infection p. 526), or inflammation at site.
- Check around neck for signs of irritation from the tracheostomy tube holder.
- Clean stoma site with gauze and normal saline.
- Apply barrier cream as necessary.
- Insert tracheostomy dressing (➙ Wound dressings p. 532) around stoma and tube.
- Apply tracheostomy holder to secure the tube in place.
- Assess patient for respiratory distress.

Inner tube
Frequency of checking and changing is dependent on individual patient requirements. Disposable inner tube should be discarded if soiled and a new one inserted. Non-disposable inner tubes should be cleaned according to manufacturer instructions and air dried. Replace with spare inner tube whilst cleaning. Assess patient for respiratory distress.

Personal care and physical activity
Patients who shower need to wear a shower guard to stop water getting into the tracheostomy. Patients must not go swimming. They should also avoid contact sports due to risk of decannulation.

Equipment
- Portable suction machine (battery and mains operated)
- Tracheal suction tubes for suctioning tracheostomy tube
- Yankeur mouth suction tubes for oral suctioning
- Suction tubing
- Suction machine liners
- Spare inner tubes
- Humidification device
- Gauze for cleaning stoma
- Normal saline for cleaning stoma
- Barrier cream for peri-stoma skin
- Tracheostomy dressings
- Tracheostomy tube holder (cotton and/or Velcro)
- Shower guard
- Gloves

Additional equipment may include nebulizer (➙ Nebulizers p. 623), manometer for checking pressure in cuffed tubes, and O_2 (➙ Long-term oxygen therapy p. 622). All provided by the NHS.

In addition to the above, every patient should be provided with a safety box for managing emergencies including decannulation or displacement, occlusion, and cardiac arrest. The following items are recommended for inclusion:[35]

- Tracheostomy tube (current patient size)
- Tracheostomy tube (one size smaller than current patient size)
- Inner tube
- Tracheostomy tube holder (cotton and/or Velcro)
- Scissors
- Water-based lubricating gel
- Gloves
- Spare humidification device

Additional contents might include a spare cuffed tracheostomy tube, a size smaller than the one *in situ* (if an uncuffed tube is *in situ*), 10ml syringe, cuff pressure manometer, bag valve mask.

Tracheostomy emergencies

An emergency algorithm should be found on the tracheostomy emergency card issued to the patient on hospital discharge. National Tracheostomy Safety Project (NTSP) have published emergency management guidelines for both tracheostomies and laryngectomies.[36,37] These need to be modified for the community setting.

References

35. East of England Trauma Network (2018) *Community tracheostomy guidelines for adults.* Available at: http://www.eoetraumanetwork.nhs.uk/docs/default-source/rehabilitation-library/east-of-england-community-tracheostomy guidelines-for-adults-final-sept-18.pdf?sfvrsn=0
36. NTSP (2016) *Emergency tracheostomy management—patent upper airway.* Available at: http://www.tracheostomy.org.uk/storage/files/Patent%20Airway%20Algorithm.pdf
37. NTSP (2016) *Emergency laryngectomy management.* Available at: http://www.tracheostomy.org.uk/storage/files/Laryngectomy%20Algorithm.pdf

Further information

e-Learning for Healthcare (*Tracheostomy safety: multidisciplinary resource for safer tracheostomy and laryngectomy care*). Available at: 🔗 https://www.e-lfh.org.uk/programmes/tracheostomy-safety/

Ear care

Nurses carrying out ear care should ensure they have received formal skills training covering:
- Understanding of anatomy and physiology of the ear, including the landmarks of a normal tympanic membrane
- The ability to carry out an ear examination using an otoscope
- Documentation (➔ Record keeping p. 86) and referral process if abnormalities identified
- Assessment of cerumen/debris in external auditory meatus, and removal management
- Referral process for patients with ear and/or hearing problems (➔ Deafness p. 696)

Ear examination

To identify normal or abnormal anatomy, the presence of infection, and cerumen/debris build-up. Should be carried out in the following cases:
- Annual checks on patients >65yrs who wear hearing aids
- Annual checks on patients who have required cerumen removal in the past: irrigation, manual removal, microsuction
- Patients presenting with ear-related symptoms (e.g. hearing loss, discharge, pain, vertigo, tinnitus, itching, and fullness in ear)
- Problems with hearing aid (i.e. whistling) or patients >60yrs with an audiology appointment

Procedure
- Take a comprehensive history.
- Examine external ear(s), checking for previous surgery/abnormalities.
- Examine ear(s) using an otoscope.
- Use a single-use speculum only, choosing a size appropriate for both comfort and adequate view.
- Examine good ear first.
- Pull pinna upwards and backwards to straighten external auditory meatus and insert otoscope.
- Hold the otoscope in a pencil grip with little finger extended to brace against patient cheek (in case of sudden movement) and turn on light.
- Assess condition of external auditory meatus. Assess whether cerumen is present, and its colour and consistency.
- Examine whether the tympanic membrane is visible, and its colour, transparency, and condition.
- Document findings.

⚠ Nurses undertaking ear examinations should be clear when and where to refer for medical or other assessments (e.g. foreign bodies (do not attempt to remove), otosclerosis, cholesteatoma). Patients >60yrs can usually be referred directly to the audiology department providing they do not suffer any other ear-related problems and there is no wax in their ears.

Cerumen/ear wax

Cerumen/ear wax is produced by the sebaceous and ceruminous glands to protect the epithelial lining of the external auditory meatus. Only needs to be removed if causing a hearing deficit and/or discomfort, or restricts the view of the tympanic membrane preventing examination. Assess colour, consistency, odour, and location (cerumen that is dull and dark in colour tends to be harder). Use clinical judgement to consider options for wax removal, assessing both the cerumen and patient suitability—first-line treatment option is softening agents to aid natural migration. Only consider irrigation when conservative methods have failed. Patients for whom irrigation is contraindicated may require referral to an ear, nose, and throat department.

Contraindications for ear irrigation

⚠. Risks include perforation to tympanic membrane, tinnitus, transient dizziness, and otitis externa (→ Clinical risk management p. 78). Contraindicated in patients with:
- A past history of tympanic membrane perforation (unless healed)
- Current or recent (<6wks) ear infection
- Previous untoward experiences following irrigation
- Previous ear surgery (e.g. mastoidectomy)
- Grommets in place or within past 18mths

There is lack of consensus as to whether best practice is not to irrigate the only hearing ear in a patient whose hearing is impaired.

Irrigation procedure

- Soften cerumen prior to removal, e.g. olive oil, one drop twice daily to the ear(s) for up to 3wks prior to treatment.
- Always use an approved electronic ear irrigator.

⚠ Syringes of any type should not be used as their design, combined with the inability to control water pressure, increases the risk of ear damage.
- Put on personal protective equipment (→ Personal protective equipment p. 100) and ensure patient is comfortable.
- Check temperature of water to ~37°C (variation may cause dizziness).
- Set water pressure to minimum and ensure single-use only jet tip applicator firmly in place.
- Gently pull pinna upwards and backwards and place tip of applicator into ear canal entrance.
- Warn patient you are about to start and to immediately report symptoms of pain, dizziness, or nausea.
- Ask patient to hold receiver under affected ear. Switch on machine and direct stream of water onto posterior superior aspect of external auditory meatus.
- Periodically inspect external auditory meatus with otoscope.

⚠ STOP irrigation if patient feels pain.
- Use a maximum of one reservoir of water per procedure per ear.
- After removal of cerumen, or when maximum volume of water is used, dry excess water from the external auditory meatus using ear mops or Jobson–Horne probe and best-quality cotton wool.
- Examine with otoscope and assess need for further treatment.
- Document procedure and condition of external auditory meatus and tympanic membrane following treatment.

Patients requiring ear irrigation should always receive education and advice, which may reduce contributory factors and therefore the need for ear irrigation in the future.

Further information

NICE (*Earwax*). Available at: ℳ http://cks.nice.org.uk/earwax

Enteral tube feeding

Feeding into the gastrointestinal tract via a tube. 1° reason dysphagia, which may result from neurological conditions (e.g. motor neurone disease (◆ Motor neurone disease p. 672), multiple sclerosis (◆ Multiple sclerosis p. 670), and stroke). Other reasons include head and neck cancer, and oesophagogastric cancer. Feeding usually initiated in hospital and patient subsequently discharged to community services.

Access route and tube type dependent on expected period of feeding, clinical condition, and anatomy. Most common are nasogastric tubes and gastrostomy tubes. Other enteral tubes involve delivery into the duodenum or jejunum, and are used if delivery into stomach is contraindicated. These are less common and beyond the scope of this section.

Nasogastric tubes

Narrow-bore tube passed into stomach via nose. Mainly for short-term support (<30 days). Common indications include early post stroke, inadequate oral intake, or acute swallowing problem. Contraindications include facial trauma and recent nasal surgery. Not generally suitable for patients with vomiting, gastro-oesophageal reflux, poor gastric emptying, ileus or intestinal obstruction (◆ Appendicitis, diverticulitis, hernias, and intestinal obstruction p. 716). Tube must be placed by appropriately trained staff. ⚠ Risk that the tube can be misplaced on insertion or move at a later stage.

Excellent standard of care is needed to avoid aspiration. Key interventions include: pH of aspirate on insertion, then prior to every tube use/ daily if fed over 24hrs to check tip position (pH 5.5 or less consistent with gastric placement); check for evidence of new or unexplained respiratory symptoms or if ↓ O_2 saturation; and check position of tube following vomiting, retching, or coughing.

Tube usually secured with tape, and changed if dirty or peeling off. Placement of a nasal retention device may be considered where other methods have failed, following discussion with patient and multidisciplinary team (◆ Teamwork p. 58).

Gastrostomy tubes

Tube passed through abdominal wall and directed into stomach. Usually placed endoscopically (percutaneous endoscopic castrostomy (PEG)) but sometimes radiologically (radiologically inserted gastrostomy (RIG)) or surgically. Generally long-term use (>30 days). Common indications include neurological disease, oesophageal pathology, head and neck cancer, and brain injury.

In adults, the most common are one-piece long tubes. Usually secured with an internal retention device (either a balloon or soft disc ('bumper')) on the inside and a firm external retention device on the outside. Some specialist self-retaining gastrostomy tubes exist, with flexible loop or 'pig-tail' which forms internal retention device.

Other types of gastrostomy tubes include low-profile devices (sometimes called 'buttons') that do not have a long tube permanently attached outside the stomach. Instead, an extension set is attached for feeding or medication administration. When the extension set is not attached, it lies flat against the body and is less easily pulled. Usually secured internally with a balloon. Less common in adults than children.

Feeding and medication administration

Choice of feed and feeding modality

Enteral feed is a sterile, specifically designed nutritional liquid that is licensed to be administered via an enteral feeding tube. Different feeds available. Dietician will determine type of feed and modality of feed. They will also order the feed.

Feeding should take place while patient is sitting or well supported, so their head and shoulders remain at a 45° angle for the entire time they are fed and for at least 30mins afterwards. Failure to maintain 45° angle will ↑ risk of reflux, vomiting, and aspiration.

Patient may be fed via a syringe (bolus feeding) or via an enteral pump (pump feeding). Only enteral syringes should be used for bolus feeding. Bolus feeds can be administered by gravity with the syringe plunger removed, or by using the plunger. Pump feeding allows feed to run continuously for up to 24hrs. Mode of administration determined by patient circumstances. Issues of gastric emptying, metabolic stability, and control of glucose levels (➔ Principles of diabetes management p. 664) may favour continuous feeding. If patient is unable to remain supported at a 45° angle, continuous overnight feeding is not recommended.

To prevent blockage, the tube should be flushed with fresh tap water before and after feeding. Tubes for patients who are immunosuppressed should be flushed with either cooled, freshly boiled water or sterile water from a freshly opened container (➔ Principles of working with someone with compromised immunity p. 466).

Medication administration via feeding tube

Most medicines are not licensed for administration via enteral feeding tube. Those prescribing, supplying, and administering them accept liability for use (➔ Prescribing p. 136; ➔ Medicines optimization p. 128). Preferred formulations are liquid solutions and soluble tablets. Crushing tablets and opening capsules are a last resort. ⚠ Some medicines should never be crushed (e.g. modified-/extended-release tablets, enteric-coated tablets, cytotoxics (➔ Oral chemotherapy in the home p. 546), and hormones). Some medicines will interact with enteral feed. Consult a pharmacist before administering medication via a feeding tube. Administer each medicine separately. Tube should be flushed with water at the beginning and end of medicines administration and between each medicine.

Equipment and supplies

Dietician usually orders all equipment (e.g. giving sets, syringes, and reservoir containers). What equipment is needed will depend on the type of tube and the feeding modality. ISO 80369 is a new standard to improve patient safety and ↓ risk of small-bore misconnections used in liquid and gas healthcare applications. Only enteral syringes and giving sets that are manufactured to this standard should be used. 50–60 ml syringes should be used to administer feed, water, and medicines. ⚠ Syringes <50ml have the potential to damage the tube.

Enteral feeding complications
• Mouth discomfort or infections (➲ Mouth and throat problems p. 698)
• Reflux, vomiting, and aspiration
• Abdominal pain and distension
• Diarrhoea
• Constipation (➲ Constipation in adults p. 512)

Patients at risk of hypoglycaemia
Hypoglycaemia is a medical emergency. Person-centred care plan should set out what action to take in the event of a hypoglycaemic event in a diabetic patient; this may include administration of glucagon injection and/or the administration of a quick-acting carbohydrate (such as Glucojuice) via the feeding tube.

Balloon gastrostomy care

Balloon gastrostomies held in place by a balloon, inflated with sterile water. Balloon volume must be checked regularly. Refer to manufacturer guidelines on frequency (usually 1–6wkly).

Most balloon gastrostomies will need to be changed every 4–9mths. Refer to manufacture guidelines on frequency. First balloon gastrostomy should be replaced in hospital. Subsequent changes can be in the community by appropriately trained staff.

Stoma care

Advance and rotate
Advance and rotate usually needs to be completed weekly for tubes, with a soft disk internal retention device ('bumper'). If not undertaken, ↑ risk that stomach lining can start to grow over the 'bumper' causing 'buried bumper syndrome'. If the 'bumper' is completely buried, it will prevent feeding.

Stoma site complications
• Infection (➲ Wound infection p. 526)
• Overgranulation
• Burns to skin from leakage of gastric contents around tube

Further information

British Association for Parenteral Nutrition (*Enteral feeding*). Available at: ℘ https://www.bapen. org.uk/nutrition-support/enteral-nutrition
National Nurses Nutrition Group (NNNG) (*Good practice guideline—changing of a balloon gastrostomy tube into the stomach for adults and children* (3rd edn)). Available at: ℘ http://www.nnng. org.uk/download-guidelines/
NNNG (*Safe insertion and ongoing care of nasogastric feeding tubes in adults* (2nd edn)). Available at: ℘ http://www.nnng.org.uk/download-guidelines/
Trend UK (*Diabetes and enteral feeding*). Available at: ℘ http://trend-uk.org/wp-content/uploads/ 2017/08/A5_Enteral_Feeding-TREND_FINAL.pdf

Care of adults with long-term conditions

Continuity of care 598

Osteoarthritis 600

Rheumatoid arthritis 602

Low back pain 604

Measuring lung function 606

Asthma in adults 608

Acute asthma in adults (asthma attacks) 612

Chronic obstructive pulmonary disease 614

Management of stable chronic obstructive pulmonary disease 616

Management of chronic obstructive pulmonary disease exacerbation 618

Drugs commonly used in the treatment of respiratory conditions 620

Long-term oxygen therapy 622

Nebulizers 623

Coronary heart disease 624

Angina 626

Hypertension 628

Hypercholesterolaemia 632

Cardiac rehabilitation 634

Heart failure 636

Abnormal cardiac rhythms 640

Atrial fibrillation 641

Patients on anticoagulant therapy 642

Drugs commonly used in the prevention and treatment of cardiovascular disease 646

Anaemia in adults 652

Varicose veins, thrombophlebitis, and deep vein thrombosis 656

Diabetes: overview 660

Principles of diabetes management 664

Multiple sclerosis 670

Motor neurone disease 672

Parkinson's disease 674

Continuity of care

Multiple comorbidities necessitate care from a number of healthcare providers → the risk of fragmentation and discontinuity of services (➔ Teamwork p. 58). Continuity of care is associated with patient satisfaction and ↑ quality of life (see Box 11.1).[1]

The 'house of care' is a co-ordinated model to deliver proactive, holistic, and patient-centred care for people with chronic illness.[2] In the complex landscape of provider services, it draws together the building blocks of integrated care to include the essential elements of continuity, including:

- Patients play an active part in determining their own care and support needs through personalized care planning.
- Collaborative relationships between patients and professionals, and shared decision making and self-management support are at the heart of service delivery.
- Each individual is engaged in a holistic care-planning process, with a single care plan regardless of how many different long-term conditions (LTCs) they have.

Box 11.1 Elements of continuity

- **Informational:** People have access to information about their conditions and how to access services; health and social care professionals have the right information and records needed to provide the right care at the right time
- **Management:** Coherent approach to the management of a person's conditions and care which spans different services; achieved through people and providers drawing up collaborative care plans
- **Relationship:** Consistent relationship between a person and one or more providers over time (and providers having consistent relationships with each other), so that people are able to go to known individuals to co-ordinate their care

---

Related topics

➔ Case management p. 114; ➔ Integrated assessment for adults p. 112; ➔ Expert patient and self-management programmes p. 340

References

1. Year of Care Partnership (2011) *Year of Care programme report from findings from the pilot programme.* Available at: https://www.yearofcare.co.uk/sites/default/files/images/YOC_Report%20-%20correct.pdf
2. King's Fund (2013) *Delivering better services for people with long-term conditions: building the house of care.* Available at: https://www.kingsfund.org.uk/sites/default/files/field/field_publication_file/delivering-better-services-for-people-with-long-term-conditions.pdf

Osteoarthritis

Osteoarthritis (OA) is the biggest cause of joint-related pain and mobility problems in adults (⊃ Common musculoskeletal problems p. 734). More ♀ affected than ♂ with onset ~50yrs. Variable condition involving the whole joint → pain, stiffness, and joint instability. Almost any joint can be affected, but most often causes problems in the knees, hips, and small joints of the hands (Herbeden's nodules). Cervical OA (neck arthritis) may present without pain or symptoms. Causes:

• Age (uncommon <45yrs)
• Obesity (strain on weight-bearing joints, especially knees and hips)
• Joint injury (e.g. sports-related or earlier operation) (⊃ Sprains, strains, and fractures p. 824)
• Occupational (e.g. physical labour)
• Family history

Symptoms and associated problems

Wide variation of experience:
• Painful and stiff joints with pain on exercise (⊃ Exercise p. 354)
• Joint may give way because of weak muscles
• Advanced OA pain is severe and constant
• Compromised mobility
• Difficulty completing activities of daily living (ADL)
• Depression (⊃ People with anxiety and depression p. 478)

OA does not always worsen, symptoms may reach a peak a few years after first onset, and plateau or lessen.

Non-pharmacological management

Assess impact on ADL (e.g. function, occupation, mood, relationships, and leisure)

• ↓ stress on joints by maintaining healthy weight (⊃ Nutrition and healthy eating p. 342; ⊃ Overweight and obesity p. 348)
• Exercise to strengthen muscles to stabilize and protect joints (consider referral to physiotherapist for advice and teaching of exercises)
• Wear flat heels and footwear with thick soft soles to act as shock absorbers
• Walking sticks can ↓ stress on hip and knee (use on opposite side to affected joint) (⊃ Assistive technology and home adaptations p. 834)
• Home modifications to avoid trips and falls, and ↓ need to bend and strain (consider occupational health referral) (⊃ Falls prevention p. 368)
• Transcutaneous electrical nerve stimulation has been shown to relieve pain in OA and ↓ need for analgesia
• Local heat and cold treatment to soothe stiff joints and tired muscles
• Expert patient and self-management programmes (⊃ Expert patient and self-management programmes p. 340)

Hip and knee replacement may be required for severe pain or immobility.

Pharmacological management

Pharmacological management will include analgesia. Usually the patient will try self-management with over-the-counter (OTC) preparations. If these are ineffective, then further analgesia and possible adjuvant therapy will be required. See local and national guidelines.

Related topics

→ Healthy ageing p. 366

Further information

Arthritis Care (*Living with osteoarthritis*). Available at: ℛ https://www.arthritiscare.org.uk/assets/000/001/893/OA_2017_Update_original.pdf?1510589554

Disabled Living Foundation (*Range of daily living equipment*). Available at: ℛ https://www.dlf.org.uk/

NICE (*Osteoarthritis: care and management (CG177)*). Available at: ℛ https://www.nice.org.uk/guidance/cg177

Rheumatoid arthritis

Rheumatoid arthritis (RA) is an inflammatory, autoimmune disease, triggered by environmental factors in patients with a genetic predisposition and characterized by inflammation of peripheral joints and tendons. Affects 0.5 to 1.1% of Northern Europeans, age onset ~55yrs; more ♀ affected than ♂. Variable disease characterized by exacerbations and remissions.

Onset and symptoms

Clinical signs may be subtle, with normal inflammatory markers:[3]
- Discomfort and intermittent swelling of distal joints
- Pain in the morning >30mins
- Fatigue, stiffness, depression (➔ People with anxiety and depression p. 478)
- Anaemia in adults (➔ Anaemia p. 652)
- Dry eyes (➔ Common problems affecting eyes p. 746)
- Rheumatoid nodules on distal joints

There is a 3mth therapeutic 'window of opportunity' from symptom onset in which treatment can delay disease progression.[4] Any patient with symptoms that might be RA should see GP for onward referral to rheumatology service within 2wks.

Examination and investigation

- Swelling and tenderness of three or more joints
- Positive squeeze test[5]
- If rheumatoid factor negative, test anti-cyclic citrullinated peptide antibodies—↑ specificity in RA
- X-ray the hands and feet early if persistent synovitis

Non-pharmacological management

- Monitor for depression and fatigue
- Exercise for function and strength (swimming recommended) (➔ Exercise p. 354). ⚠ If joints are warm, painful, or swollen, then rest should be recommended.
- Choose cushioned footwear
- Encourage healthy eating (➔ Nutrition and healthy eating p. 342)
- Monitor cardiovascular risk (➔ Coronary heart disease p. 624)
- Immunization for influenza, pneumonia, Hepatitis B (➔ Targeted adult immunization p. 392; ➔ Viral hepatitis p. 724). ⚠ Avoid live vaccines, unless recommended by rheumatologist.
- Attendance for blood tests, X-rays, and ophthalmology appointments
- Be vigilant for skin lesions (e.g. leg ulceration) (➔ Leg ulcer assessment p. 536)
- As required, surgical review to relieve trapped nerves and tendons or for joint replacement
- Physiotherapy review for exercises, joint support, and strapping
- Referral for home modifications (➔ Assistive technology and home adaptations p. 834)
- Expert patient and self-management programmes (➔ Expert patients and self-management programmes p. 340)

Pharmacological management

The basis for pharmacological treatment of RA, other than steroids to dampen down the acute inflammatory response, are drugs known as disease modifying anti-rheumatic drugs (DMARDS). There are 'conventional' DMARDS, which are agents that help to control the disease, have a slow onset of action, and can take up to 3mths to take full effect. If there is not an adequate response, then biological DMARDS or targeted synthetic DMARDS can be used as per local and national guidelines. They are protein-based drugs that target specific immune factors.

References

3. Bykerk, V. & Emery, P. (2010) Delay in receiving rheumatology care leads to long-term harm. *Arthritis & Rheumatology*, 62(12), 3519–21

4. Nishimura, K., Sugiyama, D., Kogata, Y., et al. (2007) Meta-analysis: diagnostic accuracy of anti-cyclic citrullinated peptide antibody and rheumatoid factor for rheumatoid arthritis. *Annals of Internal Medicine*, 146(11), 797–808

5. National Rheumatoid Arthritis Society (2018) *Inflammatory arthritis information pathway.* Available at: https://www.nras.org.uk/1-recognising-symptoms

Further information

Disabled Living Foundation (*Range of daily living equipment*). Available at: ℜ https://www.livingmadeeasy.org.uk/house%20and%20home/kitchen-and-household-2266/

NICE (*Rheumatoid arthritis in adults: management (NG100)*). Available at: ℜ https://www.nice.org.uk/guidance/ng100

Low back pain

Common complaint causing more disability than any other single condition (→ Common musculoskeletal problems p. 734). Low back pain is non-specific, mechanical, musculoskeletal (MSK) and simple back pain. Sciatica involves irritation of the nerve roots (radicular pain) → pain that radiates down buttocks and leg, affected by irritation of sciatic nerve. Guidelines suggest a move away from time-based definitions of acute and chronic back pain to look at low back pain as a whole, where risk of poor outcome at any time point is more important than the duration of symptoms.[6] Causes:

- Postural
- Pregnancy (→ Pregnancy p. 424)
- Prolapsed disc
- Trauma (→ Sprains, strains, and fractures p. 824; → Spinal cord injury p. 518)
- Osteoporosis
- Degenerative joint disease (e.g. osteoarthritis) (→ Osteoarthritis p. 600)
- Spinal cord compression (→ Palliative care emergencies p. 566)
- Carcinoma
- Infection
- Cauda equine syndrome

Red flag symptoms

⚠ Refer in the following circumstances:[7]

- Age of onset <20yrs
- Age of onset >55yrs
- Thoracic pain
- Loss of control of the bowel or bladder (→ Urinary incontinence p. 504; → Faecal incontinence p. 514)
- Weakness or numbness in leg or arm
- Foot drop, disturbed gait
- Fever
- Saddle anaesthesia (numbness of anus, perineum, or genitals)
- History of carcinoma
- Structural deformity

Non-pharmacological management

The Keele STarT Back Screening Tool is a simple prognostic question-naire that helps clinicians identify modifiable factors for back pain disability[8] (→ Standardized assessment tools p. 118). The resulting score stratifies patients into low-, medium-, or high-risk categories. For each category there is a matched treatment package. The overall aim is to improve self-management and manage pain:

- Provide information on low back pain
- Encourage to continue normal activities
- Consider group exercise programmes (→ Exercise p. 354)
- Consider manual therapy (e.g. massage)
- Consider psychological therapies (e.g. cognitive behavioural therapy) (→ Talking therapies p. 472))

- Encourage activities that improve back strength[9]
- Advice on correct lifting techniques
- Use chairs that support lumbar spine, firm mattresses, etc.
- Workplace assessment by occupational health department (→ Health and safety at work p. 92)
- Maintain a healthy weight (→ Nutrition and healthy eating p. 342; → Overweight and obesity p. 348)

Invasive treatments

Patient should see GP and possible orthopaedic/rheumatology referral to assess need for surgery and/or pain clinic if available locally.

Pharmacological management

In the absence of medical intervention, advice may be sought from a community pharmacist. Pharmacological management will usually involve analgesics available OTC.

References

6. NICE (2016) *Low back pain and sciatica in over 16s: assessment and management (NG59).* Available at: https://www.nice.org.uk/guidance/ng59
7. GPOnline (2008) *Red flag symptoms: back pain.* Available at: https://www.gponline.com/red-flag-symptoms-back-pain/musculoskeletal-disorders/article/798743
8. Keele University (undated) *STarT Back Screening Tool online.* Available at: https://www.keele.ac.uk/sbst/startbacktool/
9. Matsuwaka, S. & Liem, B. (2018) The role of exercise in treatment of lumbar spinal stenosis symptoms. *Current Physical and Rehabilitation Reports,* 6(1), 36–44

Measuring lung function

Early identification and management of chronic obstructive pulmonary disease (COPD) (→ Chronic obstructive pulmonary disease p. 614) requires the use of spirometry. The diagnosis and management of asthma requires the use of peak flow meters. Spirometry is also used in asthma diagnosis and management (→ Asthma in children p. 306; → Asthma in adults p. 608).

Spirometry

Measures the volume of air the patient can expel from the lungs after a maximal inspiration:[10] forced expiratory volume–one second (FEV_1) is the volume of air a patient is able to exhale in the first second of forced expiration; forced vital capacity (FVC) is the total volume of air a patient can forcibly exhale in a single breath; and FEV_1/FVC is the ratio of FEV_1 to FVC expressed as a fraction.

Measuring FEV_1 and FVC

Spirometry should only be undertaken by practitioners who have been trained and appropriately assessed as competent.[11]

- Note patient's sex, age, and height so that measurements can be compared with predicted normal values.
- Sit the patient comfortably.
- Ask patient to breathe in as deeply as possible and hold breath long enough to seal lips around mouthpiece.
- If necessary, get patient to pinch nose shut or use nose clips.
- Patient should then breathe out forcibly, as hard and as fast as possible, until there is nothing left to expel (in patients with severe COPD this can take up to 15secs).
- Repeat procedure twice until three readings of which the best two should be within 150mL or 5% of each other. Maximum of eight efforts.

Interpretation

Readings are interpreted against normal values (Table 11.1). Modern spirometers will provide predicted readings based on inputted patient data. If results are borderline normal, then repeat in a few months.[12]

Peak flow

Measures how hard and how quickly a patient can exhale. Used to monitor the progress of disease and effects of treatment for patients with asthma.

Table 11.1 Interpretation of spirometry results

Interpretation of spirometry results		
	Restrictive lung disease (e.g. interstitial lung disease)	Obstructive lung disease (e.g. COPD)
FEV_1 (% of predicted normal)	↓ (<80%)	↓ (<80%)
FVC (% of predicted normal)	↓ (<80%)	Normal or ↓
FEV_1/FVC	Normal (>70%)	↓ (<70%)

Reproduced from Simon, C., Everitt, H., van Dorp, F., & Burkes, M. (2014) Oxford Handbook of General Practice (4e). Oxford: OUP. With permission of Oxford University Press.

Peak flow meters are available on NHS prescription for self-monitoring. Patients with asthma, and all patients with severe asthma, should have an agreed written action plan and their own meter, with regular checks of technique and adherence. They should know when and how to increase their medication and when to seek medical assistance. Asthma action plans can ↓ hospitalization and deaths from asthma.

Measuring peak expiratory flow rate (PEFR)
- Measurement can be undertaken sitting or standing.
- Check indicator is at zero and track clear.
- Get patient to hold peak flow meter horizontally.
- Ask patient to take a deep breath and blow out forcefully into peak flow meter, ensuring lips are sealed firmly around mouthpiece.
- Read rate off the meter.
- Best of three attempts to be recorded.
- Consider using a low-range meter if predicted or best rate is <250L/min.

Interpretation
What is considered normal depends on age, height, and gender. Normal peak flow values charts for adults and children are available online at ℘ http://www.peakflow.com/top_nav/normal_values/index.html

References

10. Global Initiative for Chronic Obstructive Lung Disease (2010) *Spirometry for health care providers*. Available at: https://goldcopd.org/wp-content/uploads/2016/04/GOLD_Spirometry_2010.pdf
11. Association for Respiratory Technology and Physiology (2016) *Improving the quality of diagnostic spirometry in adults: the national register of certified professionals and operators*. Available at: https://arns.co.uk/wp-content/uploads/2016/09/Spirometry-v24.pdf
12. British Thoracic Society COPD Consortium (2005) *Spirometry in practice: a practice guide to using spirometry in primary care* (2nd edn). Available at: https://www.brit-thoracic.org.uk/document-library/delivery-of-respiratory-care/spirometry/spirometry-in-practice-a-practical-guide-(2005)/

Further information

NICE (*Chronic obstructive pulmonary disease in over 16s: diagnosis and management*). Available at: ℘ https://www.nice.org.uk/guidance/NG115
NICE (*Asthma: diagnosis, monitoring and chronic asthma management*). Available at: ℘ https://www.nice.org.uk/guidance/ng80
SIGN (*British guideline on the management of asthma*). Available at: ℘ https://www.sign.ac.uk/assets/sign158.pdf

Asthma in adults

A lung disease, with reversible obstruction of the airways, causing shortness of breath, wheezing, chest tightness, and cough. Characterized by
airflow limitation (usually reversible spontaneously or with treatment),
airway hyper-responsiveness to a wide range of stimuli, and inflammation
of the bronchi. During the asthma attack (🔿 Acute asthma in adults (asthma
attacks) p. 612) muscles in the bronchi contract, the lining swells, becomes
inflamed, and produces excess mucous. If left unchecked, the inflammatory
process → irreversible damage to airways. Asthma is a major cause of hospitalization and asthma attacks can be fatal.

Symptoms

Symptoms consistent with asthma include > one of the following:
- Wheeze
- Breathlessness
- Cough
- Tightness of chest
- Family history of allergies (🔿 Allergies p. 694)
- Unexplained low FEV_1 or PEFR (🔿 Measuring lung function p. 606)

Symptoms are variable, intermittent, worse at night, and provoked by trig-
gers, including:
- Exercise (🔿 Exercise p. 354)
- Household allergens, including house mites and pets
- Emotion (🔿 People with anxiety and depression p. 478)
- Weather (including fog, cold air, thunderstorms) (🔿 Weather extremes
  p. 370)
- Air pollutants (smoke and dust)

Diagnosis

Based on history, clinical examination, and objective testing including spirometry, PEFR variability, or forced exhaled nitric oxide in the breath measurement. Refer for specialist opinion when diagnosis unclear or atypical features.

Difficult to control and severe asthma

- Type 1: Wide PEFR variability (>40% diurnal variation for >50% of time
  over >150 days)
- Type 2: Sudden attacks despite asthma apparently being well controlled

Aims and principles of management

- Control symptoms and impact on everyday life.
- Restore normal or best possible long-term airway function.
- ↓ risk of severe attack.
- ↓ need for reliever medication (🔿 Drugs commonly used in the
  treatment of respiratory conditions p. 620).
- Minimize absence from work.
- Involve patient in active management (🔿 Medicine concordance and
  adherence p. 132).
- Use lowest effective doses of medications, minimizing side effects
  (🔿 Medicines optimization p. 128).

Primary care asthma services

Keep a register of asthma patients to ensure adequate follow-up (➲ General practice p. 18). Recall asthma patients at least annually for review, and after asthma attacks needing accident and emergency (A&E) attention or admission. Follow up anyone who fails to attend for review. Offer services that are flexible and reflect patient preference, e.g. telephone follow-up over clinic attendance. High-quality performance is recognized in Quality and Outcomes Framework (QOF) (➲ Quality and Outcomes Framework p. 74). ⚠ Patients who have had near fatal asthma attacks or severe asthma should always be reviewed by specialists (➲ Teamwork p. 58).

Review and monitoring

- Check and record symptoms and control since last seen; this should incorporate the three Royal College of Physicians' questions[13]
- The patient can complete the asthma control test prior to a booked appointment (🖰 https://www.asthmacontroltest.com/Europe/United%20Kingdom/en)
- Review PEFR
- Check inhaler technique (see following)
- Advise on smoking cessation (➲ Smoking cessation p. 356)
- Influenza vaccination (➲ Targeted adult immunization p. 392)
- Address any other health or psychosocial problems
- Address any problems, education needs, and queries
- Agree management plan and next review date

The medication review (➲ Principles of medication reviews p. 142) component of any review is likely to include: exploring whether the patient is overusing their short-acting beta agonist inhaler (➲ Drugs commonly used in the treatment of respiratory conditions p. 620); the number of occasions they have used oral steroids in the last year; whether they need a steroid card; use of and concordance with inhaled corticosteroids; and considering whether any dose adjustments are required to find the lowest dose to control symptoms.

Pharmacological management

See ➲ Drugs commonly used in the treatment of respiratory conditions p. 620. Follow local, national, and international guidelines for therapeutic drug regimens.

Self-management

In addition to tailored verbal and written education, all patients should be given a personal action plan. This should include information related to: prescribed treatment; areas where patient most wants improvement; recognizing and managing acute exacerbations; what to do if they have an asthma attack (e.g. when to ☎ 999 and request an ambulance (➲ Acute asthma in adults (asthma attacks) p. 612)); and allergen or trigger avoidance. Self-management will often include home monitoring of PEFR. Patients should have a patient-held record of asthma reviews (➲ Client- and patient-held records p. 90).

Secondary non-pharmacological prophylaxis

- Smoking cessation by patient and household members
- Weight reduction in obese patients to improve asthma control
  (→ Overweight and obesity p. 348; → Nutrition and healthy eating p. 342)
- Breathing exercises

Inhaler technique

The most effective inhaler is one that the patient is able to use. Inadequate technique may be mistaken for drug failure. Types of inhaler include: pressurized metered dose inhalers, breath-activated inhalers (metered dose inhalers and dry-powder inhalers), and inhalers with spacer devices. Asthma UK provide a number of short videos demonstrating proper inhaler technique (⅊ https://www.asthma.org.uk/advice/inhaler-videos/). Patients should be told explicitly of dose, frequency, and maximum number of inhalations in 24hrs in action plan. Check technique at each review.

Related topics

- → Expert patients and self-management programmes p. 340; → Asthma in children p. 306)

Reference

13. Thomas, M., Gruffydd-Jones, K., Stonham C., et al. (2009) Assessing asthma control in routine clinical practice: use of the Royal College of Physicians '3 Questions'. *Primary Care Respiratory Journal*, 18(2), 83–8

Further information

NICE (*Asthma: diagnosis, monitoring and chronic asthma management*). Available at: ⅊ https://www.nice.org.uk/guidance/ng80
SIGN (*British guideline on the management of asthma*). Available at: ⅊ https://www.sign.ac.uk/assets/sign158.pdf

Acute asthma in adults (asthma attacks)

Nurses in all settings should offer patient and carer education in managing acute asthma and asthma attacks (◆ Asthma in adults p. 608). Many deaths are preventable and delay can be fatal.

Recognition

⚠ Patients with severe life-threatening attacks may not appear distressed and may not have all the characteristic abnormalities of severe asthma. Signs that someone may be having an asthma attack include:

- Their asthma is getting worse (e.g. they are coughing or wheezing more than usual, feel more breathless, or chest feels tighter).
- They cannot breathe well and find it hard to talk, eat, or sleep.
- Their reliever inhaler is not helping as much as usual (◆ Drugs commonly used in the treatment of respiratory conditions p. 620).
- They need to use their reliever inhaler more often than usual.
- Their peak flow score is lower than normal (◆ Measuring lung function p. 606).

Asthma attacks do not usually happen suddenly; patients will notice asthma getting worse over several hours or days before the attack. Their asthma plan should advise them to seek help in such circumstances.

General guidance

See ◆ Drugs commonly used in the treatment of respiratory conditions p. 620. Follow local, national, and international guidelines for therapeutic drug regimens. Patients diagnosed with asthma should have written guidance in their action plan on what to do in the event of an acute exacerbation. General guidance to patients is:

- Take one or two puffs of reliever inhaler immediately, preferably using a spacer.
- Sit down (do not lie down), rest your hands on your knees to help support yourself, and try to slow down your breathing, as this will make you less exhausted.
- If condition is stable or improving, wait 5–10min.
- If symptoms disappear, you should be able to go back to whatever you were doing.
- If you do not start to feel better, continue to take two puffs (one at a time) of your reliever inhaler every 2min. Take up to ten puffs.
- If the reliever has no effect, ☎ 999 and request ambulance.
- Continue to take reliever inhaler every few minutes until help arrives.

⚠ This general guidance does not apply to those on MART (maintenance and reliever therapy) or SMART (symbicort maintenance and reliever therapy). These patients will get personalized exacerbation management advice.

Life-threatening asthma

In a patient with severe asthma, any one of:

- Peak expiratory flow rate <33% best or predicted
- Peripheral capillary O_2 saturation <92%

- Silent chest
- Cyanosis
- Poor respiratory effort
- Arrhythmia
- Exhaustion, altered conscious level
- Hypotension

⚠ ☏ 999 and request ambulance immediately

Risk factors for fatal or near-fatal asthma attacks

- Previous admission, especially if within 1yr
- Requires three or more classes of asthma medication
- Heavy use of beta-2 agonists
- Repeated attendance at A&E for asthma care
- Severe asthma
- Asthma poorly treated and monitored, does not have written action plans, failure to return for review, etc.
- Psychosocial problems (e.g. psychosis (**➲** People with psychosis p. 486), depression (**➲** People with anxiety and depression p. 478), and alcohol (**➲** Alcohol p. 360) or drug misuse (**➲** Substance use p. 476))
- Learning difficulties (**➲** People with learning disabilities p. 456), employment problems, income problems, social isolation, and domestic (**➲** Domestic violence p. 450), marital, or legal stress.

Related topics

- **➲** Asthma in children p. 306

Further information

NICE (*Asthma: diagnosis, monitoring and chronic asthma management*). Available at: ๛ https://www.nice.org.uk/guidance/ng80

SIGN (*British guideline on the management of asthma*). Available at: ๛ https://www.sign.ac.uk/assets/sign158.pdf

Chronic obstructive pulmonary disease

COPD is a term used to describe a number of conditions, including chronic bronchitis and emphysema. Predominantly caused by smoking and characterized by airflow obstruction (reduced FEV_1 and reduced FEV_1/FVC ratio, measured by spirometry) that is not fully reversible and is progressive over time (➔ Measuring lung function p. 606). Diagnosis relies on a combination of history, physical examination, and confirmation of airflow obstruction using spirometry. Exacerbations may occur, when there is a rapid and sustained worsening of the patient's symptoms beyond normal day-to-day variation (➔ Management of stable chronic obstructive pulmonary disease p. 616; ➔ Management of chronic obstructive pulmonary disease exacerbation p. 618).

Advanced lung destruction causes respiratory failure, i.e. disorder of such an extent that not meeting metabolic requirements. Other consequences include cor pulmonale, right-sided heart failure (➔ Heart failure p. 636), and oedema. Breathlessness can be very frightening. Patients can be very anxious and restrict activities, setting up a vicious cycle leading to further restrictions. Often also → depression (➔ People with anxiety and depression p. 478).

Indications for a diagnosis to be considered

- >40yrs
- Dyspnoea +/− exertion (Table 11.2)
- Smoker or ex-smoker (➔ Smoking cessation p. 356)
- Chronic cough, especially if producing sputum
- Recurrent lower respiratory tract infections, especially in winter
- Wheeze (controversy exists as to whether wheeze is an indicator)

Severity of airflow limitations

- Mild: cough most days, breathlessness when hurrying or walking up incline, minimal use of services, usually one exacerbation/yr, no hospitalization, FEV_1 ≥80% predicted
- Moderate: breathlessness, cough and sputum most days, stop to catch breath on level, known to GP, usually one exacerbation/yr, no hospitalization, FEV_1 50–79% predicted

Table 11.2 Medical Research Council dyspnoea scale

Grade	Degree of breathlessness related to activities
1	Not troubled by breathlessness except on strenuous exercise
2	Short of breath when hurrying or walking up a slight hill
3	Walks slower than contemporaries on level ground because of breathlessness, or has to stop for breath when walking at own pace
4	Stops for breath after walking about 100m or after a few minutes on level ground
5	Too breathless to leave the house, or breathless when dressing or undressing

- Severe: similar symptoms to 'moderate' but more frequent exacerbations or requires hospital treatment, FEV_1 30–49% predicted
- Very severe: breathless at rest, severe impact on activities of daily living, life-threatening exacerbations, very well-known to services, FEV_1 <30%

Further reading

Global Initiative for Chronic Obstructive Lung Disease (*Pocket guide to COPD diagnosis, management, and prevention*). Available at: https://goldcopd.org/wp-content/uploads/2018/11/GOLD-2019-POCKET-GUIDE-FINAL_WMS.pdf

NICE (*Chronic obstructive pulmonary disease in over 16s: diagnosis and management*). Available at: https://www.nice.org.uk/guidance/ng115

Management of stable chronic obstructive pulmonary disease

Lung damage cannot be repaired, but the symptoms and their impact can be managed. On diagnosis, patient should be coded on GP patient records (➔ General practice p. 18) and added to practice COPD register as per QOF (➔ Quality and outcomes framework p. 74). Baseline spirometry readings (➔ Measuring lung function p. 606), dyspnoea scale (➔ Management of chronic obstructive pulmonary disease exacerbation p. 618), and BMI should be recorded (➔ Adult body mass index chart p. 346). See ➔ Drugs commonly used in the treatment of respiratory conditions p. 620. Follow local, national, and international guidelines for therapeutic drug regimens.

Non-pharmacological management

- Smoking cessation: offer help to quit at every consultation (➔ Smoking cessation p. 356)
- Offer pneumococcal and seasonal influenza vaccination (➔ Targeted adult immunization p. 392)
- Weight reduction if BMI >25 (➔ Nutrition and healthy eating p. 342; ➔ Overweight and obesity p. 348)
- Enhanced calories in food and nutritional supplements if BMI <18.5 (➔ Malnutrition p. 350)
- Ensure good inhaler technique
- Referral for pulmonary rehabilitation
- Advice on action to take in an exacerbation
- Provide advice and support on living with COPD
- Referral to expert patient and self-management support groups (➔ Expert patients and self-management programmes p. 340)

Pulmonary rehabilitation

- Shown to ↓ dyspnoea, improve quality of life, and ↓ disability and use of health services irrespective of age, impairment, or smoking status. Usually, a 6wk programme led by specialist and therapy services. Includes aerobic exercise (➔ Exercise p. 354), always of lower extremities (brisk walking, cycling), and may include upper extremities. Often includes educational programme and opportunity for tailored advice on smoking cessation, nutrition, and minimizing impact on ADL and physical relationships etc.

Regular review and follow-up

Review people with mild/moderate COPD at least annually, and those with severe COPD every 6mths (Box 11.2) (➔ Principles of medication reviews p. 142). Accurate COPD registers support regular review and follow-up. People with stable severe COPD do not normally need regular hospital review, but there should be locally agreed mechanisms to allow rapid hospital assessment when necessary.

Box 11.2 Guidance on review and follow-up consultations

Mild/moderate chronic obstructive pulmonary disease (COPD)

Measurements include:

- FEV_1 and FVC
- BMI
- Medical Research Council (MRC) dyspnoea score

Assessments include:

- Smoking status/desire to quit
- Adequacy of symptom control
- Breathlessness
- Exercise tolerance
- Exacerbation frequency
- Presence of complications
- Effects of each drug treatment
- Inhaler technique
- Need for referral to specialist and therapy services and pulmonary rehabilitation

Severe chronic obstructive pulmonary disease (COPD)

Measurements include:

- FEV_1 and FVC
- BMI
- MRC dyspnoea score
- O_2 saturation of arterial blood

Assessments include:

- Smoking status/desire to quit
- Adequacy of symptom control
- Breathlessness
- Exercise tolerance
- Exacerbation frequency
- Presence of cor pulmonale
- Need for long-term O_2 therapy
- Nutritional state
- Depression
- Effects of each drug treatment
- Inhaler technique
- Need for referral to specialist and therapy services (including social services) and pulmonary rehabilitation

Further information

Global Initiative for Chronic Obstructive Lung Disease (*Pocket guide to COPD diagnosis, management, and prevention*). Available at: ℅ https://goldcopd.org/wp-content/uploads/2018/11/GOLD-2019-POCKET-GUIDE-FINAL_WMS.pdf

NICE (*Chronic obstructive pulmonary disease in over 16s: diagnosis and management*). Available at: ℅ https://www.nice.org.uk/guidance/ng115

Management of chronic obstructive pulmonary disease exacerbation

An exacerbation is defined as an acute worsening of respiratory symptoms from a stable state to one or more of the following:

• ↑ dyspnoea, use of accessory muscles at rest, pursed lip breathing
• ↑ sputum (or infected sputum)
• ↑ fluid retention
• ↑ wheeze, cough, or sore throat
• ↓ exercise tolerance (➲ Exercise p. 354)
• ↑ difficulty performing ADL
• ↑ fatigue
• Tight chest
• Acute confusion

Most common cause is respiratory infections, followed by pollutants. See ➲ Drugs commonly used in the treatment of respiratory conditions p. 620. Follow local, national, and international guidelines for therapeutic drug regimens.

Self-management of exacerbations

All patients with COPD diagnosis (➲ Chronic obstructive pulmonary disease p. 614) to be provided with a written management plan. This should include information on actions to take on identifying an exacerbation. Patients should respond quickly. At review/follow-up they may have been prescribed a 'rescue pack' containing antibiotics and oral corticosteroids. Standard advice: start oral corticosteroids if dyspnoea interferes with usual activities (unless contraindicated); start antibiotics if sputum purulent or other signs of infection; and adjust bronchodilator therapy to control symptoms (may use nebulizer). Advice should include when to contact health professional if symptoms do not improve in a specified timescale.

Referral to hospital

Decide whether to manage at home or refer to hospital based on severity, comorbidity, ability to cope at home, and availability of other services (e.g. rapid response team) (➲ Services to prevent unplanned hospital admission p. 22; ➲ Teamwork p. 58). Local care pathways inform decision making (Table 11.3). If treated at home, may require pulse oximetry to establish blood O_2 saturation levels if severe dyspnoea. Decide on optimum therapy, review, and referral to other services/therapies as appropriate.

Related topics

➲ Measuring lung function p. 606; ➲ Expert patients and self-management programmes p. 340; ➲ Management of stable chronic obstructive pulmonary disease p. 616

Table 11.3 Factors to consider when managing a chronic obstructive pulmonary disease (COPD) patient with acute exacerbation

Factor	Favours treatment at home	Favours treatment in hospital
Able to cope at home	Yes	No
Breathlessness	Mild	Severe
General condition	Good	Poor/deteriorating
Level of activity	Good	Poor/confined to bed
Cyanosis	No	Yes
Worsening peripheral oedema	No	Yes
Level of consciousness	Normal	Impaired
Already receiving long-term O_2 therapy	No	Yes
Social circumstances	Good	Living alone/not coping
Acute confusion	No	Yes
Rapid rate of onset	No	Yes
Significant comorbidity (particularly cardiac disease and diabetes)	No	Yes
O_2 saturation <90%	No	Yes
Changes on the chest radiograph	No	Present

Further reading

Global Initiative for Chronic Obstructive Pulmonary Disease (*Pocket guide to COPD diagnosis, management, and prevention*). Available at: ℘ https://goldcopd.org/wp-content/uploads/2018/11/GOLD-2019-POCKET-GUIDE-FINAL_WMS.pdf

NICE (*Chronic obstructive pulmonary disease in over 16s: diagnosis and management*). Available at: ℘ https://www.nice.org.uk/guidance/ng115

Drugs commonly used in the treatment of respiratory conditions

This section will give an overview of how drugs commonly used to treat asthma (◆ Asthma in adults p. 608; ◆ Asthma in children p. 306; ◆ Acute asthma in adults (asthma attacks) p. 612) and COPD (◆ Chronic obstructive pulmonary disease p. 614; ◆ Management of stable chronic obstructive pulmonary disease p. 616; ◆ Management of chronic obstructive pulmonary disease exacerbation p. 618) work. The purpose of having this level of understanding is that predicted benefits and potential side effects can be understood (◆ Medicines optimization p. 128). There are local, national, and international guidelines for the treatment of respiratory diseases and these should be taken into account when an individual's treatment plan is devised. The respiratory drugs can be divided into two main categories: those that help to relieve symptoms (the bronchodilators) and those that ↓ the inflammatory process (anti-inflammatory agents).

Bronchodilators

Sympathomimetic agents (beta-2 adrenergic agonists)

This group copies the sympathetic nervous system which acts on the beta-2 adrenoreceptors in the lungs and therefore dilates the bronchi by relaxing the smooth muscle in the airway. Because these agents act on the sympathetic nervous system (the 'fight or flight' response), they can also have the side effects of tachycardia, arrhythmias, palpitations (◆ Abnormal cardiac rhythms p. 640), fine tremor, and headache. Sympathomimetic agents are grouped under headings related to their duration of action: short-acting inhaled beta-2 agonists (SABAs) (e.g. salbutamol or terbutaline); and long-acting beta-2 agonists (LABAs) (e.g. salmeterol or formoterol).

Anticholinergics

The parasympathetic nervous system is the opposite to the sympathetic nervous system, and is considered to be the 'resting and digesting' response. Therefore, parasympathetic stimulation causes bronchial constriction and mucus secretion. To aid with bronchodilation, anticholinergics will block any parasympathetic stimulation at the muscarinic receptors. Again, they are grouped by their duration of action: short-acting muscarinic antagonists (SAMAs) (e.g. ipratropium bromide); and long-acting muscarinic antagonists (LAMs) (e.g. tiotropium).

Xanthine drugs

These have two distinct actions in the airways of patients with reversible obstruction: smooth muscle relaxation (i.e. bronchodilation) and suppression of the response of the airways to stimuli. These drugs include theophylline and aminophylline. They have a narrow therapeutic index and need regular monitoring and dose titration. Side effects include arrhythmias, central nervous system stimulation, and gastric irritation.

Anti-inflammatory

Corticosteroids

Act to mimic the actions of cortisol in the body. Anti-inflammatory effects ↓ bronchial hyperactivity, reducing numbers of macrophages in the airway, reducing mucus secretion. Common inhaled steroids include beclomethasone, budesonide, and fluticasone. Although 10–25% of the drugs are deposited in the airways, the remainder either stays at the back of the throat or is swallowed. More common side effects include hoarseness, loss of voice, and oral candidiasis (→ Fungal infections p. 686; → Mouth and throat problems p. 698), often avoided by rinsing the mouth after use and using a spacer device. If a patient needs high doses of inhaled corticosteroids, then a steroid card will be needed.

Sodium cromoglycate

Used as prophylactic agents. Inhibit the activation of many of the cell types involved in the development and progression of asthma. Inhibit the release of inflammatory mediators including cytokines from mast cells and ↓ the chemotactic activity of eosinophils and neutrophils. A benefit for those with asthma with an allergic basis. Side effects include headache, throat irritation, dyspepsia, and nausea (→ Dyspepsia, gastro-oesophageal reflux disease, and peptic ulceration p. 708).

Leukotriene receptor antagonists

Block the formation of leukotrienes from arachidonic acid, which is part of the body's response to inflammation, preventing bronchoconstriction and airway inflammation. An example is montelukast. Side effects include headache and gastrointestinal disturbance.

Long-term oxygen therapy

O_2 is a prescription-only (→ Prescribing p. 136) therapy for individuals with hypoxaemia (↓ blood oxygen levels). Appropriate O_2 use can prolong and enhance life, and ↓ hospitalization; however, it will not relieve breathlessness symptoms. Inappropriate use of O_2 is potentially life-threatening due to respiratory depression. ⚠ O_2 is combustible/explosive near naked flames and cigarettes (→ Smoking cessation p. 356). Inform patients and carers of risks and strongly advise not to smoke nor use E-cigarettes near O_2 supply. Also need to avoid petroleum-based emollients.

Long-term oxygen therapy (LTOT) should only be prescribed after assessment by a respiratory specialist (England, Wales, and Scotland). In Northern Ireland, either GP or specialist. Review at least 1yrly (→ Principles of medication reviews p. 142). In some areas, LTOT will not be prescribed if anyone smokes in the house.

Patients with COPD (→ Chronic obstructive pulmonary disease p. 614) and the following presentations may benefit from LTOT:[14]

- Very severe airflow obstruction (FEV_1 <30% predicted) (consider following assessment in patients with severe airflow obstruction (FEV_1 30–49% predicted) (→ Measuring lung function p. 606)
- Cyanosis
- Polycythaemia
- Peripheral oedema
- Raised jugular venous pressure
- O_2 saturations ≤92% breathing air

Ambulatory O_2 therapy

Prescribed for patients:[15]

- On LTOT who need to be away from home on a regular basis
- Not on LTOT if evidence of exercise-induced O_2 desaturation

  Specialist assessment necessary to determine need and flow rate.

O_2 services

Companies in UK provide home O_2 services for the NHS, each covering certain geographical areas. All hold contracts with the NHS (→ Commissioning of services p. 12). Arrangements can be made to have O_2 supplied to holiday destinations in England or Wales. The British Lung Foundation (BLF) website has advice on travelling with a lung condition.[16]

References

14. NICE (2010) *Chronic obstructive pulmonary disease in over 16s: diagnosis and management (NG115)*. Available at: https://www.nice.org.uk/guidance/ng115
15. NICE (2018) *Treatment summary: oxygen*. Available at: https://bnf.nice.org.uk/treatment-summary/oxygen.html
16. BLF (2018) *Going on holiday*. Available at: https://www.blf.org.uk/support-for-you/going-on-holiday

Nebulizers

Convert a prescribed drug solution into a continuous fine aerosol mist, inhaled by tidal breathing over 5–10min directly into the lungs. Patients advised not to use more frequently than prescribed or change dosage. Many patients can get the same effect by taking four to six puffs from a metered dose inhaler with a spacer. Indications for use:

- Acute exacerbations of acute asthma (➔ Asthma in adults p. 608; ➔ Asthma in children p. 306; ➔ Acute asthma in adults (asthma attacks) p. 612) and COPD (➔ Chronic obstructive pulmonary disease p. 614; ➔ Management of stable chronic obstructive pulmonary disease p. 616; ➔ Management of chronic obstructive pulmonary disease exacerbations p. 618)
- Long-term bronchodilator treatment in asthma and COPD to those shown to benefit from higher medication doses (usually after 2wk trial) (➔ Drugs commonly used in the treatment of respiratory conditions p. 620)
- When patient unable to use other inhalation devices
- Delivery of antibiotics for cystic fibrosis (➔ Cystic fibrosis p. 318) and bronchiectasis
- Delivery of pentamidine for 2° prophylaxis of pneumocystis pneumonia (➔ Pneumonia p. 750)
- Palliation of breathlessness or cough in end-of-life care (➔ Breathlessness in palliative care p. 560)

Equipment

There are four parts: face mask/mouthpiece, nebulizer chamber for the drug solution, tubing to connect to the compressor, and O_2 to drive the nebulizer chamber. Mask usually recommended method but mouthpieces may be useful for hypertonic solution in bronchiectasis or if eye irritation occurs. Most nebulizer machines are provided through respiratory services but some may require private purchase. You should always follow the instructions from the manufacturer. Chamber and masks/mouthpieces should be washed in warm soapy water after each use or at least daily. They should be rinsed and dried; 10secs of air must be blown through the system before further use to blow out any water droplets. Check manufacturer guidelines for frequency of changing masks/mouthpieces. The tubing must be kept dry and changed every 3–4mths and the compressor should be serviced yearly, and filters changed according to manufacturer's instructions. ⚠ Some patients purchase their own machines privately and, in these situations, they are responsible for ensuring maintenance, servicing, and provision of parts. In some areas, NHS prescriptions for nebulizers can only be issued to patients who have been assessed for a nebulizer by the 2° care team.

Further information

British Lung Foundation (*Nebulisers*). Available at: ℛ https://www.blf.org.uk/sites/default/files/IS16_Nebulisers_v3_2015_pdf%20download.pdf

Coronary heart disease

Sometimes called ischaemic heart disease. Describes a range of conditions including stroke (➲ Recognizing and responding to a stroke p. 830), myocardial infarction (MI)/angina (➲ Angina p. 626), hypercholesterolaemia (➲ Hypercholesterolaemia p. 632), hypertension (➲ Hypertension p. 628), and heart failure (➲ Heart failure p. 636). Coronary heart disease (CHD) is the leading cause of death in the UK and worldwide. Most deaths occur due to MI as a result of CHD. Atherosclerosis occurs when blood flow is reduced or blocked by build-up of atheroma (fatty deposits) and sclerosis (↓ elasticity) in coronary arteries.

Risk factors

Non-modifiable
- Socioeconomic status: lower status ↑ risk
- Age: risk ↑ with age
- Family history of CHD, diabetes, hypercholesterolaemia, or hypertension
- ↓ birthweight
- Ethnicity: e.g. Indian subcontinent ↑ risk
- Gender: ♂ are more likely to develop CHD at an earlier age than ♀

Modifiable
- Smoking (➲ Smoking cessation p. 356)
- Hypertension
- Hyperlipidaemia
- Diabetes (➲ Diabetes: overview p. 660; ➲ Principles of diabetes management p. 664)
- Diet (➲ Nutrition and healthy eating p. 342)
- Obesity (➲ Overweight and obesity p. 348)

Primary prevention

Calculating risk
Attempts to reduce a person's overall risk of developing cardiovascular disease (CVD) and CHD. Risk of developing CVD can be calculated using QRISK®3 (or ASSIGN in Scotland). A new version of QRISK® is produced annually to take account of changes in population characteristics etc. Check ⌘ https://qrisk.org/.

Prevention
- Smoking cessation
- Promoting healthy eating
- Taking regular exercise (➲ Exercise p. 354)
- Controlling weight and/or reducing obesity
- Controlling high BP
- Controlling raised cholesterol
- Controlling blood sugar in diabetes
- Managing stress (➲ People with anxiety and depression p. 478)
- Alcohol within recommended limits (➲ Alcohol p. 360)

Secondary prevention

Almost half of people who die from a MI are already known to have CHD. Targeting people with CHD for risk-factor modification is effective in ↓ risk of recurrent CHD.

For drugs commonly used in the treatment of CHD, see ◐ Drugs commonly used in the prevention and treatment of cardiovascular disease p. 646. Follow local and national guidelines for therapeutic drug regimens.

Management and treatment can be jointly managed between nurse and doctor (◐ Teamwork p. 58). Focus on:

- Register of patients (◐ General practice p. 18) at risk and follow up (as per QOF) (◐ Quality and Outcomes Framework p. 74)
- Providing information on how to modify risk factors (see above)
- Drug treatment and medicines optimization (◐ Principles of medication reviews p. 142; ◐ Medicines optimization p. 128)
- Blood sugar control if diabetic

Not all people need referral to a cardiologist; depends on previous history and symptoms.

Further information

NICE (*CVD risk assessment and management*). Available at: ℘ https://cks.nice.org.uk/cvd-risk-assessment-and-management#!topicsummary

Angina

Angina pectoris is the classic presentation of chest pain and is due to transient myocardial ischaemia. CHD is the most common cause (❷ Coronary heart disease p. 624). Less commonly, angina is caused by valve disease (e.g. aortic stenosis), hypertrophic obstructive cardiomyopathy, or hypertensive heart disease (❷ Hypertension p. 628). Typically caused by exertion (❷ Exercise p. 354) or emotion (❷ People with anxiety and depression p. 478), and relieved by rest. Incidence is ↑ in ♂ than in ♀, and ↑ with age. Unstable angina is angina that has become worse—symptoms develop during different (or less of same) activities, or symptoms develop at rest. This can be difficult to differentiate from MI and both together are classed as acute coronary syndrome.

Symptoms of stable angina

Typical angina presents with all three of the following features: precipitated by physical exertion; constricting discomfort in the front of the chest, in the neck, shoulders, jaw, or arms; and relieved by rest or glyceryl trinitrate (GTN) within about 5mins. Atypical angina presents with two of the aforementioned features. In addition, atypical symptoms include gastrointestinal discomfort, and/or breathlessness, and/or nausea.

⚠ Always consider possibility of MI if:
- Chest pain occurs at rest
- Discomfort lasts longer than 15mins
- Associated with nausea/vomiting, sweating, or breathlessness

If MI or acute coronary syndrome suspected, refer to hospital immediately.

Assessment

- What precipitates attack, e.g. exertion, cold weather (❷ Weather extremes p. 370), large meals, stress
- Past medical history and family history, including of CHD
- Lifestyle, e.g. smoking (❷ Smoking cessation p. 356), alcohol intake (❷ Alcohol p. 360), and drug history (❷ Substance use p. 476)
- Dietary assessment and the possibility of gastro-oesophageal reflux (❷ Dyspepsia, gastro-oesophageal reflux disease, and peptic ulceration p. 708)

Clinical examination

- Cardiorespiratory assessment (including assessment for heart murmurs, arrhythmias (❷ Abnormal cardiac rhythms p. 640), and oedema)
- Evidence of anaemia (❷ Anaemia in adults p. 652), hypercholesterolaemia (❷ Hypercholesterolaemia p. 632), and vascular disease
- BP (❷ Hypertension p. 628)
- Pulse (rate and rhythm)
- BMI (❷ Adult body mass index chart p. 346)

Investigations

Follow local protocols for diagnostic testing and referral. Arrange blood tests to identify conditions which exacerbate angina (e.g. anaemia), coronary angiography, and 12-lead electrocardiogram (ECG) (➐ Recording a 12-lead electrocardiogram p. 584).

Management and treatment of stable angina

For drugs commonly used in the treatment of angina, see ➐ Drugs commonly used in the prevention and treatment of cardiovascular disease p. 646. Follow local and national guidelines for therapeutic drug regimens.

Non-pharmacological management
- Advice and support on modifiable risk factors
- Advice and support on pacing activities, impact of stress and anxiety, physical exertion including sexual activity
- Education about angina and heart attacks (Box 11.3)
- Cardiac rehabilitation may be helpful for patients with severe angina and after surgery (➐ Cardiac rehabilitation p. 634)
- All patients should be referred for an exercise tolerance test
- Patients who drive lorries, buses, or coaches must inform DVLA
- If job requires physical labour, involve occupational health departments (➐ Health and safety at work p. 92)

⚠ If angina worsens, occurs on minimal exertion, at rest, or nocturnally, or is more frequent and with persistent pain that lasts longer than 15mins, patient at ↑ risk of MI and needs urgent hospital admission.

Unstable angina

Management is the same as for stable angina, with consideration for revascularization (coronary artery bypass grafting or percutaneous coronary intervention) if appropriate and not contraindicated.

Box 11.3 Advice for patients prescribed GTN medication

If you have symptoms consistent with angina:
- Stop what you are doing, sit down and rest.
- Take your GTN medication as prescribed.
- Take another dose after 5mins if the first does not help.

⚠ If the pain does not ease within a few minutes after your second dose, call 999 immediately.

- If you are not allergic to aspirin, take 300mg. If none available, or unsure if you are allergic to aspirin, rest until ambulance arrives.

Related topics

➐ Heart failure p. 636; ➐ Adult basic life support and automated external defibrillation p. 792

Further information

NICE (*Stable angina: management [CG126]*). Available at: ✆ https://www.nice.org.uk/guidance/cg126

NICE (*Angina*). Available at: ✆ https://cks.nice.org.uk/angina

Hypertension

In people without diabetes, hypertension is defined as a clinic blood pressure of ≥140/90mmHg and ambulatory blood pressure monitoring (APBM) daytime average or home blood pressure monitoring (HBPM) average of ≥135/85mmHg. Hypertension produces no symptoms, and is often picked up at routine screening. Occasionally, patient may complain of headache or visual disturbance.

Risk factors

Non-modifiable
- Age: risk ↑ with age
- Family history
- Ethnicity: e.g. African/African–Caribbean and South Asian at ↑ risk

Modifiable
- Smoking (→ Smoking cessation p. 356)
- Hypercholesterolaemia (→ Hypercholesterolaemia p. 632)
- Diabetes (→ Diabetes: overview p. 660; → Principles of diabetes management p. 664)
- Diet: ↑ risk with ↑ salt intake (→ Nutrition and healthy eating p. 342)
- Obesity (→ Overweight and obesity p. 348)

Severity

- Stage 1: clinic BP ≥140/90mmHg, and subsequent ABPM daytime average or HBPM average BP ≥135/85mmHg
- Stage 2: clinic BP ≥160/100mmHg, and subsequent ABPM daytime average or HBPM average BP ≥150/95mmHg
- Severe hypertension: clinic systolic BP ≥180mmHg, or clinic diastolic BP ≥120mmHg

BP measurement

- Regularly maintain and calibrate sphygmomanometer.
- Best practice is for manual sphygmomanometers.
- Always use manual sphygmomanometers if irregular pulse present (→ Abnormal cardiac rhythms p. 640).
- If using automated BP monitoring device, ensure it is validated, take at least two readings, and use lowest reading.
- Use a cuff of correct width (check manufacturer's instructions).
- Provide a relaxed, temperate setting to ↓ the 'white-coat' effect.
- Seat the patient with arm rested at the level of the heart.
- Measure BP to nearest 2mmHg.
- Measure diastolic pressure when sounds completely disappear.
- Measure BP in both arms. If the difference in readings is ≥15mmHg, repeat measurements. If difference in readings between arms remains >15mmHg, measure subsequent BP in arm with higher reading.
- If BP measured in clinic is ≥140/90mmHg, take a second measurement during consultation. If second measurement is substantially different from first, take third measurement. Record lower of the last two measurements as the clinic blood pressure
- If the clinic BP is 140/90mmHg–180/120mmHg, offer ABPM (or HBPM if not tolerated) to confirm diagnosis of hypertension.

⚠ Same-day referral if patient has:
- BP ≥180/120mmHg with signs of papilloedema and/or retinal haemorrhage
- Life-threatening symptoms such as new-onset confusion, chest pain, signs of heart failure, or acute kidney injury
- Suspected pheochromocytoma (labile or postural hypotension, headache, palpitations, pallor, and diaphoresis)

Consider referral in people with signs and symptoms suggesting a 2° cause of hypertension (➡ Teamwork p. 58).

Postural hypotension

In people with symptoms of postural hypotension (falls or postural dizziness):
- Measure BP with the person either supine or seated. Measure BP again with person standing for at least 1min prior to measurement.
- If the systolic BP falls by 20mmHg or more when person is standing, consider GP for possible referral to specialist care.

Investigations

- Calculate QRISK® (➡ Coronary heart disease p. 624)
- Urinalysis for proteinuria and haematuria
- Fasting glucose
- Electrolytes
- Creatinine
- Estimated glomerular filtration rate
- Serum total cholesterol and high-density lipoprotein (HDL) cholesterol
- 12-lead ECG (➡ Recording a 12-lead electrocardiogram p. 584)
- Examine fundi for hypertensive retinopathy

Drug treatment

For drugs commonly used in the treatment of hypertension, see ➡ Drugs commonly used in the prevention and treatment of cardiovascular disease p. 646. Follow local and national guidelines for therapeutic drug regimens. The threshold for initiating pharmacological treatment for people with diabetes is likely to be lower than for those without. ⚠ Always refer patients with severe hypertension to the GP for immediate treatment.

General practice nurse follow-up and hypertension clinics

Aim
- Monitor and treat people with hypertension
- ↓ the risk of related cardiovascular morbidity and mortality
- Identify risk factors and offer personalized advice and management

Management
- Review alcohol consumption (➡ Alcohol p. 360)
- Discourage excessive consumption of coffee/caffeine-rich products
- Encourage low or substitute sodium salt intake
- Smoking cessation advice
- Relaxation therapies can ↓ BP

- Advice on exercise and links to local initiatives, e.g. walking groups
  (➔ Exercise p. 354)
- Referral to expert patient and self-management groups (➔ Expert
  patients and self-management programmes p. 340)

Control BP to:
- <140/90mmHg for adults <80yrs
- <150/90mmHg for adults >80yrs (use clinical judgement for people
  with frailty (➔ Frailty p. 678) or multimorbidity)

Once BP controlled, regular monitoring at 3–6mthly intervals and yearly: re-
calculation of CVD risk, BP check, blood tests, and medication review
(➔ Principles of medication reviews p. 142). Maintain register for call and
recall of patients (➔ General practice p. 18) with hypertension as per QOF
(➔ Quality and Outcomes Framework p. 74).

Further information

NICE (*Hypertension in adults: diagnosis and management [NG136]*). Available at: ℘ https://www.
nice.org.uk/guidance/ng136/

Hypercholesterolaemia

Cholesterol is a fatty substance produced by the liver and cells. Vital role in cell membrane function. ↓ in cholesterol is beneficial in 1° and 2° prevention of cardiovascular disease (CVD) (Ɔ Coronary heart disease p. 624; Ɔ Angina p. 626; Ɔ Heart failure p. 636). A target cholesterol level of <5mmol/L is recommended.

Definitions

Low-density lipoprotein cholesterol (LDL)
- Atheroma-forming
- High levels associated with ↑ risk of CVD

High-density lipoprotein cholesterol (HDL)
- High levels protect against CVD
- ↓ levels associated with ↑ risk of CVD

Triglycerides
- Independent risk factor for CVD
- If >10mmol/L, refer to specialist

Non high-density lipoprotein cholesterol (non-HDL)
Combination of triglycerides, LDL, and other forms of cholesterol associated with atheroma formation. Calculated by subtracting HDL from total cholesterol.

Total cholesterol to HDL ratio
Used to predict risk. ↑ risk if ≥6mmol/L

Hypercholesterolaemia
Often referred to as high/raised cholesterol. An elevation of total cholesterol and/or non-HDL cholesterol in the blood.

Hyperlipidaemia
The elevation of triglycerides in the blood in the absence of hypercholesterolaemia, often found with abdominal obesity (Ɔ Overweight and obesity p. 348) or metabolic syndrome.

When to take a blood sample
- Aged 40–75yrs (as per NHS Health Check)
- Adults with BMI ≥30 (Ɔ Adult body mass index chart p. 346)
- Past medical history of CVD, CHD, renal disease, hypertension (Ɔ Hypertension p. 628), or diabetes (Ɔ Diabetes: overview p. 660; Ɔ Principles of diabetes management p. 664)
- Family history of CVD
- Family history (or suspected) of hypercholesterolaemia
- Take non-fasting samples, testing total blood cholesterol and non-HDL, and calculating total cholesterol:HDL ratio. Patients with a family history (or suspected) of hypercholesterolaemia will require more in-depth analysis: take fasting samples, testing total cholesterol, LDL cholesterol, HDL cholesterol, and triglycerides (TGs) Total cholesterol >6.5mmol/L may need specialist referral. Following blood tests, calculate QRISK® (or ASSIGN in Scotland).

Intervention

Aims: ↓ non-HDL and ↑ HDL; ↓ LDL to <3.0mmol/L or by 30%, whichever is lower; and ↓ total cholesterol:HDL ratio to <5mmol/L. For drugs commonly used in the treatment of hypercholesterolaemia, see → Drugs commonly used in the prevention and treatment of cardiovascular disease p. 646. Follow local and national guidelines for therapeutic drug regimens.
Lifestyle advice should include:
- ↓ overall dietary fat intake to <30% of total daily energy intake (→ Nutrition and healthy eating p. 342)
- Saturated fats <7% of total daily energy intake
- Dietary cholesterol <300mg/day
- Replace saturated fats with monounsaturated/polyunsaturated fats
- Choose wholegrain varieties of starchy food
- Aim for five portions of fruit and vegetables per day
- Aim for two portions of fish per week, including a portion of oily fish
- Smoking cessation (→ Smoking cessation p. 356)
- Alcohol within recommended limits (→ Alcohol p. 360)
- Regular exercise (→ Exercise p. 354)

Follow-up and review

Initial review after 3mths of initiating either pharmacological or non-pharmacological treatment, then at least annually (→ Principles of medication reviews p. 142).
- Check total, HDL, and non-HDL cholesterol
- Medicines optimization (→ Medicines optimization p. 128)
- Measure liver function within 3mths of pharmacological intervention and at 12mths, but not again unless clinically indicated

⚠ Advise people to seek medical advice if they develop muscle pain, tenderness, or weakness. Check bloods for creatinine kinase.

Further information

NICE (*Cardiovascular disease: risk assessment and reduction, including lipid modification [CG181]*). Available at: ✆ www.nice.org.uk/guidance/cg181

Cardiac rehabilitation

A complex intervention, delivered by the multidisciplinary team
(→ Teamwork p. 58) including cardiologist, nurse specialist, physiotherapist,
dietician, psychologist, and exercise professional. Programmes vary in location, intensity, and duration. Traditional programmes involve weekly attendance at group meetings over 6–12wks. Key elements include:[18]

- Health behaviour change and education
- Lifestyle risk factor management
- Psychosocial health
- Medical risk factor management
- Cardioprotective therapies
- Long-term management
- Audit and evaluation

Eligible patients

Patient groups who benefit include those:[17] who have had a myocardial infarction; with angina (→ Angina p. 626); with heart failure (→ Heart failure
p. 636); with heart transplant and ventricular assist device; and who
are undergoing reperfusion. About half of all eligible patients attend.[18]
Practitioners should provide a consistent message to encourage all those
who are eligible to participate.

Benefits

- ↓ mortality
- ↓ hospital admissions
- ↑ psychological well-being and quality of life
- Improved cardiovascular risk profile

References

17. Dalal, H., Doherty, P., & Taylor, R. (2015) Cardiac rehabilitation. *BMJ*, 351, h5000
18. British Heart Foundation (2018) *National audit of cardiac rehabilitation: annual statistical report 2017*. Available at: https://www.bhf.org.uk/informationsupport/publications/statistics/
national-audit-of-cardiac-rehabilitation-annual-statistical-report-2017

Further information

NICE (*Myocardial infarction: cardiac rehabilitation and prevention of further cardiovascular disease*).
Available at: ℘ https://www.nice.org.uk/guidance/CG172

Heart failure

Definitions

Heart failure

Heart failure (HF) is where the heart does not pump enough blood to meet the demands of the body, due to structural or functional abnormalities of the heart including cardiac muscle damage (systolic or diastolic dysfunction, often due to CHD) (◉ Coronary heart disease p. 624), valvular dysfunction, arrhythmias (◉ Abnormal cardiac rhythms p. 640), or other rare causes. It may affect only one side of the heart initially.

Left heart failure

→ pulmonary oedema
- Left ventricular systolic dysfunction, where the heart cannot efficiently pump blood
- HF with preserved ejection fraction, where left ventricle pumping ability intact but filling impaired

Right heart failure

→ peripheral oedema before affecting both sides

Acute heart failure

This can present as new-onset heart failure (e.g. after MI (◉ Angina p. 626)) or as acute decompensation in individuals with chronic HF. Acute HF is a leading cause of hospital admission amongst >65yrs.

Chronic heart failure

Symptoms often occur slowly and gradually worsen. Most of the evidence on treatment is for chronic heart failure due to left ventricular systolic dysfunction.

Risk factors

- CHD and previous MI
- Hypertension (◉ Hypertension p. 628)
- Heart valve disease
- Congenital heart defects (◉ Congenital heart defects p. 260)
- Lung conditions (e.g. COPD (◉ Chronic obstructive pulmonary disease p. 614))
- Alcohol (◉ Alcohol p. 360) or other substance misuse (◉ Substance use p. 476)
- Obesity (◉ Overweight and obesity p. 348)
- High cholesterol (◉ Hypercholesterolaemia p. 632)
- Pregnancy (◉ Pregnancy p. 424)

Symptoms

- Breathlessness at rest and/or on exertion
- Fatigue
- Paroxysmal nocturnal dyspnoea and orthopnoea
- Ankle, abdominal, or sacral oedema
- Abdominal discomfort from liver distention and nausea

⚠ Any patient presenting with new suspected acute heart failure should have initial treatment in 2° care.

Classification

Heart failure is usually classified using the New York Heart Association Functional Classification (Box 11.4), which is based on how much patients are limited during physical activity.[19]

Care and management in primary care

Patient may benefit from case management approach (→ Case management p. 114) and involvement of specialist nurse/community matron if newly diagnosed, recently decompensated, classified as Class III or IV, or with comorbidities (→ Teamwork p. 58). All patients with suspected heart failure should be included in practice register (→ General practice p. 18), as per the QOF (→ Quality and Outcomes Framework p. 74), and have specialist assessment. Care and management with pharmacological and non-pharmacological interventions.

Pharmacological interventions

For drugs commonly used in the treatment of heart failure, see → Drugs commonly used in the prevention and treatment of cardiovascular disease p. 646. Follow local and national guidelines for therapeutic drug regimens.

Non-pharmacological interventions

* Encourage self-management (→ Expert patients and self-management programmes p. 340)
* Refer for cardiac rehabilitation (→ Cardiac rehabilitation p. 634)
* Assess for anxiety and depression (→ People with anxiety and depression p. 478)
* Smoking cessation (→ Smoking cessation p. 356)
* Healthy eating advice (do not routinely advise ↓ sodium or fluid intake unless ↑ consumption) (→ Nutrition and healthy eating p. 342)
* Pneumococcal vaccination and seasonal influenza vaccination (→ Targeted adult immunization p. 392),
* Effective management of hypertension, diabetes (→ Diabetes: overview p. 660; → Principles of diabetes management p. 664), CHD, and high cholesterol

As part of the multidisciplinary team, review patients at least every 6mths, or more often as required. Include physical assessment, medication review (→ Principles of medication reviews p. 142), and functional ability.

Box 11.4 The New York Heart Association Functional Classification

* **Class I:** No limitation on physical activity. Ordinary physical activity does not cause undue fatigue, palpitation, or shortness of breath.
* **Class II:** Slight limitation of physical activity. Comfortable at rest. Ordinary physical activity results in fatigue, palpitation, or shortness of breath.
* **Class III:** Marked limitation of physical activity. Comfortable at rest. Less than ordinary activity causes fatigue, palpitation, or shortness of breath.
* **Class IV:** Unable to carry on any physical activity without discomfort. Symptoms of heart failure at rest. If any physical activity is undertaken, discomfort increases.

Heart failure has a poor prognosis with 30–40% mortality in first year. At the end of life, person-centred palliative care will be facilitated by advanced care planning (including advanced statements and advanced decisions) (⟴ Mental capacity p. 470; ⟴ Palliative care in the home p. 550; ⟴ Services for the dying patient p. 552).

Reference

19. Dolgin, M., New York Hearth Association, Fox, A., Gorlin, R., & Levin, R. (1994) New York Heart Association Criteria Committee. Nomenclature and criteria for diagnosis of diseases of the heart and great vessels (9th edn). Boston, MA: Lippincott Williams and Wilkins

Further information

NICE (*Acute heart failure: diagnosis and management [CG187]*). Available at: ℘ www.nice.org.uk/guidance/cg187

NICE (*Chronic heart failure in adults: diagnosis and management [NG106]*). Available at: ℘ www.nice.org.uk/guidance/ng106

Abnormal cardiac rhythms

There is considerable variation in rhythm throughout the day, and transient issues such as ectopic beats or palpitations (feeling like the heart is 'pounding' or 'thumping') are common and mostly harmless. Causes include: underlying disease, caffeine, alcohol (→ Alcohol p. 360), smoking (→ Smoking cessation p. 356), and fatigue.

Bradycardias

Slow cardiac rhythms, usually <60/min. Often present in athletes, hypothyroidism (→ Thyroid p. 702), and those taking beta blockers (→ Drugs commonly used in the prevention and treatment of cardiovascular disease p. 646). Pathological bradycardias include heart blocks (atrioventricular heart blocks or bundle branch blocks) and tachy-brady syndrome (including atrial flutter).

Tachycardias

Elevated heart rate >100/min. Occurs with stress (→ People with anxiety and depression p. 478), physical exertion (→ Exercise p. 354), dehydration, stimulants (e.g. caffeine, nicotine, amphetamines, cocaine (→ Substance use p. 476)), or medication side effects (e.g. salbutamol (→ Drugs commonly used in the treatment of respiratory conditions p. 620)). Sinus tachycardia rarely needs investigation or treatment, but recommend stopping smoking, ↓ alcohol and caffeine if appropriate. This is a fast but normal heart rhythm (e.g. what people get when they exert themselves). Other tachycardias include supraventricular tachycardia (often paroxysmal, rarely life-threatening), atrial tachycardias such as atrial flutter or atrial fibrillation (see following), ventricular tachycardia, and ventricular fibrillation. ⚠ Ventricular fibrillation is classed as cardiac arrest and requires immediate emergency treatment (→ Adult basic life support and automated external defibrillation p. 792).

Atrial fibrillation

Atrial fibrillation (AF) occurs when atria produce unco-ordinated electrical signals, resulting in irregular, often fast heartbeat (→ Atrial fibrillation p. 641). Most common sustained arrhythmia and associated with ↑ risk of stroke (→ Recognizing and responding to a stroke p. 830). Can be paroxysmal (occurs intermittently, lasts minutes to days, may resolve spontaneously) or persistent/permanent.

When investigations are required

- Symptoms include chest pain, breathlessness, diaphoresis (sweating), or hyperventilation
- Accompanied by dizziness or syncope (fainting)
- Symptoms affect driving or work
- Underlying history of cardiovascular disease (→ Angina p. 626; → Heart failure p. 636; → Coronary heart disease p. 624)

Investigations may include: 12-lead ECG (→ Recording a 12-lead electrocardiogram p. 584), blood tests, and additional cardiac investigations.

Atrial fibrillation

Risk factors

- ↑ age (particularly >65yrs)
- CHD (➲ Coronary heart disease p. 624)
- Hypertension (➲ Hypertension p. 628)
- Pre-existing cardiac conditions (e.g. cardiomyopathies, valvulopathies, heart failure (➲ Heart failure p. 636))
- Obesity (➲ Overweight and obesity p. 348)
- Alcohol (➲ Alcohol p. 360) or other substance misuse (➲ Substance use p. 476)

Symptoms

- Palpitations
- Feeling faint or dizzy
- Breathlessness
- ↓ exercise tolerance (➲ Exercise p. 354)

Care and treatment

Investigations include 12-lead ECG (➲ Recording a 12-lead electrocardiogram p. 584). All individuals should be offered treatment for rate control (e.g. medication). Referral for rhythm control (e.g. cardioversion) may be appropriate. Assess stroke risk and consider risks and benefits of anticoagulation (➲ Drugs commonly used in the prevention and treatment of cardiovascular disease p. 646; ➲ Patients on anticoagulant therapy p. 642).

- Medicines optimization (➲ Medicines optimization p. 128; ➲ Principles of medication reviews p. 142)
- Ensure patient/carer education on stroke awareness (➲ Recognizing and responding to a stroke p. 830)
- Provide information on support groups (➲ Expert patients and self-management programmes p. 340)
- Monitor mood and discuss psychological support if needed (➲ Talking therapies p. 472)
- Advise patients they may need to inform the DVLA if their symptoms are disabling or distracting
- ⚠ Holders of heavy goods vehicle and public service vehicle licences must inform DVLA.

⚠ Admit for urgent assessment if AF associated with any of the following: a rapid pulse (>150 beats per min) and/or low BP (systolic <90mmHg), loss of consciousness, severe dizziness, ongoing chest pain, or ↑ breathlessness, a complication of atrial fibrillation such as stroke, transient ischaemic attack, or acute heart failure.

Related topics

➲ Abnormal cardiac rhythms p. 640

Further information

AF Association (*Support groups*). Available online: ☍ http://www.heartrhythmalliance.org/afa/uk/support-groups

NICE (*Atrial fibrillation: management [CG180]*). Available at: ☍ www.nice.org.uk/guidance/cg180

Patients on anticoagulant therapy

Anticoagulants ↓ the formation of new blood clots and the extension of existing clots (→ Drugs commonly used in the prevention and treatment of cardiovascular disease p. 646). Most commonly used with patients with AF (→ Abnormal cardiac rhythms p. 640; → Atrial fibrillation p. 641), replacement heart valves, or following pulmonary embolism (PE) and/or deep vein thrombosis (DVT) (→ Varicose veins, thrombophlebitis, and deep vein thrombosis p. 656).

Warfarin most common anticoagulant but newer anticoagulants called non-vitamin K oral anticoagulants or direct oral anticoagulants (formerly called novel anticoagulants) now licensed. Warfarin antagonizes the effects of vitamin K, reducing total amount of clotting factors in circulation, and takes 48–72hrs to work. Non-vitamin K oral anticoagulants bind directly to specific clotting factors.

Most anticoagulants are started in 2° care or outreach clinic in 1° care. Patients on oral anticoagulants often managed by nurses working to an agreed protocol.

Patient information for both warfarin and non-vitamin K oral anticoagulants

- Take anticoagulant at same time each day
- Always carry yellow anticoagulant treatment booklet or alert card
- Medi-alert band with anticoagulant name advisable
- Inform doctor, dentist, or pharmacist about anticoagulant treatment
- Avoid aspirin or NSAIDs
- Follow missed dose and wrong dose protocols
- Avoid or use protection when undertaking activities that could cause abrasion, bruising, or cuts (e.g. contact sports, gardening, sewing)
- Take extra care when brushing teeth or shaving (consider using a soft toothbrush and an electric razor)
- Avoid insect bites and consider use of an insect repellent
- Avoid vigorous nose blowing
- Never stop medication without reference to doctor

⚠ Seek immediate help if:
- Bleeding gums
- Unexplained bruises
- Nosebleeds (→ External bleeding p. 814)
- Sudden severe back pain
- Menstrual bleeding in post-menopausal women (→ Menopause p. 364)
- Blood in urine or stool
- Subconjunctival bleeding (→ Common problems affecting eyes p. 746)
- Coughing or vomiting up blood
- Prolonged bleeding
- Head injury (due to risk of internal bleeding)

⚠ A major bleed is a serious complication of both warfarin and non-vitamin K oral anticoagulants. There are several reversal agents available for warfarin. There is a relative lack of specific reversal agents for non-vitamin K oral anticoagulants.

Additional information for patients prescribed warfarin

When the first dose of warfarin is prescribed, it does not matter how much vitamin K a patient is eating because the dosage will be based on their current blood-clotting levels. However, patients should avoid sudden changes in the amount of vitamin K they consume. Foods containing large amounts of vitamin K include green leafy vegetables, vegetable oils, and cereal grains. Avoid cranberry juice. Getting drunk or binge drinking is dangerous while taking warfarin due to ↑ risk of bleeding (➜ Alcohol p. 360). ⚠ Women must not become pregnant while taking warfarin (➜ Contraception: general p. 400). Patients should be aware of the medicines (including OTC and herbal remedies (➜ Complementary and alternative therapies p. 838)) that can interact with warfarin.

Warfarin management and international normalized ratio (INR) testing

Refer to local guidelines for dosage regimes. Normal dose varies between individuals. Therapeutic values will vary depending on warfarin indication (e.g. INR 2.5–3.0 for AF, DVT/PE).

Check INR daily and/or alternate days until within therapeutic range on two consecutive occasions. Then test twice a week for 1–2wks, followed by weekly measurements until at least two measurements are within the therapeutic range. Thereafter, depending on the stability of the INR, at longer intervals (up to 12wks, depending on local guidelines).

If INR outside range, consider:
- Medication adherence (➜ Medicine concordance and adherence p. 132)
- Sudden dietary changes
- Whether new medicines have been prescribed (➜ Prescribing p. 136)
- Use of OTC medicines (including herbal remedies)
- General health and acute illness (e.g. gastroenteritis)
- Smoking cessation (can increase the effect of warfarin) (➜ Smoking cessation p. 356)

When a drug is prescribed that may interact with warfarin, the patient's INR should be checked 3–5 days after starting treatment with the new drug.

Self-testing and management

People who require long-term anticoagulation can be considered for warfarin self-testing or self-management. Self-testing is where a person tests their own INR, but contacts a healthcare professional for dose adjustment. Self-management is where a person tests their own INR and also adjusts the dose of warfarin themselves (based on individualized algorithm).

Availability varies across the UK. May suit people that are frequently away from home, in employment, or in education, or find it difficult to travel to clinics. Previous stability of INR is not essential; people with an unstable INR may benefit from the possibility of ↑ frequency of testing. Person needs to be both physically and cognitively able to perform self-monitoring and management, or designated carer is able to do so. Supportive educational programme must be in place. Ability to self-test or self-manage must be regularly reviewed. Appropriately trained healthcare professionals must be available for ongoing support and advice.

Check to see which devices are currently recommended by NICE. Patients must purchase their own machine.

Management of non-vitamin K oral anticoagulants

There is no need to have regular blood tests to monitor INR but regular monitoring, blood tests, and review of treatment still necessary. Blood tests usually undertaken annually to monitor kidney and liver function (more frequently if indicated). Treatment usually reviewed every 3mths: medication adherence, adverse effects, and monitoring concomitant prescriptions and OTC medicine use.

Related topics

→ Medicines optimization p. 128

Further information

British Heart Foundation (*Novel anticoagulants*). Available at: ℰ https://www.bhf.org.uk/informationsupport/heart-matters-magazine/medical/drug-cabinet/novel-anticoagulants

NICE (*Anticoagulation—oral*). Available at: ℰ https://cks.nice.org.uk/anticoagulation-oral

NICE (Atrial fibrillation and heart valve disease: self-monitoring coagulation status using point-of-care coagulometers (the CoaguChek XS system) [DG14]). Available at: ℰ https://www.nice.org.uk/guidance/dg14

Drugs commonly used in the prevention and treatment of cardiovascular disease

Allergies

Oral anticoagulants

Antiplatelet

Drugs commonly used in the prevention and treatment of cardiovascular disease

This section will provide an overview of the drugs commonly used in the prevention and treatment of cardiovascular disease (CHD (➲ Coronary heart disease p. 624)), angina (➲ Angina p. 626), hypertension (➲ Hypertension p. 628), hypercholesterolaemia (➲ Hypercholesterolaemia p. 632), heart failure (➲ Heart failure p. 636), atrial fibrillation (➲ Abnormal cardiac rhythms p. 640; ➲ Atrial fibrillation p. 641), and diabetes (➲ Diabetes: overview p. 660; ➲ Principles of diabetes management p. 664). The purpose of having this level of understanding is that predicted benefits and potential side effects can be understood. It is important that nurses keep themselves updated in the use of drugs by reading research papers and international, national, and local guidelines. For doses of drugs, methods of administration, contraindications, and side effects, use a recognized formulary, in addition to any local policy. The categories to be considered are nitrates, antiplatelets, beta blockers, calcium channel blockers, angiotensin-converting enzyme (ACE) inhibitors, angiotensin II antagonists, statins, diuretics, and cardiac glycosides.

Nitrates

Used to ease and prevent angina pains. Nitrates release nitric oxide in vascular smooth muscle, resulting in relaxation and thus vasodilation. They act predominantly on the venous system, causing venodilation, which ↓ the amount of blood returning to the heart (venous return) and ↓ the preload, thereby ↓ myocardial O_2 demand. There is also some arterial dilation; coronary arteries unaffected by atherosclerotic plaques vasodilate, ↑ the blood supply to the myocardium. Peripheral arterial vasodilation ↓ the resistance against which the heart has to pump. Examples include GTN, isosorbide dinitrate, and mononitrate.

Nursing considerations

The most common side effects include flushes, headaches, and hypotension. Sublingual (SL) tablets should not be swallowed because they then become ineffective. Tolerance can develop, so 4–8hr nitrate-free period in every 24h is advised. If an attack of angina is unresponsive to a couple of doses of GTN, it could be viewed as a myocardial infarction and immediate medical assistance sought. Patients need to be informed that they can take nitrates during an episode of chest pain, but can also do so before starting any activities that are likely to precipitate chest pain, e.g. climbing stairs (➲ Exercise p. 354). Short-acting GTN tablets should be kept in their original container. Once opened, they should be discarded after 8wks as they lose their effectiveness.

Antiplatelets

Generally, this group of drugs interferes with platelet membrane function, prevents release of platelet constituents, and inhibits platelet aggregation. Aspirin, the most commonly used agent, works inside platelets, and results in the inhibition of platelet aggregation. It is used as 2° prophylaxis.

Clopidogrel and ticagrelor work by interfering with platelet function by inhibiting a different induced type of platelet aggregation. Abciximab is in a group of drugs known as glycoprotein IIb/IIIa (GPIIb/IIIa) inhibitors. GPIIb/IIIa receptors on platelets are blocked, which effectively stops platelet aggregation. This prevents further platelet or fibrinogen binding.

Nursing considerations

Administer oral drugs with food because this improves the absorption of ticlopidine and can ↓ the gastric irritation caused by aspirin. Monitor the patient for side effects including bleeding disorders, nausea, and vomiting. Can ↑ the risk of bleeding if given with anticoagulants (➔ Patients on anticoagulant therapy p. 642). A single dose of aspirin (150–300mg) is given following an ischaemic event. Ensure that the patient and family are aware that the drug is being given for its antiplatelet action and not as an analgesic. Aspirin might be stopped before surgery to ↓ the probability of post-operative bleeding. Check with medical team.

Beta blockers

May be prescribed for angina, arrhythmia, following previous heart attack (to prevent another), and for hypertension. β-blockers block β-adrenoceptors; these receptors are situated in the heart, bronchi, peripheral vasculature, pancreas, and liver. There are two β-receptor subtypes, which are identified as β_1 and β_2. The β_1 receptor subtype is found in the heart, so blocking these receptors blocks the sympathetic response and, therefore, causes ↓ cardiac output (CO), BP, and heart rate. However, although some β blockers are cardioselective, they might also block β_2 receptors. β_2 receptors are found in the lungs and, therefore, a side effect of these agents can be bronchoconstriction. Different β-blockers can be used in different clinical situations. Examples include propranolol, atenolol, metoprolol, bisoprolol, and carvedilol.

Nursing considerations

Side effects include excessive bradycardia, ↓ CO that could predispose some patients to heart failure, and excessive hypotension. Therefore, monitor patients carefully so that doses and regimens can be altered to ensure that HR, CO, and BP stay within safe limits. Moreover, ↓ CO could make a patient feel tired. Another very important side effect is bronchoconstriction; therefore, it is not advised that β-blockers (even cardioselective β-blockers) are given to patients with a history of bronchospasm (e.g. asthma (➔ Asthma in adults p. 608)) and COPD (➔ Chronic obstructive pulmonary disease p. 614). β-blockers can cause peripheral vasoconstriction and patients might suffer from coldness in their fingers and toes. These drugs can have gastrointestinal (GI) side effects, which can be ↓ if the drugs are taken before meals. Another side effect of β-blockers is that they may cause erectile dysfunction (➔ Sexual problems p. 768).

Caution should be used when giving β-blockers to patients with diabetes because the signs and symptoms of hypoglycaemia and hyperglycaemia can be masked. Therefore, monitoring of blood glucose levels is important. Patients with diabetes might also need changes to their dose of insulin or oral hypoglycaemics. Long-acting β-blockers might need to be stopped before surgery to ↓ the impact of their effects post-operatively, including bradycardia and ↓ cardiac contractility. Check with medical team. The eld-erly are more likely to be sensitive to β-blockers and therefore experience more side effects. They may also make the patient less tolerant to cold temperatures.

Calcium-channel blockers

Used in the management of hypertension, angina, and come arrhythmias. Calcium-channel blockers ↓ the flow of calcium ions into muscle cells. This calcium blockade occurs in vascular smooth muscle, myocardial cells, and the conduction system. Without calcium, muscles cannot contract, resulting in vasodilation of peripheral and coronary blood vessels, ↓ in myocardial contractility, and a ↓ in the formation and conduction of nerve impulses. Within this group of drugs there are the following subgroups:

- Dihydropyridines (e.g. nifedipine and amlodipine), which act predominantly on blood vessels and are, therefore, vasodilators with minimal effect on cardiac activity.
- Nondihydropyridines, which can be subdivided further into verapamil and diltiazem. Verapamil acts on cardiac conduction and is, therefore, administered as an antiarrhythmic. Diltiazem is intermediate between verapamil and the dihydropyridines and has some vascular and cardiac effect.

Nursing considerations

For all drugs that affect HR and BP, it is important to monitor these vari-ables. Because they are vasodilators, patients can initially suffer from flushes and headaches, which should ↓ over time. Calcium-channel blockers ↓ myocardial contractility and can interact with other drugs that ↓ contract-ility, such as β-blockers and some antiarrhythmics, which could lead to se-vere haemodynamic deterioration. Elderly patients may need to be started on lower doses as they may be more sensitive to this group of drugs than younger patients (➔ Prescribing for special groups p. 138). Verapamil can cause constipation.

Angiotensin-converting enzyme inhibitors

Used in the treatment of hypertension and heart failure. ACE inhibitors work on the renin–angiotensin–aldosterone system (RAAS). Renin is an enzyme that converts angiotensinogen into angiotensin I; angiotensin I is then converted into angiotensin II in the lungs by ACE. Angiotensin II is a powerful vasoconstrictor and stimulates the release of aldosterone, which ↑ sodium and water retention. So, by blocking the action of ACE, there is vasodilation and ↓ in fluid volume, leading to a ↓ in BP. Examples include captopril, lisinopril, enalapril, ramipril, and perindopril.

Nursing considerations

Potassium concentrations can ↑ in patients taking ACE inhibitors, which is important if patients are also taking potassium-sparing diuretics or po-tassium supplements. Hyperkalaemia can cause arrhythmias. Another side effect of ACE inhibitors is a persistent dry cough. ACE inhibitors are asso-ciated with ↓ in renal BP and thus ↓ filtration pressure, so monitor renal function. However, these drugs seem to offer renal protection in diabetic patients.

Angiotensin II antagonists

Used for hypertension, in particular to ↓ BP in patients who cannot tolerate ACE inhibitors. These agents do not block the conversion of angiotensin I to angiotensin II in the same way that ACE inhibitors do; they block the action of angiotensin II at its receptor site. Examples include losartan and candesartan. Monitoring considerations are as described for ACE inhibitors.

Statins

Used in the management of hypercholesterolaemia. Statins are 3-hydroxy-3-methyglutaryl-coenzyme A (HMG-CoA) reductase inhibitors. HMG-CoA reductase is the rate-determining enzyme in the synthesis of cholesterol. Therefore, if this enzyme is inhibited, less cholesterol is made, especially in the liver. Also ↑ the liver's ability to remove cholesterol. Examples include simvastatin, atorvastatin, and pravastatin.

Nursing considerations

Statins are more effective if taken in the evening, because the HMG-CoA reductase enzyme is most active during the night, which is, therefore, the time cholesterol is made. Contraindicated in liver disease and pregnancy (➔ Pregnancy p. 424). Can cause muscle problems ranging from myalgia (pain) to rhabdomyolysis (damaged muscles). Advise patients to report any unexplained muscle pain, weakness, or tenderness. Perform liver function test before and within 4–12wks of starting statin treatment. This should be reviewed at 6mths and 1yr because altered liver function is a potential side effect of statins.

Diuretics

Diuretics ↑ the volume of urine flow by affecting ion transport in the nephron. Diuretics are classified according to their mechanism of action:

- **Bendroflumethiazide:** belongs to the class of 'thiazide and related diuretics'. These drugs work at the beginning of the distal convoluted tubule (DCT) and inhibit sodium reabsorption. If sodium is not reabsorbed, less water is reabsorbed, causing ↑ diuresis. The drugs are moderately effective because most sodium is absorbed before it reaches the DCT. Thiazide-like diuretics are used to treat hypertension and ↓ oedema in heart failure.
- **Furosemide:** belongs to the class of 'loop diuretics' because of its site of action. Loop diuretics work primarily by blocking the sodium and potassium co-transporter system in the thick ascending limb of the loop of Henle. As a result, sodium and chloride reabsorption is inhibited, but that also means that the loss of potassium ions is ↑. These are powerful diuretics because up to 35% of NaCl is reabsorbed at this part of the loop of Henle. These agents are used to treat pulmonary oedema in left ventricular failure and also congestive heart failure.
- **Spironolactone and amiloride:** belong to the class of 'potassium-sparing diuretics', although they have different mechanisms of action. Spironolactone inhibits aldosterone, a hormone produced by the adrenal cortex, which results in not only ↑ excretion of sodium, and therefore water, but also conservation of potassium. Amiloride primarily works by inhibiting the passage of sodium into the late DCT

and collecting duct, thereby preventing the movement of potassium out into the fluid. As a result of their mechanisms of action, they are weak diuretics and are usually given with other diuretics in order to prevent hypokalaemia.

Nursing considerations

Monitoring should include vital signs and weight. It is very important to ensure that potassium levels are monitored, especially in patients who are not taking potassium-sparing diuretics. It is important to monitor blood glucose levels closely in diabetic patients because these drugs can cause hyperglycaemia. It is advised that patients take diuretics in the morning and the early afternoon to avoid having a disturbed night with frequent episodes of passing urine. Thiazide diuretics have a long duration of action (12–24hrs) so should be taken in the morning only; however, the action of furosemide only lasts up to 6hrs so it can be administered twice daily without causing sleep disturbance.

Cardiac glycosides

The most commonly used cardiac glycoside is digoxin. The drug is most useful in the treatment of supraventricular tachycardia and is used to control the ventricular rate in atrial fibrillation (AF) or atrial flutter. It can also be used for the treatment of heart failure. The therapeutic effects of cardiac glycosides are attributable to blockade of the sodium potassium ATPase pump. In AF, it slows the ventricular rate largely by ↓ the sympathetic drive and ↓ conduction across the atrioventricular (AV) node. Cardiac glycosides ↑ the force of contraction.

Nursing considerations

Side effects fall into two categories: cardiac and non-cardiac. Cardiac side effects include bradycardia, (possibly) heart block, and ventricular arrhythmias. To monitor for bradycardia, record the HR before drug administration. If the pulse is <60bpm, withhold the dose until medical team are consulted. Teach patients taking digoxin at home how to accurately take their own pulse.

Non-cardiac side effects include anorexia, nausea and vomiting, and diarrhoea. There could also be neurological side effects such as headaches, drowsiness, and confusion. Can also cause visual disturbances.

Ensure blood digoxin levels are monitored to prevent toxicity. Monitoring of blood potassium levels is also very important because hypokalaemia can ↑ the likelihood of digoxin toxicity. Therefore, caution must be taken when administering potassium-lowering drugs such as diuretics. Give either potassium-sparing diuretics or potassium supplements.

Lower doses may be required for elderly patients as they tend to be more sensitive to the effects of digoxin and are therefore more likely to experience side effects.

Anaemia in adults

A lack of sufficient red blood cells and thus haemoglobin due to ↓ red cell production or ↑ rate of destruction. Patients who become anaemic slowly may remain asymptomatic for a long time.

Classification

- ♂ aged >15yrs: Hb ↓ 130g/L
- Non-pregnant ♀ aged >15yrs: Hb ↓ 120g/L
- Pregnant ♀: Hb ↓ 110g/L (➔ Pregnancy p. 424)
- Post-partum ♀: Hb ↓ 100g/L (➔ Postnatal care p. 438)

⚠ The presence of anaemia may indicate a more serious underlying problem (e.g. malignancy).

Iron deficiency anaemia

Presentation

May include:
- Shortness of breath (SOB)
- Fatigue
- Headache
- Cognitive dysfunction
- Restless leg syndrome
- Vertigo
- Atrophic glossitis (➔ Mouth and throat problems p. 698)
- Dry and rough skin, dry and damaged hair
- Diffuse and moderate alopecia (➔ Pigmentation and hair problems p. 692)

Causes

- Lack of dietary iron
- Malabsorption
- ↑ blood loss (e.g. gastrointestinal bleeding and menstrual bleeding (➔ Menstrual problems p. 778))
- ↑ requirements (e.g. pregnancy)

Management

- Investigations may include full blood count (FBC) and ferritin levels
- Additional investigations to identify underlying cause. ⚠ If malignancy suspected, follow suspected cancer pathway. If malabsorption suspected, refer to gastroenterologist.
- Drug treatment and medicines optimization (➔ Medicines optimization p. 128)
- Dietary advice (e.g. fruit, wholemeal bread, beans, lean meat)

Vitamin B12 deficiency anaemia

Presentation

May include:
- Cognitive changes
- SOB
- Headache
- Indigestion

- Loss of appetite
- Palpitations (**➔** Abnormal cardiac rhythms p. 640)
- Tachypnoea
- Visual disturbance
- Weakness, lethargy
- Anorexia (**➔** People with eating disorders p. 474)
- Oropharyngeal ulceration
- Neurological complications

Causes

Pernicious anaemia is the main cause of vitamin B12 deficiency anaemia (see following). Other causes are rare but include drug-related causes, gastric or intestinal malabsorption, malnutrition (**➔** Malnutrition p. 350), vegan diet, some medicines, and some parasites.

Management

- Investigations may include FBC, and serum cobalamin and folate levels.
- Additional investigations to identify underlying cause ⚠ For people with neurological involvement, seek urgent specialist advice. Similarly, if the person is pregnant. If malignancy suspected, follow suspected cancer pathway. If malabsorption suspected, refer to gastroenterologist.
- Drug treatment and medicines optimization
- Dietary advice (e.g. eggs, fortified foods, meat, milk and dairy products, salmon and cod)

Folate deficiency

Presentation

May include:

- Cognitive changes
- SOB
- Headache
- Indigestion
- Loss of appetite
- Palpitations
- Tachypnoea
- Visual disturbance
- Weakness, lethargy
- Anorexia
- Oropharyngeal ulceration

Causes

- Lack of dietary folate
- Drug-related causes
- Alcoholism (**➔** Alcohol p. 360)
- Increased requirements
- Excessive urinary excretion (**➔** Renal problems p. 754)
- Liver disease (**➔** Problems of the liver, gallbladder, and pancreas p. 718)
- Malabsorption

Folate deficiency can coexist with vitamin B12 deficiency

Management
- Investigations may include FBC, and serum cobalamin and folate levels.
- Additional investigations to identify underlying cause. ⚠ For pregnant women, seek urgent specialist advice. If malignancy suspected, follow suspected cancer pathway. If malabsorption suspected, refer to gastroenterologist.
- Drug treatment and medicines optimization
- Dietary advice (e.g. asparagus, broccoli, brown rice, chickpeas, peas)

⚠ Insufficient folate at conception and early pregnancy → neural tube defects in newborns. To prevent neural tube defects ♀ who are planning a pregnancy or are pregnant should take folate supplements (➲ Preconceptual care p. 422; ➲ Neural tube defects p. 274)

Pernicious anaemia

Autoimmune disease caused by lack of intrinsic factor due to gastric atrophy. Intrinsic factor helps the absorption of vitamin B12. Usually develops in people >50yrs. Most common cause of vitamin B12 deficiency anaemia. Slow and insidious onset. See vitamin B12 deficiency anaemia presentations. Management as for vitamin B12 deficiency. Additional investigations will include tests for intrinsic factor antibodies. People with pernicious anaemia have ↑ risk of stomach cancer and should be advised to seek medical advice if they experience dyspepsia and/or stomach pain.

Related topics

➲ Coeliac disease p. 714; ➲ Inflammatory bowel disease p. 712

Further information

NICE (*Anaemia—iron deficiency*). Available online: ℜ https://cks.nice.org.uk/anaemia-iron-deficiency#!topicsummary
NICE (*Anaemia—B12 and folate deficiency*). Available online: ℜ https://cks.nice.org.uk/anaemia-b12-and-folate-deficiency

Varicose veins, thrombophlebitis, and deep vein thrombosis

Varicose veins

Veins that are swollen and enlarged, that usually occur in the legs. Occur because of incompetent valves that allow the blood to flow backwards from the deep to the superficial venous system, causing back pressure and further dilatation. Risk factors:

- Being ♀
- Family history of varicose veins
- Being older
- Obesity (➔ Overweight and obesity p. 348)
- Occupation that requires a lot of standing
- Pregnancy (➔ Pregnancy p. 424)
- History of DVT
- Pelvic tumour (➔ Gynaecological cancers p. 776)

Symptoms

In some people, varicose veins are asymptomatic or cause only mild symptoms including: cosmetic appearance of legs; aching, heavy, and uncomfortable legs; swollen feet and ankles; burning or throbbing sensation; and muscle cramps.

Complications

- Bleeding if veins are accidently cut or bumped
- Thrombophlebitis
- DVT
- Varicose eczema (➔ Eczema/dermatitis p. 684) and venous leg ulceration (➔ Leg ulcer assessment p. 536)

Care and management

- Weight management (➔ Overweight and obesity p. 348; ➔ Nutrition and healthy eating p. 342)
- Engage in light to moderate physical activity (➔ Exercise p. 354)
- Avoid standing for long periods
- Elevate legs when sitting
- Consider referral for 2° care treatments (e.g. surgical removal)
- Consider compression stockings if referral is declined or not indicated
  ⚠ Measure ankle-brachial pressure index (ABPI) using a Doppler machine to rule out arterial disease (➔ Venous leg ulcers p. 540; ➔ Compression therapy for venous leg ulcers p. 542).

Thrombophlebitis (superficial)

Occurs when a superficial vein becomes inflamed and the blood within it clots. Usually involves saphenous vein of the leg and its linked veins. Risk factors:

- Varicose veins (and trauma to varicose veins)
- IV cannulation
- Previous superficial thrombophlebitis
- Age >60yrs

- Obesity
- Smoking
- IV drug use (➔ Substance use p. 476)
- Prolonged immobility
- Pregnancy
- Oral contraceptives (➔ Combined hormonal contraceptive methods p. 402)
- Hormone replacement therapy (HRT) (➔ Menopause p. 364)
- Comorbidities (including cancer, systemic lupus erythematosus (➔ Bone and connective tissue disorders p. 738), anticardiolipin antibody syndrome, congestive heart failure (➔ Heart failure p. 636), and myocardial infarction (➔ Angina p. 626)

Symptoms
- Painful, harm lumps
- Erythema and pigmentation

Complications
- Septic thrombophlebitis (➔ Sepsis p. 826)
- DVT
- Varicose veins
- ⚠ Urgent referral for assessment if septic thrombophlebitis or DVT suspected.

Care and management
- Simple analgesia until pain and erythema have settled
- Application of local heat (e.g. warm towel to affected limb)
- Elevate legs when sitting
- Keep active to aid venous flow
- Provision of compression stockings ⚠ Measure ABPI using a Doppler machine to rule out arterial disease.
- Smoking cessation (➔ Smoking cessation p. 356)
- Weight management

> **Combined oral contraceptive pill**
> History of thrombophlebitis is a contraindication to the combined oral pill. Stop if using.

Deep vein thrombosis

Formation of a thrombus in a deep vein that partially or completely obstructs blood flow. Usually occurs in the deep veins of the calf (distal DVT) or in veins above the knee (proximal DVT). Multiple risk factors:
- Previous venous thromboembolism
- Cancer
- Increased age (>40yrs)
- Obesity
- Being ♂

- Heart failure (➔ Heart failure p. 636)
- Acquired or familial thrombophilia
- Injury to the vascular wall
- Varicose veins
- Smoking
- Immobility
- HRT
- Pregnancy
- Oestrogen-containing contraception
- Dehydration

Symptoms
- ⚠ Patient may be asymptomatic
- Unilateral pain and swelling (although both legs may be affected)
- Tenderness
- Changes to skin colour and temperature
- Vein distention

Complications
- Death due to pulmonary embolism
- Post-thrombotic syndrome (a chronic venous hypertension causing limb pain, swelling, hyperpigmentation, dermatitis, ulcers, venous gangrene, and lipodermatosclerosis)

Care and management
⚠ Refer immediately for same-day assessment and management. Following initial acute anticoagulation on heparin, oral anticoagulation will usually be prescribed and then reassessed at 3mths (➔ Patients on anticoagulant therapy p. 642). Patients with history of DVT risk recurrence in high-risk situations (e.g. surgery, pregnancy, immobility) and should receive prophylactic treatment with anticoagulants in such situations. Lifestyle advice includes smoking cessation and weight management.

Further information

NICE (*Varicose veins*). Available at: ℗ https://cks.nice.org.uk/varicose-veins#!topicsummary
NICE (*Thrombophlebitis—superficial*). Available at: ℗ https://cks.nice.org.uk/thrombophlebitis-superficial#!topicsummary
NICE (*Deep vein thrombosis*). Available at: ℗ https://cks.nice.org.uk/deep-vein-thrombosis#!topicsummary

Diabetes: overview

Diabetes is a serious chronic disease linked to premature death and disability. Classification includes Type 1 diabetes mellitus (T1DM), Type 2 diabetes mellitus (T2DM), mature onset diabetes of the young (MODY), gestational diabetes mellitus (GDM), and diabetes 2° to other causes (e.g. drugs (including steroids and thiazides), pancreatic disease (➔ Problems of the liver, gallbladder, and pancreas p. 718), and endocrine disease (including acromegaly and Cushing's disease) (➔ Adrenal disorders p. 700; ➔ Pituitary disorders p. 701). T1DM accounts for 5–10% of people with diabetes, while T2DM accounts for ~90%. A further classification is prediabetes.

Type 1 diabetes mellitus

Absolute deficiency of insulin secretion resulting from an autoimmune destruction of β-cells in the pancreas. The cause is unknown; however, environmental factors (e.g. viral infections) and genetic factors may play a part. Often occurs in childhood; although can occur at any age. ~400,000 people in the UK live with T1DM, including 29,000 children[20] (➔ Endocrine problems p. 304).

Symptoms

Typically, symptoms include: polydipsia, polyphagia, polyuria, and weight loss. Others include pruritus, blurred vision, cramping, and skin infections (➔ Bacterial skin infections p. 680; ➔ Viral skin infections p. 690). Symptoms can develop quickly in children (over a few days or weeks) but usually less quickly in adults. On symptom recognition, the patient should have a same-day appointment with their GP. Prompt diagnosis is necessary to prevent diabetic ketoacidosis (DKA). Symptoms of DKA include: ↓ appetite, nausea and vomiting, pyrexia, abdominal pain, smell of ketones on breath, and ↓ consciousness. If these symptoms are present, the patient needs urgent admission to hospital. ⚠ Untreated, DKA can be fatal.

Treatment

To ensure treatment starts immediately (➔ Principles of diabetes management p. 664), the GP will make a same-day referral to a multidisciplinary diabetes team. T1DM is always treated by insulin replacement. Macrovascular complications (coronary artery disease (➔ Coronary heart disease p. 624)), peripheral arterial disease, and stroke (➔ Recognizing and responding to a stroke p. 830) and microvascular complications (diabetic nephropathy, neuropathy, and retinopathy) also need to be managed.

Type 2 diabetes mellitus

T2DM is a chronic metabolic condition typified by insulin resistance (when the body does not respond effectively to insulin) and insufficient pancreatic insulin production, resulting in ↑ blood glucose (BG) levels. Causes include genetic factors, lifestyle factors (e.g. being overweight or obese (➔ Overweight and obesity p. 348)), and environmental factors (e.g. deprivation). People of South Asian, African Caribbean, or Black African origin are at ↑ risk. In 2013, there were ~2.88 million adults living in the UK with a diagnosis of T2DM[21] (➔ UK health profile p. 2). The number of children and young people with T2DM is reportedly increasing.

Symptoms

Symptoms are similar to those of T1DM. However, the individual is likely to have a limited number of symptoms and might think them unimportant. Diabetes in adults is usually diagnosed by an HbA1c (glycated haemoglobin) of >48mmols/mol (6.5%). HbA1c should not be used in some groups including children, young people, pregnant women, women who are 2mths post-partum, and people with symptoms for <2 months (see ᔥ https://cks.nice.org.uk/diabetes-type-2#!diagnosisSub).

Treatment

Key interventions are advice about lifestyle (physical activity (❸ Exercise p. 354), eating a healthy diet (❸ Nutrition and healthy eating p. 342), and smoking cessation (❸ Smoking cessation p. 356). Use of BG lowering therapy (which may include insulin replacement and/or oral antiglycaemics) will be dependent on an individual's HbA1c target. Macrovascular and microvascular complications also need to be managed.

Gestational diabetes mellitus

Pregnancy (❸ Pregnancy p. 424) is a period of significant maternal metabolic adaptations. Causes of insulin resistance in pregnancy are not well understood; however, excessive storage of nutrients and maternal weight gain may have adverse effects on insulin action and glucose tolerance. It can occur at any stage of pregnancy but usually >24wks. Risk factors include: BMI >30kg/m^2 (❸ Adult body mass index chart p. 346); previous baby weight >4.5kg; previous gestational diabetes; family history of diabetes; and ethnic origin with ↑ prevalence of diabetes.

Symptoms

Symptoms include polyuria, polydipsia, and ↑ tiredness. GDM will be diagnosed if ♀ has either a fasting plasma glucose level of ≥5.6 mmol/l or a 2hr plasma glucose level of ≥7.8 mmol/l.[22] GDM ↑ risk of premature birth (❸ Pre-term infants p. 176), pre-eclampsia (❸ Common problems in pregnancy p. 432), stillbirth, and the baby being born with jaundice. It can also ↑ the risk of the mother developing T2DM in the future.

Treatment

Treatment will include lifestyle and dietary advice. Treatment with BG lowering therapy will be dependent on glucose levels at diagnosis.

Maturity onset diabetes of the young

A monogenic disorder that results in a familial, young onset (<25yrs) non-insulin dependent form of diabetes. Frequently misdiagnosed as T1DM or T2DM. Most common types are: HNF1-alpha, HNF4-alpha, HNF1-beta, and glucokinase. With the exception of glucokinase, all types carry the same risk of macro and microvascular complications as T1DM and T2DM. Genetic testing often available for family members.

Prediabetes

Sometimes referred to as impaired glucose tolerance or impaired fasting glucose, it is where a person's glucose levels are raised; however, the readings do not indicate a diabetes diagnosis but do warrant intervention to prevent the development of diabetes or cardiovascular disease. Advice should be provided regarding lifestyle modification and diet. People may also be referred to a formal diabetes prevention programme (◐ Expert patients and self-management programmes p. 340).

Related topics

◐ Drugs commonly used in the prevention and treatment of cardiovascular disease p. 646; ◐ Principles of diabetes management p. 664

References

20. Juvenile Diabetes Research Foundation (2018) *Type 1 diabetes facts and figures.* Available at: ℘ https://jdrf.org.uk/information-support/about-type-1-diabetes/facts-and-figures/
21. NICE (2019) *Type 2 diabetes in adults: management [NG28].* Available at: ℘ https://www.nice.org.uk/guidance/ng28
22. NICE (2015) *Diabetes in pregnancy: management from preconception to the postnatal period [NG3].* Available at: ℘ https://www.nice.org.uk/guidance/ng3

Further information

NHS Diabetes (*The management of the hyperosmolar hyperglycaemic state in adults with diabetes*). Available at: ℘ https://diabetes-resources-production.s3-eu-west-1.amazonaws.com/diabetes-storage/migration/pdf/JBDS-IP-HHS-Adults.pdf

Principles of diabetes management

The aim of good care and management for both Type 1 diabetes mellitus (T1DM) and Type 2 diabetes mellitus (T2TD) is to improve patient experiences and disease outcomes (➲ Diabetes: overview p. 660).

1° and community care practitioners are increasingly at the forefront of diabetes care and management. These practitioners include GPs (➲ General practice p. 18), practice nurses (➲ General practice nursing p. 40), district nurses (➲ District nursing p. 50), optometrists, ophthalmologists, podiatrists, dieticians, and psychologists (➲ Teamwork p. 58). Whilst most patients will be able to work with these practitioners to achieve good diabetic care and control, specialist diabetes teams should be available to provide care and support for patients with complex needs. These include: children and young people with diabetes (➲ Endocrine problems p. 304); people newly diagnosed with T1DM; people with T1DM needing support carbohydrate counting and/or the use of insulin pumps/or continuous blood glucose (BG) monitoring; pregnant women (➲ Pregnancy p. 424) and those planning a pregnancy (➲ Preconceptual care p. 422); people with significant macrovascular or microvascular disease; and people with recurrent hypoglycaemia.[23]

Patient experiences and disease outcomes are improved when there is effective communication between practitioners across the diabetes care pathway and strong clinical partnerships are in place (➲ Continuity of care p. 598). All patients with diabetes should be recorded as diabetic on the practice register (➲ Quality and Outcomes Framework p. 74).

Principles of care and management in T1DM

Insulin replacement

All patients with T1DM will require insulin replacement. The aim of treatment is to achieve optimal BG control, while avoiding hypoglycaemic episodes. Treatment sets out to recreate normal fluctuations in circulating insulin concentrations while supporting a flexible lifestyle.

Treatment will be initiated by the specialist diabetes team. There are different types of treatment regimen, and the dose will be determined individually for each patient. The first-line regimen choice is multiple daily basal–bolus insulin injection regimens, with one or more separate daily injections of intermediate-acting insulin or long-acting insulin analogue as the basal insulin, alongside multiple bolus injections of short-acting insulin before meals. This allows flexibility to tailor insulin therapy with the carbohydrate load of each meal.

Other regimens include mixed (biphasic) regimens (involving 1–3 insulin injections per day of short-acting insulin mixed with an intermediate-acting insulin) and continuous subcutaneous insulin infusion (involving a regular or continuous amount of insulin (usually either a rapid-acting insulin analogue or soluble insulin) delivered by a pump).

Dietary management

Patients should be offered dietary advice for weight control and cardiovascular risk management (➲ Coronary heart disease p. 624). Carbohydrate counting is recommended by national guidelines.[23] This is a meal planning technique for managing BG levels by matching carbohydrate quantities to insulin doses. There are structured education programmes (e.g. DAFNE—Dose Adjustment for Normal Eating) that can help patients and their carers learn how to count the carbohydrate content of their meals and decide how much insulin they need (➔ Expert patients and self-management programmes p. 340). Patients should be made aware of the effects of alcohol (➔ Alcohol p. 360) on calorie intake and ↑ the risk of hypoglycaemia. Do not advise adults with T1DM to follow a low glycaemic index diet for glucose control.

Physical activity

Patients should be advised that regular physical activity (➔ Exercise p. 354) is important to reduce cardiovascular risk. Whilst mild to moderate exercise poses a low risk, there is a risk of hypoglycaemia during or up to 24hrs after exercise. Strategies to ↓ the likelihood of exercise-induced hypoglycaemia include nutritional supplementation and insulin dose adjustment.

Blood glucose management

Adults with T1DM should monitor their blood glucose level (BGL) >4 times/day, aiming for: a fasting BGL of 5–7 mmol/L on waking, and a BGL of 4–7 mmol/L before meals at other times of the day.[23] An individualized HbA1c target will be agreed, considering daily activities, risk of complications, comorbidities, occupation, and history of hypoglycaemia. Adults will usually aim for a HbA1c level of ≤48 mmol/mol (6.5%).[23] HbA1c should be measured every 3–6mths in adults with T1DM (or more frequently if indicated).

Hypoglycaemia awareness

Hypoglycaemia occurs with BGL <3.5mmol/L. It can be caused by an overdose of insulin or oral hypoglycaemics, delayed meals, exercise, and alcohol. Symptoms include sweating, fatigue, feeling dizzy, feeling hungry, tachycardia, blurred vision, confusion and convulsions. Hypoglycaemia awareness decreases over time and with ageing. ⚠ In extreme cases, hypoglycaemia can → coma and death. Initial treatment involves oral consumption of 10–20g glucose, repeated after 10–15mins if necessary. Thereafter, if next meal is not due, a carbohydrate snack should be provided. If the patient is unconscious, administer injectable glucagon.

Diabetic ketoacidosis

DKA is a medical emergency. Ketone monitoring is a key part of management for prevention and early detection of DKA. When testing the blood, a ketone result of: <0.6mmols/L is normal; 0.6–1.5mmol/L indicates a slightly ↑ risk and the test should be repeated in 2hrs; 1.6–2.9mmol/L indicates an ↑ risk and the diabetes team or GP should be contacted as soon as possible; and >3mmol/L indicates a very ↑ risk ☎ 999. Similarly, ketones are dangerously high if >2+ in the urine.

Pregnancy

♀ of childbearing age will be informed of the benefits of preconception glycaemic control and of any risks, including medication, that may harm the unborn child. ♀ who are pregnant or who are planning a pregnancy should be referred to the specialist diabetes team (➔ Prescribing for special groups p. 138).

Cardiovascular risk

Assess cardiovascular risk factors annually including albuminuria, smoking (Ⓔ Smoking cessation p. 356, BG control, BP (Ⓔ Hypertension p. 628), full lipid profile (Ⓔ Hypercholesterolaemia p. 632), and abdominal adiposity. Pharmacological treatment will be considered for patients with angina or other ischaemic heart disease (Ⓔ Drugs commonly used in the prevention and treatment of cardiovascular disease p. 646). Similarly, pharmacological treatment will be considered for hypertensive patients.

Managing complications

These include eye disease, diabetic kidney disease, diabetic foot problems, erectile dysfunction (Ⓔ Sexual problems p. 768), and psychological problems (Ⓔ People with anxiety and depression p. 478). All patients with T1DM should have eye screening within 3mths of diagnosis and routinely reviewed annually (Ⓔ UK screening programmes p. 362; (Ⓔ Common problems affecting the eyes p. 746). In relation to kidney disease, an early morning urine sample should be collected and serum creatinine tested once a year (Ⓔ Renal problems p. 754). People who are at risk of foot ulceration should be referred for regular review by foot protection team. Patients should be offered the seasonal influenza vaccination and pneumococcal vaccination (Ⓔ Targeted adult immunization p. 392).

Consideration of specific situations

Patients should be provided with information about how to inform the DVLA of their diagnosis.

For further information and advice on self-management, see Diabetes UK (℘ https://www.diabetes.org.uk/).

Principles of care and management in T2DM

Drug treatment

Some patients will be managed with lifestyle and diet. Drug treatment is dependent on agreed individualized HbA1c target. Standard-release metformin is usually offered as the initial drug treatment for adults with T2DM. Thereafter, follow algorithm for BG lowering therapy in adults with T2DM.[24] Insulin may be recommended if HbA1c rises to 58mmol/mol (7.5%) or if the person is symptomatically hyperglycaemic.

Dietary management

Patients should be offered dietary advice that is applicable for the general population for weight control and cardiovascular risk management. Individualize recommendations for carbohydrate and alcohol intake, and meal patterns. Reducing the risk of hypoglycaemia should be an aim for people using insulin and oral antihyperglycaemic drugs.

Physical activity

Patients should be advised that regular physical activity is important to reduce cardiovascular risk. For patients using insulin and oral antihyperglycaemic drugs, see precautions relating to physical activity in people with T1DM.

Blood glucose management

For adults managed either by lifestyle and diet, or by lifestyle and diet together with a single drug not associated with hypoglycaemia, a HbA1c of 48mmol/mol (6.5%) is recommended; whilst for adults on a drug associated with hypoglycaemia, a HbA1c level of 53mmol/mol (7.0%) is recommended.[25] For frail older adults (➲ Frailty p. 678), those with impaired hypoglycaemia awareness, those at risk of falls (➲ Falls prevention p. 368), or with significant comorbidities, HbA1c limits may be relaxed on a case-by-case basis.

Macro and microvascular complications will need to be managed. Self-monitoring of BGL is not routinely offered unless the person is on insulin, experiencing hypoglycaemic episodes, is at risk of hypoglycaemic episodes while driving or operating machinery, or is pregnant or planning to get pregnant.

Hypoglycaemia awareness

For patients using insulin and oral antihyperglycaemic drugs, see information pertaining to hypoglycaemia awareness in people with T1DM.

Diabetic ketoacidosis

DKA is more common in T1DM; however, people with T2DM who produce very little of their own insulin may also be at risk. See information pertaining to DKA in people with T1DM.

Hyperglycaemic hyperosmolar state

Hyperglycaemic hyperosmolar state (HSS) can occur in people with T2DM who experience very ↑ BGL. It develops over a number of days/weeks through illness (e.g. infection) and dehydration. ⚠ HSS is a medical emergency associated with ↑ risk of myocardial infarction, stroke, and peripheral arterial thrombosis. Symptoms include those associated with dehydration and hyperglycaemia. Urgent admission to hospital is required.

Pregnancy

For patients who are pregnant or planning a pregnancy, see information on pregnancy in people with T1DM.

Cardiovascular risk and managing complications

See managing cardiovascular risk in people with T1DM and managing complications in people with T1DM.

Consideration of specific situations

See consideration of specific situations in people with T1DM.

Structured education programmes

Patients with T2DM should be referred to structured education programmes (e.g. DESMOND) to learn more about the condition, the complications associated with the disease, the importance of medication concordance, food choices, and physical activity. For further information and advice on self-management, see Diabetes UK (⌨ https://www.diabetes.org.uk/).

Personalized care plan

All patients with either T1DM or T2DM should have a personalized care plan (PCP) which sets out self-monitoring and HbA1c targets. The PCP should be shared with other relevant and involved teams and practitioners.

Annual review

Focused on individualized care, education, and lifestyle advice, and identifying and managing complications. Many organizations have clinical review protocols for the management of diabetes and templates for the annual review (◆ Principles of medication reviews p. 142).

References

23. NICE (2015) *Type 1 diabetes in adults: diagnosis and management [NG17]*. Available at: https://www.nice.org.uk/guidance/ng17/chapter/Key-priorities-for-implementation
24. NICE (2018) *Algorithm for blood glucose lowering therapy in adults with type 2 diabetes*. Available at: https://www.nice.org.uk/guidance/ng28/resources/algorithm-for-blood-glucose-lowering-therapy-in-adults-with-type-2-diabetes-pdf-2185604173
25. NICE (2019) *Type 2 diabetes in adults: management [NG28]*. Available at: https://www.nice.org.uk/guidance/ng28

Multiple sclerosis

Multiple sclerosis (MS) is a chronic, incurable neurological disorder characterized by autoimmune damage to neural tissue (patches of demyelination) that usually → increasing levels of disability. Cause is unknown, but there is a marked geographical variation in prevalence increasing with latitude. Four different types of MS:

- **Relapsing remitting:** commonest form of the disease. Acute relapses punctuated by periods of stability. Each relapse leads to ↑ disability. Over time, remissions are less complete and residual disability increases.
- **Benign:** between 10–20% of cases. Involves occasional relapses and limited disability.
- **Secondary progressive:** after ~15yrs of relapsing remitting form of the disease, 60% of people will be in the 2° progressive phase. They have fewer or no relapses, but their disability increases.
- **Primary progressive:** ~10% of cases. Disease gradually advances, without relapse or remission.

Symptoms

- Fatigue
- Vision problems
- Numbness and tingling
- Muscle spasms, stiffness, and weakness
- Mobility problems
- Pain
- Problems with thinking, learning, and planning
- Depression and anxiety (⊃ People with anxiety and depression p. 478)
- Sexual problems (⊃ Sexual problems p. 768)
- Bladder problems (⊃ Urinary incontinence p. 504)
- Bowel problems (⊃ Faecal incontinence p. 514; ⊃ Constipation in adults p. 512)
- Speech and swallowing difficulties

Diagnosis

MS is difficult to diagnose and can take about a year to confirm due to presentation of various individual symptoms of visual and sensory disturbances, limb weakness, gait problems, bladder and bowel symptoms. The 2017 McDonald criteria is widely used for diagnosis in clinical practice.[26]

Progression

Due to the varied and unpredictable nature of MS, it is not possible to predict the progress of disability across the disease. The Expanded Disability Status Scale is used to quantify disability in MS and monitor changes over time.[27]

Care and management

The team around the patient will include: MS nurse, neurologist, physiotherapist, occupational therapist, continence advisor, speech and language therapist, dietician, psychologist, and GP (⊃ Teamwork p. 58).

Drug treatment may include a short course of steroid medication for treating relapses of MS symptoms and disease-modifying therapies to reduce the number of relapses.

Patients should be encouraged to quit smoking (→ Smoking cessation p. 356) as evidence suggests smoking is a risk factor in the progression of MS. Regular activity is important and has specific benefits for reducing fatigue and improving strength and mobility (→ Exercise p. 354).

Patients should be made aware of local expert patient and self-management programmes (→ Expert patients and self-management programmes p. 340). Family and carer (→ Carers p. 458) needs should be considered. At the end of life, person-centred palliative care will be facilitated by advanced care planning (including advanced statements and advanced decisions) (→ Mental capacity p. 470).

References

26. Thompson, A., Banwell, B., Barkhof, F., et al. (2017) Diagnosis of multiple sclerosis: 2017 revisions of the McDonald criteria. *Lancet Neurology*, 17(2), 162–73

27. Kurtzke, J. (1993) Rating neurological impairment in multiple sclerosis: an expanded disability status score. *Neurology*, 33(11), 1444–52

Further information

National Institute of Health and Care Excellence (NICE) (*Multiple sclerosis in adults*). Available at: ℛ https://www.nice.org.uk/guidance/cg186/chapter/Introduction

Motor neurone disease

Motor neurone disease (MND) refers to a group of incurable, rapidly progressive, neurodegenerative diseases affecting the nerves in the brain and spinal cord. Onset usually 55–79yrs. Causes largely unknown; possible genetic and environmental (~one in ten people have a family history of MND). Main types of MND:
- Amyotrophic lateral sclerosis (ALS): ~50% of cases
- Progressive bulbar palsy (PBP): ~25% of cases
- Progressive muscular atrophy (PMA): ~25% of cases

Life expectancy

Varies depending on form:
- ALS: ~2–5yrs
- PBP: ~6mths–3yrs
- PMA: usually >5yrs

Symptoms

Presentation varies according to type of disease. Symptoms can include:
- Muscle weakness, wasting, and cramps
- Small involuntary contractions of skeletal muscles
- Weight loss
- Weak grip
- Stumbling
- Emotional lability
- Dysarthria and dysphasia with nasal speech
- Poor swallow and regurgitation if upper motor neurons are involved

Cognition

Experience varies:
- No cognitive changes
- Mild cognitive and/or behavioural change
- Frontotemporal dementia (diagnosed at the same time or after MND) (● People with dementia p. 498)
- People with frontotemporal dementia who go on to develop MND

Care and management

Referral to neurologist for diagnosis and management. Care by the multidisciplinary team (including specialist nurses, physiotherapists, speech and language therapy (SaLT), and dieticians) (● Teamwork p. 58) to maintain quality of life by symptom management and support. Maintain emotional, physical, social, and financial support throughout course of disease for patient, family, and carers (● Carers p. 458). MND Association can help with information, advice, and support.

Dysarthria

Can → isolation, frustration, increased fear and anxiety (● People with anxiety and depression p. 478), and low self-esteem. SaLT to assess needs. Use of different forms of augmentative and alternative communication (● Adults and children with additional communication needs p. 122).

Dysphagia

Can → drooling, dehydration, weight loss, and aspiration and recurrent chest infections. Assess nutritional intake, hydration, and weight. Control of head position with pillows, collar, or head support. Modify diet and use thickened fluids. Also, possibility of gastrostomy feeding depending on patient wishes (● Enteral tube feeding p. 594).

Respiratory function

Respiratory muscle weakness occurs eventually in everyone with MND. Respiratory function should be assessed every 2–3mths or more frequently if indicated (● Measuring lung function p. 606). Assessment should include consideration of sleep-related respiratory symptoms. Referral to specialist respiratory team for management, which may include positioning, relaxation and anxiety management, breathing techniques, and O_2 therapy (● Long-term oxygen therapy p. 622). Also, potential option of assisted ventilation, depending on patient wishes.

Saliva problems

Assess volume and viscosity, respiratory function, swallowing, diet, posture, and oral care. Provide advice on swallowing, diet, posture, positioning, and oral care. Suction or medication to ↓ production may be required.

Pain

Due to factors including joint immobility, spasm, and cramps. Consider simple analgesia for joint pain. Physiotherapy can provide advice on positioning to relieve discomfort, passive exercise programme (● Exercise p. 354), prevention of contractures, maintenance of joint mobility, etc. Seek advice on pharmacological interventions for cramps and spasms.

Planning for end of life

At the end of life, person-centred palliative care will be facilitated by advanced care planning (including advanced statements and advanced decisions) (● Mental capacity p. 470).

Further information

MND Association (*Cognitive change, frontotemporal dementia and MND*). Available at: ℛ https://www.mndassociation.org/wp-content/uploads/PX018-Cognitive-change-frontotemporal-dementia-and-MND.pdf

MND Association (*Motor neurone disease: a guide for GPs and primary care teams*). Available at: ℛ https://www.mndassociation.org/wp-content/uploads/px016-motor-neurone-disease-a-guide-for-gps-and-primary-care-teams.pdf

MND Association (*A professional's guide to end of life care in MND*). Available at: ℛ https://www.mndassociation.org/wp-content/uploads/px012-a-professional-guide-to-end-of-life-care-in-mnd-v1-0-jan16-web.pdf

National Institute of Health and Care Excellence (NICE) (*Motor neurone disease: assessment and management [NG42]*). Available at: ℛ https://www.nice.org.uk/guidance/ng42/chapter/Recommendations

Parkinson's disease

Parkinson's disease (PD) is a chronic, incurable, progressive, degenerative, neurological disorder. Young onset can appear from 40yrs. More commonly, onset is from 50yrs. Causes are largely unknown but evidence of genetic susceptibility (e.g. seen in identical twins where one twin has early onset PD). Environmental risk factors include exposure to herbicides, pesticides, heavy metals, proximity to industry, and rural residence. Repeated head trauma also a risk factor.

Parkinsonism are Parkinson's symptoms that are seen in other conditions (e.g. multi-systems atrophy, progressive supranuclear palsy, Lewy body dementia (➜ People with dementia p. 498), encephalitis, and the side effect of some medications (e.g. haloperidol and chlorpromazine (➜ People with psychosis p. 486)).

There is poor specificity of a clinical diagnosis of PD in the early stages. Diagnosis should be made by a specialist and based on the UK PD Society Brain Bank Clinical Diagnostic Criteria (see ℘ http://www.toolkit.parkinson.org/sites/toolkit.parkinson.org/files/resources/UK%20Brain%20Bank%20Diagnostic%20Criteria.pdf).

Pathology

Degeneration of dopaminergic neurons in the substantia nigra, which is part of the basal ganglia (region of the brain that controls voluntary movement). In 80–90% of cases symptoms are due to depletion of dopamine in the substantia nigra. The brain can also have Lewy bodies.

Symptoms

Slow insidious onset

Motor symptoms

PD is diagnosed by the presence of two or more of the following:
- Rigidity and stiffness (resulting in typical shuffling walk)
- Bradykinesia
- Resting tremor
- Postural instability (usually later in the disease trajectory)

Non-motor symptoms

Many and varied, including:
- Orthostatic or postural hypotension
- Constipation (➜ Constipation in adults p. 512)
- Bladder dysfunction (➜ Urinary incontinence p. 504)
- Pain
- Sleep disorders and fatigue
- Restless leg syndrome
- Seborrhoea
- Hyperhidrosis
- Dysphagia
- Slurred speech
- Depression

Cognitive impairment

Whilst PD can coexist with other forms of dementia (e.g. vascular dementia), cognitive impairment and dementia are ↑ recognized as features of PD. When severe, may surpass motor symptoms as a major cause of disability and mortality. Characterized by executive function deficits, attention difficulties, visuospatial dysfunction, slowed thinking, word-finding difficulties, and difficulties learning and remembering information.

Psychosis

Key neuropsychiatric feature of PD. Associated with a significant degree of disability. Symptoms include hallucinations, delusions, and paranoid beliefs. May be exacerbated by drug treatments for PD.

Care and management

Multidisciplinary approach (➔ Teamwork p. 58) including neurologist, GP, specialist nurses, physiotherapist, occupational therapist, speech and language therapist, and psychologist.

Early stages

In the early stages, focus on maintaining physical functioning and quality of life. Pharmacology treatment is the main disease management. Monitor progression of the disease and possible side effects of medications (e.g. impulse control disorders associated with dopamine agonists). Falls prevention important (➔ Falls prevention p. 368). Patients should be made aware of local expert patient and self-management programmes (➔ Expert patients and self-management programmes p. 340). Parkinson's UK can provide information and advice. Family and carer (➔ Carers p. 458) needs should be considered across the disease trajectory.

Later stages

As the disease progresses, motor fluctuations occur and are described using the terms 'on' (symptoms are controlled) and 'off' (symptoms are not controlled). Over time, the 'on' periods become shorter. Deterioration is usually gradual, unless caused by an infection or acute illness. Identifying motor fluctuations is important to ensure people remain mobile for as long as possible. Also monitor non-motor symptoms and intervene as indicated.

⚠ Timings of medications are critical to adequate symptom control; delayed administration can have significant effects including a decline in physical functioning.

Planning for end of life

At the end of life, person-centred palliative care will be facilitated by advanced care planning (including advanced statements and advanced decisions) (➔ Mental capacity p. 470).

Further information

NICE (*Parkinson's disease in adults (NG71)*). Available at: ℌ https://www.nice.org.uk/guidance/ng71
Parkinson's UK (*Treatment and therapies*). Available at: ℌ https://www.parkinsons.org.uk/information-and-support/treatments-and-therapies
Parkinson's UK (*Side effects of Parkinson's drugs*). Available at: ℌ https://www.parkinsons.org.uk/information-and-support/side-effects-parkinsons-drugs
SIGN (*Diagnosis and pharmacological management of Parkinson's disease*). Available at: ℌ https://www.sign.ac.uk/assets/sign113.pdf

Adult health problems

Frailty 678

Bacterial skin infections 680

Skin cancer 682

Eczema/dermatitis 684

Fungal infections 686

Psoriasis 688

Viral skin infections 690

Pigmentation and hair
problems 692

Allergies 694

Deafness 696

Mouth and throat problems 698

Adrenal disorders 700

Pituitary disorders 701

Thyroid 702

Hyper- and hypocalcaemia 704

Anal conditions 706

Dyspepsia, gastro-oesophageal
reflux disease, and peptic
ulceration 708

Irritable bowel syndrome 710

Inflammatory bowel disease 712

Coeliac disease 714

Colorectal cancer 715

Appendicitis, diverticulitis, hernias,
and intestinal obstruction 716

Problems of the liver, gallbladder,
and pancreas 718

Viral infections 720

Methicillin-resistant staphylococcus
aureus (MRSA) 722

Viral hepatitis 724

Pandemic influenza 726

Tuberculosis 728

Food-borne disease 730

Common musculoskeletal
problems 734

Bone and connective tissue
disorders 738

Seizures and epilepsy 740

Migraine 744

Common problems affecting
eyes 746

Blindness and partial sight 748

Pneumonia 750

Lung cancer 751

Occupational lung disease 752

Renal problems 754

Urinary tract infection 756

Prostate problems 758

Sexual health: general issues 760

Sexual health consultations 762

Sexually transmitted infections 764

Sexual problems 768

Sexual health and adults with a
learning disability 770

Breast problems 772

Breast cancer 774

Gynaecological cancers 776

Menstrual problems 778

Problems of the ovaries and
uterus 780

Hysterectomy 782

Problems with fertility 784

Vaginal and vulval problems 786

Termination of pregnancy 788

Frailty

Distinguishing older people living with frailty from those who remain fit is of key importance to ensure that fit people are supported to remain fit while those with established frailty are supported on the basis of their needs. Frailty can be defined as a precarious balance between the assets maintaining health and the deficits threatening it.[1] With age, physical, cognitive, emotional, and social factors become ↑ interdependent, influencing health and well-being, and often overlap with multi-morbidity and polypharmacy. Frailty may appear suddenly (e.g. an individual who has been coping can have multiple needs following a single incident (such as illness)). Frailty is predictive of ill health, a move to care home (Ⓢ Care homes p. 32), and death. ~25–50% of 85yr olds are frail.

Indicators consistent with frailty in older people

- Extreme fatigue, unexplained weight loss, and frequent infections
- Immobility/poor physical strength
- Falls: balance and gait impairment present. Spontaneous falls occur in more severe frailty when vision, balance, and strength affect ability to walk
- Sensitivity to drug reactions (Ⓢ Prescribing for special groups p. 138)
- Delirium: rapid onset of fluctuating confusion /impaired awareness

Frailty assessments

- NHS checks to prevent and identify dementia, disability, and frailty
- Ask the patient to walk 4m, taking ≥5secs may indicate frailty
- Do they stop walking whilst talking on the way from the waiting room?
- Edmonton Frail Scale[2] and PRISMA-7[3] are multidimensional assessment instruments
- Electronic frailty index (eFI) is embedded in software packages in 1° care[4]

The use of frailty tools may improve: identification of individuals requiring complex care; the way in which health and social care practitioners co-ordinate their goals and care plans (Ⓢ Teamwork p. 58; Ⓢ Continuity of care p. 598); evaluation of care according to person-centered outcomes, rather than disease or care outcomes; monitoring of the effects of interventions; and charting of significant changes in individual's well-being and vulnerability.

Interventions

Interventions that may help ↓ the impact of frailty include: strength and balance training to ↑ muscle strength and functional abilities (Ⓢ Falls prevention p. 368); nutritional interventions to address impaired nutrition and weight loss (Ⓢ Malnutrition p. 350); strengthening of social networks and support (Ⓢ Social support p. 28); advice for carers (Ⓢ Carers p. 458); and identifying patients at end of life.

References

1. Clegg, A., Young, J., Iliffe, S., et al. (2013) Frailty in elderly people. *Lancet*, 381, 752–62
2. Rolfson, D., Majumdar, S., Tsuyuki, R., et al. (2006) Validity and reliability of the Edmonton Frail Scale. *Age & Ageing*, 35, 526–9
3. Raîche, M., Hébert, M., & Dubois, M. (2008) PRISMA-7: A case finding tool to identify older adults with moderate to severe disabilities. *Archives of Gerontology and Geriatrics*, 47, 9–18
4. Clegg, A., Bates, C., Young, J., et al. (2016) Development and validation of an electronic frailty index using routine primary care electronic health record data. *Age and Ageing*, 45(3), 353–60

Further information

NICE (*Multimorbidity: clinical assessment and management [NG56]*). Available at: ℗ https://www.nice.org.uk/guidance/ng56

NICE (*Dementia, disability and frailty in later life—midlife approaches to delay or prevent onset [NG16]*). Available at: ℗ https://www.nice.org.uk/guidance/ng16

SIGN (*Polypharmacy*). Available at: ℗ https://www.sehd.scot.nhs.uk/publications/DC20150415polypharmacy.pdf

Bacterial skin infections

Impetigo

Contagious superficial cutaneous infection caused by Staphylococcus aureus (STA) and/or beta-haemolytic Streptococcus. Symptoms include vesicles that rupture easily, producing golden yellow exudates which form a crust when dry. Commonly occur on face and neck, but can be more extensive. Can occur as a 2° infection to other skin conditions (e.g. eczema (→ Eczema in childhood p. 284; → Eczema/dermatitis p. 684) and scabies). Children who live in overcrowded conditions (→ Homes and housing p. 26) and/ or with poor hygiene at ↑ risk. Localized infection should be treated with topical antibiotic cream. Before initial application, ask patient to soak and remove crusty areas (unless too painful). For extensive areas or if patient has a fever, prescribe oral antibiotics and use saline soaks to cleanse areas and remove crusts. Encourage good hygiene practice to limit the spread of infection (e.g. not sharing towels, flannels, or clothes). Exclude from nursery or school until 48hrs after starting treatment and crusts improving. If no significant improvement in 7 days, swab for a bacterial culture.

Infection of the hair follicles

Follicullitis

Superficial active pustular inflammation caused by STA. Triggered by shaving, waxing, and tar- or oil-based ointments. Some cases will heal without intervention but topical antibiotics may be indicated.

Furuncle (boil)

Deep infection caused by STA. Methicillin-resistant Staphylococcus aureus (MRSA) (→ Methicillin-resistant Staphylococcus aureus p. 722) and Panton Valentine Leukocidin Staphylococcus aureus (PVL-SA) can also be responsible. Characterized by inflammation and nodule with peeling of overlying skin. Common areas affected are those that sweat and/or are exposed to friction (e.g. nose, face, axilla, and buttocks). Patients who are immunosuppressed (→ Principles of working with someone with compromised immunity p. 466) or have diabetes (→ Diabetes: overview p. 660) are more prone. Most heal without intervention. To speed up healing, apply a warm, moist cloth for 10–20mins, three or four times a day. When boil ruptures, cover with sterile dressing (→ Wound dressings p. 532). Use analgesia as required. Antibiotics indicated if the person is pyrexial, develops a 2° skin infection (e.g. cellulitis), or boil is on face. Some boils will need to be drained in either general practice (→ General practice p. 18) or 2° care. Further investigation if patient is experiencing recurrent boils.

Carbuncle

Deep infection of a group of hair follicles by STA. Commonly found in nape of neck. Characterized by dome-shaped area of erythema developing into a deep and painful abscess. Patients who are immunosuppressed or diabetic more prone. Carbuncles always require oral antibiotics. Large carbuncle or in a sensitive area may require incision. Refer to 2° care if not responding to treatment. Rule out diabetes and weakened immunity (if not already diagnosed). Further investigation if patient experiencing recurrent carbuncles.

⚠ An active boil or carbuncle is contagious, with potential to spread to other parts of the body or other people. Encourage good hygiene practice and keep area covered.

Cellulitis

Infection of the subcutaneous tissues with Streptococcus pryrogenes. Most commonly on the lower legs. Organism enters the tissues through a fissure caused by eczema (➲ Eczema/dermatitis p. 684), tinea pedis, leg ulceration (➲ Leg ulcer assessment p. 536), although an entry port may not be found. Erythematous, oedematous, and painful. Blistered areas occur. It is often a recurrent problem. Eron classification summarized in Box 12.1.[5] Types IV and III require hospitalization. Will also require hospitalization if has severe or rapidly deteriorating cellulitis, is aged <1yr or is frail (➲ Frailty p. 678), is immunocompromised, has lymphoedema (➲ Lymphoedema p. 548), has facial cellulitis, or has suspected orbital or periorbital cellulitis. Type II may require admission depending on services to administer intravenous anti-biotics in the community. Type I managed with oral antibiotics at home. If a recurrent problem, prophylactic antibiotics.

Box 12.1 Eron Clinical Classification System Cellulitis

Class I: no signs of systemic toxicity, have no uncontrolled comorbidities
Class II: systemically ill or systemically well, but with a comorbidity
Class III: significant systemic upset such as acute confusion, tachycardia, tachypnoea, hypotension, or unstable comorbidities, or have a limb-threatening infection due to vascular compromise
Class IV: sepsis or severe life-threatening infection (e.g. necrotizing fasciitis)

Reference

5. Eron, L. (2000) Infections of skin and soft tissues: outcome of a classification scheme. *Clinical Infectious Diseases*, 31, 287

Further information

NICE (*Impetigo*). Available at: ℘ https://cks.nice.org.uk/impetigo
NICE (*Boils, carbuncles and staphylococcal carriage*). Available at: ℘ https://cks.nice.org.uk/boils-carbuncles-and-staphylococcal-carriage
NICE (*Cellulitis: acute*). Available at: ℘ https://cks.nice.org.uk/cellulitis-acute

Skin cancer

This 1° cutaneous cancer is most commonly of the keratinocytes or melanocytes. Caused by genetic factors, exposure to sunlight, and sometimes exposure to carcinogens (❺ Skin cancer prevention p. 374; ❺ Cancer prevention p. 372). Two main types: malignant melanoma (majority) and non-melanoma skin cancer (basal cell carcinoma (BCC) and squamous cell carcinoma (SCC)).

ABCDEFG of melanoma

A useful guide for determining which moles are potential melanomas:
- Asymmetry: an unusual shape or a non-symmetrical shaped mole requires further evaluation
- Border: a benign mole will usually have a smooth, clearly demarcated border; a mole with an ill-defined or irregular border requires further evaluation
- Colour: pigment variation is indicative of malignancy and requires further evaluation
- Diameter: most melanomas are >6mm
- Elevated/evolutionary changes: in colour, size, symmetry, surface characteristics, and symptoms
- Firm
- Growing: for >1mth

These changes usually take place over a relatively short time from weeks to months. Other signs can include mole or growth that crusts, bleeds, or is itchy, or a sore that will not heal.

Malignant melanoma (or cutaneous melanoma)

Good prognosis depends on early detection and treatment. Four types:
- Superficial spreading malignant melanoma: an enlarging brown/black macular/popular lesion, may be irregular with colour variation
- Nodular melanoma: a pigmented papule that enlarges and ulcerates
- Acral melanoma: brown/black macules on the non-hair-bearing skin of the palms, soles, and nail beds
- Lentigo maligna melanoma: an irregularly shaped, flat, pigmented lesion on sun-damaged skin. Most frequently occurs on the face or other sun-exposed sites
- Nodular melanoma: a pigment papule that enlarges and ulcerates

Treatment
All suspected cases of melanoma referred to 2° care. Surgical removal of suspected lesion to establish the histological diagnosis. May require further surgery to ensure adequate margins around the excised lesion. Laser therapy and immunotherapy also used. Patient assessed for the presence of metastatic disease. Patient is followed up by 2° care for at least 5yrs.

Non-melanoma skin cancer

Basal cell carcinoma
Most common type of skin cancer. Also known as rodent ulcer. Locally invasive, low-grade tumours of the basaloid cells that rarely metastasize.

Usually occur on sun-exposed skin of older patients, but can affect younger patients. There are different types of basal cell carcinoma:
- Nodular basal cell carcinoma (BCC): slow-growing with a characteristic translucent or pearly surface. Dilated vessels may be visible. The area may ulcerate
- Cystic BCC: similar to nodular but there will be more dilated vessels
- Superficial spreading BCC: thin lesions that gradually ↑ in surface area. They may be reddened, slightly raised, with some scaling
- Morphoeic BCC: white/yellow morphoeic plaques resembling an enlarging scar. Ulceration and crusting are usual

Squamous cell carcinoma

An invasive tumour of the keratinocytes that can metastasize. There are different types of SCC:
- Actinic keratosis: these are premalignant lesions. If left untreated, a small % will develop into SCC. Appear in sun-exposed sites as tiny, palpable lesions
- Bowen's disease (SCC *in situ*): may appear on non-sun-exposed sites. Appears as a persistent, erythematous, indurated plaque
- Nodular SCC: hard nodule which ↑ rapidly in size
- Ulcerated SCC: nodular area on the edge of an ulcer or an ulcer on a scar

Treatment for non-melanoma skin cancer

All suspected BCC and SCC are referred to dermatology. Treatment is dependent on the type and size of lesion but may include: cryosurgery, curettage and electrosurgery, fluorouracil topically applied, excision, radiotherapy, surgery, photodynamic therapy.

Further information

Cancer Research (*Skin cancer*). Available at: ℘ https://www.cancerresearchuk.org/about-cancer/skin-cancer

Macmillan Cancer Support (*Melanoma*). Available at: ℘ https://www.macmillan.org.uk/information-and-support/melanoma

Macmillan Cancer Support (*Skin cancer: non-melanoma*). Available at: ℘ https://www.macmillan.org.uk/information-and-support/skin-cancer

NICE (*Skin cancers: recognition and referral*). Available at: ℘ https://pathways.nice.org.uk/pathways/suspected-cancer-recognition-and-referral

NICE (*Melanoma assessment and management [NG14]*). Available at: ℘ https://www.nice.org.uk/guidance/ng14/evidence

Eczema/dermatitis

An acute and/or chronic pruritic inflammation of the skin.

Clinical features

Atopic eczema

Usually presents at 3–12mths of age (⮢ Eczema in childhood p. 284). Often an inherited predisposition to eczema, allergic rhinitis (hay fever), and asthma (⮢ Asthma in adults p. 608; ⮢ Allergies p. 694). It may start on the face and scalp in young children. In older children and adults, often localized to the flexures. Can continue through into adulthood.

Seborrhoeic dermatitis

Associated with an overgrowth of pityrosporum ovule yeast in adults. The distribution is characterized by pink, orange/brown, scaly patches on the scalp, eyebrows, eyelashes, nasolabial folds, external ear, and centre of the chest and back.

Discoid (nummular) eczema

Characterized by well-demarcated, round, scaly plaques. There may be numerous vesicles present that produce exudate and crusting.

Contact dermatitis

Three types: allergic contact dermatitis or irritant (patch testing for diagnosis); irritant contact dermatitis; and phototoxic dermatitis (activated by sunlight).

Pompholyx

Eczema on the hands and feet may present as crops of vesicles with severe itching. There may be peeling and cracking of the skin.

Gravitational (venous, varicose, stasis) eczema

Occurs on the lower legs of patients with venous hypertension.

Management

Emollients

Patients with eczema usually have dry skin and therefore should be prescribed an emollient package of bath additive, soap substitute, and moisturizer. Moisturizers should be applied after bathing and then frequently throughout the day. ⚠ Additives may make the bath slippery (⮢ Falls prevention p. 368)

Topical steroids

There are different strengths of topical steroids (mild, moderate, potent, and very potent). Some need prescription. The weakest steroid that is effective should be the steroid of choice. Administered in finger-tip units. Advice on side effects (including thinning of the skin). Should not be mixed with emollient (applied 30mins after emollient).

Topical immunomodulators

Recommended if the eczema has not responded to topical steroids or is severe. They are prescribed by dermatology specialists. The treatment acts by blocking the molecular mechanisms of inflammation. The patient may experience burning or stinging of the skin for about 20mins when the treatment is applied.

Antihistamines

Useful for short-term use in acute phases of the eczema for their sedative effect. They are to be taken 1hr before bedtime.

Infection

Bacterial: Staphylococcus aureus

Characterized by yellow crusting or weeping pustules. Flare-up of eczema not responding to usual treatment. Treat with oral antibiotics.

Viral herpes simplex

Painful, small, umbilicated vesicles. Requires medical assessment as widespread infection (eczema herpeticum) may be life-threatening. The patient will be unwell and will require systemic antiviral treatment as an inpatient.

General advice

Avoid the use of soaps and detergents on the skin. Extremes of temperature, cold winds, or hot environments with ↓ humidity may exacerbate eczema. Cotton clothing should be worn next to the skin. Nails should be kept short to ↓ damaging from scratching. Dietary manipulation, under the direction of a dietician, is indicated if there is a history of specific food allergy.

Further information

National Eczema Society (*Treatments*). Available at: ℘ http://www.eczema.org/basic-treatment
NICE (*Eczema: atopic*). Available at: ℘ https://cks.nice.org.uk/eczema-atopic
SIGN (*Management of atopic eczema in primary care*). Available at: ℘ https://www.sign.ac.uk/assets/sign125.pdf

Fungal infections

Fungal infection in humans is largely attributable to two groups: dermatophytes (multicellular filaments or hyphae) and yeasts (unicellular forms replicating by budding). Infection can occur from direct contact with infected animals, humans, or soil, or contact with a contaminated object (e.g. shared towels).

Dermatophyte (tinea) infections

Tineas are superficial infections in keratinized tissue (hair, nails, stratum corneum). Three types: trichophyton, microsporum, and epidermophyton. Diagnosis usually clinical, but can be confirmed by skin scrapings or nail clippings sent for laboratory examination. Give advice on good hygiene.

Tinea corporis (ringworm)

Single or multiple pink, scaly plaques on trunk or limbs, which gradually ↑ in size. As expands, the centre clears to look like a ring. Treatment is by application of topical antifungal creams but, in extensive or difficult to treat cases, systemic treatment with oral medication may be required after confirmation of diagnosis from laboratory examination.

Tinea cruris (ringworm in the groin)

Common in young ♂ and may be associated with tinea pedis. Itchy, pink, scaly patches with central clearing on insides of thigh; scrotum rarely affected. Treated with antifungal creams as advised by healthcare professional.

Tinea pedis (athlete's foot)

Five patterns of tinea pedis on the feet: itchy scaling and maceration between toes, usually fourth and fifth toes; plaques of tinea pedis, similar to tinea corporis, on dorsum of foot; white itchy scaling on the soles of one or both feet; scaling on the sides of the foot; and vesicles on the instep, usually on one foot. Treated with an antifungal preparation. Oral treatment if widespread, severe, or topical treatment failed.

Tinea manium

Affects hands with powdery scaling. Uncommon. Antifungal treatment will be required.

Tinea unguium

Nail(s) becomes thickened, discoloured white or yellow. Treated if patient requests or is causing other recurrent infections. Diagnosis by laboratory examination from nail clippings. Antifungal treatment available over the counter (OTC).

Tinea capitis (scalp ringworm)

Most common in children, rarely seen in adults. Causes discrete bald areas with short broken-off hairs. The underlying skin is scaly and red. Treatment with oral antifungal.

Sometimes also a kerion, red, boggy swelling discharging pus. Treated by softening crusts with olive oil. Take a swab for laboratory examination. Treat with antibiotics if microbiology suggest to do so.

Yeast infections

Candida (thrush) skin infections

Caused by the opportunistic pathogen Candida albicans. Advise good skin hygiene and allowing air to circulate. Commonly seen as a result of a broad-spectrum antibiotic or poor nappy hygiene (→ Baby hygiene and skin care p. 194). Also seen in patients with diabetes (→ Diabetes: overview p. 660) and patients who are immunosuppressed (→ Principles of working with someone with compromised immunity p. 466). Usually flexures are affected and pattern is symmetrical. Adults should be treated with a topical antifungal cream.

Cheilitis topical

Infections causing inflamed and cracked grooves at corner of mouth. Commonly seen in people wearing poorly fitting dentures. Advise to clean dentures after meals, sterilize at night, and get a dental review.

Oral candidiasis

Seen as white plaques on the mouth, tongue, and gums. Plaques do not wipe off. Commonly seen in babies, the elderly, and following a course of antibiotics. Treat with oral antifungal. Ensure baby teats and bottles being used are sterilized (→ Bottle feeding p. 186). Patients with dentures need to treat them at the same time as mouth.

Genital candidiasis

♂ can present with redness, sore glans penis, and/or ulceration of fore-skin. ♀ see → Vaginal and vulval problems p. 786. Not usually transmissible. Treat with good hygiene, cotton underwear, and antifungal cream.

Intertrigo

Usually in skin folds due to heat and humidity. Frequently seen in overweight people. The area will be red and painful with red satellite lesions. Treat with combined antifungal and steroid cream.

Paronychia

Infection of nail fold and loss of cuticle → chronic infection. To induce growth of new cuticle, advise to keep hands dry by wearing cotton gloves inside rubber gloves. Apply petroleum jelly to affected nail several times a day to protect the area.

Pityrosporum skin infections

Pityriasis versicolor

A scaly rash that occurs most commonly in young adults due to pityrosporum orbiculare. Characterized by pigmentary skin changes, either hypo- or hyper-pigmented, and occasionally red patches. If localized, treat with antifungal cream. If extensive, refer to dermatology. Reassure the patient that the pigmented areas will take ~3mths to go.

Further information

British Association of Dermatologists (*Patient information leaflets*). Available at: ℘ www.bad.org.uk/for-the-public/patient-information-leaflets

NICE (*Candida oral*). Available at: ℘ https://cks.nice.org.uk/candida-oralInfections

NICE (*Candida: skin*). Available at: ℘ https://cks.nice.org.uk/candida-skin

NICE (*Scalp: fungal skin infections*). Available at: ℘ https://cks.nice.org.uk/fungal-skin-infection-scalp

Psoriasis

Chronic, relapsing, inflammatory, hyperproliferative skin disease. Affects 1.3–2.2% of the population (white population more than other ethnic backgrounds). Onset most commonly between 20–30yrs. Genetically predetermined, but also caused by infection, stress (➲ Managing stress p. 358), drugs (e.g. lithium, antimalarials, beta blockers, systemic glucocorticoids), and the environment. Clinical features summarized in Table 12.1.

Management

Management depends on type and severity of psoriasis and the impact it has on the person. Also consider previous therapies and the ability of the patient to apply topical treatments. Provide lifestyle advice including weight loss (➲ Nutrition and healthy eating p. 342), smoking cessation (➲ Smoking cessation p. 356), and alcohol reduction (➲ Alcohol p. 360). Treatments for psoriasis fall into three groups.

Table 12.1 Clinical features of psoriasis

Type	Features
Chronic plaque psoriasis	Well-demarcated, raised pink plaques; dry silver/white scales. Commonly on elbows, knees, scalp, behind ears, trunk, buttocks, periumbilical area, extensor surfaces, and lower back.
Scalp psoriasis	75–90% of cases. May be dry and scaly or, in more severe cases, inflamed, scaly, well-demarcated plaques. It can also present as non-scarring alopecia or severe alopecia (see erythrodermic psoriasis).
Guttate psoriasis	Multiple red papules and small psoriatic lesions. Usually on the trunk and proximal limbs in a 'raindrop' distribution, commonly following a streptococcal infection. Can be first presentation of psoriasis.
Flexural psoriasis	Can present as lesions affecting areas such as the groin, genital area, axillae, inframammary folds, abdominal folds, sacral and gluteal cleft. Lesions often red and glazed in appearance with possible fissures in skin creases.
Pustular psoriasis (localized or generalized)	Localized: multiple small, sterile (brown/yellow) pustules, with erythema and hyperkeratosis on the palms and soles. As they dry, brown patches develop. Generalized: multiple tiny pustules on generalized erythrodermic skin. The skin is unstable and requires emergency dermatology care (potentially life-threatening emergency). Systemic symptoms such as: fever, tachycardia, malaise, weight loss, and arthralgia.
Erythrodermic psoriasis	Involves ~90% of skin surface. Lesions may feel warm, and may be associated with systemic illness.
Facial psoriasis	Well-demarcated plaques on face. Lesions can also affect hairline. Can also have possible mild scaling around the eyebrows and nasolabial folds.
Nail psoriasis	Nail pitting, discolouration, subungual hyperkeratosis, onycholysis, and complete nail dystrophy.

Topical treatments

Used for mild to moderate psoriasis, or with other therapies:

- Emollients: regular use ↓ scaling and itching, and ↑ penetration of other topical medications
- Vitamin D3 analogues: effective in plaque psoriasis. Colourless and odourless.
- Coal tar: ↓ in use as concerns about oncogenic potential. Have a strong smell so are not acceptable to all patients. Used in shampoos, bath emollient, lotions, and scalp treatments
- Retinoid: used for mild-to-moderate psoriasis
- Dithranol: short-term contact cream preparations available for home use. Only applied to the plaques as local irritation to non-affected skin. Leaves an unwanted staining on the skin
- Keratolytics: ↓ scale, greater penetration of other drugs
- Corticosteroids: may be used in combination with aforementioned products. Important to explain side effects to prevent misuse

Phototherapy

Natural sunlight may be beneficial. Phototherapy (artificial sunlight) in-dicated for moderate-to-severe psoriasis, administered in dermatology clinic. Commercial sunbeds are not an alternative. The long-term effects of phototherapy include ageing of the skin and ↑ risk of certain skin cancers (→ Skin cancer p. 682).

Systemic treatments

Considered when 10–15% body coverage, patient not responded to other treatments, or causing severe negative impact on quality of life. Treatments are under the supervision of the dermatology consultant, although care may be shared with 1° care. There are two sorts of systemic treatment: systemic non-biological therapy (requiring ↑ levels of monitoring); and systemic bio-logical therapy. Only considered if the patient is unresponsive or intolerant to all other treatments or has life-threatening psoriasis.

Further information

NICE (*Psoriasis*). Available at: ℘ https://cks.nice.org.uk/psoriasis
NICE (*Psoriasis: assessment and management [CG 153]*). Available at: ℘ https://www.nice.org.uk/guidance/cg153
Psoriasis Association (*Psoriasis and treatments*). Available at: ℘ https://www.psoriasis-association.org.uk/psoriasis-and-treatments/

Viral skin infections

Warts (verrucae)

Warts appear as firm, rough, pink- or brown-coloured papules with black pinpoint dots on the surface. Benign, cutaneous tumours caused through the infection of the epidermal cells with human papillomavirus (HPV). Characterized by hyperkeratosis and thickening of the epidermis. Common in children.

Treatment and advice

The majority will resolve with no treatment within 2yrs. Topical wart treatments may be bought OTC or prescribed. The topical treatments need to be used for 3mths or until it resolves. Patients can use a swimming sock to cover any warts on their feet to ↓ the risk of spreading the virus.

Molluscum contagiosum

Discrete, umbilicated, pearly white or pink papules caused by the pox virus. Common in children and young adults. Most commonly seen on the face and neck, but can occur on any part of the skin.

Treatment and advice

The lesions will resolve spontaneously within 6–24mths. Picking and squeezing the lesions may cause the lesions to spread.

Herpes simplex

1° infection with Type I occurs either in the epidermis or buccal mucosa, usually within the first 5yrs of life. The virus remains dormant in dorsal root ganglion until reactivated. A recurrence commences with a prodromal sensation of itching, burning, or tingling. A few hours later, there will be small grouped vesicles. These will burst, crust, and heal in 7–10 days. Triggers for reactivation include fever, sunlight, menstruation, and stress. Eczema herpeticum occurs when eczema becomes secondarily infected with the herpes simplex virus. The patient will be unwell.

Treatment and advice

Usually no treatment is required. Topical antiviral treatment applied at start of episode will ↓ duration of the episode, but will not prevent future attacks. Patients with eczema herpeticum will require systemic antiviral treatment.

Genital herpes

See ⊃ Sexually transmitted infections p. 764

Herpes varicella zoster (chickenpox)

It usually affects children <10yrs of age but adults can also be affected. Infectious droplet infection from the upper respiratory tract. There is a prodromal illness that is often mild; first signs of infection are lesions. Characterized by pink macules which develop into papules, tense vesicles, pustules, and then crusts. The condition is very itchy. Antihistamine and calamine lotion may ↓ irritation. Pock-like scarring can occur.

Treatment and advice

Treatment is not usually required unless immunocompromised (❸ Principles of working with someone with compromised immunity p. 466) or pregnant (❸ Pregnancy p. 424). These groups should urgently see GP. Pregnant ♀ should be referred to an obstetrician with expertise in this areas.

Herpes zoster (shingles)

Reactivation of the varicella zoster virus, allowing replication and migration along nerve endings—prodromal phase of pain and tenderness. May occur at any age but more common in >50yrs and in immunocompromised patients. The acute phase is characterized by erythema and vesicles, followed by weeping and crusting. Healing occurs within 3–4wks; however, the pain may continue for months or years (particularly in older people).

Treatment and advice

Skin hygiene advice and non-adherent dressings on rash (❸ Wound dressings p. 532). Antiviral drugs used only for groups at risk of complications (e.g. >50yrs or immunocompromised) who present within 72hrs of rash onset. Calamine lotion and regular analgesia may reduce discomfort during prodromal phase. Post-herpetic neuralgia pain can be severe and debilitating, and nerve painkillers will be required on the advice of pain specialists. If the skin around the eye is affected, patients are referred to an ophthalmologist. Shingles vaccine is available within the NHS to those aged 70–78yrs (❸ Targeted adult immunization p. 392).

Related topics

❸ Infectious diseases in childhood p. 290

Further information

British Association of Dermatologists (*Eczema herpeticum*). Available at: ℘ www.bad.org.uk/shared/get-file.ashx?id=197&itemtype=document

NICE (*Chickenpox*). Available at: ℘ https://cks.nice.org.uk/chickenpox

NICE (*Herpes simplex-ocular*). Available at: ℘ https://cks.nice.org.uk/herpes-simplex-ocular

NICE (*Warts and verrucae*). Available at: ℘ https://cks.nice.org.uk/warts-and-verrucae

Pigmentation and hair problems

Albinism

Rare genetic condition in which melanocytes produce ↓ or no pigment in skin, hair, and eyes. Affects all races. Two main types: ocular-albinism (affects just eyes), and oculo-cutaneous albinism (affects skin, eyes, and hair). Associated with vision problems such as photophobia, nystagmus, and strabismus, requiring specialist follow-up and support (➔ Blindness and partial sight p. 748). It requires ↑ level skin protection in sun (➔ Skin cancer prevention p. 374; ➔ Skin cancer p. 682).

Vitiligo

Vitiligo appears as white patches due to loss of melanocytes in skin. It affects 1 in 100 people. 50% start <20yrs of age. It is thought to be autoimmune response; 30% have a family history (FH). Areas most commonly affected include face, neck, hands, arms, elbows, and knees. A small % of people repigment. Some people will decide on treatment to arrest spread or restore original skin colour. Others will use skin camouflage, whilst others will embrace what makes them different.

Alopecia or hair loss

♂ pattern baldness is common. Alopecia means hair loss. May be due to side effects of other therapies (e.g. cytotoxic therapy) or other conditions such as ringworm (➔ Fungal infections p. 686).

Alopecia areata

Thought to be an autoimmune response of the hair. Sometimes FH. Three types, named according to severity: alopecia areata (mild patchy hair loss on the scalp); alopecia totalis (loss of all scalp hair); and alopecia universalis (loss of scalp and all body hair). If <50% hair loss, then 80% chance of regrowth. Severe cases referred to dermatology. Some wigs may be available on the NHS.

Hirsutism or excess hairiness

Additional hair in ♂ pattern on face, torso, and limbs. Affects one in ten ♀. Mostly idiopathic, although may be associated with therapies (e.g. steroids) or syndromes (e.g. polycystic ovary syndrome (➔ Problems of the ovaries and uterus p. 780)). Patients are referred to a specialist as required. Topical treatments available on consultant prescription. Advice to those with idiopathic hirsutism includes home therapies of cosmetic bleaching, removal by creams, shaving, waxing, and electrolysis. Laser therapy is available in some areas for those with severe problems.

Hypertrichosis

Excess hairiness in non-male pattern. Often caused by drug therapies, (e.g. ciclosporin). If idiopathic, advice as for hirsutism.

Further information

Albinism Fellowship (*Living well with albinism*). Available at: ℰ https://www.albinism.org.uk/living-well-with-albinism/

Alopecia UK (*Working to improve the lives of those affected by alopecia*). Available at: ℰ https://www.alopecia.org.uk/

British Association of Dermatologists (*Guidelines for the treatment of alopecia areata*). Available at: ℰ http://www.bad.org.uk/shared/get-file.ashx?id=68&itemtype=document

British Association of Dermatologists (*Information leaflet on hirsutism*). Available at: ℰ http://www.bad.org.uk/shared/get-file.ashx?id=89&itemtype=document

Changing Faces (*Helping everyone with a scar, mark or condition on their face that makes them look different*). Available at: ℰ www.changingfaces.org.uk

Vitiligo Society (*Information and support*). Available at: ℰ https://www.vitiligosociety.org.uk/index.php/information-support.html

Allergies

An allergic reaction is an exaggerated response by the immune system to an allergen. Antibodies are naturally produced by the body when it first meets an invading organism, but this sometimes results in adverse effects. Common allergens are house dust mite excreta, grass and tree pollen, molds, pet hair, wasp and bee stings, industrial and household chemicals, medicines (e.g. penicillin), and foods (e.g. milk and eggs). Less common allergens include latex, nuts, and fruit. In subsequent exposures, the allergens attach to the immunoglobulin E (IgE) antibodies and the cell releases histamines, causing widened blood vessels, leakage of fluid into tissues, and muscle spasms. Common symptoms include itching, watering eyes, sneezing, swelling, urticaria, and wheezing. Conditions associated with allergic problems include asthma (⟴ Asthma in children p. 306; ⟴ Asthma in adults p. 608). There are four classifications when referring to hypersensitive reactions (Table 12.2).

Assessment and management

Investigations

Depends on the type and severity of symptoms and associated conditions (e.g. asthma). Refer to specialist allergy clinic if diagnosis in doubt, and for investigation and management of anaphylaxis, food allergies, occupational allergies (⟴ Health and safety at work p. 92).

Allergen avoidance

Exclude pets, check documentation of medication allergies (⟴ Record keeping p. 86), avoid pollen (keep windows shut, avoid grass in pollen season, wear wraparound sunglasses, wash hair after being out, cover bed during day), and check food labels for food allergens.

Table 12.2 Reaction classification

Type	Reaction
Type 1 (atopic)	IgE primed mast cells react when exposed to the allergen causing rapid release of histamine and inflammation. If severe, this can amount to anaphylaxis.
Type 2 (cytotoxic)	Antigens in the system are detected by the immune system causing either an immunoglobulin G (IgG) or immunoglobulin M (IgM) response. IgG is found in all body fluids, and IgM in blood and lymph fluid. IgG protects against bacterial and viral infections, and IgM any new infection. IgG or IgM response can occur within minutes or hours. Treatment includes the use of anti-inflammatory and immunosuppressive agents.
Type 3 (immune complex hypersensitivity)	Reaction can be generalized or localized to specific organs. Response to an allergen usually takes between 3 and 10hrs. Treatment includes the use of anti-inflammatory medications.
Type 4 (cell mediated)	Also identified as cellular hypersensitivity, reactions can occur up to 72hrs following exposure to an antigen. Contact dermatitis is an example of this condition which occurs in response to T-cell and macrophage sensitization.

Antihistamines

Histamine has a key role in the body's defence mechanism. It is located in mast cells in the skin, lungs, and gut and is present in circulating basophils. Histamine is released following exposure to physical or chemical injury. On release, it causes inflammation as a reaction to injury; if this is excessive, antihistamines are used.

Allergen immunotherapy

Called desensitization treatment. Involves giving increasing doses of an allergen by injection or drops under tongue. Works by re-programming the immune system to prevent allergy symptoms. Should be performed under the supervision of a doctor.

Anaphylaxis

See ➔ Anaphylaxis p. 810

Allergic rhinitis (including hay fever)

Characterized by an irritation and inflammation of nose and eyes. Common disorder, often seasonal or perennial, and triggered by allergens. Affects ~20% of the UK population. Hay fever is an allergic rhinitis caused by pollen. For allergic rhinitis, low-dose steroid nasal sprays and nose drops, but need to be used daily. Decongestants also helpful, but short-term use only. For hay fever, systematic antihistamine and/or topical nasal spray and/or eye drops may be helpful. Severe symptoms may require a short course of oral steroids. Treatment should begin 2–3wks before pollen season.

Bee/wasp sting allergy

~3 in 100 people who are stung have some kind of allergic reaction (few have a severe reaction). Local or mild generalized reactions treated with antihistamine. Anaphylactic reactions treated with adrenalin.

Food allergies and intolerances

Affect ~5–7% of children (➔ Food and the under-fives p. 212). Less in adults. Foods causing allergic reactions include nuts, wheat, eggs, fish, shellfish, and cows' milk. Some provoke an anaphylactic reaction. There are other types of food intolerances that do not involve an allergic response but symptoms such as rashes, abdominal pain, vomiting, and diarrhoea. Referred to specialist allergy clinic for identification and management. Advice for prevention of food allergy or intolerances includes breastfeeding (➔ Breastfeeding p. 182), appropriate weaning (➔ Weaning p. 188), and avoiding preservatives and additives in food.

Further information

Allergy UK (*Information and advice*). Available at: ℘ https://www.allergyuk.org/information-and-advice

NICE (*Allergic rhinitis*). Available at: ℘ https://cks.nice.uk/allergic-rhinitis

Deafness

Hearing impairments are categorized as: mild (difficulty following speech in noisy situations); moderate (difficulty following speech without a hearing aid); severe (lip reading used to supplement use of hearing aid); and profound deafness (little ability to hear sounds and British Sign Language (BSL) will be first language, along with lip reading, to aid communication). There are multiple possible causes:

- Age: >50% of people >60yrs have a hearing loss
- Noise: prolonged and repeated exposure to loud noise at work/leisure (e.g. listening to loud music through headphones)
- Conduction problems: cerumen (ear wax) (➔ Ear care p. 590), trauma, perforated ear drum, and inflammation/infection
- Genetic: 1 in 1,000 babies born moderately/profoundly deaf; 50% are thought to be due to genetic causes (➔ Hearing screening p. 163; ➔ Deafness in children p. 268)

Presentation in adults

Slow onset with ↑ difficulties in understanding people (e.g. when there is background noise). Questions to ask as part of assessment: Do people seem to be mumbling? Are you often saying pardon? Do you always hear a phone/doorbell? Are conversations sometimes difficult to follow? Do other family members complain that the TV is too loud?

Management

Check that problem not caused by ear wax or presence of infection. Referral for audiology or specialist ear, nose, and throat services for assessment of cause of deafness, to quantify hearing loss, and to assess for hearing aid. Cochlear implant surgery for sensorineural hearing loss. For principles in working with people with hearing loss, see ➔ Adults and children with additional communication needs p. 122).

Tinnitus

A ringing or buzzing heard in the ear or head. For some this will be severe and interfere with life and the ability to sleep. The cause is largely unknown. If continues long term can → distress and depression (➔ People with anxiety and depression p. 478). Management includes: masking with background music/radio; referral to ear, nose, and throat services for a white noise aid; and referral for cognitive behavioural therapy (CBT) (➔ Talking therapies p. 472).

Further information

Royal Association for Deaf People (*Together with deaf people; creating a better more accessible future*). Available at: ℬ www.royaldeaf.org.uk

Mouth and throat problems

Mouth ulcers

Common problems can make it difficult to eat, drink, and talk. Causes include:

- Trauma (e.g. toothbrushing or a minor burn from a hot drink). Should heal <1wk unless trauma ongoing (e.g. badly fitting dentures).
- Apthous ulcers: painful white ulcers commonly seen in people who are stressed and/or of poor health (❯ Managing stress p. 358). May first appear at puberty (❯ Puberty and adolescence p. 228) or pregnancy (❯ Pregnancy p. 424) due to hormonal changes, and take longer to heal and likely to recur unless there is an improvement in health.
- Ulcer caused by herpes infection (❯ Viral skin infections p. 690), inflammatory bowel disease (❯ Inflammatory bowel disease p. 712), coeliac disease (❯ Coeliac disease p. 714), and Behcet's disease. Usually linked to other symptoms.
- Iron or vitamin B12 deficiency (❯ Anaemia in adults p. 652).

Other differential diagnosis of hand, foot, and mouth disease or oral lichen planus should be considered.

All red or white patches in the mouth and ulcers persisting for >3wks need medical assessment by a doctor or dentist to exclude malignancy.

Care and management

Advise on dental hygiene (❯ Dental health in older children p. 226) and regular dental check-ups. Healthy diet avoiding food and drink that may exacerbate symptoms (e.g. highly spiced foods). OTC medication can speed up healing, prevent infection, and ↓ pain.

Gingivitis

Inflammation of the gums which often occurs with a build-up of plaque (bacteria) and hardened plaque (tartar). In mild cases, patients may only have reddened gums. Causes also include: trauma to gums, pregnancy, diabetes (❯ Diabetes: overview p. 660), smoking, stress, diet (❯ Nutrition and healthy eating p. 342), or a side effect of medication (e.g. phenytoin). Can → receding gums, halitosis, infection, abscesses, and loss of teeth. Acute ulcerative gingivitis will need antibiotics.

Care and management

Care and management is the same as for mouth ulcers, plus antiseptic toothpaste and mouth washes. If a smoker, advise quitting (❯ Smoking cessation p. 356).

Sore throat (including laryngitis and tonsillitis)

70% of sore throats have a viral cause and 90% will resolve in a week. Patients complain of pain on swallowing and a fever. Adolescents with persistent sore throat need review to exclude glandular fever. In 5–15yr olds consider adenoids, otitis media (glue ear), and strep throat (a bacterial throat infection). Also consider tonsillitis. Anyone with stridor, breathing difficulty, or dehydration needs urgent medical assessment.

Care and management

Antibiotics are unnecessary for most patients; although they will be indicated if patient has a past history of rheumatic fever, immunodeficiency (➲ Principles of working with someone compromised immunity p. 466), or is a child with diabetes (➲ Endocrine problems p. 304). Exclude sepsis (➲ Sepsis p. 826). OTC analgesia. ↑ fluid intake to avoid dehydration. Rest voice and steam inhalation for laryngitis. Severe tonsillitis four to six times in a year, consider referral for a tonsillectomy.

Unilateral peri-tonsillitis, consider referral to exclude squamous cell carcinoma or lymphoma. Persistent sore throats may be a symptom of throat cancer. HPV (the cervical cancer virus) is becoming more prevalent. Prevent by using condoms when having oral sex (➲ Cancer prevention p. 372).

Sinusitis

An acute or chronic inflammation of sinuses. Maxillary sinusitis will usually clear in a week without antibiotics. Frontal sinusitis is associated with brain abscess and cavernous sinus thrombosis and should be treated with antibiotics. Sinusitis is more common in adults with nasal abnormalities, cystic fibrosis (➲ Cystic fibrosis p. 318), allergic rhinitis (➲ Allergies p. 694), and smokers. Acute sinusitis may follow an upper respiratory tract infection. Some will be a result of dental problems. Sinusitis is characterized as: acute headache and facial pain, worse on bending or coughing, fever; blocked nose; thick nasal mucus; purulent discharge; and loss of smell and taste.

Care and management

Advise to stop smoking and avoid smoky environments. OTC analgesia and decongestant nose drops or sprays. Steam inhalation may be helpful. Refer chronic sufferers to ear, nose, and throat for surgical assessment.

Further information

NICE (*Aphthous ulcer*). Available at: ℘ https://cks.nice.org.uk/aphthous-ulcer
NICE (*Sinusitis*). Available at: ℘ https://cks.nice.org.uk/sinusitis
NICE (*Sore throat: acute*). Available at: ℘ https://cks.nice.org.uk/sore-throat-acute
SIGN (*Management of sore throat and indications for tonsillectomy*). Available at: ℘ https://www.sign.ac.uk/assets/sign117.pdf

Adrenal disorders

Adrenal glands are situated above each kidney and produce hormones such as adrenaline and steroids such as cortisol. These hormones and steroids play important roles in a number of biological functions.

Cushing's syndrome

This is caused by ↑ levels of adrenocortical hormones. In the majority of cases this is the result of the administration of prednisolone or other corticosteroids. Other rare causes include a pituitary adenoma or tumour in the adrenal glands. Signs and symptoms include: redistribution of body fat to create a moon face and truncal obesity, hypertension (➔ Hypertension p. 628), hirsutism (➔ Pigmentation and hair problems p. 692), acne (➔ Acne vulgaris p. 300), bruising and striae, osteoporosis, glycosuria, and hyperglycaemia. Children may exhibit growth cessation but ↑ weight.

Diagnosis and management

Cortisol levels are measured in urine or blood. Steroids are reduced or stopped. If the cause is not due to prescribed steroids, then other causes such as adenoma might be treated and the patient is referred to an endocrinologist.

Addison's disease

This is the result of adrenal cortical insufficiency, primarily caused by destruction of the adrenal cortex (1° adrenal insufficiency). Problems with the immune system account for most cases. Other causes include: TB (➔ Tuberculosis p. 728), infections, haemorrhage, cancer, amyloidosis, surgery, and adrenoleukodystrophy.

Management and treatment

Patient referred to endocrinology. Treatment usually involves replacing deficient steroids. Advise patients to tell any health professional treating them about their condition and to wear a warning bracelet in case of emergency (use of MedicAlert, steroid treatment card, and emergency crisis letter). Patients can apply for a medical exemption for NHS prescriptions (➔ Help with costs of medicines p. 134).

Further information

NICE (*Addison's disease*). Available at: ℘ https://cks.nice.org.uk/addisons-disease
Pituitary Foundation (*Cushing's disease*). Available at: ℘ https://www.pituitary.org.uk/information/pituitary-conditions/cushings-disease/

Pituitary disorders

Pituitary gland secretes many hormones—adrenocortitrophic hormone (ACTH), anti-diuretic hormone (ADH), growth hormone, melanocyte-stimulating hormones (MSH), follicle-stimulating hormone (FSH), luteinizing hormone (LH), thyroid-stimulating hormone (TSH), oxytocin, and prolactin—and affects the function of most other glands in the endocrine system. Pituitary disorders are relatively rare in the UK.

Hypopituitarism

↓ production of all pituitary hormones. Caused by tumour, surgery, trauma, and necrosis from post-partum haemorrhage. Signs and symptoms include: hypogonadism, hypothyroidism, debility, and ↓ weight. Patients are referred to neurology or endocrinology. Treatment is lifelong HRT supervised by a specialist.

Pituitary tumours

These can affect any part of the pituitary and be either malignant or non-malignant. Signs and symptoms are associated with the pressure effects on surrounding structures: chronic headaches; visual disturbances; hypopituitarism; hyperprolactaemia with associated galactorrhoea; ↓ libido (➔ Sexual problems p. 768); menstrual disturbances (➔ Menstrual problems p. 778); and ↓ fertility (➔ Problems with fertility p. 784). Patients are referred to neurology. Treatment options include surgery and radiotherapy. Prolactinomas will be treated medically.

Acromegaly

Hypersecretion of the growth hormone. Has an insidious course over many years. Signs and symptoms include: headaches; changes in appearance (oily skin, change in facial appearance with coarsening of features, ↑ foot size, and ↑ teeth spacing); deepening of voice; sweating; paraesthesiae; proximal muscle weakness; progressive heart failure (➔ Heart failure p. 636); and goitre (➔ Thyroid p. 702). Patients are referred to endocrinologist. Treatment options include surgery, radiotherapy, and medication.

Diabetes insipidus

Impaired water reabsorption by the kidney caused either by ↓ ADH secretion or by trauma, tumour, or inherited. Signs and symptoms include: polydipsia, polyuria, dilute urine, and dehydration. It is managed according to the cause.

Further information

Pituitary Foundation (*Information*). Available at: ♒ https://www.pituitary.org.uk/information/

Thyroid

The thyroid concentrates iodine in order to produce the hormones thyroxine (T_4) and triiodothyronine (T_3). Thyroxine controls many body functions, including heart rate, temperature, and metabolism. It also plays a role in the metabolism of calcium in the body.

Enlargement or lumps in the pre-tracheal neck region require medical assessment. Solitary thyroid nodules can be benign or malignant. Goitres are enlarged thyroid glands that can be:
• Physiological (associated with teenagers, pregnancy (⊃ Pregnancy p. 424)): do not require treatment
• Nodular: do not require treatment unless thyrotoxic, compressing other structures, or cosmetically unacceptable
• Toxic or inflammatory: require treatment and referral to an endocrinologist

Hyperthyroidism

Causes, signs, and symptoms

Graves' disease is the most common cause of hyperthyroidism. It is an autoimmune disease associated with smoking and stressful life events in which antibodies to the thyroid stimulating hormone (TSH) receptor are produced. Other causes include: thyroiditis, amiodarone, kelp ingestion, and toxic nodular goitre (older ♀ with past history of goitre). Signs and symptoms include:
• Weight loss (⊃ Adult body mass index chart p. 346)
• Tremor
• Palpitations
• Hyperactivity
• Eye changes (bulging of the eye)
• Atrial fibrillation (⊃ Atrial fibrillation p. 641)
• Emotionally labile
• Infertility (⊃ Problems with fertility p. 784)

In older people, symptoms may be less obvious and include confusion, dementia (⊃ People with dementia p. 498), apathy, and depression (⊃ People with anxiety and depression p. 478).

Management

Refer to an endocrinologist (and ophthalmologist if eye problems). Treatment options include: pharmacological control of symptoms, radioactive iodine, and surgery.

Hypothyroidism (myxoedema)

A deficiency of thyroid hormones which results in a lowered rate of all metabolic processes.

Causes, signs, and symptoms

Chronic autoimmune thyroiditis, that occurs after treatment with radioactive iodine, thyroidectomy. Onset tends to be insidious and may go undiagnosed for years.

Patients with hypercholesterolaemia, infertility, depression, dementia, obesity, other autoimmune diseases, Turner's syndrome, or congenital hypothyroidism are screened using thyroid function tests (TFTs).

Non-specific symptoms may include:

- Depression
- Fatigue
- Lethargy or general malaise
- Weight gain
- Constipation (➲ Constipation in adults p. 512)
- Hoarse voice or dry skin/hair
- Mental dulling

Management

Depending on TSH concentrations, thyroxine may be started. If a decision is made to treat, check TSH 2mths after starting and adjust the dose accordingly. Once TSH has normalized, TFTs should be measured at least annually thereafter.

Related topics

➲ Hyper- and hypocalcaemia p. 704

Further information

British Thyroid Foundation (*Information*). Available at: ℗ http://www.btf-thyroid.org/information
NICE (*Hypothyroidism*). Available at: ℗ https://cks.nice.org.uk/hypothyroidism

Hyper- and hypocalcaemia

Most of the calcium in the body is in bone and needed for constant re-newal. Calcium is important in normal neuromuscular activity and blood coagulation. There is debate as to whether venepuncture to check calcium levels should be performed without a tourniquet (⊃ Venepuncture p. 580). Assessment of serum calcium concentration includes consideration of serum albumin levels

Hypocalcaemia

↓ level of serum calcium. Causes include: hypoparathyroidism (may be 2° to thyroid or parathyroid surgery) (⊃ Thyroid p. 702); insensitivity to parathyroid hormone; osteomalacia; over-hydration; and pancreatitis (⊃ Problems of the liver, gallbladder, and pancreas p. 718). Signs and symptoms include tetany, neuromuscular excitability, and carpo-pedal spasm (wrist flexion and fingers drawn together). Management includes calcium supplements prescribed and referral to specialist for investigation of cause.

Hypercalcaemia

↑ level of serum calcium. Causes include: 1° hyperparathyroidism, malig-nancy, and chronic renal failure (⊃ Renal problems p. 754). More rarely: familial benign hypercalcaemia, milk alkali syndrome (↑ use of antacids for indigestion), thyrotoxicosis, and vitamin D treatment. Signs and symptoms are often very non-specific, but can include: lethargy, weakness, weight loss, low mood, mild aches and pains, and nausea. Management is dependent on the cause.

Related topics

⊃ Common musculoskeletal problems p. 734

Further information

NICE (*Hypercalcaemia*). Available at: ℔ https://cks.nice.org.uk/hypercalcaemia

Anal conditions

Embarrassment can be a barrier to help-seeking behaviour. Whilst most are benign, maintain ↑ index of suspicion for colorectal cancer (● Colorectal cancer p. 715).

Haemorrhoids

Occur when the veins in the lower part of the rectum and anus distend and swell. Risk factors include: constipation (● Constipation in adults p. 512), ageing, heavy lifting, chronic coughing, and pregnancy (● Pregnancy p. 424). Classed as external or internal. External haemorrhoids can be itchy and painful. Both types can cause bleeding. Internal haemorrhoids are graded: first-degree (project into the lumen of the anal canal but do not prolapse); second-degree (prolapse on straining but ↓ spontaneously when straining is stopped); third-degree (prolapse on straining and require manual reduction); and fourth-degree (prolapsed and incarcerated and cannot be reduced).

Complications include: ulceration, maceration of the perianal skin, is-chaemia, thrombosis, gangrene, perianal sepsis (● Sepsis p. 826), and anaemia (● Anaemia in adults p. 652). Thorough history and clinical examination required to confirm diagnosis and exclude serious pathology. Refer if the diagnosis unclear or serious pathology suspected. Otherwise, management includes: avoiding constipation, maintaining good anal hygiene, offering simple analgesia and/or topical haemorrhoid preparations. Refer if person does not respond to treatment.

Anal fissure

Defined as a tear or ulcer in the lining of the anal canal, immediately within the anal margin. Most cases occur in patients with constipation. Other risk factors include: persistent diarrhoea, inflammatory bowel disease (● Inflammatory bowel disease p. 712), pregnancy and childbirth (● Complicated labour p. 436), sexually transmitted infections (such as syphilis or herpes) (● Sexually transmitted infections p. 764), and colorectal cancer. Fissures are classified as: acute (present for <6wks); chronic (present for ≥6wks); 1° (no clear underlying cause); 2° (has a clear underlying cause (e.g. constipation, persistent diarrhoea)).

Symptoms include pain, rectal bleeding, and anal spasm. Thorough history and clinical examination required as per haemorrhoids. Refer if diagnosis unclear or serious pathology suspected. Management for all types includes: dietary and lifestyle advice to soften stools (● Nutrition and healthy eating p. 342), offering simple analgesia and/or a topic anaesthetic, and maintaining good anal hygiene. Management also includes management of the underlying cause of 2° fissures. Adults with 1° fissures should be reviewed after 6–8wks (sooner if required) and children with 1° fissures after 2wks (sooner if required).

Refer at the point of review if, despite adherence to dietary and lifestyle recommendations, fissures have not healed. For patients with 2° fissures, review dates depend on underlying condition.

Anal cancer

Most common is squamous cell carcinoma. Risk factors include: HPV infection; HIV (➔ Human immunodeficiency virus p. 462); immune suppression in transplant patients, use of immunosuppressants (e.g. long-term corticosteroids); autoimmune disorders (➔ Principles of working with someone with compromised immunity p. 466); and smoking. Commonly presents as bleeding. May also present as a mass, non-healing ulcers around anus, itching, discharge, faecal incontinence, and fistulae. If anal cancer is suspected, refer to a specialist.

Anal abscess

Usually occur in one of the glands that lubricate the anus. There are four types: perianal, ischiorectal, intersphincteric, and supralevator. Risk factors include: inflammatory bowel disease, smoking, and HIV. Signs and symptoms associated with superficial abscesses include tender, localized swelling with redness. Deeper abscesses can be harder to diagnose and may present with perianal or pelvic pain. On rare occasions, anal abscesses may present with sepsis. Complications include fistula formation. Both abscesses and fistulas will require further investigation and referral, the former for surgical drainage and the latter for surgical repair.

Pilonidal sinus

Caused by the forceful insertion of hairs into the skin of the natal cleft in the sacrococcygeal area, which initiates a chronic inflammatory reaction, causing a chronic sinus tract. Risk factors include ♂ aged 15–40yrs, being white, hirsutism, and obesity (➔ Overweight and obesity p. 348). If the patient has no symptoms, they will normally be advised to keep the area clean and to dry well after washing. Acute infection may → a pilonidal abscess, requiring urgent surgical drainage. Chronic infection is when the infection keeps coming back after drainage, with referral needed for surgical excision.

Further information

Glynne-Jones, R., et al. (2014) Anal cancer: ESMO-ESSO-ESTRO clinical practice guidelines for diagnosis, treatment and follow up. *Annals of Oncology,* 25(Supplement 3), iii10–20

NICE (2016) (*Clinical knowledge summaries: haemorrhoids*). Available at: https://cks.nice.org.uk/haemorrhoids#!topicsummary

NICE (2016) (*Clinical knowledge summaries: anal fissure*). Available at: https://cks.nice.org.uk/anal-fissure#!topicsummary

Red Whale (2017) *Perianal abscess.* Available at: https://www.gp-update.co.uk/SM4/Mutable/Uploads/pdf_file/Perianal-abscess.pdf

Dyspepsia, gastro-oesophageal reflux disease, and peptic ulceration

Dyspepsia

Very common. Characterized by recurrent epigastric pain, heartburn, or acid regurgitation. Can include bloating, nausea, and vomiting. Cause often unknown, but can be due to gastric oesophageal reflux disease, gastric and peptic ulceration, or rarely cancer. Can also be exacerbated by: medication (e.g. Ca^{2+} (calcium ions) agonists, nitrates, theophyllines, bisphosphonates, *selective serotonin reuptake inhibitors*, corticosteroids, and NSAIDs) and previous gastric surgery or history of ulceration.

People presenting with indigestion may in fact have cardiac pain.

Requires urgent medical assessment if any of the following with dyspepsia: bleeding and/or iron deficiency (anaemia) (● Anaemia in adults p. 652); dysphagia (actual difficulty swallowing); and recurrent vomiting and/or weight loss.

Helicobacter pylori (H. pylori) bacteria (major cause of gastric ulceration) present in ~40% of UK population, so does not always trigger disease. In patients with non-specific symptoms, consider urea breath test, faecal antigen test, and eradication therapy by antibiotics and antisecretory medication according to set regimen.

Care and management

Review with patient possible triggers to avoid (e.g. medication, particular foods or actions such as bending etc.). Lifestyle advice including weight loss (● Nutrition and healthy eating p. 342), smoking cessation (● Smoking cessation p. 356), and ↓ alcohol (● Alcohol p. 360). Eating smaller meals, not eating before bed, and propping up bedhead can help control symptoms. OTC medication for symptom relief (e.g. antacids and alginates). If H. pylori has been excluded, then patient may be prescribed low-dose proton pump inhibitor for a month. Also refer patients with unresolved/ongoing symptoms to 2° care.

Gastro-oesophageal reflux disease

Heartburn is common symptom of gastro-oesophageal reflux disease (GORD). Can also experience reflux of acid in the mouth, nausea and vomiting, nocturnal cough. Symptoms caused by regurgitation of gastric contents irritating oesophagus. GORD can cause oesophagitis, oesophageal strictures, oesophageal haemorrhage, and anaemia. Risk factors include: diet rich in fatty foods, alcohol, smoking, hiatus hernia, Barrett's oesophagus (intestinal metaplasia), obesity, and pregnancy (● Pregnancy p. 424). Care and management as for dyspepsia.

Gastritis

Inflammation of the stomach mucosa when there is no ulcer present, although may → subsequent ulceration if H. pylori is the cause. Vitamin B12 deficiency (● Anaemia in adults p. 652) can cause symptoms as can certain medications (e.g. NSAIDs). Care and management as for dyspepsia.

Hiatus hernia

Hiatus hernia is a common problem. Many people with hiatus hernia will also have GORD. Occurs when proximal stomach herniates/protrudes through a tear or weakness in the diaphragm into the thorax. Major risk factor is obesity. Two types of hiatus hernia: sliding hiatus hernia (most common) and rolling hiatus hernia (also called paraoesophageal hiatus hernia). Care and management as for dyspepsia and GORD.

Peptic ulceration

Peptic ulceration includes gastric ulceration (GU) and duodenal ulceration (DU). GU may be asymptomatic or complain of epigastric pain made worse with food, but helped with antacids and/or lying flat. DU may be asymptomatic or relapse and remit, and associated epigastric pain is typically relieved by food and worse at night. Risk factors include H. pylori (main cause in both types of ulcer), NSAIDs, and alcohol. Complications include bleeding, perforation (requiring emergency admission), and pyloric stenosis (scarring from chronic DU). Pyloric stenosis results in unrelieved and copious vomiting of food which requires medical assessment and referral for surgery. Care and management includes investigation and treatment as for dyspepsia. If possible, stop NSAIDs, lower dose, or safer option (e.g. paracetamol). Medication may include proton pump inhibitors (PPIs) or H2 receptor agonist. Lifestyle advice as described earlier; eat little and often, avoid eating 3hrs before bed. Referred to 2° care if symptoms persist/unrelieved.

Further information

Guts UK (*Conditions*). Available at: ℅ https://gutscharity.org.uk/advice-and-information/conditions/

NICE (*Gastro-oesophageal reflux disease and dyspepsia in adults: investigation and management*). Available at: ℅ https://www.nice.org.uk/guidance/cg184

Irritable bowel syndrome

Irritable bowel syndrome (IBS) is a common gastrointestinal problem. Stress/food intolerance/infection precipitate symptoms. Characterized by abdominal pain that is relieved by defecation and two of the following: altered stool passage, abdominal bloating, symptoms made worse by eating, and passage of mucus.

Patients should see their GP for confirmation of diagnosis of IBS and discount other possible causes such as inflammatory bowel disease (IBD) (→ Inflammatory bowel disease p. 712), infection, and endometriosis (→ Problems of the ovaries and uterus p. 780). ⚠ Be cautious about making a new diagnosis of IBS in a patient >50yrs: think about colorectal cancer (→ Colorectal cancer p. 715) or ovarian cancer (→ Gynaecological cancers p. 776). The symptoms of IBS and IBD can overlap. Faecal calprotectin is a useful test to differentiate between IBS and IBD. If cancer is suspected, refer via urgent 2wk wait NHS pathway.

Care and management

Review with patient possible triggers (e.g. particular foods, social situations) and plan how to avoid. For some, exclusion diets are successful (e.g. exclude dairy products, citrus, caffeine, alcohol, gluten, and eggs). Consider referral to dietician for low FODMAP (fermentable oligosaccharides, disaccharides, monosaccharides, and polyols) diet. Some patients find small and frequent meals help ↓ symptoms. It may be helpful to limit intake of ↑ fibre foods. Probiotics often recommended ≥4wks. Encourage smoking cessation (→ Smoking cessation p. 356), ↑ exercise (→ Exercise p. 354), and attending self-management programmes (→ Expert patients and self-management p. 340). For specific symptoms:

- Constipation, if diet insufficient: consider bulk-forming laxatives
- Abdominal pain: peppermint oil and antispasmodics
- Diarrhoea: anti-diarrhoeal

Specialist referral if symptoms are severe, change, and/or do not respond to treatments.

Further information

Irritable Bowel Syndrome Network (*Self-care programme*). Available at: ℘ https://www.theibsnetwork.org/the-self-care-programme/

NICE (*Irritable bowel syndrome in adults: diagnosis and management [CG6]*). Available at: ℘ https://www.nice.org.uk/Guidance/CG61

NICE (*Faecal calprotectin diagnostic tests for inflammatory diseases of the bowel: diagnostics guidance [DG11]*). Available at: ℘ https://www.nice.org.uk/guidance/dg11

Inflammatory bowel disease

Ulcerative colitis (UC) and Crohn's disease (CrD) are chronic, relapsing, inflammatory, non-infectious conditions of the gut. Cause is unknown, although environmental and genetic factors, infections, and possibly foods are thought to adversely affect susceptible individuals. Symptoms are described in Box 12.2. All patients with suspected UC or CrD should be referred to specialist gastroenterology for assessment. Consider testing faecal calprotectin before referral for colonoscopy in patients who may have inflammatory bowel disease (IBD) or irritable bowel syndrome (IBS) (➔ Irritable bowel syndrome p. 710).

⚠ Emergency referral to hospital by GP if any of the following are present: severe abdominal pain, severe diarrhoea >8 days and bleeding, dramatic weight loss, and signs of systemic infection.

Box 12.2 Ulcerative colitis (UC) and Crohn's disease (CrD) symptoms vary according to extent and severity of inflammation

Ulcerative colitis
- At any time 50% will be asymptomatic.
- *Mild:* 30% have mild symptoms, usually limited to rectum (proctitis), with diarrhoea and/or rectal bleeding. May be mistaken for haemorrhoids.
- *Moderate:* symptoms more severe, with frequent stools with blood (4–6 liquid stools a day), and pain relieved with defecation. General tiredness, fatigue, weight loss. Other symptoms may occur: skin rashes, uveitis, arthritis, inflammation of the liver.
- *Severe:* profuse diarrhoea, bleeding, ↑ fever, abdominal tenderness and distention, tenesmus (constant desire to defecate), ↓ appetite and weight, fatigue.
- Severe episodes uncommon, but can cause serious illness. Danger of perforation or haemorrhage (requiring surgical intervention).
- Patients with UC at ↑ risk of developing cancer.

Crohn's disease
- Diarrhoea, often with blood and mucous, mouth ulcers.
- Abdominal pain, weight loss.
- Fever and general tiredness.
- Perianal sores and/or abscess with discharge (may be first indication of CrD).
- Can also have related symptoms that include: uveitis, pain, arthritis, skin rashes, liver inflammation.
- Complications include: strictures caused by scar tissue impede the passage of food, leading to pain and vomiting.
- Perforation of the gut wall (potentially life-threatening).
- Creation of fistulas (often perianal between colon and other organs, leading to leakage).
- People with CrD have a small ↑ risk of cancer.

Care and management

Both conditions are lifelong and characterized by flare-ups and periods of remission. Patients can become socially isolated and depressed (➔ People with anxiety and depression p. 478). UC is also linked to other autoimmune diseases. Most patients have ongoing hospital follow-up and the multidisciplinary team (MDT) always provides care across 1° and 2° care settings (➔ Teamwork p. 58).

- UC: most patients will have symptoms controlled by medication to ↓ the impact of inflammation and prolong periods of remission.
- CrD: patients receive similar medication regimen plus antibiotics and monoclonal antibodies ⚠ NSAIDs can exacerbate symptoms,
- Surgery: for CrD to remove damaged part of the colon and/or as for UC when symptoms cannot be managed medically → ilestomy/ileo-anal pouch (➔ Stoma care p. 516)

Advise patients:
- Side effects of medication including steroid therapy
- Cancer risk and surveillance (➔ Colorectal cancer p. 715)
- Importance of fluid intake during bouts of diarrhoea
- Possible need for dietary supplements (including enteral nutrition (➔ Enteral tube feeding p. 594; ➔ Malnutrition p. 350)
- Smoking cessation (➔ Smoking cessation p. 356)
- Those who have had ileal resection will have B12 levels checked and possible supplementation (➔ Anaemia in adults p. 652)
- Contraception must be used if taking monoclonal therapies or methotrexate and for 6mths after stopping (➔ Contraception: general p. 400)
- Combined oral contraceptive not advised due to malabsorption (➔ Combined hormonal contraceptive methods p. 402)
- Fertility may be suboptimal in ♀ (➔ Problems with fertility p. 784) and pregnancy has to be planned when IBD is controlled (see earlier regarding medication) (➔ Preconceptual care p. 422)
- Refer to self-management and expert patient groups (➔ Expert patients and self-management programmes p. 340)
- Encourage screening for colonoscopy 10yrs from diagnosis and monitoring with blood tests for side effects of drugs

Further information

Crohn's and Colitis UK (*Self help for people with IBD*). Available at: ℬ https://www.crohnsandcolitis. org.uk/research/projects/self-help-for-people-with-ibd

NICE (*Crohn's disease: management [CG152]*). Available at: ℬ https://www.nice.org.uk/guidance/CG152

NICE (*Ulcerative colitis: management [CG166]*). Available at: ℬ https://www.nice.org.uk/Guidance/CG166

Coeliac disease

A common autoimmune gastrointestinal (GI) disease. Lifelong inflammatory disease of the upper small intestine triggered by eating gluten (protein found in wheat, rye, and barley). It occurs at any age, causing villous atrophy → malabsorption problems. Peak occurrence in childhood and then further peak in mid-adulthood. Risk factors are environmental and family history.

Presentation

Patients are often either asymptomatic or have non-specific symptoms. All people with suspected symptoms of coeliac disease will need referral for specialist assessment and confirmation of diagnosis. The following summarizes how coeliac disease can present (can be mistaken for irritable bowel syndrome (→ Irritable bowel syndrome p. 710) or wheat intolerance).

Babies being weaned may fail to thrive, suffer from diarrhoea and vomiting, and be generally pale and irritable with swollen abdomen (→ Weaning p. 188). Older children may present with loss of appetite, anaemia and vitamin deficiencies (→ Anaemia in adults p. 652), and may have steatorrhoea. Lack of growth may be most significant symptom. In adults, the majority complain of tiredness and fatigue, weight loss, and bowel symptoms (e.g. constipation, diarrhoea, and flatus (→ Constipation in adults p. 512)). May have mouth ulcers and a sore tongue and mouth (→ Mouth and throat problems p. 698). Some patients develop dermatitis herpetiformis (itchy skin condition) (→ Eczema/dermatitis p. 684) and/or osteoporosis-related bone pain.

Care and management

Gluten-free diet gives complete remission from symptoms within weeks. Patient will need to remain gluten-free for life. May initially need vitamin supplements. ♀ planning a family should take folic acid until 12wks gestation (→ Preconceptual care p. 422; → Neural tube defects p. 274). Skin symptoms can take up to a year to settle.

Due to malabsorption of calcium, ↑ risk of osteoporosis. Link between coeliac disease and Type 1 diabetes (→ Diabetes: overview p. 660) and hypothyroidism (→ Thyroid p. 702). Small ↑ risk of gastrointestinal malignancy (reduced after gluten-free diet for 3–5yrs). Lactose intolerance is common pre-diagnosis; however, once established on a gluten-free diet, lactose digestion returns to normal.

Further information

Coeliac UK (*Live well gluten free*). Available at: ℘ www.coeliac.co.uk
NICE (*Coeliac disease: recognition, assessment and management [NG20]*). Available at: ℘ https://www.nice.org.uk/guidance/ng20

Colorectal cancer

Fourth most common cancer in the UK. Incidence ↑ with age and 99% occurs in people >40yrs. Risk factors include: ♂ sex, ↑ age, family history, inflammatory bowel disease (● Inflammatory bowel disease p. 712), diabetes (● Diabetes: overview p. 660), obesity (● Overweight and obesity p. 348), alcohol use (● Alcohol p. 360), and smoking. Prevention includes: diet ↑ in fibre (● Nutrition and healthy eating p. 342), exercise (● Exercise p. 354), and smoking cessation (● Smoking cessation p. 356). Some evidence that low-dose aspirin from age 55yrs is protective[6] (● Cancer prevention p. 372). Important to participate in bowel screening (● Bowel cancer screening p. 376).

Symptoms and investigations

Patients should have a medical assessment if they experience: change in bowel habit; abdominal pain; rectal bleeding, or complain of abdominal or rectal mass; and/or experience weight loss, anaemia, or malaise (especially if they have a family history of bowel cancer). Suspicious lower GI tract symptoms to be urgently referred to specialist. Investigations include: colonoscopy; CT colon and barium enema.

Care and management

Treatment is usually surgical; also radiotherapy and/or chemotherapy care provided by multidisciplinary team (● Teamwork p. 58).

Reference

6. García Rodríguez, L., Soriano-Gabarró, M., Bromley, S., et al. (2017) New use of low-dose aspirin and risk of colorectal cancer by stage at diagnosis: a nested case-control study in UK general practice. *BMC Cancer,* 17, 637

Further information

Bowel Cancer UK (*About bowel cancer*). Available at: ℘ https://www.bowelcanceruk.org.uk/about-bowel-cancer/

NICE (*Colorectal cancer: diagnosis and management [CG131]*). Available at: ℘ http://guidance.nice.org.uk/CG131

NICE (*Suspected cancer: recognition and referral [NG12]*) Available at: ℘ https://www.nice.org.uk/guidance/ng12/chapter/1-Recommendations-organised-by-site-of-cancer#lower-gastrointestinal-tract-cancers

Appendicitis, diverticulitis, hernias, and intestinal obstruction

Appendicitis

Appendicitis is an infection in the appendix. It is the most common surgical emergency in the UK, affecting mainly people aged 10–30yrs. It always requires emergency admission (although 50% suspected appendicitis admissions turn out to be something else such as urinary tract infection (UTI) (➔ Urinary tract infection p. 756), food poisoning (➔ Food-borne disease p. 730), ectopic pregnancy (➔ Pregnancy p. 424), or diverticulitis). Complications include peritonitis from perforation, abscess, and ♀ infertility. Signs and symptoms include abdominal colicky pain becoming progressively worse, more constant, and localizing in right iliac fossa, worse on walking and movement (may walk stooped). Tenderness and guarding when palpated. Dysuria; may be blood or leucocytes in urine. Nausea and vomiting. Fever and generally flushed and unwell. It requires medical assessment and emergency referral.

Diverticulosis

When the colon wall is weaker in some areas than others and small 'pouches' (i.e. diverticula) are forced outwards through the outer layer of the colonic wall. Common in people >60yrs; however, the majority have no or only mild symptoms. Diagnosis confirmed through endoscopy or barium enema. Predisposing factors include low-roughage diet, history of constipation (➔ Constipation in adults p. 512), and increasing age. Encourage patients to: ↑ fibre and fluid intake (may benefit from bulk-forming agents); ↑ activity to ↓ constipation (➔ Exercise p. 354); and antispasmodic medication and peppermint oil can ↓ colicky pain.

Diverticulitis

Occurs when there is infection and inflammation precipitated by faeces trapped in the diverticula and bacterial infection. Complication of diverticulitis is peritonitis. Patients complain of: altered bowel habit, abdominal colicky pain, and nausea and flatulence (may be improved with defecation). Patients require medical assessment. Acute diverticulitis treated with antibiotics, painkillers, antispasmodics, laxatives, and diet. In severe cases or patients at higher risk (e.g. older person, someone who is immunosuppressed), may be admitted to hospital. Diverticulitis recurs in about a third of cases. Advise on diet and prevention as for diverticulosis.

Hernias

Occur when there is an abnormal protrusion of peritoneal contents through a weakness in the abdominal wall. Common problem: inguinal hernia most common and occurs at any age. It may be precipitated by a chronic cough, constipation, urinary obstruction, heavy lifting, previous abdominal surgery. Patient complains of lump in the groin which in ♂ can track down into the scrotum, and discomfort when straining or standing for long periods.

Hernias require medical assessment. Usually requires surgery because otherwise hernia may enlarge and ↑ discomfort, risk of strangulation → emergency surgery. Trusses are used for patients who are a poor surgical risk or are awaiting surgery. Lifestyle advice: to maintain ideal weight, healthy diet, and learn correct lifting and handling procedures. For hiatus hernia, see ➲ Dyspepsia, gastro-oesophageal reflux disease, and peptic ulceration p. 708.

Incisional hernia (post-abdominal surgery)

Bulging at the side of operation site occurs when there is a breakdown of the muscle closure at an abdominal wall. It may have been preceded by wound infection (➲ Wound infection p. 526) or haematoma. It does not always need surgical intervention. If causing pain, discomfort, or risk of obstruction or strangulation, then referred to 2° care for surgical review/treatment.

Umbilical hernia

Most common in infants; in adults may present as a bulge next to the umbilicus. It requires medical assessment and may be referred for surgical assessment, as ↑ risk of strangulation or obstruction.

Intestinal obstruction

Arises from mechanical obstruction or failure of peristalsis. Patients complain of anorexia, nausea, vomiting, abdominal pain and distention, no guarding or rebound but uncomfortable and restless. Requires urgent medical assessment/referral for surgical intervention. Types:

- Obstruction external to bowel: including adhesions, volvulus, external malignancy, and strangulated hernia
- Obstruction internal to the bowel: including cancer of the bowel (➲ Colorectal cancer p. 715), infarction, inflammatory bowel disease, and diverticulitis
- Obstruction in the lumen: including constipation/impaction, large polyps, intussusception, swallowed foreign body, and gallstone ileus
- Ileus functional obstruction: post-operatively, uraemia, and anticholinergic drugs

Further information

NICE (*Appendicitis*). Available at: ℛ https://cks.nice.org.uk/appendicitis
NICE (*Diverticulosis*). Available at: ℛ https://cks.nice.org.uk/diverticular-disease#!scenario
NICE (*Diverticular disease*). Available at: ℛ https://cks.nice.org.uk/diverticular-disease#!scenario:2
Scottish Palliative Care Guidelines (*Bowel obstruction*). Available at: ℛ https://www.palliativecareguidelines.scot.nhs.uk/guidelines/symptom-control/bowel-obstruction.aspx

Problems of the liver, gallbladder, and pancreas

Cirrhosis

Cirrhosis develops progressively as a result of damage to the liver. It is characterized by fibrosis/scarring of the liver. Also described as compensated (liver can still function effectively) and decompensated (cannot function adequately). Causes and risk factors include:

- Excessive alcohol intake (➜ Alcohol p. 360)
- Chronic Hepatitis B or C infection (➜ Viral hepatitis p. 724)
- Obesity (➜ Overweight and obesity p. 348)
- Type 2 diabetes (at risk if they have non-alcoholic fatty liver disease) (➜ Diabetes: overview p. 660)
- Autoimmune conditions (autoimmune hepatitis, 1° biliary cholangitis, and 1° sclerosing cholangitis)
- Active hepatitis
- 1° biliary cirrhosis and other chronic diseases of the bile duct (e.g. biliary atresia in children)
- Congenital disease
- Prolonged exposure to drugs or toxins (e.g. methotrexate)
- Vascular disease or Budd–Chiari syndrome.

Patients with cirrhosis can be asymptomatic, but they may experience: lack of appetite; lethargy, fatigue, and general feeling of being unwell; and nausea and vomiting. In the later stages of the disease: jaundice; itching; ascites and oedema; haematemesis; confusion arising from encephalopathy; weight loss; and hepatomegaly. Complications include: portal hypertension; ascites; hepatic encephalopathy; haemorrhage from oesophageal varices; infection; hepatorenal syndrome; hepatocellular carcinoma; portal hypertensive gastropathy; portal vein thrombosis; and cirrhotic cardiomyopathy.

Care and management

Refer to a specialist in hepatology. For decompensated liver disease, refer immediately to a hepatologist or to a gastroenterologist with an interest in hepatology. Ongoing care includes: avoiding alcohol; smoking cessation (➜ Smoking cessation p. 356); advice on diet and nutrition (➜ Nutrition and healthy eating p. 342); considering ability to continue driving; ensuring flu and pneumococcal immunization (➜ Targeted adult immunization p. 392); and follow-up and monitoring.

Portal hypertension

A consequence of chronic liver disease. Other rarer causes are parasitic disease (schistosomiasis), pancreatic disease, and clotting disorders. BP ↑ in portal vein which carries blood from bowel and spleen to liver → collateral circulation. It causes oesophageal varices, which can ooze blood causing anaemia (➜ Anaemia in adults p. 652), maleana, or haemorrhage and/or haematemesis. Other signs are ascites and encephalopathy. Early treatment of varices can be very effective, but bleeding is a medical emergency.

Gallstones

Made of cholesterol and bile pigments. Associated with obesity, ♀ with children, use of hormone replacement therapy (HRT) (**⊃** Menopause p. 364), and smoking. Can be asymptomatic or complain of vague intermittent discomfort. Patient with obstructed, inflamed, infected bile duct may experience:

• Biliary colic: most common complication. Severe upper abdominal pain causing jaundice, nausea, and vomiting. Requires medical assessment for analgesia and possible emergency admission.
• Acute cholecystitis: pain and tenderness in epigastrium. Can progress to perforation and fistula formation. Requires medical assessment for antibiotics, analgesia, and possible referral to 2° care.

Care and management

↓ fat in diet, maintain ideal weight, and avoid trigger foods. Patients referred to 2° care may be offered lithotripsy, endoscopic retrograde cholangiopancreatography, or cholecystectomy. Post-surgery patients may still experience symptoms that may settle over time.

Pancreatitis (inflammation of the pancreas)

Acute pancreatitis

Sudden onset of acute epigastric pain often with nausea and vomiting. Range of possible causes including: alcohol, gallstones, and medication (e.g. thiazide diuretics). Admit as medical emergency. To avoid further attacks, advise: to avoid triggers (e.g. alcohol); to eat a lower-fat diet; and address avoidable causes (e.g. gallstones).

Chronic pancreatitis

Causes gradual destruction and fibrosis with loss of pancreatic function → malnutrition and diabetes. Alcohol is the commonest cause; also cystic fibrosis (**⊃** Cystic fibrosis p. 318). It is characterized by: chronic ill health; fatigue; weight loss; frequent pain radiating to the back, sometimes relieved by sitting forwards; steatorrhoea; jaundice; pain and vomiting; and diabetes mellitus. Care and management: advice on diet (↓ fat, ↑ protein, ↑ calories with fat-soluble vitamins); pancreatic enzyme supplementation and corticosteroids (autoimmune treatment); no alcohol; pain relief; and referred to 2° care for possible surgery.

Further information

British Liver Trust (*Cirrhosis of the liver*). Available at: ℘ https://www.britishlivertrust.org.uk/liver-information/liver-conditions/cirrhosis/
NICE (*Pancreatitis—chronic*). Available at: ℘ https://cks.nice.org.uk
NICE (*Pancreatitis—acute*). Available at: ℘ https://cks.nice.org.uk/pancreatitis-chronic

Viral infections

Viruses are the smallest known type of infectious agent and consist of genetic material surrounded by one or two protective protein shells. Viruses enter through mucous membranes, latch on or enter cells, and then multiply. Spread can be airborne (coughing, sneezing), passed on by touch, or through body fluids (e.g. blood, saliva, semen (❯ Sexually transmitted infections p. 764; ❯ Viral skin infections p. 690)). The body's own immune system then has to deal with the virus. Vaccinations have been developed for many common viral infections, which sensitize the immune system to rapidly produce antibodies to destroy those viruses (❯ Travel vaccinations p. 399; ❯ Targeted adult immunization p. 392; ❯ Childhood immunization schedule (UK) p. 166).

Viral infections are the usual causes of colds, rashes, diarrhoea, influenza, sore throats, cold sores, etc. Most are mild and short-lasting, but can cause the person to feel very unwell. They do not respond to antibiotics (❯ Antimicrobial stewardship p. 146). More serious if the person is immunocompromised or vulnerable in some other way. Immunocompromised people (❯ Principles of working with someone with compromised immunity p. 466) and pregnant ♀ (❯ Pregnancy p. 424) should seek medical advice if exposed to conditions such as chickenpox or parvovirus infection.

Self-help advice for viral infections

- Keep comfortable, warm, and rested
- Avoid unnecessary contact with others to ↓ spread
- Drink plenty of liquids
- Take OTC medication for aches, pains, and fevers
- Seek medical advice if illness appears to be getting worse after a few days, or complications (e.g. ear infection, sinusitis (❯ Mouth and throat problems p. 698), exacerbation of asthma (❯ Asthma in adults p. 608; ❯ Asthma in children p. 306), COPD (❯ Chronic obstructive pulmonary disease p. 614))

⚠ Specific NHS advice about coronavirus (COVID19), including symptoms, and what to do if you suspect someone is infected, can be found at ℘ https://www.nhs.uk/conditions/coronavirus-covid-19/

Seasonal influenza

Three main types: C causes a mild form, like a cold, and provides immunity for life; A and B alter to produce new strains. Symptoms: fever, headache, muscle ache, weakness, and mucus in respiratory tract. Patients are at risk of severe symptoms if COPD, diabetes (❯ Diabetes: overview p. 660), coronary heart disease (❯ Coronary heart disease p. 624), immunosuppressed, and older people. Pre-winter vaccination available for at-risk groups.

It is treated by rest, fluids, and OTC medication. Antivirals used with ↑-risk groups (>65yrs, pregnant, those with LTCs, immunocompromised) when flu incidence ↑ to shorten duration of symptoms and ↓ risk of complications. Public Health England (PHE) monitors incidence of influenza and alerts practitioners when antivirals can be used. Complications treated as required. 2° chest infection common.

Herpes virus

Of the more than a hundred known herpes viruses, eight routinely infect humans: herpes simplex virus types 1 and 2 (cold sores and genital herpes); varicella zoster virus (causing chickenpox and shingles); cytomegalovirus; Epstein–Barr virus (causing glandular fever); human herpes virus 6 (variants A and B); human herpes virus 7; and Kaposi's sarcoma virus or human herpes virus 8.

Related topics

➔ Infections in children p. 288

Further information

NICE (*Influenza—seasonal*). Available at: ℘ https://cks.nice.org.uk/influenza-seasonal
NICE (*Glandular fever*). Available at: ℘ https://cks.nice.org.uk/glandular-fever-infectious-mononucleosis
PHE (*Seasonal influenza*). Available at: ℘ https://www.gov.uk/government/collections/seasonal-influenza-guidance-data-and-analysis

Methicillin-resistant Staphylococcus aureus (MRSA)

Staphylococcus aureus

Gram-positive bacterium which is carried as a skin commensal by about 30% of the population, usually in moist sites such as nose (anterior nares), axillae, and perineum. Causes infections such as boils (◑ Bacterial skin infections p. 680) and styes, and is the commonest cause of wound infections (◑ Wound infection p. 526). Most strains are resistant to penicillin and some strains are resistant to several classes of antibiotics (including methicillin); these latter are known as MRSA. Overuse of antibiotics has played a significant part in ↑ resistance to them (◑ Antimicrobial stewardship p. 146).

MRSA

Infection with MRSA does not present a risk to healthy people in the community. MRSA is carried by about 2% of the population, although most are not infected. The proportion of people colonized by MRSA tends to be higher in hospitals and nursing homes (◑ Care homes p. 32) because of the more widespread use of antibiotics that wipe out a person's normal skin microbes, leaving gaps for the MRSA to occupy.
- Most MRSA occurs in those who have had direct contact with hospitals, care homes, or other healthcare facilities.
- Some strains of MRSA have a particular ability to spread and cause epidemics (referred to as EMRSA).
- Very occasionally, there is no history of healthcare contact; these strains are referred to as community-associated MRSA (CA-MRSA).
- Mandatory reporting to PHE is currently required for all healthcare-associated infection, including those caused by MRSA.
- Prevention of transmission from those affected by MRSA is very important.
- Patients who are colonized with MRSA can come home from hospital or go to a care home if their general condition allows. 1° healthcare and care home staff should be informed of patient's status.

MRSA treatment

Only on advice of local microbiologist or member of local infection-control team. Most asymptomatic, requiring no treatment.

MRSA decolonization

May be required for those screened positive prior to hospital admission and may involve:
- Applying antibacterial cream inside the nose three times/day for 5 days
- Washing with an antibacterial shampoo daily for 5 days
- Changing towels, clothes, and bedding every day during treatment (the resulting laundry should be washed separately from other people's and at a ↑ temperature) (◑ Home food safety and hygiene p. 352)

MRSA in care homes

In the UK, 20% of older residents in care homes are colonized with MRSA, but clinical infections in such settings are uncommon. The local infection control team can help to evaluate the risk to other residents and provide advice on infection control measures. Staff who require treatment for MRSA carriage (carry MRSA without infection) should follow local policies and be referred to their GP.

Infection control measures

The spread of MRSA can be prevented by:

- Handwashing, handwashing, and more handwashing (with liquid soap), especially after giving patient care, and after removing protective clothing (gloves and aprons) (❯ Hand hygiene p. 98; ❯ Personal protective equipment p. 100)
- Judicious use of antibiotics (according to local policy)
- Aseptic handling of catheters or any invasive device/procedure
- Cleaning equipment after use
- Covering patients' wounds, pressure sores, and skin lesions on staff or patients with an impermeable dressing (❯ Wound dressings p. 532)
- Controlled handling of contaminated dressings (❯ Managing healthcare waste p. 106) and linen
- Washing laundry at ↑ temperatures

Further information

MRSA Action UK (*About MSRA*). Available at: ℘ http://mrsaactionuk.net/MRSA.html

NICE (*MRSA in primary care*). Available at: ℘ https://cks.nice.org.uk/mrsa-in-primary-care#!scenario

PHE (*Summary of antimicrobial prescribing guidance: managing common infections*). Available at: ℘ https://assets.publishing.service.gov.uk/government/uploads/system/uploads/attachment_data/file/777505/Common_Infect_-_PHE_context_references_and_rationale_Feb_2019.pdf

Viral hepatitis

Hepatitis is inflammation of the liver. Viral infection (➔ Viral infections p. 720) is responsible for around half of all cases of acute hepatitis and is a notifiable disease (➔ Infectious disease notifications p. 104). Chronic infection is a problem with both Hepatitis C and Hepatitis B (the former being more common).

Hepatitis A (HAV)

Spread via faecal–oral route. Patients are infectious 2wks before feeling ill. Incubation 2–7wks (~4wks). Risk factors: travel to ↑-risk areas (➔ Travel healthcare p. 394), living or working in an institution (➔ Health and safety at work p. 92), poor hand hygiene, poor access to toilet and handwashing facilities, intravenous (IV) drug use (➔ Substance use p. 476), and ↑-risk sexual practices (➔ Sexually transmitted infections p. 764).

Signs and symptoms

May be asymptomatic (especially young children), fever, ↓ appetite, nausea +/− vomiting, pale stools +/− diarrhoea, fatigue, jaundice, dark urine, and abdominal pain. Investigations include liver function tests (LFTs) and hepatitis serology.

Management

Management is supportive. Advised to avoid alcohol (➔ Alcohol p. 360) until LFTs are normal. Most recover in <2mths. There is no carrier state and hepatitis A does not cause chronic liver disease (➔ Problems of liver, gallbladder, and pancreas p. 718). After infection, immunity is lifelong.

Prevention

Vaccination is indicated for travellers to ↑-risk areas, people with chronic liver disease, or working in ↑-risk situations (➔ Targeted adult immunization p. 392). Hepatitis A vaccine (combined with typhoid) is a single dose with booster 6–12mths later.

Hepatitis B (HBV)

Common. It is endemic in much of Asia and the Far East. Spread via blood and bodily fluids. Incubation 6–23wks (~17wks). Risk factors: travel to ↑-risk areas; babies of infected mothers; sexual partners of infected patients or patients with ↑-risk sexual practices; IV drug users; and healthcare workers (➔ Occupational exposure to blood-borne viruses p. 102).

Signs and symptoms

May be asymptomatic or present with fever, malaise, fatigue, arthralgia, urticaria, pale stools, dark urine, and/or jaundice. Investigations include LFTs and hepatitis serology (looking for the so-called 'surface' antigen or antibody or other markers of disease, e.g. the e-antigen) (see Box 12.3).

> ### Box 12.3 Hepatitis B (markers of disease)
> - Hepatitis B surface antibody is present from 1–6mths post exposure
> - If present >6mths after the acute episode, defines carrier status
> - Hepatitis B surface antibodies appear >10mths after infection: imply immunity

Management

Management is to avoid alcohol and referral for specialist advice. Treatment is supportive for acute illness. Chronic hepatitis is treated with antiviral medication to slow the spread and damage to the liver. ~85% recover fully, 10% develop carrier status, 5–10% develop chronic hepatitis (may → cirrhosis and/or liver carcinoma).

Prevention

All pregnant (➔ Pregnancy p. 424) ♀ in the UK are offered screening (➔ Antenatal care and screening p. 426). Advise patients regarding safe sex practices. ↑-risk groups (including health workers, travellers to ↑-risk areas) should be immunized. Men who have sex with men offered immunization at first visit to sexual health services. Passive immunization with human immunoglobulin is used to protect non-immune ↑-risk contacts of infected patients.

Hepatitis C (HCV)

Most common type and a major cause of liver damage. Most patients are unaware they have it. Spread via contact with infected blood. Mother to baby spread is uncommon and only at birth. Not easily spread through sexual contact. Incubation 2–25wks (~8wks). Patients at ↑ risk of infection should be offered HCV test: unexplained jaundice; ever an IV drug user; blood transfusion pre-1992 or blood products pre-1986; had dental or medical treatments in countries with poor infection control; child of HCV mother; regular sex with HCV+ person; accidental exposure to blood; and has had tattoos, piercings, acupuncture, etc. where infection control poor.

Signs and symptoms

As for HBV. Often asymptomatic. Anti-HCV antibody detectable 3–4mths post infection. Positive antibody results are followed by blood tests that look for the genetic material of the HCV virus. If positive antibody test, advised not to donate blood or carry organ donor card.

Management

Referred to specialist for treatment, which includes a combination of different antiviral drugs. Successful in clearing virus in about 90% of people. Advised to avoid alcohol and how to avoid infecting others.

Hepatitis E (HEV)

Spread via faeco–oral route. Incubation 2–9wks (~40 days). Risk factors: travel to developing countries (especially pregnant ♀). Symptoms and clinical presentation similar to HAV infection. Diagnosis is made after serological confirmation. Treatment is supportive. There is no chronic state. No vaccine exists. Mortality in pregnancy can be as high as 20%

Further information

Hepatitis C Trust (*Information*). Available at: ℺ http://www.hepctrust.org.uk/information
PHE (*Hepatitis A, B, C, E*). Available at: ℺ https://www.gov.uk/topic/health-protection/infectious-diseases

Pandemic influenza

Influenza pandemics are unpredictable but recurring events. Such an event is ↑ on the list of threats to the UK. Pandemic influenza is different from seasonal influenza; it is caused by the emergence of a novel virus which is markedly different from recently circulating strains (⊃ Viral infections p. 720). Few people are likely to have immunity → rapid spread and more serious illness than seasonal influenza. Production of a vaccine can only start when the virus is identified and may take 4–6mths to develop. A pandemic can occur in one wave, or a series of waves. Each wave may last 12–15wks. A worst-case scenario in the UK is described in Box 12.4.[7]

Preparedness

The UK Influenza Pandemic Preparedness Strategy[8] is aimed at guiding and supporting integrated contingency planning and preparations in health and social care organizations, and more widely across government and public and private sector organizations (⊃ Public health in the NHS and beyond p. 14). Objectives: minimize the potential health impact; minimize the potential impact on society and the economy; and instil and maintain trust and confidence.

Detection

Commences with the World Health Organization (WHO) declaring a public health emergency of international concern: intelligence gathering from countries affected; enhanced surveillance in the UK; development of diagnostics specific to new virus; and information and communication to public and professionals.

Assessment

Commences on identification of the novel virus in patients in the UK: collection and analysis of information on early cases, on which to base early estimates of likely impact and severity in the UK; and reducing the risk of transmission within the local community by active case finding, encouraging self-isolation of confirmed and suspected cases, treatment of confirmed and suspected cases, and possible use of antiviral prophylaxis for close/vulnerable contacts.

Treatment

Commences with evidence of sustained community transmission. Followed by treatment of individual cases and population treatment through routine NHS services, including the potential for using the National Pandemic Flu

---

Box 12.4 Worst-case scenario (UK)

Clinical attack rate: 50% of the population, spread over one or more waves
Peak clinical attack rate: 10–12% of the local population per week
Hospitalization: 1–4% of those who are symptomatic
Case fatality rate: 2.5% of those who are symptomatic (~750,000)
Peak absence rate: 15–35% of the workforce

Service (NPFS) if 1° care is under excessive pressure. The NPFS is an online and telephone self-assessment service where people are assessed by non-clinicians using protocols, which determine whether the person is eligible for antiviral medication or not. At the same time, enhancement of public health measures to disrupt transmission (e.g. localized school closures) and preparing for targeted vaccination as the vaccine becomes available.

Escalation

Commences when demand for services start to exceed capacity: escalation of surge management arrangements in health and other sectors; and prioritization and triage of service delivery with the aim of maintaining essential services.

Recovery

Commences when infection rate is significantly reduced: normalization of services; catch up with activity scaled down during escalation; post-incident review and lessons learnt; and planning and preparation for a resurgence in influenza activity.

References

7. Cabinet Office (2013) *Preparing for pandemic influenza: guidance for local planners.* Available at: https://assets.publishing.service.gov.uk/government/uploads/system/uploads/attachment_data/file/225869/Pandemic_Influenza_LRF_Guidance.pdf
8. Department of Health (2011) *UK influenza pandemic preparedness strategy 2011* Available at: https://assets.publishing.service.gov.uk/government/uploads/system/uploads/attachment_data/file/213717/dh_131040.pdf

Further information

Cabinet Office (2017) *National risk register of civil emergencies.* Available at: ✍ https://assets.publishing.service.gov.uk/government/uploads/system/uploads/attachment_data/file/644968/UK_National_Risk_Register_2017.pdf
WHO (2013) (*Pandemic influenza risk management: WHO interim guidance*). Available at: ✍ http://www.who.int/influenza/preparedness/pandemic/GIP_PandemicInfluenzaRiskManagementInterimGuidance_Jun2013.pdf

Tuberculosis

Tuberculosis (TB) is caused by the inhaling of the bacteria Mycobacterium TB complex. Pulmonary TB affects the lungs. Extra-pulmonary TB presents outside the lungs with symptoms specific to site of infection. Latent TB is where someone has been infected with the TB bacteria but does not have any symptoms of active infection. Pulmonary TB is highly infectious, but more likely amongst:

- Socially excluded groups in deprived areas
- People born in areas of the world with ↑ prevalence (40 per 100,000 population/year) of TB
- Homeless people and people living in prisons (● Homeless people p. 446)
- People with a history of living in overcrowded areas
- Problem drug (● Substance use p. 476) or alcohol misuse (● Alcohol p. 360)
- People with HIV (● Human immunodeficiency virus p. 462) or people who are immunocompromised (● Principles of working with someone with compromised immunity p. 466)
- Previous (especially incomplete) treatment of TB

Key issues

- Need to prevent the emergence of multi-drug resistant TB.
- TB is highly stigmatizing, and patients can feel isolated and find it difficult to communicate their problems.

Prevention

Bacillus–Calmette–Guerin (BCG) immunization (● Targeted adult immunization p. 392; ● Childhood immunization schedule (UK) p. 166) now recommended for:

- All infants (0–12mths) living in areas where TB incidence ≥40 per 100,000
- Infants whose parents or grandparents were born in a country where TB incidence ≥40 per 100,000
- Previously unvaccinated new immigrants from a country where TB incidence ≥40 per 100,000
- Those at risk: due to their occupation (healthcare workers and veterinary staff); due to contact with known cases; and because intending to work or travel in a country where TB incidence >40 per 100,000

Prior to vaccination, those at risk will be offered tuberculin skin test (Mantoux test). Those with a positive result will be investigated for TB by a specialist team; those with a negative test will be vaccinated.

Common symptoms

- Persistent productive cough, night sweats, fever, loss of appetite, weight loss, and fatigue and malaise
- TB of the lymph glands will cause enlargement of the glands
- TB affecting other parts of the body (commonly the kidneys, bones, or joints) will cause other symptoms

Children may not have such specific symptoms, but may present with symptoms such as limited growth, ↓ energy levels, or persistent fever.

Investigations

Suspected pulmonary TB
Chest X-ray and sputum samples.

Suspected extra-pulmonary TB
Computerized tomography (CT) scan, magnetic resonance imaging (MRI) scan, or ultrasound scan of the affected part of the body. Endoscopy or laparoscopy of the affected part of the body. Urine and blood tests. A biopsy from the affected area. Lumber puncture if suspected infection of the central nervous system.

Suspected latent TB
Mantoux test and interferon gamma release essay (IGRA) blood test.

Management

Referred to the local TB service. TB is a notifiable disease (◆ Infectious disease notifications p. 104) and contact tracing/testing will need to take place. Patients with pulmonary TB will be prescribed ≥6mth course of a combination of antibiotics. Following 2wks' treatment or three negative sputum samples, most cases are non-infectious.

Patients with extra-pulmonary TB will be prescribed a similar combination course of antibiotics and a shorter course of steroids to reduce inflammation and swelling, depending on the location of the infection.

People with latent TB and aged ≤65yrs will be treated with a 3–6mth course of antibiotics; however, the antibiotics used to treat TB can cause liver damage in older adults.

People with TB and comorbidities and coexisting conditions (including pregnancy (◆ Pregnancy p. 424) and breastfeeding (◆ Breastfeeding p. 182)) will be managed by a specialist multidisciplinary team. All patients on TB antibiotics should be monitored for side effects. Adherence to treatment for the whole length of treatment is very important (◆ Medicine concordance and adherence p. 132) to prevent further transmission and drug resistance (◆ Antimicrobial stewardship p. 146). Non-adherence is best managed by directly observed therapy.

Further information

British Lung Foundation (*Tuberculosis*). Available at: ℜ https://www.blf.org.uk/support-for-you/tuberculosis

NICE (*Tuberculosis*). Available at: ℜ https://cks.nice.org.uk/tuberculosis

Food-borne disease

Food-borne disease is an important issue. Incidents are under-reported. Food poisoning is defined by the Food Safety Act (1990) as 'any disease of an infectious or toxic nature caused by or thought to be caused by the consumption of food or water'.

Factors which most commonly contribute to outbreaks

- Preparation of food more than half a day in advance of needs
- Storage at ambient temperature
- Inadequate cooling
- Inadequate reheating
- Use of contaminated processed food
- Undercooking
- Contaminated canned food
- Inadequate thawing
- Cross-contamination from raw to cooked food
- Infected food handlers and poor hygiene

People do not play a significant role in outbreaks except in Staphylococcus aureus food poisoning; they tend to be victims, not sources. Meat and poultry account for 75% of outbreaks (➔ Home food safety and hygiene p. 352).

Notification

All cases of suspected food poisoning are statutorily notifiable to the environmental health department of the LA (➔ Environmental health services p. 27; ➔ Infectious disease notifications p. 104). Providing information about food eaten, signs, symptoms, and incubation period (Table 12.3) may suggest the micro-organism involved.

Personal care

- Give symptomatic care and treat signs such as dehydration.
- Do not advise anti-diarrhoea drugs as contraindicated in children and rarely needed in adults (can aggravate nausea and vomiting and occasionally ileus).
- Antibiotics are rarely indicated; may prolong the carrier state.

Infection control measures

- Handwashing before and after contact with patient and vomit/urine/faeces is essential (applies to family members) (→ Hand hygiene p. 98).
- If handling contaminated material, wear **personal protective equipment** (→ Personal protective equipment p. 100).
- Discard excreta directly into the drainage system.
- Anyone with gastroenteritis should not attend work or school until free from diarrhoea and vomiting for 2 days and, if necessary, clearance tests have been completed.
- Obtain faeces for microscopy and culture if the patient has been abroad, is severely ill, comes from an institution or works as a food handler, or has symptoms for >1wk.

Table 12.3 Causes and characteristic clinical features of food poisoning

Organism	Common source	Incubation period	Signs and symptoms						Duration
			Vomiting	Diarrhoea	Abdominal pain	Prostration	Pyrexia	Other	
Bacillus cereus (toxin in food)	Inadequately heated rice	1–16hrs	Profuse	Slight	Often present	Moderately severe	Absent		12–24hrs
Campylobacter jejuni (infection)—most common	Undercooked poultry and meat; unpasteurized milk	3–5 days	Slight	Often profuse	Often severe	Often severe	Often present	Blood-stained faeces often	Days or weeks
Clostridium botulin (toxin in food)	Contaminated canned food	12–96hrs, usually 8–36hrs	Slight	Absent	Absent	Severe	Absent	Nausea, vertigo, aphonia, respiratory paralysis and death can occur	Death in 24hrs–8d, or slow convalescence over 6–8mths
Clostridium perfringens (toxin in intestine)	Spores on contaminated meat	8–22hrs	Absent	Moderate	Colicky pains often present	Slight	Absent		24–48hrs
E.coli (infection and toxin)—common	Undercooked beef and beef products, milk, and vegetables	12–72hrs	Slight	Moderate	Slight	Slight	Absent	E.coli 0157—bloody diarrhoea	1–7 days

Listeria monocytogenes	Freshly cut salads, paté, soft cheeses	48hrs–3wks	Slight	Slight	Often present		Present	Pregnant ♀ especially vulnerable	Few days
Norovirus—common	Contaminated water and food, especially shellfish	24–48hrs	Moderate	Moderate	Not usually		Present	Person-to-person spread common via contact with faeces and vomit	
Salmonella (infection)—common	Meat, poultry, eggs, dairy products	6–36hrs, usually 12–24hrs	Slight	Moderate	Often present	Possibly in later stages	Often present	Blood-stained faeces in up to 25% cases	1–7 days
Staphylococcus aureus (toxin in food)	Cooked food (meat, poultry, fish) and dairy products (custards, creams, trifles)	2–6hrs	Profuse	Slight	Often present	Often severe	Absent		6–24hrs
Vibrio parahaemolyticus (infection)	Seafood	2–48hrs, usually 12–18hrs	Moderate	Moderate	Often present	Slight	Absent		2–5 days
Vibrio cholera	Water, seafood	24–72hrs	Slight	Profuse	Often present	Often severe	Often present		

Common musculoskeletal problems

Sporting-related injuries

Can often be avoided with suitable equipment, warm-up routines, gradual build-up of activity, trainers, proper training, and supervision. For treatment, see strains and strains (→ Sprains, strains, and fractures p. 824). Muscle and ligament injuries may need referral to GP and/or physiotherapist.

Neck problems

Most neck pain is acute, but self-limiting within days or weeks. Patients with persistent pain should be referred to GP. Causes can be multifactorial (e.g. arthritis (→ Osteoarthritis p. 600; → Rheumatoid arthritis p. 602), infection). ⚠ Any significant neck trauma requires neck immobilization with a hard collar and referral to emergency department (→ Spinal cord injury p. 518).

Cervical spondylosis

Degenerative disease of the cervical spine, characterized by intermittent pain often related to exercise and decreased movement. Can cause nerve root pain. Will need diagnosis confirmed. Usual treatment is analgesia.

Torticollis

Relatively common. Can be triggered by poor posture and sleeping awkwardly. A sudden onset of pain due to muscle spasm that immobilizes the neck. Self-limiting. Treat with heat, gentle mobilization, and analgesia.

Whiplash injuries

Often after road traffic accident (RTA). Sudden extension of neck → stretches or tears cervical muscles. Pain may occur hours or days after injury, and can radiate to head, shoulders, and arms. Medical assessment to exclude other causes. Treatment includes analgesia, early mobilization, and a collar initially. Recovery often slow.

Back pain

See → Low back pain p. 604.

Shoulder problems

Always consider the possibility of pain being referred from elsewhere, (e.g. neck, cardiac ischaemia, pulmonary embolism, gallbladder problems, subphrenic abscess).

Frozen shoulder (adhesive capulitis)

Cause unknown. More common in people with diabetes (→ Diabetes: overview p. 660). Painful stiff shoulder with very restricted movement; pain often worse at night. Care includes NSAIDs and referral to physiotherapist. May benefit from steroid injections. Recovery is often slow with uncertain outcome.

Dislocated shoulder

Usually because of a fall. Referred to emergency department for reduction. Recurrent dislocation can occur in teenagers with no history of injury but general joint laxity: referral to physiotherapy and/or GP.

Elbow, wrist, and hand problems

Pulled elbow

Common in children <5yrs. A traction injury often occurs when child pulled up suddenly by the hand. Child stops using the arm. Refer to GP.

Golfer's elbow and tennis elbow

Characterized by pain and tenderness: tendon inflammation caused by repeated strain. Patient should avoid trigger movements and take NSAIDs. Often resolves with rest. Physiotherapy and/or local steroid injection may help.

Repetitive strain injury

Work-related upper limb pain often in arm and wrist (e.g. related to computer keyboard use) (➜ Health and safety at work p. 92). Suggest patient reviews working posture and involve occupational health to review office equipment. Advise rest from aggravating activities and then gradually reintroduce. May help to have physiotherapy assessment.

Carpal tunnel syndrome

Pain, numbness, pins and needles in the fingers due to nerve compression. Often worse at night. Symptoms are improved by shaking wrist. Can occur with pregnancy (➜ Pregnancy p. 424), hypothyroidism (➜ Thyroid p. 702), obesity (➜ Overweight and obesity p. 348), and carpal arthritis. Symptoms can be helped with night splints and steroid injections. Surgery an option in moderate to severe pain.

Growing pains

Term used for non-specific and diffuse pain in children. May involve child waking at night with leg or arm pain. Rubbing the affected limb brings rapid relief. Resolves spontaneously.

Leg cramps

Transient involuntary episode of pain lasting for a few minutes (10min maximum). Cause unknown. Care and management: check not on drugs with side effects of cramps; reassure benign; passive stretching and massaging of affected muscle. If cramps persist, refer to GP (check for peripheral artery disease).

Ankle and foot problems

Ruptured Achilles tendon

Patient complains of sudden pain in back of ankle during activity. Walks with a limp and cannot raise heel from floor or stand on tiptoe. Urgent orthopaedic referral.

Plantar fasciitis (bursitis)

Common cause of heel pain. Worst when person gets out of bed. Suggest shoes with soft padding and support. If pain persistent, refer to GP for review.

Flat feet

Normal in young children. Painless flat foot where arch is restored when standing on tiptoe. D-oes not need treatment. Needs referral if painful and/or not restored on tiptoe.

Hammer and claw toes

If causing pain, footwear or mobility problems will need surgery.

Bunion (hallux valgas)

Lateral deviation of the big toe exacerbated by wearing high heels and tight-fitting shoes. Arthritis pads can help, but severe deformation will need surgery.

Ingrowing toe nail

Most common in big toe, caused by ill-fitting shoes and poor nail care. Nail grows into skin causing pain and inflammation. If infected, will need antibiotics. Advise to cut nails straight and with edges beyond the flesh and refer to podiatry. Persistent problems may need referral to podiatrist for surgery.

Further information

NICE (*Carpel tunnel syndrome*). Available at: https://cks.nice.org.uk/carpal-tunnel-syndrome
NICE (*Leg cramps*). Available at: https://cks.nice.org.uk/leg-cramps
NICE (*Neck pain: acute torticollis*). Available at: https://cks.nice.org.uk/neck-pain-acute-torticollis
NICE (*Plantar fasciitis*). Available at: https://cks.nice.org.uk/plantar-fasciitis
NICE (*Shoulder pain*). Available at: https://cks.nice.org.uk/shoulder-pain
NICE (*Tennis elbow*). Available at: https://cks.nice.org.uk/tennis-elbow

Bone and connective tissue disorders

Paget's disease of bone

Metabolic disorder of unknown cause that can be asymptomatic. Affects bone growth, bone deformity, weakness, and risk of fracture. Many people will be asymptomatic and only a small proportion experience severe symptoms. Signs and symptoms include:

- Pain or dull ache aggravated by weight bearing (can persist at rest)
- Deformity of the bone (skull may ↑ in size and spine may curve)
- Bowing of weight-bearing bones (e.g. femur)
- Nerve compression and pain; disturbed vision and dizziness
- Fractures (➔ Sprains, strains, and fractures p. 824) as 2° complication, and osteoarthritis (➔ Osteoarthritis p. 600)

Patient will need rheumatology referral for treatment and ongoing management. Pain managed with analgesia.

Rickets/osteomalacia

Caused by vitamin D deficiency. Rickets is the term used for children and osteomalacia for adults. Characterized by:

- Widespread bone pain, muscle weakness, and muscle cramps
- Deformity (e.g. bow legs, pigeon chest, and pelvic deformities)
- Pathological fractures
- Dental caries and delayed teeth formation
- Impaired growth and short stature (may not be reversible)
- Low calcium → numbness of extremities (hands and feet)

People most at risk include: older people, especially >80yrs and those in residential care (➔ Care homes p. 32); people with deficient diet and/or little access to sunshine; immigrants with pigmented skin; and people with chronic kidney disease (➔ Renal problems p. 754), coeliac disease (➔ Coeliac disease p. 714), and other absorption problems.

Following diagnosis by blood test, majority treated with vitamin supplements.

Osteomyelitis

An infection of the bone requiring urgent referral to 2° care. May follow systemic infection and/or injury. Children and people with diabetes mellitus (➔ Diabetes: overview p. 660) most susceptible. Complications include: septic arthritis (➔ Sepsis p. 826), chronic osteomyelitis chronic infection, bone deformity, and pathological fracture. Characterized by:

- Pain and reluctance to move affected limbs
- Warmth and effusion in affected joints
- Fever and malaise

Treatment is with intravenous and then oral antibiotics for several weeks, and surgery to drain abscesses.

Systemic lupus erythematosus (SLE)

A rare autoimmune connective tissue disease. Higher prevalence in African Caribbean and Far East Asian populations. No cure. It affects multiple systems. Majority of patients have skin and joint involvement, and often complain of severe fatigue:

- Joints: arthritis and arthralgia
- Skin: hypersensitivity, facial butterfly rash, vasculitis, hair loss (➔ Pigmentation and hair problems p. 692)
- Lungs: pleurisy, pneumonitis (➔ Pneumonia p. 750), and alveolitus
- Kidneys: proteinuria, hypertension, glomerulonephritis, and renal failure (➔ Renal problems p. 754)
- Heart: pericarditis and endocarditis
- Central nervous system: depression (➔ People with anxiety and depression p. 478), psychosis (➔ People with psychosis p. 486), myocardial infarction, and fits (➔ Seizures and epilepsy p. 740).

Patients will need specialist rheumatology treatment and ongoing care.

Recommend patients to avoid direct sunlight (can exacerbate rash). Medications include: NSAIDs, disease-modifying anti-rheumatic drugs, steroids, and immunosuppressants. Hormonal contraception and HRT may aggravate symptoms.

Raynaud's syndrome

Intermittent ischaemia of the fingers, precipitated by cold and/or emotion. Cause unknown. Fingers very painful, numb, tingle, ache, and become pale; then blue and red on being warmed. Minority may go on to develop other rheumatic diseases (e.g. SLE). Advise on keeping warm. Patients with mild symptoms should use thermal gloves, avoid cold and draughts. Promote smoking cessation (➔ Smoking cessation p. 356). More severe symptoms treated with medication (e.g. vasodilators and serotonin reuptake inhibitors) and specialist referral.

Related topics

➔ Osteoarthritis p. 600; ➔ Rheumatoid arthritis p. 602

Further information

Lupus UK (What is lupus?). Available at: ℗ www.lupusuk.org.uk/home
Paget's Association (Paget's disease). Available at: ℗ www.paget.org.uk
Scleroderma and Raynaud's UK (About us). Available at: ℗ https://www.sruk.co.uk/about-us/

Seizures and epilepsy

A seizure or fit is when there is a sudden disturbance of neurological function associated with an abnormal neuronal discharge. All children, young people, and adults with a recent-onset suspected seizure should be seen urgently by a specialist. The term 'seizure' is used to avoid the emotive term of epilepsy, unless a specialist diagnosis has been made.

Epilepsy

Recurrent seizures other than febrile convulsions (→ Febrile convulsions and epilepsy p. 280). 60% of adult epilepsy starts in childhood. Suspected cases are referred to neurologists. Diagnosis made on history, clinical examination, and electroencephalogram (EEG). The cause of epilepsy is often not found, but the known causes include:

- Genetic factors
- Physical factors: head trauma, space-occupying lesions, raised BP
  (→ Hypertension p. 628), and stroke
- Metabolic factors: alcohol withdrawal (→ Alcohol p. 360),
  drug-related (→ Substance use p. 476), hyper-/hypoglycaemia
  (→ Diabetes: overview p. 660), hypoxia, and electrolyte disturbance
- Infective causes (e.g. encephalitis)

Focal epilepsy

Involves one part of the body and may progress to other parts, becoming generalized (Jacksonian epilepsy).

Grand mal epilepsy

Generalized seizure with sudden onset of tonic contraction of the muscles, often associated with a cry or a moan, and falling to the ground. The tonic phase gives way to clonic convulsive movements occurring bilaterally and synchronously, which slow and stop, followed by a variable period of unconsciousness and gradual recovery.

Myoclonic epilepsy

A variant of petit mal epilepsy, characterized by atonic drop attacks.

Petit mal epilepsy

A pause in speech or other activity, with the patient unaware of the episode.

Temporal lobe epilepsy

A disorder with seizures originating from the temporal lobe with numerous, bizarre presentations which can include altered perception and oral and auditory hallucinations.

Status epilepticus

A generalized convulsion, lasting 30mins or longer, or when successive convulsions occur between which the patient does not recover consciousness.

Management and support

Structured person-centred care plan is agreed in 2° and 1° care, and review undertaken at least annually with specialist.

Medication

It is controlled by antiepileptic drugs (AED):

- Treatment individualized by seizure type, epilepsy syndrome, comorbidity, lifestyle, and preference.
- Adherence to treatment is important (**→** Medicine concordance and adherence p. 132).
- Usually started at a low dose; dose ↑ until fits are controlled or side effects occur.
- Buccal midazolam (first-line treatment) or rectal diazepam prescribed for prolonged seizures and convulsive status epilepticus.
- Once stable and management straightforward, continuing AED therapy is prescribed in 1° care.
- Once seizure-free for >2yrs, specialist (with patient's/parents' consent) may decide to gradually withdraw AED.

Information and education

- Specifics of diagnosis and prognosis
- AED and side effects (include side effects for contraception (**→** Contraception: general p. 400), pregnancy (**→** Pregnancy p. 424), childcare, and menopause (**→** Menopause p. 364))
- Risk management: life should be as normal as possible, avoiding risks (e.g. swimming or cycling alone) but not being overprotective
- Possible triggers for seizures (e.g. stress (**→** Managing stress p. 358), drugs and alcohol, antidepressants (**→** People with anxiety and depression p. 478), tiredness, flickering lights, menstruation, and illness)
- Counselling services (**→** Talking therapies p. 472), voluntary organizations (e.g. Epilepsy Action ℜ https://www.epilepsy.org. uk/), and expert patient programmes (**→** Expert patients and self-management programmes p. 340)
- Need to ensure that school staff are aware of the diagnosis, but are careful not to stigmatize or overprotect children
- DVLA restrictions apply (patient to notify DVLA and insurer) (see ℜ https://www.gov.uk/epilepsy-and-driving)
- Employer should be aware and some occupations are precluded for people with epilepsy (e.g. pilot and train driver)

Key principles for managing a seizure

⚠ Keep the person safe from harm and stay with them as they recover afterwards.

- Note the time the seizure started
- Only move them if they are in danger (e.g. by a busy road)
- If they are in a safe place, leave them, cushion head if on ground
- Loosen any tight clothing around their neck

- Do not place anything in the mouth
- After seizure has stopped, place in recovery position (❥ Recovery position for babies, children and adults p. 796)
- Stay and reassure the person as they recover
- Do not offer food or drink until fully recovered

⚠ ☎ 999 for an ambulance if: you know it is their first seizure; they are fitting for >5mins; they do not regain full consciousness; they have several seizures without regaining consciousness; or they are seriously injured during the seizure.

Further information

NICE (*Epilepsy [CG137]*). Available at: ℅ https://www.nice.org.uk/guidance/cg137

Migraine

Signs and symptoms

Management

Further information

Migraine

A syndrome characterized by periodic headaches with complete resolution between attacks. Most common cause of recurrent disabling headache in the population. Triggers include: emotional and/or physical stress; diet/food (e.g. sugary foods or long breaks without food; environmental factors (e.g. bright lights (including computer visual display units)); and hormonal factors. Most patients can successfully manage the condition.

Signs and symptoms

An attack can include all or some of the following stages:
- Prodrome: change in mood or appetite before migraine onset
- Some people experience aura before onset of headache (e.g. visual disturbance or motor or sensory disturbance)
- Headache (common migraine): often pulsatile and unilateral, lasts 4–72hrs; moderate/severe intensity may be associated with symptoms of nausea and vomiting, photophobia, phonophobia, and aggravated by movement

Management

Prevention

Identify and avoid trigger factors. Keep a migraine diary to help identify triggers. Recommend: regular sleep pattern and dietary pattern; ↓ caffeine and alcohol intake (➔ Alcohol p. 360); and drinking 2 litres water a day. Refer to GP to discuss use of prophylactic medications. ♀ with focal aura are contraindicated for combined hormonal methods (➔ Combined hormonal contraceptive methods p. 402).

Management of acute attack

First-line treatments should be taken early in an attack and will include OTC analgesia. If such treatment inadequate, refer to GP for second-line treatments including antiemetics. Consider referral to migraine clinic.

Further information

Migraine Trust (*Living with migraine*). Available at: ℛ www.MigraineTrust.org
NICE (*Migraine*). Available at: ℛ https://cks.nice.org.uk/migraine

Common problems affecting eyes

Conjunctivitis

Inflammation of the conjunctiva, the cause of which can be infective irritant or allergic. Can be unilateral (often if infection present) or bilateral. Most common condition seen in 1° care. Characterized by:

- Red sore eye
- Discharge
- Swollen eyelids
- Eyes stuck together after sleep
- Linked to seasonal changes and contact with allergen (➔ Allergies p. 694)
- Close contact with another affected person (infective)
- Presence of upper respiratory infection (infective)

Care and management

In neonates <28 days old with purulent discharge, possibility of sexually transmitted infection from the mother (➔ Sexually transmitted infections p. 764). Seek urgent GP appointment (➔ General practice p. 18) and take swabs for chlamydia and Neisseria gonorrhoeae.

Most symptoms self-limiting and resolve in 2–5 days. Maintain good eye hygiene. If symptoms persist, may benefit from topical antibiotics. Whilst these may be purchased OTC, the pharmacist will need to be satisfied they are clinically beneficial (e.g. bacterial conjunctivitis rather than viral) (➔ Antimicrobial stewardship p. 146). For people with allergic conjunctivitis, treat with antihistamines or topical anti-inflammatory. If infective conjunctivitis, advise on not sharing towels, pillows, or face cloths, and on good hand hygiene. School and group childcare exclusion until treated. Avoid wearing contact lens until no symptoms.

Blepharitis

Causes are unknown. A chronic persistent condition, usually bilateral. May be characterized by:

- Sore inflamed eyelids, red-rimmed eyes
- Eyelids may stick together in the morning (consider possibility of infection)
- Eyes may feel gritty
- May have scales on eyelashes
- Complain of dry eyes, blurred vision
- Unable to tolerate contact lens

Care and management

Good eye hygiene, at least once a day, is the mainstay of treatment:

- Soak a clean flannel or cotton wool in warm water.
- Place on eye for 10mins.
- Gently massage eyelids for ~30secs.
- Clean eyelids using cotton wool or cotton bud.
- May help to use a small amount of baby shampoo in water.

Advise patients to avoid eye make-up or to use water-soluble eyeliner. Do not use contact lens. Avoid rubbing eyes. If eyes are persistently dry, may benefit from artificial tears. If persists, may need specialist referral.

Floaters

Small shapes (e.g. spots and shadowy strands) caused by debris floating in the eye's vitreous humour. Occur with ↑ age, but may be a sign of retinal detachment. If sudden onset or ↑ with white flashes, the person should visit the optician immediately.

Subconjunctival haemorrhage

A painless localized haemorrhage visible at the front of the eye that occurs spontaneously. Common in older people. Clears in 1–2wks. Consider referral to specialist if history of trauma or edges of haemorrhage cannot be seen (● Eye trauma p. 818).

⚠ Red-eye symptoms that are potentially dangerous should have same-day referral to doctor/specialist if one or more of following are present:
- Moderate to severe pain (non-surface irritation) and/or photophobia
- ↓ visual acuity
- Inability to move eye
- Visibly dilated blood vessels seen between white of eye and iris
- Loss and/or affected sight
- Corneal damage (often only visible after fluroscein staining)
- Absent or sluggish pupil response
- Eye involvement when patient has shingles (herpes zoster)
- History of trauma or post-operatively

Related topics

● Blindness and partial sight p. 748

Further information

NICE (*Blepharitis*). Available at: ℬ https://cks.nice.org.uk/blepharitis
NICE (*Conjunctivitis: infective*). Available at: ℬ https://cks.nice.org.uk/conjunctivitis-infective
NICE (*Conjunctivitis: allergic*). Available at: ℬ https://cks.nice.org.uk/conjunctivitis-infective

Blindness and partial sight

Adults aged 18–60yrs should have an eye exam every 2yrs; older adults should have annual exams. ⚠ Sudden loss of vision is an emergency needing specialist attention via A&E.

Visual acuity is measured by a Snellen chart. To be certified severely sight impaired (blind) or sight impaired (partially sighted) see Box 12.5.

Age-related macular degeneration (AMD)

Bilateral disease affecting one eye more than the other. Characterized by deterioration of central vision affecting reading, face recognition, and ability to see colour. Types of AMD include wet AMD and dry AMD. Wet AMD is caused by growth of abnormal blood vessels at the back of the eyes. Dry AMD is caused by a build-up of a fatty substance at the back of the eyes. Generally, no treatment for dry AMD. Treatment for wet AMD may include eye injections.

Cataracts

Occurs when the lens of an eye becomes cloudy. Develops gradually. Experienced as blurred vision, spots, or halos around bright lights and being dazzled by car lights. Affects distance judgement. Treatment when interferes with everyday life: routine surgery day-case operation. Cloudy lens is removed and is replaced with an artificial plastic lens. Patient will need glasses to adjust for refractive changes.

Chronic simple glaucoma

↑ in eye pressure causes damage to the optic nerve. Initially, asymptomatic as peripheral vision is the first to be affected. People often present late. Symptoms include visual loss and sausage-shaped blind spots. Treatment intended to ↓ eye pressure and prevent further damage to optic nerve. Achieved through eye drops and potential surgery.

Box 12.5 Definitions of certifiable blindness and sight impairment

Severely sight impaired (blind)

Sight has to fall into one of the following (while wearing any glasses or contact lenses as necessary):
- Visual acuity of less than 3/60 with a full visual field
- Visual acuity between 3/60 and 6/60 with a severe reduction of field of vision (e.g. tunnel vision)
- Visual acuity of 6/60 or above but with a very reduced field of vision, especially if a lot of sight is missing in the lower part of the field

Sight impaired (partially sighted)

Sight has to fall into one of the following (while wearing any glasses or contact lenses as necessary):
- Visual acuity of 3/60 to 6/60 with a full field of vision
- Visual acuity of up to 6/24 with a moderate reduction of field of vision or with a central part of vision that is cloudy or blurry
- Visual acuity of 6/18 or better if a large part of field of vision (e.g. a whole half of vision) is missing or a lot of peripheral vision is missing

Retinal detachment

Relatively rare condition: painless loss of vision, like a curtain coming across the vision. 50% have some premonition with flashing lights, spots, or floaters. ⚠ Should attend optician immediately for eye assessment as may need to be referred for urgent treatment to secure retina.

Diabetic retinopathy

Complication of diabetes, caused by high blood sugar levels damaging the retina. People with diabetes should have an eye exam annually. Important to control blood sugar levels (➲ Principles of diabetes management p. 664). Treatment options include laser treatment, injections into the eye, and possible surgery.

Registering as sight impaired

Referred to consultant ophthalmologist for assessment. Once registered, social services (➲ Social services p. 30) should undertake an assessment to determine what help and advice the person needs to maintain independence (e.g. access to equipment such as talking clocks, home modifications such as bright lights (➲ Assistive technology and home adaptations p. 834), and training in Braille). Concessions for people who are registered as sight impaired may include a reduction on the TV licence, help with NHS costs, help with Council Tax, tax allowances, leisure discounts, and free public transport.

Health promotion to prevent sight loss

- Protect eyes from bright sunlight with sunglasses
- Eat fruits and green leafy vegetables (➲ Nutrition and healthy eating p. 342)
- Monitor BP (➲ Hypertension p. 628)
- Smoking cessation (➲ Smoking cessation p. 356)
- Moderate alcohol intake (➲ Alcohol p. 360)
- Regular eye exam
- Measures to prevent or control diabetes

Related topics

➲ Common problems affecting eyes p. 746; ➲ Eye trauma p. 818

Further information

Macular Disease Society (*Understanding macular disease*). Available at: ℅ https://www.macularsociety.org/

Royal National Institute for the Blind (*Sight loss advice*). Available at: ℅ https://www.rnib.org.uk/advice

Pneumonia

Infection of lung tissue. Rates of pneumonia ↑ during winter months. Two types: hospital-acquired pneumonia (HAP) and community-acquired pneumonia (CAP). HAP is pneumonia which occurs ≥48hrs after admission. CAP can affect anyone, but is more common and usually more serious in: the very young; the very old; smokers; anyone with long-term illness; and those who are immunocompromised. Streptococcus pneumoniae is the commonest cause of CAP. Those less seriously affected are managed in the community, but up to 42% need hospital admission, with a mortality rate of 5–14%. Preventative interventions include smoking cessation (➔ Smoking cessation p. 356) and pneumococcal and influenza vaccination (➔ Targeted adult immunization p. 392).

Symptoms

Acute illness characterized by: flu-like symptoms (e.g. fevers, shivers, aches, ↑ temperature, and nausea and vomiting); cough with sputum production; dyspnoea and/or tachypnoea; tachycardia; some have pleural chest pain; and older people may have acute confusion and/or walking difficulties and/or loss of appetite.

Assessment

Clinical assessment in 1° care is based on symptoms and signs of lower respiratory tract infection. Severity needs to be assessed and a CRB65 score is calculated by giving one point for: confusion (abbreviated mental test score ≤8); raised respiratory rate (>30 per min); low BP (diastolic <60mmHg, systolic <90mmHg); and age ≥65. A score of 0 = low risk (less than 1% mortality risk); 1 or 2 = intermediate risk (1–10% mortality risk); and 3 or 4 = ↑ risk (more than 10% mortality risk). Score of 0 can be treated at home, and score >2 to consider hospital treatment. Diagnosis testing may include blood and sputum cultures, chest X-ray, and pneumococcal and legionella urinary antigen tests.

Treatment and management at home

Will include a course of antibiotics. Duration and possible combination will depend on severity. Symptoms should improve within 48hrs although rate of improvement depends on individuals. Patient should be reviewed at this point and, if deteriorating or not improving, considered for hospital referral. Provide advice on: completing course of antibiotics (➔ Antimicrobial stewardship p. 146); smoking cessation; plenty of fluids; and simple analgesia as required.

Further information

British Thoracic Society (*Guidelines for the management of community acquired pneumonia in adults*). Available at: ℬ https://www.brit-thoracic.org.uk/quality-improvement/guidelines/pneumonia-adults

Lung cancer

Lung cancer is the third most common cancer and is the leading cause of cancer death in the UK (➲ UK health profile p. 2). Caused mostly by smoking and passive smoking. Other cases due to exposure to radioactive gases, occupational exposure, and pollution. Two main groups: small-cell lung cancer and non-small-cell (mainly squamous cell carcinoma, adenocarcinoma, or large-cell carcinoma). Signs and symptoms include: persistent cough; dyspnoea; haemoptysis; chest/shoulder pain; finger clubbing; unexplained weight and appetite loss; and persistent tiredness and lack of energy. Symptoms can be unnoticeable, which has an impact on prognosis.

Diagnosis

Investigations include: chest X-ray; CT/PET (positron emission tomography)-CT scan; and bronchoscopy and biopsy.

Stages of lung cancer

Non-small-cell lung cancer has four main stages: localized cancer in lung with slow-growing cells (stage 1); cancer in lung and nearby lymph nodes (stage 2); cancer spread to chest wall or surrounding tissue (stage 3); and metastases (stage 4). Small-cell lung cancer has two stages: limited disease (to nearby lymph nodes) (stage 1); and extensive disease (metastases) (stage 2).

Treatment and management

Depends on type of cancer and may include: surgery (rarely suitable for small-cell lung cancer), radiotherapy, and chemotherapy (standard for small-cell lung cancer). Other treatments that are sometimes used include: biological therapies, radiofrequency ablation, cryotherapy, and photodynamic therapy. If in advanced stage, palliative care offered (➲ Palliative care in the home p. 550).

Related topics

➲ Smoking cessation p. 356; ➲ Cancer prevention p. 372

Further information

British Lung Foundation (*Lung cancer*). Available at: ℘ https://www.blf.org.uk/support-for-you/lung-cancer

Cancer Research UK (*Stages and grades*). Available at: ℘ https://www.cancerresearchuk.org/about-cancer/lung-cancer/stages-types-grades

NICE (*Lung cancer: diagnosis and management [CG122]*). Available at: ℘ https://www.nice.org.uk/guidance/ng122

Occupational lung disease

Occupational asthma

More than 200 substances known to produce asthma-like symptoms and treated as such (→ Asthma in adults p. 608). Vehicle spray painters and bakers have ↑ rates. Employers should seal off hazardous substances, fit extractor fans, and provide personal protective equipment.

Work-related asthma

People with pre-existing asthma whose symptoms are worsened by exposure to irritants at work (e.g. dust, chlorine, air temperature variation, or ↓ humidity).

Pneumoconiosis

A group of lung diseases caused by inhalation and retention of mineral dust, resulting in fibrosis of the lungs. Takes up to 20yrs from exposure to develop disease, so current laws about working conditions should prevent most workers from developing pneumoconiosis in the future. Types include: coal worker's pneumoconiosis from coal dust; asbestosis and related lung cancer (e.g. mesothelioma from asbestos fibres); and silicosis from silica dust in iron foundries, pottery factories, and quarries. Patient should not be further exposed to substance, and should stop smoking (→ Smoking cessation p. 356). Symptoms managed as for COPD (→ Chronic obstructive pulmonary disease p. 614), lung cancer (→ Lung cancer p. 751), and palliative care (→ Palliative care in the home p. 550).

Hypersensitivity pneumonitis

Inflammation of alveoli, caused by allergic response to external substances. Also known as extrinsic allergic alveolitis. At-risk groups include: farmers (lung-inhaled fungal spores); metal workers (metal-working fluids); and bird fanciers (lung-inhaled avian protein). Treatment involves steroids and avoiding exposure.

Notification of occupational disease

GP, with patient's permission (→ Consent p. 82), informs employer in writing of any legally notifiable occupational illness, and the employer must report it according to Reporting of Injuries, Diseases, and Dangerous Occurrences Regulations (RIDDOR) (→ Health and safety at work p. 92).

Benefits and compensation

The patient may be eligible for government industrial injuries benefit scheme and compensation. Can also make a personal injury claim.

Further information

Health and Safety Executive (*Prevent work-related lung disease*). Available at: ℜ http://www.hse.gov.uk/lung-disease/index.htm

Renal problems

Glomerulonephritis

Inflammation of both kidneys, primarily affecting all or part of the kidney's glomeruli (the tiny bundle of arterioles at the beginning of the nephron, where the urine is initially formed). It is most common in children, young adults, and ♂. Can be acute or chronic, but can cause renal damage with long-term consequences. Patient may be initially asymptomatic or have vague symptoms (e.g. tiredness). More acute symptoms include proteinuria, oliguria, haematuria, oedema, anorexia, and hypertension (➲ Hypertension p. 628). Suspected cases need urgent referral to specialist.

Nephrotic syndrome

When proteinuria is severe and → oedema and hypoalbuminaemia. Patients can have ascites, swelling of the face, peripheral oedema fatigue, anorexia due to kidney damage arising from:

• Glomerulonephritism of various sorts
• Scarring of glomeruli (focal segmental glomerulopnephritis)
• Diabetes mellitus (➲ Diabetes: overview p. 660)

Suspected cases referred to specialist. Prognosis depends on cause (e.g. children with minimal change disease respond well to treatment).

Renal stones

Passage of a stone in the ureter or kidney or bladder that causes acute, severe pain that comes in waves (renal colic). Patients may have haematuria and appear pale and sweaty. Believed incidence of stones ↑ because of Western diet and obesity. Often no underlying cause. Severity of pain unrelated to size of stone. Risk factors:

• People with recurrent UTIs (➲ Urinary tract infection p. 756)
• People with neuropathic bladder dysfunction (➲ Spinal cord injury p. 518)
• People on certain medication (e.g. loop diuretics, thiazides, antacids, aspirin, calcium, vitamin D, steroids)
• People with congenital kidney abnormalities that cause urinary stasis
• Dehydration
• Patient with ileostomy → ↑ alkali loss from gut (➲ Stoma care p. 516)
• Family history of renal stones

Prompt referral (same day if possible) for urogram or kidney–bladder ultrasound and X-ray. Stones usually pass spontaneously. Priority is good pain control and ↑ fluid intake. Patient may be prescribed an alpha blocker to speed their passage. Patient will need an emergency hospital admission if they are pregnant (➲ Pregnancy p. 424) or have only one kidney, a fever, uncontrolled pain, have not passed urine, and/or symptoms have persisted for >24hrs.

Chronic kidney disease (CKD) and end-stage renal disease

CKD is progressive loss of renal function over time. Prevalence ↑ in people of South Asian and African Caribbean ethnicity. Hypertension and diabetes are the main causes. Other risk factors include recurrent UTIs, urinary obstruction, and family history of cardiovascular disease. Most widely used methods for screening for CKD are: an analysis of a random urine sample for albumin/creatinine ratio (ACR), and a serum creatinine measurement to calculate an estimate glomerular filtration rate (eGFR)—an indication of functioning kidney mass (see Box 12.6).

> ### Box 12.6 Stages of chronic kidney disease
> **Stage 1:** Normal eGFR (above 90ml/min), but other tests have detected signs of kidney damage
> **Stage 2:** Slightly reduced eGFR (60–89ml/min), with other signs of kidney damage
> **Stage 3a:** eGFR of 45–59ml/min
> **Stage 3b:** eGFR of 30–44ml/min
> **Stage 4:** eGFR of 15–29ml/min
> **Stage 5:** eGFR below 15ml/min, meaning the kidneys have lost almost all of their function

Care and management

In 1° care, aim is to detect CKD early, take measures to slow disease progression, and provide timely referral to a nephrologist. Measures to slow down progression include stopping nephrotoxic drugs (e.g. NSAIDs) and treating hypertension. Patient should also be advised: to quit smoking (➲ Smoking cessation p. 356); eat ↓ fat ↓ salt diet (➲ Nutrition and healthy eating p. 342); take regular exercise (➲ Exercise p. 354); and limit alcohol consumption (➲ Alcohol p. 360). Patients with stage 3a and 3b disease will need monitoring for anaemia and early bone disease. They should also have their kidney function checked every 6–12mths. Those patients with stage 4 or 5 disease should be referred to a specialist. See national guidelines on indications to start renal replacement therapy.[9]

Two types of dialysis: haemodialysis and continuous ambulatory peritoneal dialysis (CAPD). CAPD may be performed at home. Automated peritoneal dialysis uses a machine, and can be performed overnight. Common problems include: peritonitis, infection of the exit site, and catheter blockage (requires admission to hospital as emergency).

Patients are eligible for the influenza, Hepatitis B, and pneumococcal immunizations (➲ Targeted adult immunization p. 392).

Reference

9. NICE (2018) *Renal replacement therapy and conservative management [NG107]*. Available at: https://www.nice.org.uk/guidance/ng107/chapter/Recommendations

Urinary tract infection

Urinary tract infections (UTIs) are a consequence of the presence and multiplication of micro-organisms in the urinary tract (bladder, urethra, or kidneys). Depending on the location of the infection, different clinical syndromes may develop. UTIs may be asymptomatic.

Types and symptoms

- Lower UTI (including cystitis): frequency, urgency, dysuria, polyuria, suprapubic pain, fever, flank or back pain
- Upper UTI (including pyelonephritis): fever, rigor, vomiting, loin pain and tenderness, acute renal failure

Differentiation between the two types is important. Diagnostic tools include dipstick urine specimen for laboratory examination, and vital signs.

Patients who are catheterized may complain of suprapubic pain and discomfort and have cloudy and foul-smelling urine (➲ Indwelling urinary catheter care p. 508). Older people who appear confused and disorientated may have a UTI. Children appear generally unwell (babies may be irritable, not feed properly, and have a high temperature), wet the bed or themselves, and deliberately avoid passing urine due to a burning sensation.

Management of a lower UTI

Majority of untreated, acute, uncomplicated cystitis will usually resolve in 3 days. Current guidance advises antibiotics should only be used when evidence that eradicating a bacterial infection will result in health gains (e.g. symptom relief).[10] Management plans differs between ♂, ♀, pregnant ♀ (➲ Pregnancy p. 424), and children. Bacteriuria common in asymptomatic older patients and treating can do more harm than good. Those with an infection may benefit from pain relief. If a patient has indwelling catheter, current evidence suggests it may be beneficial to change catheter if it has been in place for >7 days. All children <3mths should be referred urgently to 2° care. Pregnant ♀ should be monitored carefully. Patients with recurrent UTIs should be further investigated. Similarly, patient is referred to specialist 2° care if symptoms unresolved.

Management of an upper UTI

Manage with antibiotics. Monitor for signs of more serious illness (e.g. renal failure and sepsis (➲ Sepsis p. 826)). If no improvement in general condition within 48hrs, refer to 2° care.

Prevention

- Drink plenty of fluids.
- Void after intercourse.
- ♀ wipe from front to back after going to the toilet.
- Following investigation, ♀ with recurrent UTIs may need prophylactic antibiotics or have a prescription in readiness for prompt treatment when first have symptoms.
- Menopausal ♀ may benefit from HRT (➲ Menopause p. 364).

Reference

10. SIGN (2012) *Management of suspected bacterial urinary tract infection in adults.* Available at: https://www.sign.ac.uk/assets/sign88.pdf

Further information

NICE (*Urinary tract infection (lower): men*). Available at: ℛ https://cks.nice.org.uk/urinary-tract-infection-lower-men

NICE (*Urinary tract infection (lower): women*). Available at: ℛ https://cks.nice.org.uk/urinary-tract-infection-lower-women

NICE (*Urinary tract infection: children*). Available at: ℛ https://cks.nice.org.uk/urinary-tract-infection-children

Prostate problems

Benign prostatic hyperplasia

Benign prostatic hyperplasia (BPH) is also sometimes known as benign prostate enlargement (BPE). Very common in ♂ >50yrs. The prostate enlarges with ageing → narrowing of urethra and partially obstructs the flow of urine. Symptoms often initially mild but become more severe. Signs and symptoms:

- Poor and ↓ stream: taking longer to empty bladder
- Hesitancy: having to wait before urine flows
- Dribbling of urine soon after finishing micturition
- Feeling of incomplete bladder emptying
- Frequency, urgency, and nocturia

Complications

- Recurrent UTIs (◗ Urinary tract infections p. 756)
- Acute urinary retention
- Chronic urinary retention
- Overflow incontinence (◗ Urinary incontinence p. 504)
- Haematuria
- Erectile dysfunction pain on ejaculation (◗ Sexual problems p. 768)

Care and management

The International Prostate Symptom Score (IPSS) is a patient-completed questionnaire, which provides a useful baseline measure of severity and impact on quality of life. A bladder diary can also be useful. Assessing flow rate and post-void residual urine volume are simple tests often performed in urology clinics.

Patients with mild to moderate symptoms: strategy of watchful waiting, reassurance, education, and advice on ↓ caffeine and alcohol intake (◗ Alcohol p. 360), avoiding constipation (◗ Constipation in adults p. 512), ↓ fat intake in diet (◗ Nutrition and healthy eating p. 342), and bladder retraining. Plan ahead and ↓ fluid intake before important events, but important to maintain good fluid intake of minimum 1.5L per day. Control urgency with distraction and relaxation techniques.

Patients with mild to moderate symptoms may benefit from drug treatment (e.g. alpha blockers and/or 5-alpha reductase inhibitors). Surgery is considered for ♂ with ongoing symptoms despite medical management, and those who have episodes of retention. A long-term catheter is another option for men unwilling or unfit for surgery (◗ Indwelling urinary catheter care p. 508).

Prostatitis

Prostatitis refers to inflammation of the prostate gland. Often caused by an infection, it can be considered as a complicated UTI. Symptoms can include difficulty passing urine, fevers, and pain or discomfort in the testicle, back passage, lower back, or abdomen. It is treated initially with a prolonged course of antibiotics.

Prostate cancer

Prostate cancer is the most common cancer in ♂. Risk factors include: ↑ age; family history; ethnic group (some evidence to suggest more aggressive disease in African Caribbean men); obesity (➋ Overweight and obesity p. 348); and diet (e.g. ↑ fat/meat diet may predispose to the condition). Early cancer is symptomless. Patient may present with:

- Haematuria
- Urinary retention/obstruction
- Erectile dysfunction
- Lower back pain and or bone pain (from metastases)
- Weight loss

Prostate-specific antigen (PSA) testing

England has introduced an informed choice approach to PSA testing in general practice (➋ General practice p. 18). The PSA test has poor sensitivity and specificity, and many ♂ with raised levels will not have clinically relevant prostate cancer. If the PSA level is slightly raised, the GP undertakes further clinical assessment (excluding an infection) and performs a digital rectal examination. On the basis of this or higher levels of PSA, the GP will refer to a urology specialist.

Care and management

Management for localized disease should be directed by the prognostic significance of the cancer, taking into account the patient's age and life expectancy. Options include: active surveillance (careful monitoring of the PSA, repeat imaging, and/or biopsies); watchful waiting (less intensive monitoring); radical prostatectomy (potential for cure but risks and complications associated with surgery including impotence and incontinence); radiotherapy (potential for cure, usually given alongside hormone therapy); and hormone monotherapy (predominantly reserved for metastatic disease, or patients unfit for other options).

Further information

NICE (*Prostate cancer: diagnosis and treatment [CG175]*). Available at: ℘ https://www.nice.org.uk/guidance/cg175

NICE (*The management of lower urinary tract symptoms in men [CG97]*). Available at: ℘ https://www.nice.org.uk/guidance/cg97

PHE (*Prostate cancer risk management programme overview*). Available at: ℘ www.cancerscreening.nhs.uk/prostate/

Sexual health: general issues

With rising diagnoses of sexually transmitted infections (STIs) and the ability to prevent HIV transmission through HIV treatment and pre-exposure prophylaxis (→ Human immunodeficiency virus p. 462), the need to provide access to a range of prevention, diagnostic, and treatment opportunities remains important. Target groups include young adults (<25yrs), men who have sex with men (MSM), and Black and African ethnic minorities (BME), as these tend to be higher-risk and marginalized groups.

Treatment of STIs should be in accordance with national clinical guidelines and free of prescription charges. People at risk of STIs should have their care managed by appropriately trained staff in a range of 'open access' services, including 1° care. There has been a reduction of 'level 3' services due to changes in commissioning, which is now done by LAs (→ Commissioning of services p. 12). Expenditure has ↓ as public health money is no longer ring-fenced and has been reduced (→ Public health in the NHS and beyond p. 14). Integrated services incorporating contraception (→ Contraception: general p. 400) and sexual health/STIs have been introduced. E-screening has been introduced for those without symptoms to refer suspected cases of STIs and HIV to the local sexual health (SH)/sexual and reproductive health (GUM) clinic.

Confidentiality

People have the right to confidentiality regardless of where they access care (→ Confidentiality p. 89). Concerns over confidentiality can be overcome by developing a sensitive and non-judgemental culture. Non-discrimination and confidentiality statements should be displayed for patients to see (→ Anti-discriminatory healthcare p. 81). NHS organizations have an obligation to keep secure any information about STIs obtained by healthcare workers. Information should be regarded as confidential and not communicated except to other healthcare practitioners for the purposes of treatment or prevention. In exceptional circumstances, information may need to be shared in the interests of the patient or public, as set out in guidance documents (e.g. local safeguarding policies (→ Adults at risk from harm and abuse p. 454)). See Fraser guidelines for confidentiality in relation to people aged <16yrs. For further information about consent and confidentiality in sexual health services for clients <16yrs, please see ℐ https://www.fpa.org.uk/factsheets/under-16s-consent-and-confidentiality-sexual-health-services

Partner notification

- All services should instigate partner notification (PN) as part of STI management.
- Explain to the patient that PN is essential (except for candida and bacterial vaginosis) to ↓ risk of reinfection to self, and to stop the spread of infection to other sexual partners.
- Encourage patient to notify recent sexual partner(s) of their STI, and advise them to seek treatment.
- For complex cases, seek advice or refer to health advisers or other SH/GUM staff. Health advisers can perform provider referral PN, whereby the index patient provides information on partner(s) to a health adviser, who then confidentially traces and notifies the partner(s) directly.

Sexual assault

Disclosure of non-consenting sex should never be ignored. People who have been sexually assaulted or raped can be referred as urgent cases to designated sexual assault referral centres (SARCs or Havens) that can provide medical care, forensic examination, and liaison with the police, as and if requested by the patient. Patients can self-refer to SARCs. Patients can be seen in SH/GUM services but are offered referral if the assault is recent. Non-consenting sex in <16yrs requires local child protection procedures to be followed (➔ Child protection processes p. 252).

Health promotion

Sexual health should be proactively and positively promoted as an important aspect of an individual's overall health and well-being. Specific interventions should focus on safer sex skills acquisition, enhancing communication skills and ↑ motivation to adopt safer sex behaviours.

- Promote consistent condom use for vaginal and anal sex, plus water-based lubricant (lube) for anal sex.
- Provide free condoms and lube, or suggest where client can access these. Demonstrate condom use as required.
- Discuss regular contraception and promote awareness of emergency contraception (➔ Emergency contraception p. 420) and long-acting reversible contraception.
- Promote awareness of STI signs and symptoms.
- Provide sexual health leaflets, web links, and helpline numbers.
- Where there is an ongoing risk of HIV transmission, discuss HIV post-exposure prophylaxis (PEP) and pre-exposure prophylaxis (PrEP).
- Refer to sexual health services for specialist intervention on risk reduction.

Related topics

➔ Sexually transmitted infections p. 764; ➔ Sexual health consultations p. 762; ➔ Sexual health and adults with learning disability p. 770)

Further information

British HIV Association (*HIV testing and management guidelines*). Available at: ℘ www.bhiva.org

PHE (*STIs: surveillance, data, screening and management*). Available at: ℘ https://www.gov.uk/government/collections/sexually-transmitted-infections-stis-surveillance-data-screening-and-management

Royal College of General Practitioners (*E-learning on sexual health in primary care*). Available at: ℘ http://elearning.rcgp.org.uk/course/info.php?id=179&popup=0

Sexual health consultations

Practitioners should ensure that the consultation is undertaken in a sensitive and non-judgemental manner. Ensure privacy and reassure confidentiality (➔ Confidentiality p. 89), unless the person is at risk. When undertaking care of under-18s and vulnerable adults, follow local and national guidance on safeguarding (➔ Adults at risk from harm and abuse p. 454; ➔ Safeguarding children p. 248).

Sexual history assessment

Degree of assessment depends on practitioner skill and competence. Good practice suggests:
- Ask about symptoms (location, type, severity, duration, aggravation/ alleviating factors, self-treatment)
- Recent sexual partner(s) (gender, type of sex, condom use)
- Contraception use
- Past STIs, HIV status, and testing history, and cervical cancer screening in ♀ (➔ Cervical cancer screening p. 380)

Physical examination

Degree of examination is dependent on practitioner competence. Referral to medical colleagues or SH/ GUM service may be required if not competent, equipment not available, or history indicates complex problems. If performing an examination, offer a chaperone (➔ Chaperones p. 84). Good practice suggests an examination should include:
- Observe external genital area for ulceration, rashes, warts, and other abnormal lesions/growths, other dermatoses, pubic lice, scabies; palpate for lymphadenopathy
- ♂: observe for urethral discharge (colour, consistency), palpate testicles for irregularities, pain, epididymal tenderness and other abnormalities
- ♀: speculum examination for abnormal discharge (colour, consistency, odour, pH), internal warts or ulcers, cervical erosion, or contact bleeding. Palpate for lower abdominal tenderness. Bimanual examination for adnexal tenderness and cervical excitation (if competent).

STI testing

- Undertaken in 1° care according to commissioned pathway (➔ Commissioning of services p. 12), availability of skilled staff, equipment, and diagnostic capability.
- Practices and clinics preparing to undertake testing should confirm with local laboratory the testing methods available, required samples, transport medium, and how soon samples should reach the laboratory, as these often differ between services.
- Local treatment and referral pathways determined by local SH clinical networks.
- Opportunistic chlamydia self-taken swab or urine screening widely available for <25yrs in GP, family planning clinics, high-street pharmacies, youth centres.
- Other STI tests performed according to signs and symptoms.
- Genital sites for STI testing dependent on signs and symptoms, and sexual behaviour/orientation.

HIV testing

- All nurses have the communication skills required to engage patients in a pre-HIV test discussion, supported with leaflets and information on availability of testing.
- Local policies will determine if practice or clinic provides HIV antibody tests, including rapid point-of-care tests.
- Where ↑ risk of HIV infection, the patient may require support before or after testing, which can be provided in SH/GUM clinics.

Referral to GUM clinics

- Patients should be referred if equipment and/or diagnostic technology not available, diagnosis unclear, specialist investigation or treatment required, or according to local care pathways.
- Complex partner notification should be managed by GUM clinic specialists.
- Referral letter useful if investigations have already been performed and treatment commenced.
- Patients can self-refer to GUM clinics and SARCs.

Related topics

➔ Sexually transmitted infections p. 764; ➔ Sexual health: general issues p. 760; ➔ Sexual health and adults with learning disability p. 770

Sexually transmitted infections

Bacterial vaginosis

See ➔ Vaginal and vulval problems p. 786

Candidiasis (thrush)

See ➔ Fungal infections p. 686; ➔ Vaginal and vulval problems p. 786

Chlamydia

- ♀: mostly asymptomatic or ↑ vaginal discharge, post-coital or intermenstrual bleeding (➔ Menstrual problems p. 778), dysuria, lower abdominal pain, dyspareunia
- ♂: often asymptomatic or mild to moderate clear or whitish urethral discharge, dysuria
- Rectal: ↑ in men who have sex with men (MSM). Mucopurulent blood-stained rectal discharge, rectal pain, and tenesmus (a continual or recurrent inclination to evacuate the bowels). Sexual and reproductive health clinic (GUM) referral essential for management of potential lymphogranuloma venereum.
- Pharyngeal: ↑ MSM, although incidence and natural history unclear

Investigations
- ♀: vaginal self-swab (VVS) preferable or endocervical swab/urine for nucleic acid amplification test (NAAT)
- ♂: urine for NAAT

Treatment
Antibiotics

Genital herpes

Presents as blistering and ulceration, usually painful, multiple, and clustered. Systemic flu-like symptoms may be present. ⚠ Specialist advice required if in third trimester of pregnancy (➔ Pregnancy p. 424).

Investigations
Swab base of lesion(s) and place in appropriate viral transport medium.

Treatment
Advise saline bathing and analgesia for symptom relief. Oral antiviral drugs indicated within 5 days of the start of the episode and while new lesions are still forming.

Genital warts

External anogenital skin lesions. Also found on vagina, cervix, urethral meatus, and anal canal. Soft and fleshy, or firm and irregular growths. Single or multiple, raised or flat. Usually non-painful, sometimes itchy.

Diagnosis
Clinical observation in most cases. Refer to GUM if in doubt.

Treatment
Some home treatments available. Other treatments are available in GUM clinic.

Gonorrhoea

- ♀: Majority asymptomatic or ↑ vaginal discharge, dysuria, intermenstrual bleeding
- ♂: 90% urethral infection, yellow/green purulent discharge, dysuria within 2–5 days of sexual contact
- Rectal: ↑ MSM. Often asymptomatic. Mucopurulent discharge, pain, tenesmus, bleeding, constipation, anal pruritus
- Pharyngeal: ↑ MSM. Usually asymptomatic; occasionally pharyngitis

Investigations

Exposed sites (VVS endocervical, urethral, pharyngeal, rectal) sampled and sent for NAAT (nucleic acid amplification tests) or culture (essential in positive results as ↑ rates of antimicrobial resistance). Rapid diagnosis is available in GUM.

Treatment

IM antibiotic injection or oral antibiotics (as per local guidelines).

HIV

See ➔ Human immunodeficiency virus p. 462.

Hepatitis A/B/C

See ➔ Viral hepatitis p. 724.

Lymphogranuloma venereum (LGV)

Anorectal syndrome presents with anal discharge, pain, and tenesmus. Inguinal syndrome presents with genital ulceration, painful inguinal adenopathy.

Investigation and treatment

Refer MSM with anorectal symptoms to GUM for management.

Non-gonococcal urethritis (NGU)

♂ only: mild to moderate clear or whitish urethral discharge +/– dysuria. Chlamydia is the cause in 30–50% of cases.

Investigations

Diagnosis relies on microscopy, usually only available in GUM clinics. Urine for gonorrhoea and chlamydia NAAT. ↑ significance of mycoplasma genitalium, with availability for testing in only some GUM clinics.

Treatment

Oral antibiotics, but can be resistant to many antibiotics.

Pubic lice

See ➔ Insects and infestations p. 294.

Syphilis

By the 1980s, syphilis had largely been eradicated in the UK. However, it has since re-emerged, including a substantial ↑ in MSM. Incubation 9–90 days. Refer to GUM for investigation, treatment, and PN. Presents in four stages:

- 1° syphilis: usually a solitary, painless, indurated ulcer (chancre) at point of sexual contact (genital, oral, rectal).

- 2° syphilis: 2–4wks after chancre. Non-itchy, macular or papular rash, may affect palms and soles. Systemic symptoms: fever, malaise, generalized lymphadenopathy.
- Latent syphilis: asymptomatic period between untreated 2° and tertiary stages.
- Tertiary syphilis: very rare in UK. Cardiovascular or neurological manifestations up to 30yrs after untreated infection.

Treatment
Dependent on stage. Refer to GUM for management.

Trichomonas vaginalis (TV)

- ♀: ↑ vaginal discharge (discoloured, offensive, frothy), vulval soreness, dyspareunia, dysuria. Can be asymptomatic.
- ♂: rarely diagnosed in ♂, but should always treat if a sexual contact.

Investigations
Usually swab from posterior vaginal fornix sent in transport media (e.g. Amies, Stuarts) to laboratory within 6hrs. Refrigerate while awaiting transportation. NAAT available in some areas. Rapid diagnosis is available in GUM clinics.

Treatment
Oral antibiotics

Related topics

➲ Sexual health: general issues p. 760; ➲ Sexual health consultations p. 762

Further information

British Association for Sexual Health and HIV (*Standards for the management of STIs*). Available at:
   🔊 https://www.bashh.org/about-bashh/publications/standards-for-the-management-of-stis/
Royal College of General Practitioners (*E-learning on sexual health in primary care*). Available at:
   🔊 http://elearning.rcgp.org.uk/course/info.php?id=179&popup=0
Family Planning Association (FPA) (*FPA busts sexually transmitted disease myth*). Available at:
   🔊 https://www.fpa.org.uk/news/fpa-busts-sexually-transmitted-infection-myths

Sexual problems

Can be physical or psychogenic in origin, but are commonly a mix of both. They can have a considerable effect on quality of life and relationships. Careful, non-judgemental history taking is important. Encourage the patient to seek help from their GP (➲ General practice p. 18) who can then refer for specialist assessment and management as needed. Various self-help books and videos available, plus general counselling (➲ Talking therapies p. 472), which can help resolve hidden conflicts, deal with various emotions, and explore relationship issues. Psychosexual therapy provides more specialist intervention.

History taking

Define the exact nature of the problem and consider key clues as to its origin. Take full medical history, mental health history, medications (past and present), and alcohol (➲ Alcohol p. 360) and recreational drug use (➲ Substance use p. 476). Also social and relationship history including life events associated with the sexual problem. Explore: Why is the patient seeking treatment now, and what do they hope to achieve? What does the patient think is the cause and what have they tried? Does the patient's partner know?

Sexual problems in women

Dyspareunia, vulvodynia, and vaginismus can all be separate sexual problems in ♀ but can often overlap, and are referred to in some guidelines as a sexual pain syndrome. Repeated sexual pain from any cause can set up a cycle, in which fear of pain → avoidance of the sexual activity that produces it, in turn leading to lack of arousal, failure to achieve orgasm, and loss of sexual desire. These problems can be from sexual debut (1°) or arise at any point in a woman's life (2°).

Dyspareunia

Recurrent genital or pelvic pain associated with sexual activity. Causes of pain in the vagina include infection, dryness, vaginismus, irritation, and psychogenic. Causes of pain in the pelvis include pelvic inflammatory disease (PID), endometriosis, fibroids (➲ Problems of the ovaries and uterus p. 780), irritable bowel syndrome (➲ Irritable bowel syndrome p. 710), or psychogenic.

Vaginismus

An involuntary reflex spasm of the muscles surrounding the entrance to the vagina. It may prevent any form of vaginal penetration (difficulty with inserting tampons, cervical smear tests (➲ Cervical sample taking p. 384), sexual intercourse).

Vulvodynia

Persistent pain in the vulva. It can be provoked, only occurring when touched in a particular area, or unprovoked, where more generalized pain is experienced.

Management

A full medical history is important to establish any underlying conditions. Examination is facilitated when done sensitively. An infection screen may be needed. Psychosexual therapy aims to tailor treatment to the individual needs of the ♀. Treatment can include topical analgesia, relaxation techniques, physiotherapy, and sensate focus. Use of vaginal trainers and biofeedback can also be useful. A ♀ can have treatment alone or with their partner.

Loss of libido

Libido varies from person to person and can change through life. During pregnancy (➲ Pregnancy p. 424), breastfeeding (➲ Breastfeeding p. 182), and the menopause (➲ Menopause p. 364) there may a physiological reduction in libido. It may be a result of physical illness, hormonal changes, medication side effects, and psychological problems (depression, anxiety, stress, tiredness, and body image (➲ People with anxiety and depression p. 478)). Sexual pain syndromes can → loss of libido. Loss of libido may also indicate underlying relationship issues. Identify and treat physical causes and/or refer for counselling.

Sexual problems in men

Loss of libido in ♂ has similar underlying causes to ♀. Dyspareunia in ♂ can be a result of physical problems: penile problems (e.g. phimosis, balanitis, and urethritis); prostate problems (e.g. prostatitis (➲ Prostate problems p. 758)); and testicular problems (e.g. epididymo-orchitis). More commonly, ♂ present with difficulties with getting and/or sustaining erections and ejaculation.

Erectile dysfunction

Failure to achieve or maintain satisfactory erection. This can be as a result of physical or psychogenic causes or a mix of both. It may be the first sign of cardiovascular disease. It is more common in patients with diabetes (➲ Diabetes: overview p. 660). It can be an adverse effect of medication (some antidepressants, antihypertensives) and also recreational drug use, or performance-enhancing drugs such as anabolic steroids and testosterone. Hormonal evaluation is often requested. Treatment includes oral phosphodiesterase-5 inhibitors taken prior to sex. Counselling may be of benefit for psychogenic causes.

Ejaculation problems

Premature ejaculation is ejaculation before the person or partner wishes. Delayed ejaculation is difficulty in achieving ejaculation. History taking is important to identify a cause (depression, anxiety, relationship difficulties, medications (e.g. antidepressants, antihypertensives, antipsychotics)). Squeeze/stop-start technique common approach to controlling premature ejaculation—intercourse is halted and penis is firmly squeezed at base of glans when man feels close to ejaculation/orgasm. Sex can then resume until point of ejaculation is reached again, when squeeze/stop-start repeated. Other treatments include formal psychosexual counselling and pharmacotherapy prescribed by sexual dysfunction specialist.

Sexual health and adults with a learning disability

Sexual health needs of people with a learning disability (LD) (€ People with learning disabilities p. 456) will vary, but are very much the same as anyone else, although they may need help in understanding:

- Relationship guidance and counselling: boundary setting, differentiating good and bad touch, giving and withholding consent (€ Consent p. 82) to sexual activity, keeping safe, emotional health, and feelings such as love, friendship, etc.
- Bodily awareness and information on sexual functioning and management: the mechanics of sex, erections, masturbation, oral, vaginal, and anal sex, etc.
- Contraception: the use of and access to barrier and hormonal contraceptives (€ Contraception: general p. 400)
- Pregnancy (€ Pregnancy p. 424), childbirth (€ Birth options and labour p. 434), and information on termination/abortion (€ Termination of pregnancy p. 788)
- Information on and access to vital, routine health screening services such as cervical smear testing (€ Cervical cancer screening p. 380) and breast screening (€ Breast cancer awareness and screening p. 378)
- Information on and access to sexual and reproductive health clinic (GUM) services (€ Sexual health: general issues p. 760)
- How can they report concerns, assault, or abuse? Is there a safeguarding team? (€ Adults at risk from harm and abuse p. 454)

Fundamental elements in service provision

- Liaise with the community learning disability nursing or social work teams to acquire background knowledge.
- Involve family and carers when appropriate (€ Carers p. 458), but maintain confidentiality whenever possible (€ Confidentiality p. 89). Try to speak with the client alone if at all possible.
- Communicate directly with the client. Be aware of sensory impairment. Sometimes informed consent (€ Consent p. 82) may be difficult to achieve (€ Mental capacity p. 470).

Attitudes of professionals and carers

Many people with a learning disability are sexually active, and their families and carers may not know or want to acknowledge or consider this. Consider your clients sexuality, sexual orientation, and/or gender issues. They may be lesbian, *gay*, bisexual, transgender, questioning, and *plus* (which represents other sexual identities including pansexual, asexual, and omnisexual). Be vigilant for signs of abuse and listen to what the client tells you. This could be domestic, sexual, financial, psychological, or emotional abuse. Make sure you know what to do if someone reports abuse to you.

Consent versus co-operation

When a client cannot give verbal consent, their capacity will need to be assessed to ascertain if the treatment is in their best interests. Where verbal consent is not possible, and there is reason to believe that the client is sexually active or has been exposed involuntarily to sexual activity, you will need to inform the safeguarding lead and get contact details of any involved professionals. Consider the consequences to the client of withholding the treatment/service when making a decision. Always try to seek advice and back-up when making a best interests decision

Time and place

People with LDs may need more time: plan the visit and try to allocate a double appointment accordingly.

- Try to allocate an appointment suitable for the client and supporter(s).
- Avoid crowded, rushed, or noisy situations.
- Have a quiet area put aside if no separate waiting area is available.
- Inform staff involved in advance, if possible, of need for reasonable adjustments.
- Ensure that your service is fully accessible.

Further information

British Institute of Learning Disabilities (BILD) (*Resources: dating to sex*). Available at: ℘ http://www.bild.org.uk/resources/relationships/dating-to-sex/

Mencap (*Sexuality*). Available at: ℘ https://www.mencap.org.uk/learning-disability-explained/research-and-statistics/sexuality

Breast problems

⚠ ♀ should consult or be referred to GP if they report:
- Lump: new, discrete lump; breast abscess; refilling/recurrent cyst
- Pain: associated with a lump; persistent pain
- Nipple discharge
- Nipple retraction, distortion, or nipple eczema
- Change in skin contour
- Family history of breast cancer
GP assessment includes need for referral to specialist.

Breast cysts

Firm, rounded lump of any size, single or multiple. Occurs pre-menopause, and not associated with skin changes. Refer to GP.

Fibro-adenoma

Majority of all benign breast neoplasms. Common in ♀ <35yrs. Giant fibro-adenomas may occur in older ♀. Presents with painless, hard, extremely mobile lump. It is usually removed.

Breast problems associated with breastfeeding

Mastitis, breast abscess (➔ Breastfeeding p. 182).

Breast pain (mastalgia)

Many ♀ experience breast pain. Most common in ♀ 30–50yrs. Cause un-known. It can present as cyclical pain associated with menstruation or be non-cyclical. For some it is also associated with a lump or diffuse lumpi-ness that changes size through the cycle (known as benign mammary dys-plasia). Refer to GP for assessment. Once serious problems ruled out, pain managed by:
- Wearing a well-supporting bra 24hrs, especially approaching period
- Reducing caffeine intake and eating a low-fat diet
- Simple analgesics
- Combined oral contraceptives (➔ Combined hormonal contraceptive methods p. 402) and HRT can make pain worse (➔ Menopause p. 364)
- Topical NSAIDs can be helpful
- Oestrogen-reducing medicine may be used for severe, cyclical, persistent pain, but side effects include weight gain and menorrhagia (➔ Menstrual problems p. 778)

Related topics

➔ Breast cancer awareness and screening p. 378; ➔ Breast cancer p. 774

Further information

NICE (*Breast pain–cyclical*). Available at: ℬ https://cks.nice.org.uk/breast-pain-cyclical#!topicSummary

Breast cancer

Risk factors

Prevention

Presentation

Management

Classification

Breast cancer

Breast cancer is the commonest cancer in the UK, where ♀ have a one in eight lifetime risk of developing the disease. Rare in ♂.

Risk factors

- Age: ♀ >50yrs
- Early menarche or late menopause (➲ Menopause p. 364); late age at first birth
- Current and recent use of combined oral contraceptives (➲ Combined hormonal contraceptive methods p. 402) (excess risk disappears >10yrs after stopping) and use of HRT
- Obesity (➲ Overweight and obesity p. 348), smoking, and alcohol consumption (➲ Alcohol p. 360)
- Taller ♀ and ♀ with denser breasts
- Exposure to ionizing radiation
- Previous breast disease (either benign or malignant breast disease)
- First-degree relative with breast cancer (mother or sister) (but most ♀ with breast cancer have no family history)

Prevention

- ↓ alcohol intake, maintain a healthy weight (➲ Adult body mass index chart p. 346), ↑ physical activity (➲ Exercise p. 354), and stop smoking (➲ Smoking cessation p. 356)
- Avoid exogenous sex hormones (e.g. HRT)
- Breastfeed (➲ Breastfeeding p. 182)

If several family members with early onset breast cancer, ♀ referred for genetic screening. If BRCA1 or BRCA2 genes are identified, options may include chemoprevention (e.g. tamoxifen) and prophylactic surgery.

Presentation

Clinical presentation includes: breast lump; breast pain; nipple skin change; skin contour change; and nipple discharge. In older people, breast cancer may grow slowly and present with extensive local lesions. Alternatively, no visible abnormalities but cancer detected at breast screening (➲ Breast cancer awareness and screening p. 378).

Management

Referred for urgent assessment to a breast surgeon. Specialist investigation includes ultrasound scan; mammography +/− fine-needle aspiration or biopsy; investigations to evaluate spread (e.g. CT, liver, ultrasound, and bone scan).

Classification

Virtually all breast cancers are adenocarcinomas. The stage of cancer (1–4) describes the size of cancer and how far it has spread. Stage 1 cancers are smaller and have limited lymph node spread. Stage 4 cancers are cancers that have metastasized to other parts of the body, such as distant lymph nodes (beyond those under the arm), lungs, bone, liver, or brain.

Treatment

Treatment includes surgery (lumpectomy +/− axillary clearance, mastectomy) and other treatments (radiotherapy, hormonal therapy, biological therapy, and/or chemotherapy).

Post surgery

- Pain: some ♀ find that their breast and arm are sore for up to a year after the treatment. Encourage appropriate pain relief.
- Arm and shoulder stiffness, tingling: encourage exercise as per physiotherapy advice.
- Pins and needles, burning, numbness or darting sensations in the chest area and down the arm is quite common and can persist for weeks,
- Cording: feels like a tight cord running from armpit, down arm, through to the back of hand. Can appear 6–8wks after surgery. Thought to be hardening of lymph vessels. May resolve or may need physiotherapy.
- A lightweight foam prosthesis (sometimes called a 'cumfie' or 'softie') given to be worn inside bra post surgery. When wound healed (6–8wks) (➔ Post-operative wound care p. 524), can be fitted for a worn silicone prosthesis. Breast care nurse provides advice on type and care. Several types available from the NHS.
- Possibilities of reconstructive surgery discussed with specialists.

Lymphoedema

All patients who have breast surgery are at risk (➔ Lymphoedema p. 548). Injury to the arm on the surgery side may precipitate/worsen lymphoedema. Do not take blood from that limb (➔ Venepuncture p. 580) or BP measurement; and do not use it for intravenous access or vaccination (➔ Immunization administration p. 390).

Psychological impact

Depression and anxiety (➔ People with anxiety and depression p. 478), and sexual problems (➔ Sexual problems p. 768) are common. Psychological support should be offered (➔ Talking therapies p. 472).

Further information

Breast Cancer Care (*Information and support*). Available at: ℬ www.breastcancercare.org.uk
Cancer Research UK (*Breast cancer*). Available at: ℬ www.cancerresearchuk.org/about-cancer/breast-cancer
NICE (*Early and locally advanced breast cancer: diagnosis and management [NG101]*). Available at: ℬ https://www.nice.org.uk/guidance/ng101

Gynaecological cancers

The possibility, as well as the diagnosis of cancer provokes fear and anxiety. Most ♀ feel shocked and upset by the idea of having treatment to the most intimate parts of their body. Psychological support is important, as well as clear information about investigations, treatments, and effects (including on sex life). Treatment may involve surgical removal of part or whole organs that many ♀ feel are important parts of their female identity. The most common cancers are ovarian, cervical, and uterine.

Cervical cancer

Incidence dropping due to screening programme (➔ Cervical cancer screening p. 380) and introduction of human papilloma virus (HPV) vaccination (➔ Childhood immunization schedule (UK) p. 166). Symptoms include abnormal smear test, post-coital bleeding, vaginal bleeding and/or discharge. Referred to gynaecologist. Diagnosis is by colposcopy or cone biopsy. Treatment dependent on stage. Localized early cancerous changes destroyed by electrocoagulation, diathermy, laser treatment or cryosurgery, or cone biopsy. Later stage cancer requires surgery and radiotherapy.

Ovarian cancer

Risk factors include increasing age, family history, and null parity. Symptoms include vaginal bleeding, abdominal discomfort and bloating, and ascites. Treatment includes surgery. The extent of surgery depends on stage and sometimes adjuvant chemotherapy.

Uterine cancer

Endometrial cancer is the most common form. Risk factors include: increasing age, obesity (➔ Overweight and obesity p. 348), null parity, late menopause (➔ Menopause p. 364), diabetes mellitus (➔ Diabetes: overview p. 660), and family history of breast (➔ Breast cancer p. 774), ovary, or colon cancer (➔ Colorectal cancer p. 715). Symptoms include abnormal vaginal bleeding, dyspareunia, and post-menopausal bleeding. Treatment includes surgery (usually hysterectomy (➔ Hysterectomy p. 782)), radiotherapy, progesterone treatment, and/or chemotherapy.

Vaginal cancer

Rare. More common as a 2° cancer. Squamous cell carcinoma (SCC) most common. Adenocarcinoma rare. Symptoms include vaginal bleeding, dyspareunia, and problems with micturition. Treatment includes surgery and/or radiotherapy and/or chemotherapy. Type of surgery depends on the position and size of cancer. May affect part or whole vagina. Sometimes possible for vaginal reconstruction using tissue from other parts of the body. May also need hysterectomy. Radiotherapy may be external or internal.

Vulval cancer

Rare. Risk factors include increasing age, vulval intraepithelial neoplasia, and HPV. Symptoms include skin colour or texture change, itching, burning, lump, or swelling. Treatment involves surgery: radical, wide, local excision; radical partial vulvectomy (this may include the labia and clitoris); or radical vulvectomy (including the inner and outer labia, and possibly the clitoris and some lymph nodes). Treatment may also include radiotherapy and/or chemotherapy.

Further information

The Eve Appeal (Gynaecological cancers). Available at: ℘ https://eveappeal.org.uk/gynaecological-cancers/

Menstrual problems

Menstruation

This is the periodic shedding of the endometrium. Day 1 of bleeding is the start of the menstrual cycle. Follicle stimulating hormone (FSH) stimulates the egg follicle to mature, secreting oestrogen which thickens the endometrium. Luteinizing hormone (LH) causes egg release (ovulation). Some ♀ feel a pain (known as mittelschmerz). The egg is viable for about 2 days in the fallopian tube. Empty egg follicle produces progesterone. If egg is not fertilized, oestrogen and progesterone production stops. This causes the endometrium lining to shed, about 14 days after ovulation. Normal cycle length 21–40 days, average 28 days. Normal bleeding is for 2–8 days, average 4–5 days. In cycle, changes in consistency of cervical mucus, cervix position, body temperature, breasts, abdominal pain, and mood. Menstrual blood loss is ~80ml a month. ♀ use internal tampons or external pads for containment. Mooncup is a reusable silicone menstrual cup used internally. It addresses environmental concerns, financial issues, and concerns about bleaches in internal tampons.

Toxic shock syndrome

Very rare, acute illness caused by toxins from staphylococci or streptococci. Symptoms include: pyrexia; flu-like symptoms; nausea and vomiting; diarrhoea; widespread sunburn-like rash, with the whites of the eyes, lips, and tongue turning bright red; dizziness or fainting; breathing difficulties; and drowsiness and confusion. Toxic shock syndrome is a medical emergency. Association with tampons unclear, but tampon absorbency thought to be a factor. Preventative advice includes frequent changes, occasional use of pads, and not to use two tampons at once.

Premenstrual syndrome (PMS)

A collection of symptoms and bodily changes that occur on a regular basis. Lasting for anything from a few days to weeks before a period and ceasing with its arrival. Commonest symptoms are nervous tension, mood swings, irritability, weight gain, abdominal bloating, breast tenderness, and headache. Advice on maintaining a healthy diet (◆ Nutrition and healthy eating p. 342), smoking cessation (◆ Smoking cessation p. 356), alcohol reduction (◆ Alcohol p. 360), exercise (◆ Exercise p. 354), and stress reduction (◆ Managing stress p. 358). Conflicting evidence on complementary and alternative therapies (◆ Complementary and alternative therapies p. 838). Treatments include NSAIDs for cramping and pain. For moderate PMS, use of the combined oral contraceptive may be indicated (◆ Combined hormonal contraceptive methods p. 402). For severe PMS, selective serotonin reuptake inhibitors may be considered.

Menorrhagia/heavy periods

Bleeding >7 days and >80mL. In most cases, cause unexplained. Other causes include intrauterine devices (IUD) (◆ Contraception: intrauterine devices and systems p. 414), fibroids, endometriosis (◆ Problems of the ovaries and uterus p. 780), cancer (◆ Gynaecological cancers p. 776), and blood-clotting disorder. Following examination and investigations, if does not require or wish hormonal contraception, then treated with non-hormonal medication (e.g. NSAIDs or tranexamic acid). If requires contraception as well, offered combined oral contraceptive or long-acting progesterone or intrauterine system (IUS). If has an IUD, this is changed to IUS. Patient is referred to gynaecologist if symptoms indicate or treatment failure.

Dysmenorrhoea/painful periods

Tends to start 6–12mths after menarche when ovulatory cycles are established. Tends to improve after adolescence (➲ Puberty and adolescence p. 228) and after childbirth. Uterine hypercontractility (associated with prostaglandin production) and ischaemia of the uterine wall causes pain. It occurs in the first 1 or 2 days of each period. Lower abdominal cramps +/− backache. It may be associated with gastrointestinal disturbance (e.g. constipation, diarrhoea/vomiting). Can interfere with ability to go about daily life, attend school, work. Self-help advice includes OTC analgesia, exercise to relieve cramps, and hot-water bottles or self-heating patches. If pain still a problem, mefenamic acid may be indicated. Can be treated by combined oral contraception or IUS insertion. Some evidence for acupuncture. Pain that still does not respond may have underlying pathology and requires medical investigation.

Amenorrhea

1° amenorrhea is when menstruation delayed. 2° amenorrhea is the absence of menses in ≥6mths in a previously menstruating woman. Causes may be pregnancy (➲ Pregnancy p. 424), menopause (➲ Menopause p. 364), stress, low nutritional intake (e.g. anorexia (➲ People with eating disorders p. 474)), ↑ levels of exercise, disease of the brain, thyroid (➲ Thyroid p. 702), adrenal glands (➲ Adrenal disorders p. 700), and ovaries (➲ Problems of the ovaries and uterus p. 780). Treatment or action based on cause.

Further information

Mooncup (Why mooncup?). Available at: ℘ https://www.mooncup.co.uk/why-mooncup/
NICE (Premenstrual syndrome). Available at: ℘ https://cks.nice.org.uk/premenstrual-syndrome#!topicSummary
NICE (Heavy menstrual bleeding [NG88]). Available at: ℘ www.nice.org.uk/guidance/ng88

Problems of the ovaries and uterus

Ovarian problems

Ovarian cysts

A growth on, or inside, the ovary. Very common. Functional cysts are the most common type. Many ♀ experience no symptoms. Dependent on size and position may cause discomfort and pain. If <5cm diameter usually resolve spontaneously; >5cm referred to gynaecologist. Laparoscopic fenestration can be used to drain contents, or laparotomy for removal. Acute severe pain and vomiting caused by bleeding into the cyst, rupture, or torsion, and needs medical assessment urgently.

Polycystic ovary syndrome

A polycystic ovary is larger than normal, with multiple cysts around the edge, disrupting hormonal cycle and inhibiting release of eggs. Common in premenopausal ♀. Cause unknown. Associated with ↑ risk of cardiovascular disease and endometrial cancer (⊃ Gynaecological cancers p. 776). ♀ may be asymptomatic or have any or all of the following symptoms: acne (⊃ Acne vulgaris p. 300), obesity (⊃ Overweight and obesity p. 348), infertility (⊃ Problems with fertility p. 784), irregular periods, insulin resistance, and hirsutism (⊃ Pigmentation and hair problems p. 692). It is diagnosed on history, pelvic ultrasound scan, and blood tests. Treatment dependent on symptoms. Encouraged to maintain weight in BMI range 19–25 (⊃ Adult body mass index chart p. 346). Oligomenorrhoea may be treated with progestogens. Synthetic ovulation stimulants may be used.

Uterine problems

Endometriosis

Fragments of the endometrium (lining of the uterus) located in other areas of the body, usually pelvic cavity. Fragments under hormonal control, so breakdown and bleeding each month. It → inflammation, pain, and scar tissue. Most common in ♀ 25–40yrs. Cause unclear. May cause heavy menstrual bleeding (⊃ Menstrual problems p. 778), severe abdominal pain, dyspareunia, bowel and bladder symptoms, and infertility. Patient is referred to gynaecologist and diagnosis confirmed on laparoscopy. Treatment involves either hormonal treatment to stop ovulation and allow the endometrial deposits to regress, or surgery (e.g. local ablation using laser during laparoscopy, or more radical surgery), dependent on symptoms.

Fibroids

Benign, often multiple, tumours of the uterus. Fibroids are oestrogen-dependent, so more common in premenopausal ♀ and then shrink post menopause. Usually asymptomatic but may cause heavy periods (in turn cause anaemia (⊃ Anaemia in adults p. 652)), pelvic discomfort, backache, pressure on bladder. It is diagnosed by pelvic ultrasound scan. Referred to gynaecologist if symptomatic. Treatment may be medical or surgical. Medical treatment includes: use of the combined oral contraception; gonadotropin-releasing hormone analogues may shrink the fibroid but can only be used for 6mths; or insertion of intrauterine system. Surgical options include: myomectomy (removing fibroids individually), hysterectomy, or uterine artery embolization (blocking blood supply).

Pelvic organ prolapse

Very common, particularly in older ♀. Caused by poor pelvic muscle tone and weakness of pelvic ligaments. Risk factors include childbirth and menopause (➔ Menopause p. 364). Aggravated by obesity. Prevention includes pelvic floor exercises (➔ Urinary incontinence p. 504), weight management in normal BMI range, and avoiding constipation (➔ Constipation in adults p. 512). Types of prolapse: bladder and anterior vaginal wall (cystocoele); urethra (urethrocoele); rectum and posterior vaginal wall (rectocoele); herniation of the top of the vagina (enterocoele); and uterine prolapse. Treatment according to severity and symptoms.

Uterine prolapse

Uterine prolapse most common type. Uterus descends into the vagina. Classified by degree: first-degree (cervix remains in the vagina); second-degree (cervix protrudes from vagina on coughing/straining); and third-degree (procidentia) (uterus lies outside the vagina and may ulcerate).

Signs and symptoms include a dragging sensation. Often gets worse if standing for a long time, coughing, or straining. May be associated with bowel and bladder problems (e.g. stress incontinence).

Treatment depends on severity. In 1° care, pelvic floor exercises and weight reduction are encouraged, plus treatment of coexisting problems (e.g. constipation). Refer to gynaecologist. Sometimes HRT prescribed to help. Second- and third-degree prolapse may be treated with surgical repair or hysterectomy (➔ Hysterectomy p. 782). Vaginal ring pessaries are used to hold uterus in place while waiting for surgery or if surgery not appropriate.

Further information

Endometriosis UK (*Information*). Available at: ℔ www.endometriosis-uk.org/

Royal College of Obstetricians and Gynaecologists (*Pelvic organ prolapse*). Available at: ℔ https://www.rcog.org.uk/globalassets/documents/patients/patient-information-leaflets/gynaecology/pi-pelvic-organ-prolapse.pdf

Verity (About polycystic ovary syndrome). Available at: ℔ https://www.verity-pcos.org.uk/about-us.html

Hysterectomy

One of the most common operations for women. Majority are in ♀ 40–50yrs. Most commonly undertaken:
- Electively for painful menorrhagia, endometriosis, fibroids causing pain and bleeding, prolapsed uterus, or pelvic inflammatory disease (PID) or adhesions which cause pain that is not controlled by other means (◗ Problems of the ovaries and uterus p. 780; ◗ Menstrual problems p. 778)
- For cancer of the uterus, ovaries, fallopian tube/s, or cervix (◗ Gynaecological cancers p. 776)
- For emergencies such as rupture/puncture of the uterus during other surgery

In elective situations, women should have counselling to help them make informed an choice, based on understanding alternatives, benefits, risks, and long-term consequences. Such consequences can include: loss of menstruation and ability to have a child; immediate menopause if surgery also removes ovaries (and 50% who have ovaries intact post surgery experience menopause within 5yrs of operation, regardless of age); and some women have strong emotional response to the loss of the organ, whilst others feel liberated and relieved after years of severe pain and heavy bleeding. Endometrial ablation and resection is a surgical alternative. Techniques include lasers, microwaves, electricity, balloons filled with hot water, freezing, and heated loops.

Types of hysterectomy
- Subtotal hysterectomy removes the uterus leaving the cervix in place (cervical smears still required (◗ Cervical cancer screening p. 380)).
- Total hysterectomy (most common) removes uterus and cervix.
- Total hysterectomy with bilateral or unilateral salpingo-oophorectomy removes body of uterus, cervix, fallopian tube(s), and ovary/ies.
- A radical hysterectomy removes the uterus, cervix, part of the vagina, fallopian tubes, peritoneum, the lymph glands, and fatty tissue of the pelvis, and possibly one or both ovaries.

Performed either through an incision in the lower abdomen, or through an incision in the top of the vagina, or vaginal surgery with laparoscope (keyhole surgery).

Post hysterectomy
- Takes about 6–8wks for abdominal muscles and tissues to heal. Advice to remain off work for this period, take gentle exercise, avoid strenuous exercise or lifting.
- Vaginal discharge for up to 6wks. Sanitary pads rather than tampons used to reduce risk of infection.
- Sex can be resumed after a minimum of 6wks/post-surgery check. Many have no problems with sex, but some find the surgery has shortened their vagina and slightly changed its angle. May also find their vagina is dry and would benefit from a lubricant.
- HRT often prescribed for those whose ovaries removed.

More general advice

- Advice not to drive until comfortable wearing a seatbelt and can safely perform an emergency stop.
- Avoid any lifting or housework for the first few weeks.
- Avoid heavy lifting for ~3mths.
- Avoid standing for long periods.
- Do the exercises recommended by hospital physiotherapist for pelvic floor and abdominal muscle strengthening.
- Ensure a balanced diet and fluids to avoid constipation (➔ Constipation in adults p. 512).

Further information

Hysterectomy Association (*Information*). Available at: ℘ www.hysterectomy-association.org.uk

Royal College of Obstetricians and Gynaecologists (*Hysterectomy*). Available at: ℘ https://www. rcog.org.uk/en/patients/menopause/hysterectomy/

Problems with fertility

♀ trying to conceive are aided by additional information on the most fertile time in the menstrual cycle, but should be encouraged to have sex two or three times a week throughout the cycle. Timing of intercourse using temperature charts or hormone detection kits causes stress and does not improve conception rates, so not recommended. ♀ and ♂ should be given lifestyle advice on alcohol intake (➔ Alcohol p. 360), weight management, and smoking (➔ Smoking cessation p. 356), as well as preconception care (➔ Preconceptual care p. 422). ♀ fertility ↓ significantly >35yrs. Sperm function also ↓ >55yrs but less markedly.

Infertility

Affects around one in seven couples. Causes psychological distress. Infertility defined as absence of pregnancy after 1yr of regular unprotected intercourse. Infertility is classed as 1° in couples who have never conceived and 2° in couples who have previously conceived. Investigated earlier if other factors present (e.g. ♀ aged >36yrs). Usually, health consultations and investigations dealt with as a couple. This may be in 1° care by GP or referred to specialists. Investigations follow the same pathway: checking ♀ partner is ovulating normally; checking ♂ partner has a normal semen analysis; and confirming normality of ♀ genital tract.

Treatment

Types of treatment dependent on problems identified: medicines to assist with ovulation; surgical treatment (e.g. tubal surgery to remove obstruction); or assisted conception. Assisted conception includes: intrauterine insemination; donor insemination (DI); *in vitro* fertilization (IVF); intracytoplasmic sperm injection (ICSI); oocyte donation stimulation; and embryo donation. Usually, only specialist infertility clinics offer IVF, ICSI, and DI. National and local guidelines apply in terms of what NHS treatments are available and to whom. Many couples may need counselling (➔ Talking therapies p. 472).

Repeated miscarriages

Recurrent miscarriage is defined as three times, <20wks gestation. Maternal age and previous miscarriages are independent risk factors. All couples with recurrent miscarriages tested for chromosome abnormalities. At subsequent pregnancy, ♀ is referred to early pregnancy clinic at hospital (➔ Pregnancy p. 424).

Further information

Human Fertilization and Embryology Authority (Treatments). Available at: ℛ https://www.hfea.gov.uk/treatments/

Miscarriage Association (*Information*). Available at: ℛ https://www.miscarriageassociation.org.uk/information/

NICE (*Fertility problems: assessment and treatment [CG156]*). Available at: ℛ https://www.nice.org.uk/guidance/cg156

Vaginal and vulval problems

Vaginal discharge

All ♀ produce vaginal discharge. It is part of the physiological changes in sexual activity, pregnancy (**⊃** Pregnancy p. 424), and menstrual cycle. It is affected by age and stress and use of combined oral contraceptive (**⊃** Combined hormonal contraceptive methods p. 402). In the menstrual cycle, secretions change in texture and colour. At the fertile part of the month (luteal phase), secretions are thinner, colourless, and slippery. In the infertile part, the secretions become whiter, thicker, and stickier. Discharge may become yellow on contact with air. The amounts of discharge vary between ♀.

Abnormal discharge

Only abnormal when it is different from individual ♀'s normal discharge. Abnormal discharge mostly caused by Candida albicans (thrush), bacterial vaginosis, Tricomonas vaginalis, and cervicitis (**⊃** Sexually transmitted infections p. 764; **⊃** Fungal infections p. 686).

Bacterial vaginosis

Commonest cause of abnormal discharge. An offensive, fishy-smelling, thin, white, homogeneous vaginal discharge. Not usually associated with soreness, itching, or irritation. 50% are asymptomatic. Bacterial vaginosis can be recurrent and generally not sexually transmissible. Can be diagnosed by clinical signs/symptoms alone plus ↑ pH of vaginal fluid. No culture available. Diagnosis by use of microscopy. Advise to avoid vaginal douching and use of shower gels and soaps, and to use antiseptic agents in the bath. Treatment includes antibiotics.

Candida albicans (thrush)

Vulval pruritus and soreness, curdy white discharge, superficial dyspareunia, superficial dysuria. It can be recurrent. Generally not sexually transmissible. Diagnosis by clinical observation in most cases. High-vaginal swab for microcopy sensitivity and culture. Advise to avoid vaginal douching and use of shower gels and soaps, and to use antiseptic agents in the bath. Treatment includes antifungals. ⚠ Topical treatments may cause condoms to split.

Atrophic vaginitis

Post-menopausal changes create dryness that presents as vaginal soreness and dyspareunia (**⊃** Menopause p. 364). Treated short term with topical oestrogen as pessaries or vaginal ring, and advise lubricants during sexual intercourse.

Bartholins gland swellings

Two glands with ducts opening into vulva, which in sexual arousal secrete lubricant. Obstruction of the ducts leads to vulval swelling and cyst formation. Cysts resolve spontaneously. If infected, an abscess results that may respond to antibiotics or need surgical drainage.

Genital warts and herpes

See **⊃** Sexually transmitted infections p. 764.

Vulval swelling

Can be due to venous or lymphatic obstruction. Causes include: 2° to malignancy in the pelvis; dependent oedema with prolonged sitting in bed (address positioning and movement); and pregnancy, where varicosities may appear (resolves at end of pregnancy). With bruising, may be trauma of a sexual nature (➔ Victims of crime p. 452).

Vulval itching (pruritus)

May be caused by infection, infestations, vulval atrophy, dystrophy, carcinoma (➔ Gynaecological cancers p. 776), allergic response to perfumed soaps, etc. (➔ Allergies p. 694). Aim of care is to identify cause and treat.

Vulval skin changes

The vulva can be affected by dermatitis (lichen simplex) (➔ Eczema/dermatitis p. 684) and by another skin disease (lichen planus), which can cause pain, and by simple post-menopausal atrophy. Most vulval conditions can cause dyspareunia. Lichen sclerosus is uncommon. Skin appears thin, white, and crinkly, and is more likely in post-menopausal women. It is sometimes treated with powerful steroid ointments. Vulval intraepithelial neoplasia (VIN) is similar to precancerous changes that can occur in the cervix. It needs diagnosis and treatment by specialists.

Psychosexual problems

♀ who have any chronic genital disorders may lose interest in sexual activity and have psychosexual problems. Important to give patients the opportunity to express concerns on their sexual function and to offer referral or information on psychosexual counselling (often via community family planning service and sexual health services) (➔ Talking therapies p. 472; ➔ Sexual health: general issues p. 760).

Further information

Relate: The Relationship People (*Relationship help*). Available at: ♫ https://www.relate.org.uk/relationship-help

Termination of pregnancy

UK Law

The 1967 Abortion Act and 1990 Human Fertilization/Embryology Act govern abortion (also known as termination of pregnancy (TOP)) in England, Wales, and Scotland. TOP allowed up to 24wks of pregnancy if two doctors agree that it is necessary because of one or more of the following:

- Continuation of pregnancy involves ↑ risk to the life of the ♀
- Continuation would cause injury to the mother's physical or mental health (90% TOPs are carried out under this clause)
- Continuation would cause injury to the physical or mental health of the mother's existing children
- Baby is at substantial risk of being physically or mentally handicapped

Upper gestation limit does not apply if mother's life threatened or serious injury or fetal handicap.

The 1967 Abortion Act did not extend to Northern Ireland (NI) where TOP was only lawful where there was a real and serious risk to the ♀'s mental and physical health, and the risk was permanent or long-term. Consequently, many ♀ from NI travelled to England for TOP. Terminations in NI were decriminalised in 2020 and NI's Department of Health instructed health trusts that abortions could be carried out lawfully.

Consultations in primary care

All health professionals should ensure ♀ are treated non-judgementally and have access to full information, irrespective of professionals' own personal views. This may mean offering another professional for that consultation or referring ♀ elsewhere to receive counselling of options and full information to make an informed choice.

Unplanned and unwanted pregnancy

♀ need to talk through their emotions and choices with partners and/or relatives and/or close friends. 1° care and contraceptive services are often the first health services consulted to confirm pregnancy and advise on options and processes for TOP.

Prenatal diagnosis of abnormality

♀ undergoing routine antenatal screening may be told that their baby has a serious risk of physical and mental impairment and TOP should be considered (➲ Antenatal care and screening p. 426). Requires specialist support in counselling on options (➲ Talking therapies p. 472).

Main areas of information

- ♀ has right to confidentiality (➲ Confidentiality p. 89). GPs are not informed of TOPs unless the ♀ has given permission. In terms of <16yr olds, social services will only be informed if there is the significant risk of sexual abuse or emotional or physical harm (➲ Safeguarding children p. 248).
- ♀ alone gives consent (➲ Consent p. 82). If the ♀ is <16yrs or has learning difficulties, her consent can be taken if doctors believe the ♀ has understanding of the situation (➲ Mental capacity p. 470).

- TOPs safer earlier in pregnancy (risks of all procedures include haemorrhage, failure and ongoing pregnancy, infection, and psychological impact).
- TOPs available through the NHS (GPs and sexual health services) and private organizations (self-referral and payment). All carried out in NHS hospitals or special licensed clinics.
- Process in all organizations ensures a counselling/assessment visit to help ♀ reach the decision that is right for her and then time before the TOP visit to change mind.

Types of TOP

<9 weeks' pregnancy

Early medical induction. Involves two appointments. Involves taking medication that causes the breakdown of the lining of the womb and the early pregnancy to detach. A vaginal pessary or tablet is given 2 days later. This opens and softens the entrance to the womb, causing the womb to contract and the pregnancy to be passed out.

<14 weeks' pregnancy

Early surgical abortion. The contents of the womb are removed by suction using a pump or a syringe. This can be carried out under local anaesthetic or general anaesthetic (GA). Up to 14 days after the abortion there will be some bleeding and pain.

>9–20 weeks' pregnancy

Late medical induction undertaken as early medical induction but uses more medication. It may take longer and often requires overnight stay. For around a week afterwards there may be some bleeding and pain.

>15 weeks' pregnancy

Surgical dilation and evacuation under GA. Contents of the womb are removed by narrow forceps and suction. The procedure is carried out under GA. For up to 14 days after the abortion there might be some pain and bleeding.

Late abortion: 20–24 weeks' pregnancy

Either two-stage surgical procedure under GA or medically induced labour, followed often by surgical procedure to ensure uterus is empty.

All TOP have a follow-up visit to clinic or GP 2wks later. After TOP, menstrual cycle returns to normal and can conceive again within 2wks. Contraception options to be considered as part of pre-TOP counselling (⊃ Contraception: general p. 400).

Further information

British Pregnancy Advisory Service (*Considering abortion?*). Available at: ℛ www.bpas.org/

Chapter 13

First aid and emergencies

Adult basic life support and automated external
  defibrillation 792
Recovery position for babies, children and adults 796
Adult choking 798
Child basic life support 800
Child choking 806
Anaphylaxis 810
External bleeding 814
Burns and scalds 816
Eye trauma 818
Hypothermia 820
Poisoning and overdoses 822
Sprains, strains, and fractures 824
Sepsis 826
Recognizing and responding to a stroke 830

Adult basic life support and automated external defibrillation

Adult basic life support (BLS) and automated external defibrillation (AED) are critical to saving lives in the event of a cardiac arrest.

The Resuscitation Council (UK) describes the steps for community responders to follow when assessing and treating an adult who is unresponsive.[1] The adult BLS algorithm is summarized in Fig. 13.1. These guidelines should be read in conjunction with the Resuscitation Council UK Statement on COVID19 in relation to CPR and resuscitation in first aid and community settings (⊕ https://www.resus.org.uk/covid-19-resources/covid-19-resources-general-public/resuscitation-council-uk-statement-covid-19).

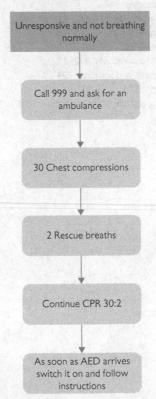

Fig. 13.1 Adult basic life support algorithm.

Reproduced with the permission of the Resuscitation Council UK (2015). Available at: https://www.resus.org.uk/resuscitation-guidelines/adult-basic-life-support-and-automated-external-defibrillation/

Safety

Check you, the patient, and bystanders are safe.

Response

Check the patient for a response; if there is none, follow the steps below.

Airway

Open the airway (see Fig. 13.2):
- Turn the patient onto their back.
- Place your hand on their forehead and gently tilt their head back.
- With your fingertips under their chin, lift the chin to open the airway.

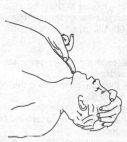

Fig. 13.2 Opening the airway

Breathing

Keeping the airway open, look, listen, and feel for normal breathing for no more than 10secs. In the first few minutes after cardiac arrest, a person may be barely breathing, or taking infrequent, slow, and noisy gasps. This is not normal breathing. If you have any doubt whether breathing is normal, act as if the patient is not breathing normally and prepare to start cardiopulmonary resuscitation (CPR).

Dial 999

Ask helper to ☏ 999. If no helper is available, stay with the patient and call emergency services using speaker function on phone.

Send for AED

Send helper to get an AED. If no helper is available, start CPR. Defibrillators are available where: large numbers of people congregate (e.g. railway stations); there is ↑ risk of cardiac arrest (e.g. gyms); and access to emergency services may be delayed (e.g. aircraft). When you ☏ 999, the call handler will identify the nearest available defibrillator and provide you access details.

Circulation

Start chest compressions:
- Kneel beside the patient.
- Place heel of one hand in the centre of the patient's chest.
- Place the heel of your other hand on top of the first hand.
- Interlock fingers.
- Keep your arms straight.
- Do not apply any pressure over the upper abdomen or bottom end of the bony sternum.
- Position your shoulders vertically above the patient's chest and press down on the sternum to a depth of 5–6cm.
- After each compression, release all the pressure on the chest without losing contact between your hands and the sternum.
- Repeat at a rate of 100–120/min.

Give rescue breaths

After 30 compressions, open the airway again (see previous description) and give two rescue breaths:
- Pinch the soft part of the nose closed, using the index finger and thumb of your hand on the forehead.
- Allow the mouth to open, but maintain chin lift.
- Take a normal breath and place your lips around the patient's mouth, ensuring you have a good seal.
- Blow steadily into the mouth while watching the chest visibly rise, taking about 1sec as in normal breathing.
- Maintaining head tilt and chin lift, remove your mouth and watch the chest fall as air expelled.
- Repeat for a second breath.
- Mouth-to-nose ventilation may be indicated if the patient's mouth is seriously injured or cannot be opened. Mouth-to-tracheostomy ventilation may be used for a patient with a tracheostomy tube (➜ Tracheostomy care p. 586).

Do not interrupt compression for more than 10secs to deliver two breaths. Then return to give a further 30 chest compressions. Continue at a ratio of 30 chest compressions to two rescue breaths. If you are unable to do rescue breaths, give continuous chest compressions only.

Arrival of automated external defibrillation

If AED arrives, follow Box 13.1.

Continue CPR

Continue resuscitation efforts until the patient is definitely waking up, moving, opening eyes, and breathing normally, or you become too exhausted to continue, or further qualified help arrives.

Recovery position

If you are certain the patient is breathing normally but is still unresponsive, place in the recovery position (➜ Recovery position for babies, children, and adults p. 796). Be prepared to restart CPR if the patient deteriorates or stops breathing normally.

Box 13.1 How to use a defibrillator
- Turn the defibrillator on.
- Follow the spoken/visual instructions.
- Attach the electrode pads on the patient's bare chest (if a helper is available, they should continue CPR whilst the pads are being placed).
- Once the pads have been attached, stop CPR and do not touch the patient whilst the defibrillator analyses the patient's heart rhythm.
- If a shock is needed, the defibrillator will tell you to press the shock button. Do not touch the patient while they are being shocked.
- The defibrillator will tell you when the shock has been delivered and whether you need to continue CPR.

Related topics
➔ Child basic life support p. 800

Reference
1. Resuscitation Council (UK) (2015) *Adult basic life support and automated external defibrillation*. Available at: https://www.resus.org.uk/resuscitation-guidelines/adult-basic-life-support-and-automated-external-defibrillation/

Further information
British Heart Foundation (*How to use a defibrillator*). Available at: ℛ https://www.bhf.org.uk/how-you-can-help/how-to-save-a-life/defibrillators/how-to-use-a-defibrillator

Recovery position for babies, children and adults

If someone is unconscious but breathing, and has no other life-threatening conditions, they should be placed in the recovery position. This will: maintain a good airway, ensure the tongue does not cause obstruction, and minimize the risk of inhalation of gastric contents.

Holding a baby in the recovery position

Cradle them in your arms with their head tilted downwards. Whilst waiting for emergency assistance, keeping monitoring breathing, pulse, and level of response.

Recovery position for adults and children

- Remove patient's glasses if worn.
- Kneel beside patient and make sure that both legs are straight.
- Place arm nearest to you out at right angles to body, elbow bent, with hand palm uppermost.
- Bring far arm across chest, and hold back of hand against patient's cheek nearest to you.
- With other hand, grasp far leg just above knee and pull it up, keeping foot on ground.
- Keeping patient's hand pressed against their cheek, pull on leg to roll patient towards you onto their side.
- Adjust upper leg so that both hip and knee are bent at right angles.
- Tilt head back to make sure airway remains open. Adjust hand under cheek, if necessary, to keep head tilted.
- Check breathing regularly.

Suspected spinal injury

If spinal cord injury is suspected (e.g. the person has sustained a fall or has been struck on the head or neck), take care to maintain alignment of head, neck, and chest (➔ Spinal cord injury p. 518). A spinal board and/or cervical collar should be used if available. To open their airway, instead of tilting their neck, place your hands on either side of their head and gently lift their jaw with your fingertips to open the airway.

Related topics

➔ Adult basic life support and automated external defibrillation p. 792;
➔ Child basic life support p. 800

Further information

Resuscitation Council (UK) (*Adult basic life support and automated external defibrillation*). Available at: ℘ https://www.resus.org.uk/resuscitation-guidelines/adult-basic-life-support-and-automated-external-defibrillation/
St John Ambulance (*Recovery position*). Available at: ℘ http://www.sja.org.uk/sja/first-aid-advice/first-aid-techniques/the-recovery-position.aspx

Adult choking

Choking usually results from airway obstruction by a foreign body. Usually occurs when the person is eating or drinking. Early recognition is key. Important not to confuse with fainting, heart attack, stroke (**⟳** Recognizing and responding to a stroke p. 830), or other conditions which may cause sudden respiratory distress, cyanosis, or loss of consciousness.

Foreign bodies may cause either mild or severe airway obstruction. Ask the conscious patient: Are you choking? If the person is able to speak, cough, and breath, it is likely they have a mild obstruction. If the person is unable to speak, has a weakening cough, is struggling or unable to breath, they have a severe airway obstruction.

The Resuscitation Council (UK) describes the steps for community responders to follow when managing an adult who is choking.[2] The adult choking algorithm is summarized in Fig. 13.3.

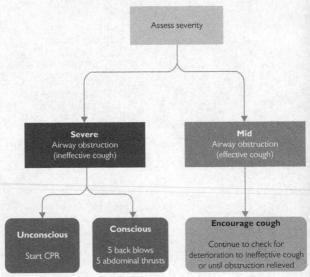

Fig. 13.3 Adult choking algorithm.

Reproduced with the permission of the Resuscitation Council UK (2015). Available at: https://www.resus.org.uk/resuscitation-guidelines/adult-basic-life-support-and-automated-external-defibrillation/

Suspect choking

Be alert to choking, especially if the person is eating.

Encourage to cough

Tell the person to cough.

Give back blows

If obstruction is not cleared by coughing, administer up to five back blows:
- Stand to the side and slightly behind the person.
- Support the chest with one hand and lean the person forwards so that when the obstruction is dislodged it comes out of the mouth.
- Administer five sharp blows between the shoulder blades with the heel of your hand. (The aim is to relieve the obstruction with each blow rather than administer all five.)

Give abdominal thrusts

If obstruction is not cleared by back blows, administer up to five abdominal thrusts:
- Stand behind the person and put both your arms round the upper part of the abdomen.
- Lean the person forwards.
- Clench your fist and place between the umbilicus and the ribcage.
- Grasp this hand with your other hand and pull sharply inwards and upwards.
- Repeat up to five times. (The aim is to relieve the obstruction with each thrust rather than administer all five.)

If the obstruction is still not relieved, continue alternating five back blows with five abdominal thrusts.

Commence CPR

If the person becomes unresponsive, support them to the ground.
☎ 999 and begin CPR with chest compressions (➲ Adult basic life support and automated external defibrillation p. 792).

Aftercare

Abdominal thrusts can potentially cause internal injuries and everyone who is successfully treated following this procedure should be examined afterwards for injury. Patients on antiplatelet or anticoagulant drugs are at ↑ risk of intra-abdominal haemorrhage and require a senior clinical opinion (➲ Patients on anticoagulant therapy p. 642).

Related topics

➲ Child choking p. 806

Reference

2. Resuscitation Council (UK) (2015) *Adult basic life support and automated external defibrillation*. Available at: https://www.resus.org.uk/resuscitation-guidelines/adult-basic-life-support-and-automated-external-defibrillation/

Child basic life support

Child cardiopulmonary arrest is uncommon. The causes include: upper or lower airway disease (e.g. croup, bronchiolitis, pneumonia, asthma (● Asthma in children p. 306)), trauma (e.g. near drowning, electrocution, poisoning), sudden infant death syndrome (● Sudden infant death syndrome p. 278), congenital heart disease (● Congenital heart defects p. 260), respiratory depression caused by prolonged convulsions (● Febrile convulsions and epilepsy p. 280), or drug overdose (● Poisoning and overdoses p. 822; ● Accident prevention p. 168).

Modified sequence for non-specialists

To promote paediatric basic life support (BLS) by the general public, the Resuscitation Council (UK) states that using the adult BLS sequence for a child is better than doing nothing (● Adult basic life support and automated external defibrillation p. 792). Therefore, they describe a modified sequence for non-specialists:[3] give five initial rescue breaths before starting chest compression; if you are on your own, perform CPR for 1min before going for help; and compress the chest by at least a third of its depth (~4cm for an infant and ~5cm for an older child) using two fingers for an infant and one or two hands for a child. The compression rate should be 100–120/min. These guidelines should be read in conjunction with the Resuscitation Council UK Statement on COVID19 in relation to CPR and resuscitation in first aid and community settings (✆ https://www.resus.org.uk/covid-19-resources/covid-19-resources-general-public/resuscitation-council-uk-statement-covid-19).

Sequence for those with a duty to respond to paediatric emergencies

The Resuscitation Council (UK) describes the steps those with a duty to respond to paediatric emergencies should follow when assessing and treating an infant or child who is unresponsive.[3] The paediatric BLS algorithm is summarized in Fig. 13.4. These guidelines should be read in conjunction with the Resuscitation Council UK Statement on COVID19 in relation to CPR and resuscitation in first aid and community settings (✆ https://www.resus.org.uk/covid-19-resources/covid-19-resources-general-public/resuscitation-council-uk-statement-covid-19).

Safety
Make sure you, the child, and bystanders are safe.

Response
Gently stimulate the child and check for a response. If the child does not respond, ask a helper to ✆ 999. If you are on your own, perform CPR for 1min before getting help.

Airway
Open the airway (see Fig. 13.2):
• Turn the child onto their back.
• Place your hand on their forehead and gently tilt their head back.
• With your fingertips under their chin, lift the chin to open the airway.
• Do not push on the soft tissues under the chin as this may block the airway.

If you have difficulty opening the airway, try the jaw thrust method: place the first two fingers of each hand behind each side of the child's mandible and push the jaw forwards.

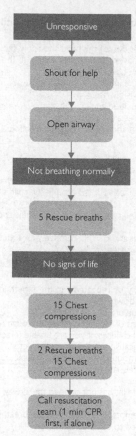

Fig. 13.4 Paediatric basic life support algorithm.

Reproduced with the permission of the Resuscitation Council UK (2015). Available at: https://www.resus.org.uk/resuscitation-guidelines/paediatric-basic-life-support/

Breathing

Keeping the airway open, look, listen, and feel for normal breathing for no more than 10secs. In the first few minutes after cardiac arrest, a child may be barely breathing, or taking infrequent, slow, and noisy gasps. This is not normal breathing. If you have any doubt whether breathing is normal, act as if they are not breathing normally. If breathing is not normal or absent:

• Carefully remove any obvious airway obstruction.

Box 13.2 Rescue breaths for infants and children

For an infant <1yr

- Ensure a neutral position of the head and apply chin lift.
- Take a breath and cover the mouth and nose of the infant with your mouth, ensuring you have a good seal.
- Blow steadily into the infant's mouth and nose about 1sec, sufficient to make the chest visibly rise.
- Maintaining head position and chin lift, remove your mouth, and watch for the chest to fall as air is expelled.
- Take another breath and repeat this sequence four more times.

For a child >1yr

- Ensure head tilt and chin lift.
- Pinch the soft part of the child's nose closed.
- Open the child's mouth a little, but maintain the chin lift.
- Take a breath and place your lips around the child's mouth, making sure you have a good seal.
- Blow steadily into their mouth about 1sec, sufficient to make the chest visibly rise.
- Maintaining head tilt and chin lift, remove your mouth and watch the chest fall as air is expelled.
- Take another breath and repeat this sequence four more times.

⚠ Do not poke blindly or repeatedly in the mouth in case you push any foreign object further down.
- Give five initial rescue breaths (Box 13.2).
- Observe for any signs of life including gag or cough response.
- For both infants and children, if you are unable to achieve an effective breath, it may be because the airway is obstructed:
  - Open the child's mouth and remove any visible obstruction.
  - Ensure there is adequate head tilt and chin lift, but the neck is not overextended.
  - If head tilt and chin lift has not opened the airway, try the jaw thrust method.
- Make up to five attempts to achieve effective breaths but if still unsuccessful, proceed to chest compression

Circulation

Look for signs of life (e.g. movement, coughing, and normal breathing). This step should take a maximum of 10secs. If checking the pulse, feel the carotid pulse in the neck in a child and the brachial pulse in the inner aspect of the upper arm in an infant. The femoral pulse in the groin can be used for both infants and children. If you are confident that you can detect signs of circulation within 10secs, continue rescue breathing if necessary and until the child is able to breath effectively and independently. Thereafter, move into the recovery position (⊃ Recovery position for babies, children, and adults p. 796). If there are no signs of life, start chest compressions, and combine rescue breathing and chest compressions (see Boxes 13.3 and 13.4, and Fig. 13.5).

Box 13.3 Rescue breaths and chest compressions for all children

Compress the lower half of the sternum.

- To avoid compressing the upper abdomen, locate the xiphisternum by finding the angle where the lowest ribs join in the middle; compress the sternum one finger's breadth above this.
- Compression should be sufficient to depress the sternum by at least one third of the depth of the chest, which is ~4cm for an infant and ~5cm for a child.
- Release the pressure completely, then repeat at a rate of 100–120/min.
- Allow the chest to return to its resting position before starting the next compression.
- After 15 compressions, tilt the head, lift the chin, and give two rescue breaths.
- Continue compressions and breaths at a ratio of 15:2.

Box 13.4 Chest compressions

For an infant

The lone rescuer should compress the sternum with the tips of two fingers. If there are two or more rescuers, use the encircling technique (see Fig. 13.5):

- Place both thumbs flat, side by side, on the lower half of the sternum, with the tips pointing towards the infant's head.
- Spread the rest of both hands, with the fingers supporting the infant's back.
- Press down on the lower sternum with your two thumbs to depress it at least a third of the depth of the infant's chest (~4cm).

For a child >1yr

- Place the heel of one hand over the lower half of the sternum.
- Lift the fingers to ensure that pressure is not applied over the child's ribs.
- Position yourself vertically above the child's chest and, with your arm straight, depress the sternum by at least a third of the depth of the chest (~5cm).
- In larger children, or for small rescuers, this may be achieved most easily by using both hands with the fingers interlocked.

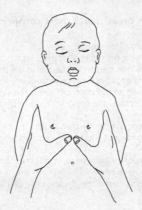

Fig. 13.5 Encircling technique for infants under one year old.

Continue resuscitation until the child shows signs of life, or you become too exhausted to continue, or further qualified help arrives.

Automated external defibrillation

Shockable rhythms are very unusual in the paediatric population.[4] Therefore, in the community setting, the focus should not be on automated external defibrillation (AED) but ↑ quality CPR. Guidance states that if using an AED on a child <8yrs, paediatric attenuated shock energy should be used if possible.

References

3. Resuscitation Council (UK) (2015) *Paediatric basic life support*. Available at: https://www.resus. org.uk/resuscitation-guidelines/paediatric-basic-life-support/
4. Resuscitation Council (UK) (2015) *Frequently asked questions: defibrillators*. Available at: https:// www.resus.org.uk/faqs/faqs-defibrillators/

Child choking

Foreign body aspiration is asphyxia, suffocation, or inhalation of food and non-food items into the respiratory tract. Aspiration of foreign bodies is an important and preventable cause of morbidity in children <3yrs. ↑ incidence in this age group is attributed to the absence of molar teeth (◆ Development and care of teeth for young children p. 196) which ↓ their ability to properly chew food (◆ Food and the under-fives p. 212), and exploring the world through putting objects into their mouth, meaning that small objects such as marbles, beads, and button batteries can get stuck in the respiratory tract (◆ Accident prevention p. 168).

The signs and symptoms of a child choking are set out in Box 13.5.

Box 13.5 Recognizing when a child is choking
General signs of choking
- Person present who witnessed episode
- Coughing or choking
- Sudden onset
- Recent history of playing with or eating small objects

Ineffective coughing
- Unable to vocalize
- Quiet or silent cough
- Unable to breathe
- Cyanosis
- ↓ level of consciousness

Effective coughing
- Crying or verbal response to questions
- Loud cough and able to take breaths between coughing
- Fully responsive

First aid for a child who is choking

The Resuscitation Council (UK) describes the steps that should be followed when a child is choking.[5] The paediatric choking algorithm is summarized in Fig. 13.6.

Conscious child with choking

If the child is conscious but has absent or ineffective cough, give back blows (Box 13.6). If back blows are ineffective and do not relieve choking, administer chest thrusts to infants or abdominal thrusts to children (Box 13.7).

Unconscious child with choking

If the child is unconscious or becomes unconscious:
- Place them on a firm, flat surface.
- Ask helper to confirm that an ambulance has been requested.
- Open the mouth and look for any obvious object.
- If one is seen, attempt to remove it with a single finger sweep.

⚠ Do not poke blindly or repeatedly in case you push the foreign object further down.
- Administer five rescue breaths and if there is no response, proceed immediately to chest compressions.
- Follow paediatric BLS pathway (◆ Child basic life support p. 800).

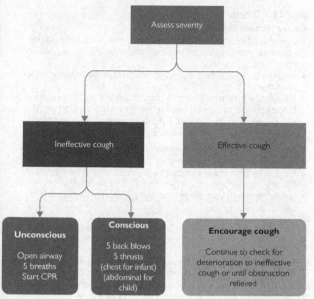

Fig. 13.6 Paediatric choking algorithm.

Reproduced with the permission of the Resuscitation Council UK (2015). Available at: https://www.resus.org.uk/resuscitation-guidelines/paediatric-basic-life-support/

Box 13.6 Back blows

In an infant

- Support the infant in a head-downwards, prone position; allow gravity to help with removal of the foreign object.
- If you are seated or kneeling, you should be able to support the infant safely across your lap.
- Support the infant's head by placing the thumb of one hand at the angle of the lower jaw, and one or two fingers from the same hand at the same point on the other side of the jaw. ⚠ Do not compress the soft tissues under the infant's jaw as this will exacerbate the airway obstruction.
- Deliver up to five sharp back blows with the heel of one hand in the middle of the back; discontinue if the obstruction is relieved before administering all five back blows.

In a child

- Position child head down.
- A small child may be placed across your lap; if this is not possible, support the child in a forward-leaning position.
- Deliver up to five sharp back blows with the heel of one hand in the middle of the back; discontinue if the obstruction is relieved before administering all five back blows.

Box 13.7 Thrusts

Chest thrusts for infants

- Turn the infant into a head-downwards supine position by placing your free arm along the infant's back and encircling the occiput with your hand.
- Support the infant down your arm, which is placed down or across your thigh.
- Identify the landmark for chest compression and deliver five chest thrusts (similar to chest compressions but sharper and delivered at a slower rate); discontinue if the obstruction is relieved before administering all five compressions.

Abdominal thrusts for children

- Stand or kneel behind the child.
- Place your arms under the child's arms and encircle their torso.
- Clench your fist and place it between the umbilicus and sternum.
- Grasp hand with your other hand and pull sharply inwards and upwards.
- Repeat up to five times.

Aftercare

Even if the foreign object has been removed, seek medical assistance as part of the object may be left behind. Abdominal thrusts can also potentially cause internal injuries and everyone who is successfully treated following this procedure should be examined afterwards for injury.

Related topics

➔ Adult choking p. 798

Reference

5. Resuscitation Council (UK) (2010) *Paediatric basic life support: choking*. Available at: https://www.resus.org.uk/resuscitation-guidelines/paediatric-basic-life-support/#choking

Anaphylaxis

Anaphylaxis is a severe, lifethreatening, generalized or systemic hypertensive reaction[6] (→ Allergies p. 694). Common causes of the reaction include:

- Insect stings
- Nuts: including peanuts, walnuts, almonds, brazils, and hazelnuts
- Food: including milk, eggs, fish and shellfish, sesame seeds and oil, bananas, kiwis, grapes and strawberries
- Antibiotics: including penicillin, cephalosporin, amphotericin, ciprofloxacin, and vancomycin
- Anaesthetic drugs
- Other drugs: including NSAIDs
- Vaccinations (→ Travel vaccinations p. 399; → Childhood immunization p. 164; → Childhood immunization schedule (UK) p. 166; → Immunization administration p. 390; → Targeted adult immunization p. 392)
- Contrast media
- Proteins in transfused blood components
- Latex (→ Personal protective equipment p. 100; → Indwelling urinary catheter care p. 508; → Wound dressings p. 532)
- Hair dye
- Idiopathic anaphylaxis

Exercise-induced (→ Exercise p. 354) anaphylaxis is a phenomenon in which anaphylaxis occurs during or after physical activity.[7] Different types including: anaphylaxis during or following exercise; food-dependent exercise-induced anaphylaxis; aspirin plus exercise; and food plus exercise plus aspirin.

Nurses involved in the administration of injections (→ Injection techniques p. 576) and other procedures in the home and/or clinic should carry/have direct access to emergency adrenaline and be aware of local guidelines on the treatment of anaphylaxis. Adrenaline should be checked at least weekly to ensure that it is suitable for injection (e.g. expiry date and presence of discoloration). Community psychiatric nurses administering depot injections (→ People with psychosis p. 486) should check local guidelines as to whether or not they are required to carry adrenaline.

Clinical features

Types of anaphylactic reaction (AR):

- Uniphasic: symptoms develop quickly and rapidly worsen, but once successfully treated do not return (until triggered by a subsequent exposure)
- Biphasic: symptoms may be mild or severe at the onset of the AR, followed by a period when there are no symptoms, and then increasing symptoms
- Protracted: where symptoms last several days

Clinical presentation

According to the Resuscitation Council UK,[6] anaphylaxis is likely when all of the following three criteria are met:
- Sudden onset and rapid progression of symptoms
- Life-threatening airway and/or breathing and/or circulation problems
- Skin and/or mucosal changes (flushing, urticarial, angioedema)

Exposure to a known allergen for the patient supports the diagnosis. ⚠ It is important to note that skin and mucosal changes can be subtle or absent in AR. There can also be gastrointestinal symptoms (including, abdominal pain, nausea and vomiting, and diarrhoea).

Treatment

Anaphylaxis is a medical emergency and requires immediate treatment:
- ☎ 999 and tell the operator there is a suspected case of anaphylaxis.
- Rapidly assess airway, breathing, circulation, disability, and exposure (ABCDE).

Patient positioning
- If patient is having difficulty breathing, sit them up.
- If the patient is hypotensive, lie them flat with their legs elevated.
- If patient is breathing and unconscious, lie them in the recovery position (➔ Recovery position for babies, children, and adults p. 796).

Remove trigger
- Stop the suspected drug.
- Remove the stinger after a bee sting.

⚠ Do not delay treatment if removing the trigger is not feasible.

Cardiorespiratory arrest following an anaphylactic reaction
Commence CPR (➔ Child basic life support p. 800; ➔ Adult basic life support and automated external defibrillation p. 792).

Administer adrenaline
Adrenaline should be given to all patients with potentially life-threatening symptoms. If the symptoms are not present but there are other symptoms of systemic allergic reaction, the patient needs careful observation and systemic treatment using the ABCDE approach.[6] When indicated, adrenaline should be administered by the intramuscular route. The preferred site is the anterolateral of the middle third of the thigh. Administration of adrenaline should be repeated if there is no improvement in the patient's condition (at ~5min intervals). See Fig. 13.7.

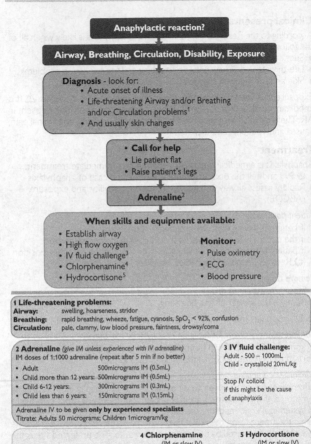

Fig. 13.7 Anaphylaxis algorithm.

Reproduced with the permission of the Resuscitation Council UK (2012). Available at: https://www.resus.org.uk/anaphylaxis/emergency-treatment-of-anaphylactic-reactions/

Oxygen

Should be given as soon as possible, initially at the highest concentration possible (10–15L/min) using a mask.

Aftercare

Even if symptoms have reversed, the patient should be encouraged to go to hospital for a period of observation in case they experience a biphasic AR.

Preventing anaphylaxis

All those suspected of having an AR should be referred to an NHS allergy clinic and to their GP for discussion about the prescription of an adrenaline auto-injector (such as Epipen®, Jext®, or Emerade®). If a trigger has been identified, steps should be taken to avoid exposure to the trigger in the future (e.g. checking food labels, telling restaurant staff and healthcare practitioners about the allergy, and using insect repellent). Write a personalized crisis plan to ensure family, friends, and school staff (➔ Working in schools p. 44) know how to handle an emergency. Personalized allergy action plan templates for children are available from the British Society for Allergy and Clinical Immunology (see ⅏ https://www.bsaci.org/about/download-paediatric-allergy-action-plans).

References

6. Resuscitation Council UK (2008) *Emergency treatment of anaphylactic reactions: guidelines for healthcare providers.* Available at: https://www.resus.org.uk/anaphylaxis/emergency-treatment-of-anaphylactic-reactions/
7. Anaphylaxis Campaign (2016) *Fact sheet: exercise induced anaphylaxis.* Available at: https://www.anaphylaxis.org.uk/wp-content/uploads/2015/06/Exercise-induced-anaphylaxis-V7-formatted.pdf

External bleeding

Types of external bleeding

- Capillary: blood oozes from capillaries, usually not serious, and generally easy to control
- Venous: occurs when a vein is severed, blood flows steadily, and most veins collapse when cut, which aids control of bleeding
- Arterial: life-threatening, requires urgent attention, blood spurts with each heartbeat, and difficult to control

Preventing cross infection

Some diseases such as Hepatitis B (➔ Viral hepatitis p. 724) are transmitted through the exchange of body fluids. To minimize the risk of infection, wear disposable gloves and, where appropriate, a mask and goggles or visor (➔ Personal protective equipment p. 100; ➔ Principles of working with someone with an infectious disease p. 467).

First aid for light external bleeding

Wash superficial wounds with warm soapy water to remove any obvious debris or dirt, and apply a sterile dressing (➔ Wound dressings p. 532). Apply direct pressure to the wound with thumb and fingers over the dressing.

First aid for a nose bleed

For a child, check whether or not there is a foreign body present. If an object is present, do not attempt to remove it but refer to GP. If bleeding is due to a head injury, ☎ 999 and ask for an ambulance as soon as possible. Otherwise, encourage the patient to sit down and to hold their head well forward and breath through the mouth while pinching the entire soft part of the nose for 10–20mins. If bleeding is severe or lasts more than 30mins, ☎999 and ask for an ambulance.

First aid for heavy external bleeding

Expose the wound. Check whether there is anything embedded in the wound. If nothing present, apply and maintain firm pressure over the wound using a clean bulky pad (if a dressing is not available, use a clean handkerchief, towel, piece of clothing, or your hand alone). ⚠ If there is a foreign body in the wound, do not attempt to remove it but apply pressure on either side of it with a pad or fingers to push the edges together.

☎ 999 and ask for an ambulance as soon as possible. Encourage the person to lay down. If you have no reason to suspect a spinal injury (➔ Spinal cord injury p. 518) or fracture (➔ Sprains, strains, and fractures p. 824), elevate the legs so that they are above the level of the heart. Continue to apply pressure until help arrives. Secure the pad with a bandage that maintains the pressure but does not cut off circulation. If the bleeding continues through the pad, apply another pad over the top and bandage it in place. Continually check level of patient responsiveness. If patient becomes unresponsive, open airway and check breathing (➔ Adult basic life support and automated external defibrillation p. 792; ➔ Child basic life support p. 800).

Application of tourniquets and haemostatic dressings

Whilst catastrophic external haemorrhage from a limb is rare and most bleeds can be controlled with direct pressure, the European Resuscitation Council First Aid Guidelines[8] state that haemostatic dressings and tourniquets should be used when direct pressure is either not possible or not effective (e.g. stabbings, firearms incidents, and industrial accidents). However, tourniquets and haemostatic dressings must be used correctly to avoid complications. Training is required to ensure application is safe and effective.

Amputation

Recover the severed part and place in a plastic bag and seal. The sealed bag should be kept in a cold environment and transferred to hospital with the patient.

Reference

8. European Resuscitation Council (2015) *Summary of the 2015 first aid guidelines.* Available at: https://ercguidelines.elsevierresource.com/european-resuscitation-council-guidelines-resuscitation-2015-section-9-first-aid#Introduction

Further information

St John Ambulance (*Severe bleeding*). Available at: ℜ http://www.sja.org.uk/sja/first-aid-advice/bleeding/severe-bleeding.aspx

St John Ambulance (*Nose bleeds*). Available at: ℜ http://www.sja.org.uk/sja/first-aid-advice/bleeding/nosebleeds.aspx

Burns and scalds

Burns and scalds are damage to the skin usually caused by heat. Both are treated the same way. A burn is caused by dry heat (e.g. an iron or fire) and a scald is caused by something wet (e.g. hot water or steam).

Depending on how serious a burn is, it may be possible to treat it at home. More serious burns require an emergency response and specialist treatment in hospital:

- Chemical and electrical burns
- Large burns (any burn bigger than the injured person's hand)
- Deep burns
- Burns that cause white or charred skin of any size
- Burns on the face, hand, arms, feet, legs, or genitals causing blisters
- Severe frostbite

The British Burn Association,[9] makes first aid recommendations for thermal, chemical, electrical, tar and bitumen, and cold burns (see the following).

First aid for thermal burns

Think—stop, remove, cool, warm, and cover.

Stop the burning process

Remove person from the source of the burn once safe to do so. Extinguish burning process using water. Alternatively, use the stop, drop, and roll method (see Box 13.8).

> ### Box 13.8 Stop, drop, and roll method
> - STOP where you are.
> - DROP to the ground; cover your eyes and mouth with your hands.
> - ROLL over and back and forth until the flames are out.

Remove clothing and jewellery

Remove any burned/contaminated/damp/constricted clothing. Remove any nappies, jewellery, and contact lenses near the burned area if able to do so. Leave any molten/adherent clothing in place.

Cool the burn

Do not delay cooling. Cool the burn immediately with cool running water for 20mins and within 3hrs of injury. (⚠ Do not use iced water.) Aim to complete 20mins of cooling (further attempts may induce hypothermia, especially in children and older people, and where large burns are present).

Warm the patient

Cool the burn but warm the patient to prevent hypothermia (➲ Hypothermia p. 820). Cover non-burned areas during cooling.

Cover the burn

Cover the cooled burn with loose longitudinal strips of cling film or non-adherent dressing (➲ Wound dressings p. 532). (⚠ Do not wrap cling film circumferentially around limbs or burned areas, and do not apply cling film to facial burns.)

First aid for chemical burns

Wear appropriate personal protective equipment (⊃ Personal protective equipment p. 100) to ↓ cross-contamination. Brush off dry powders, remove fragments of solid chemical substances, and discard contaminated clothing. Urgently irrigate skin and eyes with copious amounts of room-temperature running water for at least 20mins (⊃ Eye trauma p. 818). Treatment to be initiated by urgent response unit or specialist burns centre. Will include: accessing National Poisons Information Service/TOXBASE for agent-specific decontamination and treatment information; administering antidote treatment for specific agents if appropriate; and managing any systemic toxicity or expected side effects of a chemical agent (⊃ Poisoning and overdoses p. 822).

First aid for electrical burns

Ensure the electrical source has been controlled. Prioritize and manage life-threatening conditions as per standard adult basic life support or child basic life support. Cool the injury site immediately with cool running tap water for 20mins within 3hrs of the injury.

First aid for tar and bitumen burns

Cool the molten agent and injury site with cool running tap water for 20mins within 3hrs of injury, or until it is completely cooled. Tar removal is not an emergency and may be delayed until arrival at the burns unit.

First aid for cold burns

Prioritize management of hypothermia. In the pre-hospital care of cold injury, only begin rewarming of injury if refreezing will not occur in transit. (⚠ Do not rub or massage the affected areas.)

Reference

9. British Burn Association (2018) *First aid clinical practice guidelines*. Available at: https://www.britishburnassociation.org/wp-content/uploads/2017/06/BBA-First-Aid-Guideline-24.7.18.pdf

Eye trauma

Eye injuries can have sight-threatening consequences. Employers should undertake workplace risk assessments (⊃ Health and safety at work p. 92) and provide eye protection to people in the construction, manufacturing, chemical, and pharmaceutical industries (⊃ Personal protective equipment p. 100). At home, eye protection should be worn during activities such as drilling, sawing, sanding, and hammering, and when using lawn mowers and strimmers. Caution advised when using household and garden chemicals (e.g. fertilizer, drain and oven cleaners, limescale removers, bleach, solvents and fixatives) (⊃ Accident prevention p. 168). Eye protection is recommended during racquet sports (e.g. squash) (⊃ Exercise p. 354). Welders, sunbed users, and skiers must protect their eyes against UV light.

Assessment

Practitioners should recognize their limitations and, where necessary, seek further advice or refer the patient elsewhere. History taking will include inquiry about trauma (time and mode), previous similar episodes, systemic illness, eye disease, contact lens use, medication, and symptoms (e.g. pain, watering, altered vision). Examination of the eyes and vision will include tests of visual acuity, visual fields, pupils, and eye movements. Ophthalmoscopy should also be performed. Check for discharge from the eyes. Serious and potentially sight-threatening presentations are listed in Box 13.9.

> **Box 13.9 Serious and potentially sight-threatening presentations**
> * ↓ visual acuity
> * Deep pain within the eye
> * Unilateral red eye
> * Contact lens use
> * Photophobia
> * Penetration injuries
> * ↑ velocity injuries
> * Chemical injuries
> * Ciliary injection (redness all around the edge of the cornea)
> * Fluorescein staining
> * Pupil abnormalities

Common injuries

Corneal abrasion

Often caused by small sharp objects (e.g. finger nail). Important to exclude penetrating injury and presence of foreign bodies. Symptoms include pain, eyelid twitch, photophobia, watering, and redness. May only be visible using magnification equipment and fluorescein stain with cobalt blue light illumination. Anti-inflammatory or antibiotic eye drops may be recommended. Abrasions usually heal quickly.

Superficial foreign bodies

Small pieces of grit and eyelashes. Symptoms include foreign body sensation, pain, watering, blurred vision, and red eye. If metal or penetrating injury is suspected, refer to eye casualty. Superficial foreign bodies can usually be washed out or removed with a moistened tip of a cotton bud. If foreign body cannot be removed using these methods, refer to eye casualty.

Penetrating trauma

Partial or full-thickness injury of outer wall of eye caused by sharp object. Symptoms include history of trauma, pain, and visual loss. Refer urgently to eye casualty if penetrating injury is a possibility. ⚠ Do not attempt to remove large foreign bodies.

Blunt trauma

Following a blow to the eye (e.g. a fist or squash ball). Symptoms include pain, watering, visual loss, photophobia, possible double vision. Mild cases may result in bruising and swelling around the eye, which will not require intervention. More severe cases include orbital fracture, internal bleeding, or raised eye pressure, which will require urgent referral to eye casualty.

Chemical injuries

Cause significant damage (➲ Burns and scalds p. 816). Symptoms include pain, redness, watering, and visual loss. Must be treated immediately by holding the eyelids open and bathing the eyes with copious amounts of water. May require a topical anaesthetic to help keep affected eye open. Refer urgently to eye casualty.

Photokeratitis

Damage caused by exposure to UV light. Delay of 6–12hrs between exposure and symptoms, which include pain, redness, photophobia, eyelid twitch, and blurred vision. Treatment may include cold compresses and rest with eyes closed. Analgesia and eye lubricants may be recommended for symptom relief. Symptoms should resolve within 48hrs.

Corneal ulcer and contact lens-related red eye

Inflammation of the cornea. Symptoms include pain, watering, red eye, blurred vision, discharge, and photophobia. May only be visible using magnification equipment and fluorescein stain with cobalt blue light illumination. A bacterial or fungal infection of the cornea is a sight-threatening emergency requiring urgent referral to eye casualty.

Related topics

➲ Common problems affecting eyes p. 746; ➲ Blindness and partial sight p. 748

Further information

College of Optometrists (*Clinical management guidelines*). Available at: ℜ https://www.college-optometrists.org/guidance/clinical-management-guidelines.html

Moorfields Eye Hospital (*Common eye condition management*). Available at: ℜ https://www.moorfields.nhs.uk/sites/default/files/GP%20Handbook%20-%20Common%20eye%20condition%20management.pdf

Hypothermia

Hypothermia is a medical emergency. It is defined by a core body temperature <35°C. Below this temperature, the body loses more heat than it generates. Acute hypothermia occurs with immersion in cold water or exposure to cold weather (➲ Weather extreme p. 370). Chronic hypothermia occurs with certain diseases, ageing, or prolonged exposure to cold temperatures. People with long-term conditions, homeless people (➲ Homeless people p. 446), older people, and young children are at risk of hypothermia. Symptoms of hypothermia are listed in Box 13.10.

> **Box 13.10 Symptoms of hypothermia**
> **Adults**
> - Shivering
> - Pallor
> - Drowsiness, confusion, irrational behaviour
> - Slow and shallow breathing
> - Slow pulse
>
> **Infants**
> - Bright red, cold skin
> - ↓ energy levels
> - Babies may be limp, quiet, and refuse to feed

First aid for hypothermia

- ☎ 999 and ask for an ambulance as soon as possible.
- Move person to a warm building.
- Remove wet clothing and cover person with dry or warm blanket.
- If the person is conscious and able to swallow properly, provide warm drinks (⚠ Do not give alcohol) and ↑-energy foods such as chocolate.
- ⚠ Do not rub or massage skin or apply direct heat.

Continually check level of patient responsiveness. If patient becomes unresponsive, open airway and check breathing (➲ Adult basic life support and automated external defibrillation p. 792; ➲ Child basic life support p. 800).

Further information

British Red Cross (*Learn first aid for someone who has hypothermia*). Available at: ℜ https://www.redcross.org.uk/first-aid/learn-first-aid/hypothermia

Poisoning and overdoses

Poisoning is defined as exposure to a substance that is dangerous to health or life.[10] A poison may be a drug, household product, industrial chemical, or plant or animal derivative. Examples include alcohol (→ Alcohol p. 360), laundry products, carbon monoxide, and snake venom. Poisoning can be accidental or intentional (→ Suicidal intent and deliberate self-harm p. 494).

Overdose is the use of a quantity of drug in excess of its intended or prescribed dose.[10] It may be accidental or intentional and involve the use of over-the-counter, prescribed, or illicit drugs (→ Substance use p. 476). Routes include ingestion, inhalation, injection, skin/eye contamination, and bites.

Accidental poisoning with a substance found at home is common in children <5yrs (→ Accident prevention p. 168). Deliberate poisoning is part of the spectrum of deliberate self-harm or a form of Munchausen syndrome by proxy. Accidental overdose may result from errors in drug administration (→ Medicine concordance and adherence p. 132). When referring to drugs of misuse, overdose may mean adverse effects that occur when the drug is used, or when quantities are used that are larger than can be physically tolerated.

Prognosis depends on the type of poison or drug, the quantity taken, and associated comorbidity.

Signs and symptoms

Some people will self-report accidental or intentional poisoning or overdose. In other cases, poisoning or overdose will be reported by parents or friends. On other occasions, people may present with symptoms for which there is no obvious cause. Signs and symptoms depend on the substance and amount taken. They may include:

- Altered behaviour
- Acute confusion
- Hypoglycaemia
- Unexplained seizures (→ Seizures and epilepsy p. 740)
- Abnormal bleeding
- Headaches and dizziness
- Nausea and vomiting
- Hyperventilation
- Respiratory depression
- Reduced consciousness
- Dilated pupils
- Tachycardia or bradycardia (→ Abnormal cardiac rhythms p. 640)
- ↓ O_2 saturation
- Hypothermia (→ Hypothermia p. 820 or hyperthermia)

Information regarding symptoms and signs of drugs that are commonly involved in poisoning or overdose is available in the British National Formulary (BNF).

First aid for poisoning and overdose

Call NHS ☎111 for advice if a person has been poisoned or has taken an overdose but does not appear to be ill. It is important to seek advice as serious illness may be delayed (e.g. people who have ingested paracetamol are frequently asymptomatic or have only mild gastrointestinal symptoms at initial presentation).

Helping someone who is conscious

If you think someone has been poisoned or has taken an overdose and is ill or is likely to become ill, ☎ 999 and request an ambulance as soon as possible, and ↓ absorption of poison if possible. For example, if carbon monoxide is suspected, open windows or move the person to open air; if the poison has been swallowed, encourage the person to spit out anything remaining in their mouth; if the harmful substance has been splashed onto the skin or clothes, remove contaminated items and wash skin with copious amounts of water (➲ Burns and scalds p. 816). Continually check level of patient responsiveness. If patient becomes unresponsive, open airway and check breathing.

Helping someone who is unconscious

- ☎ 999 and request an ambulance as soon as possible.
- ↓ absorption of poison if possible (as stated earlier).
- Move person into the recovery position (➲ Recovery position for babies, children, and adults p. 796).
- Continually check level of patient responsiveness and breathing.
- If the person is not breathing, begin CPR (➲ Adult basic life support and automated external defibrillation p. 792; ➲ Child basic life support p. 800).

⚠ Do not perform mouth-to-mouth resuscitation if the person's mouth or airway is contaminated with poison: perform hands-only CPR.

Reference

10. NICE (2017) *Poisoning or overdose*. Available at: https://cks.nice.org.uk/poisoning-or-overdose#!topicSummary

Further information

National Poisons Information Service (NPIS) (*TOXBASE: clinical toxicology database of the NPIS*). Available at: ℘ http://www.npis.org/toxbase.html

Sprains, strains, and fractures

Sprains are injuries to the ligaments (commonly wrists, ankles, thumbs, and knees) and strains are injuries affecting the muscles (commonly knees, feet, legs, and back). A fracture is a broken or cracked bone. A closed fracture is when the fractured bone does not break the skin. An open fracture is when the fractured bone breaks the skin. Unless the bone is protruding, the initial symptoms of a sprain, strain, and fracture are very similar (see Box 13.11).

> ### Box 13.11 Symptoms of sprains, strains, and fractures
> **Sprains and strains**
> - Pain or tenderness
> - Swelling or bruising
> - Inability to weight bear
> - Muscle spasms
> - Muscle cramping
>
> **Fractures**
> - Pain or tenderness
> - Swelling or bruising
> - Deformity
> - Inability to weight bear
>
> Person may report hearing or feeling a snap or grinding noise as the injury happened. The person may also exhibit signs of shock.

Treating sprains or strains
- Rest: stop any exercise (➔ Exercise p. 354) and avoid putting weight on the injury.
- Ice: apply an ice pack to the injury for up to 20mins every 2–3hrs.
- Compression: wrap a bandage around the injury to support it.
- Elevation: keep the limb raised on a pillow as much as possible.

First aid for fractures
If a broken bone is suspected, medical attention should be sought. If it is a broken toe or finger, the person can go to a minor injury unit or urgent care centre. For a broken arm or leg, the patient should go to A&E. If the injury is severe, ☎ 999. Very severe suspected breaks, such as a broken neck or back, should always be treated by ☎ 999. Whilst awaiting emergency services:
- Cover open fracture with a sterile dressing (➔ Wound dressing p. 532).
- Provide first aid for heavy external bleeding (➔ External bleeding p. 814).
- ⚠ Do not move the person unless they are in immediate danger.
- Support the injured area to reduce movement (e.g. an arm sling).
- Continually check level of patient responsiveness. If patient becomes unresponsive, open airway and check breathing (➔ Adult basic life support and automated external defibrillation p. 792; ➔ Child basic life support p. 800).

Sepsis

A life-threatening condition caused by the body's immune response to a bacterial or fungal infection (➔ Bacterial skin infections p. 680; ➔ Fungal infections p. 686; ➔ Urinary tract infections p. 756; ➔ Infections in children p. 288; ➔ Wound infection p. 526; ➔ Pneumonia p. 750). Without quick treatment, sepsis can → septic shock, multiple organ failure, and death.

Risk factors for sepsis

Risk factors include:[11]
- The very young (<1yr) and older people (>75yrs) or people who are very frail
- People who have impaired immune systems because of illness or drugs
- Women who are pregnant (➔ Pregnancy p. 424), have given birth (➔ Postnatal care p. 438), or had a termination (➔ Termination of pregnancy p. 788) or miscarriage in the past 6wks.

Symptoms of sepsis

Initial symptoms are often non-specific. As the illness progresses, any combination of the following may develop:
- Shivering, fever, or feeling very cold
- Extreme pain or discomfort
- Clammy or sweaty skin
- Confusion or disorientation
- Shortness of breath
- High heart rate

Early symptoms of sepsis often resemble a viral illness (➔ Viral infections p. 720). However, in the context of a presumed infection, there are a number of red flag criteria indicating a ↑ risk of deterioration and amber flag criteria indicating an intermediate risk of deterioration. These criteria were developed by the UK Sepsis Trust and are supported by NICE Guidelines.[12–15] See Boxes 13.12–13.15.

Responding to red flags

⚠ If any one red flag symptom present, ☎ 999 and arrange blue-light transfer. Write a brief, clear handover including observations and antibiotic allergies (➔ Allergies p. 694) where present. Ensure crew pre-alert as 'red flag sepsis'.[12–15] Prompt recognition and initiation of treatment for all patients suspected of having sepsis are vital within the hour.[16]

Box 13.12 Symptoms in children 0–4 yrs
Red flag criteria
- Doesn't wake when roused or won't stay awake
- Looks very unwell to healthcare professional
- Weak, high pitched or continuous cry
- Severe tachypnoea
- Severe tachycardia
- Bradycardia
- Non-blanching rash/mottled/ashen/cyanotic
- Temperature <36°C
- If under 3mths, temperature 38°C +
- SPO_2 <90% on air or increased O_2 requirements

Amber flag criteria
- Not responding normally/no smile
- Reduced activity/very sleepy
- Moderate tachypnoea
- Moderate tachycardia
- SPO_2 <92% or increased O_2 requirements
- Nasal flaring
- Capillary refill time 3secs or more
- Reduced urine output
- Leg pain or cold extremities
- Parental or carer concern

Box 13.13 Symptoms in children aged 5–11yrs
Red flag criteria
- Objective evidence of new or altered mental state
- Doesn't wake when roused/ won't stay awake
- Looks very unwell to healthcare professional
- Severe tachypnoea
- Severe tachycardia
- Bradycardia
- SpO_2 <90% on air
- Non-blanching rash/mottled/ashen/cyanotic

Amber flag criteria
- Behaving abnormally/not wanting to play
- Parental or carer concern
- Moderate tachypnoea
- Moderate tachycardia
- SpO_2 < 92% on air
- Capillary refill time 3 secs or more
- Reduced urine output
- Temperature <36°C
- Leg pain

Box 13.14 Symptoms in adults and children and young people 12 years and over

Red flag criteria

- Objective evidence of new or altered mental state
- Systolic BP ≤ 90 mmHg (or drop of >40 from normal)
- Heart rate ≥ 130 per minute
- Respiratory rate ≥ 25 per minute
- Needs O_2 to keep SpO_2 ≥ 92% (88% in COPD)
- Non-blanching rash/mottled /ashen/cyanotic
- Recent chemotherapy
- Not passed urine in 18 hours (<0.5ml/kg/hr if catheterized)

Amber flag criteria

- Relatives concerned about mental status
- Acute deterioration in functional ability
- Immunosuppressed
- Trauma/surgery/procedure in last 8wks
- Respiratory rate 21–24
- Systolic BP 91–100 mmHg
- Heart rate 91–130 or new dysrhythmia
- Temperature <36°C
- Clinical signs of wound infection

Responding to amber flags

If any amber flag symptoms present, immediately escalate to the most senior healthcare professional (GP or medical team). They will use clinical judgment to determine whether the patient can be managed in the community. If treated in the community, second assessment should be planned and may include blood. Patient should be given specific safety netting advice. For example, ☎ 999 if any of the following: slurred speech or confusion; extreme shivering; passing no urine; severe breathlessness; I feel like I might die; or skin mottled, ashen, blue or very pale. ⚠ If immunity impaired in the presence of any amber flags, treat as red flag sepsis (➲ Principles of working with someone with compromised immunity p. 466).

Related topics

➲ Indwelling urinary catheter care p. 508; ➲ Wound assessment p. 522; ➲ Oral chemotherapy in the home p. 546; ➲ Palliative care emergencies p. 566

Box 13.15 Symptoms in pregnancy or up to 6wks post-pregnancy

Red flag criteria
- Objective evidence of new or altered mental state
- Systolic BP ≤ 90 mmHg (or drop of >40 from normal)
- Heart rate ≥ 130 per minute
- Respiratory rate ≥ 25 per minute
- Needs O_2 to keep SpO_2 ≥ 92% (88% in COPD)
- Non-blanching rash/mottled/ashen/cyanotic
- Not passed urine in 18 hours (<0.5ml/kg/hr if catheterized)

Amber flag criteria
- Behavioural/mental status change
- Acute deterioration in functional ability
- Respiratory rate 21–24
- Heart rate 100–129 or new dysrhythmia
- Systolic BP 91–100 mmHg
- Has had invasive procedure in last 6 weeks (e.g. caesarean, forceps delivery, evacuation of retained products of conception, cerclage, chorionic villus sampling, miscarriage, termination)
- Temperature <36°C
- Has diabetes or gestational diabetes
- Close contact with Group A streptococcal infection
- Prolonged rupture of membranes
- Bleeding/wound infection
- Offensive vaginal discharge

References

11. UK Sepsis Trust (2017) *The sepsis manual* (4th edn). Available at: https://www.e-lfh.org.uk/wp-content/uploads/2018/02/Sepsis_Manual_2017_final_v7.pdf
12. UK Sepsis Trust (2019) *Sepsis screening tool general practice: under 5*. Available at: https://sepsistrust.org/wp-content/uploads/2020/02/Sepsis-GP-Under-5-Version-1.2.pdf
13. UK Sepsis Trust (2019) *Sepsis screening tool general practice: age 5–11*. Available at: https://sepsistrust.org/wp-content/uploads/2020/02/Sepsis-GP-5-11-Version-1.3.pdf
14. UK Sepsis Trust (2019) *Sepsis screening tool general practice: age 12+*. Available at: https://sepsistrust.org/wp-content/uploads/2019/10/Sepsis-GP-12-v3.2.pdf
15. UK Sepsis Trust (2019) *Sepsis screening tool general practice: pregnant or up to 6 weeks post-pregnancy (or after the end of pregnancy if pregnancy did not end in a birth)*. Available at: https://sepsistrust.org/wp-content/uploads/2020/02/Sepsis-GP-Pregnant.-Version-1.3.pdf
16. Royal College of Nursing (undated) *Sepsis*. Available at: https://www.rcn.uk/clinical-topics/infection-prevention-and-control/sepsis

Further information

NICE Guidelines (*Sepsis: recognition, diagnosis and early management*). Available at: ℘ https://www.nice.org.uk/guidance/ng51

Recognizing and responding to a stroke

There are two main types of stroke: ischaemic and haemorrhagic. The 1° difference is that ischaemic strokes are caused by a lack of blood flow to the brain, and haemorrhagic strokes are caused by bleeding in the brain. A transient ischaemic attack (TIA) is sometimes referred to as a 'mini stroke' and is caused by a temporary disruption in the blood supply to part of the brain.

A stroke is a medical emergency. The sooner the person arrives at a specialist stroke unit, the sooner they will receive appropriate treatment to ↓ the risk of severe brain injury, disability, and death. In the early stages of a TIA, it is not possible to tell if a person is having a TIA or a full stroke; therefore, they should always be treated as if they are having a full stroke.

Risk factors

- Hypertension (⊃ Hypertension p. 628)
- Increased cholesterol (⊃ Hypercholesterolaemia p. 632)
- Atrial fibrillation (⊃ Atrial fibrillation p. 641)
- Diabetes (⊃ Diabetes: overview p. 660; ⊃ Principles of diabetes management p. 664)

Symptoms of a stroke (FAST)

See Box 13.16.
- Face: facial weakness
- Arms: arm weakness
- Speech: slurred speech
- Time: to ☎ 999 if you notice any of these signs

> **Box 13.16 Symptoms of a stroke**
> - Sudden onset
> - Paralysis of one side of the body
> - Sudden loss or blurring of vision
> - Slurred speech
> - Dizziness
> - Confusion
> - Poor balance and co-ordination
> - Dysphagia
> - Sudden headache
> - Loss of consciousness

Responding to a stroke

If the patient has any of the aforementioned symptoms, ☎ 999. Whilst waiting for help, keep checking the person's breathing, pulse, and level of response. If they are unconscious, place in the recovery position (⊃ Recovery position for babies, children, and adults p. 796).

Useful information

- Telehealth and telecare *832*
- Assistive technology and home adaptations *834*
- Complementary and alternative therapies *838*
- Death confirmation and certification *840*
- Registration of births, marriages, and deaths *842*

Telehealth and telecare

Telecare

Defined as technologies in patients' homes and communities to minimize risk and provide urgent notification of adverse events.[1] Include: personal alarms, activity monitors, bed and chair occupancy sensors, bogus caller buttons (➲ Victims of crime p. 452), carbon monoxide monitors (➲ Poisoning and overdoses p. 822), epilepsy sensors (➲ Seizures and epilepsy p. 740), fall detectors (➲ Falls prevention p. 368), fire and smoke alarms, flood detectors, gas shut-off valves, incontinence sensors (➲ Urinary incontinence p. 504; ➲ Faecal incontinence p. 514), medication prompt devices (➲ Medicine concordance and adherence p. 132), property exit sensors, and temperature extreme sensors (➲ Weather extremes p. 370).[2] People who may find telecare helpful include: older people (➲ Healthy ageing p. 366; ➲ Frailty p. 678), adults with mental health or learning disabilities (➲ People with learning disabilities p. 456), adults with physical disabilities, people with dementia (➲ People with dementia p. 498), people with epilepsy, and children with disabilities.

Telehealth

Defined as remote monitoring of patients in their own homes to anticipate exacerbations early and build their self-care competencies.[1] Include: blood pressure monitors, pulse oximeters, glucose meters, and body weight scales. People who may find telehealth helpful include: women with high-risk pregnancies (➲ Pregnancy p. 424) and people with long-term conditions such as diabetes (➲ Diabetes: overview p. 660; ➲ Principles of diabetes management p. 664), chronic obstructive pulmonary disease (➲ Chronic obstructive pulmonary disease p. 614; ➲ Management of stable chronic obstructive pulmonary disease p. 616; ➲ Management of chronic obstructive pulmonary disease exacerbation p. 618), and heart failure (➲ Heart failure p. 636).

Access to telecare and telehealth

Levels of investment differ between local authorities (LAs) and clinical commissioning groups (CCGs). In some areas, telecare and telehealth are central to the health and social care integration agenda. People who choose to buy their own telecare service, product, or device should be encouraged to do some research (see the consumer standards organization Which? ℬ https://www.which.co.uk/).

Related topics

➲ Homes and housing p. 26; ➲ Assessment by remote consultation p. 124

References

1. NHS Commissioning Assembly (2015) *Technology enabled care services: resource for commissioners*. Available at: ℬ https://www.england.nhs.uk/wp-content/uploads/2014/12/TECS_FinalDraft_0901.pdf

2. TEC Services Association (undated) *Telecare and telehealth*. Available at: ℬ https://www.tsa-voice.org.uk/consumer-services/telecare-and-telehealth

Assistive technology and home adaptations

Definitions

Assistive technologies (ATs) are devices intended to compensate for, or alleviate, an injury, disability, or illness or to replace physical function.[3] They include equipment to aid daily living and to meet health-related needs, such as:

- Toileting equipment (e.g. raised toilet seats and commodes)
- Bathing and showering equipment (e.g. bath chairs and bath steps)
- Mobility aids (e.g. furniture raisers, wheelchairs, and walking sticks)
- Communication and hearing aids (⊃ Adults and children with additional communication needs p. 122; ⊃ Blindness and partial sight p. 748; ⊃ Deafness in children p. 268; ⊃ Deafness p. 696; ⊃ Communication and learning problems p. 224)
- Posture management systems
- Pressure area management systems (e.g. mattresses and turning tables) (⊃ Pressure ulcer prevention p. 520)
- Moving and handling systems (e.g. hoists and slide sheets) (⊃ Patient moving and handling p. 96)
- Hospital and community beds
- Special educational needs equipment (e.g. dyslexia software) (⊃ Children with special educational needs p. 242)
- Therapy equipment (e.g. suction machines (⊃ Tracheostomy care p. 586) and nebulizers (⊃ Nebulizers p. 623))

Some forms of AT will be classified as medical devices. A medical device is a healthcare product or piece of equipment that a person uses for a medical purpose (but not a medicine or drug).[4] They can be used to diagnose, monitor, or treat disease and to help people with physical impairments become more independent. By law, medical devices must have a CE mark. Examples of medical devices include blood glucose meters (⊃ Principles of diabetes management p. 664) and wheelchairs. If the 1° purpose of the equipment is personal hygiene, rather than medical or mobility (e.g. a shower chair or a commode), it will not usually be classified as a medical device.

Home adaptations are changes that can be made to the home to make it easier and safer to move around and perform activities of daily living. Examples of such adaptations include: installing stairlifts, fitting grab rails, widening doorways, lowering kitchen worktops, and putting in an outdoor ramp.

Assessment and provision of assistive technology

It should be noted that the system for public provision and public funding is complex, and grey areas exist. Different LAs and CCGs have different arrangements for assessment and provision (⊃ Commissioning of services p. 12; ⊃ Social support p. 28; ⊃ Social services p. 30).

Equipment and home adaptations to aid daily living

If a person needs equipment and/or home adaptations to aid daily living, they should contact their LA and ask for a care needs assessment. If the person is found to have eligible needs, the LA has a duty to ensure they are met. The assessment will usually be carried out by a social worker or occupational therapist. The outcome of the assessment should be agreed with the person and set down in a care and support plan, which must include a personal budget figure showing the cost to the LA of meeting the agreed needs.

LAs should not charge for the provision of disability equipment and minor adaptations that assist with nursing at home or aid daily activities. Different mechanisms exist for the provision of disability equipment. For example, it might be supplied on loan from a community equipment store or the person may be encouraged to buy the equipment themselves with their direct payments. In some areas, 'prescriptions' are issued for simple aids to daily living (e.g. raised toilet seats) so they can have more choice by exchanging them at an accredited retailer.

A minor adaptation is defined as one costing ≤£1,000. For major home adaptations, some people may be eligible for a disabled facilities grant or a charitable grant from Independence at Home (➲ Homes and housing p. 26).

Equipment to meet health-related needs

Equipment to meet health-related needs will typically include hospital and community beds, pressure area management systems, and therapy equipment. Provision will be dependent on a health needs assessment by a healthcare professional. This may be part of an assessment for continuing healthcare or immediate care services. Equipment to meet assessed health-related need is usually free (➲ NHS Entitlements p. 10). Some items of equipment will be provided on loan by a community equipment store. Other items (such as devices for blood glucose measurement) may be available on FP10 prescription (➲ Prescribing p. 136).

Complex equipment

Complex equipment requiring regular servicing and maintenance, such as mobile hoists, electric beds, and therapy equipment, is always delivered and fitted. It is provided on loan, with the LA or NHS retaining responsibility for it. Responsibility will include training in the use of the device, and repair and maintenance. Local policies (e.g. medical devices policies) apply.

Wheelchair services

NHS wheelchair services provide wheelchairs for people of all ages with a long-term disability that affects their mobility, necessitating a wheelchair and/or specialist postural seating. The way services are delivered varies between areas. Services comprise: referral, assessment, prescription, purchase/provision of equipment, equipment delivery and collection, repair service, reassessment, and service user training.

Buying and hiring disability equipment

People who choose to buy their own disability equipment should be encouraged to do some research (see the consumer standards organization

Which? $\Re$ https://www.which.co.uk/). Equipment for a disabled child or adult attracts a zero rate of VAT. Visit HM Revenue and Customs for further details ($\Re$ https://www.gov.uk/financial-help-disabled/vat-relief).

Some organizations provide short-term loan or hire of disability equipment (e.g. wheelchairs after an operation or for holidays). One such organization is the Red Cross.

Equipment for education and employment

LAs and schools provide equipment and adaptations for special educational needs. The Equality Act 2010 states that employers must make reasonable adjustments, which includes modified equipment to accommodate the needs of disabled employees.

Related topics

➜ Falls prevention p. 368; ➜ Children with complex health needs and disabilities p. 238

References

3. MHRA (2018) Assistive technology: definition and safe use. Available at: $\Re$ https://www.gov.uk/government/publications/assistive-technology-definition-and-safe-use
4. MHRA (2019) Medical devices: information for users and patients. Available at: $\Re$ https://www.gov.uk/guidance/medical-devices-information-for-users-and-patients

Further information

Age UK (*Disability equipment and home adaptations: factsheet 42*). Available at: $\Re$ https://www.ageuk.org.uk/globalassets/age-uk/documents/factsheets/fs42_disability_equipment_and_home_adaptations_fcs.pdf
Contact a Family (*Aids, equipment, and adaptations*). Available at: $\Re$ https://contact.org.uk/media/829408/aids_adaptations_and_equipment.pdf
Independence at Home (*How to apply*). Available at: $\Re$ http://www.independenceathome.org.uk/how-to-apply.html

Complementary and alternative therapies

Acupuncture

Aromatherapy

Contraindications

Herbal medicine

Homeopathy

Hypnotherapy

Complementary and alternative therapies

There are a wide range of healthcare practices, products, and therapies that are used by the public as an alternative or complementary to evidence-based healthcare and medicine (➲ Evidence-based healthcare p. 72). Key issues are the lack of evidence for efficacy, lack of regulation of practitioners (except osteopaths and chiropractors) (➲ Professional accountability p. 83), and potential toxicity associated with some topical and ingested products (➲ Poisoning and overdose p. 822). The following are examples of some types of complementary and alternative therapies.

Acupuncture

Derived from ancient Chinese medicine, the western version of acupuncture involves the use of needles to alleviate symptoms or cure disease. Fine needles are inserted at certain sites in the body, stimulating the body to produce substances such as endorphins, which produce beneficial effects. It is used in many general practices, as well as pain clinics and hospices. NICE[5] recommends acupuncture for migraine (➲ Migraine p. 744) or chronic tension-type headaches. It is used to treat musculoskeletal conditions (➲ Low back pain p. 604; ➲ Common musculoskeletal problems p. 734) and chronic pain, but with less evidence of effectiveness.

Aromatherapy

Inhaling aromatic plant oils or applying them to the skin for physical or emotional benefit. No medical evidence that it can prevent, treat, or cure disease. Oils are very strong, may cause skin irritation (➲ Eczema/dermatitis p. 684), and can be poisonous if ingested. The oils may be as potent as any other drug, and their safety and interactions with other medications are unknown.

Faith healing

Founded on the belief that people and places have the power to heal through a connection to a supreme being. No evidence of effectiveness.

Herbal medicine

Use of plants for medicinal purposes. Some herbal compounds have some evidence of effectiveness: e.g. St John's wort (for depression) (➲ People with anxiety and depression p. 478), Echinacea (for the common cold) (➲ Viral infections p. 720), and feverfew (for migraine prophylaxis). However, herbal remedies may have potent side effects and interactions with other drugs.

Homeopathy

Practitioners 'treat' using extremely dilute substances. There is no evidence that it works better than placebos.[6]

Hypnotherapy

Consists of training the patient to relax very deeply. Used to treat conditions or change habits. Evidence is weak. May have some value in managing anxiety, symptom control in irritable bowel syndrome (➲ Irritable bowel syndrome p. 710), and smoking cessation (➲ Smoking cessation p. 356), but should not be used if patient has psychosis (➲ People with psychosis p. 486) or personality disorder. Not available on the NHS.

Osteopathy and chiropractic

Physical treatments aimed at restoring alignment of the joints and improving functioning of the body. In the UK, they are distinguished from other complementary and alternative therapies by being under statutory regulation. All osteopaths and chiropractors have to undergo training, and after that time are registered with their governing body that enforces a code of standards and discipline (➲ Professional conduct p. 80). They must have professional indemnity insurance. Manual therapy is most effective, alongside exercise (➲ Exercise p. 354), for lower back pain. There is limited evidence for treatment of neck, shoulder, lower-limb pain, and recovery after knee and hip operations. There is no good evidence of effectiveness for health conditions unrelated to the musculoskeletal system.

Reflexology

Considers that a representation of the body is found on the foot. Treatment consists of massaging points on the foot or applying acupressure to relieve symptoms. There is no evidence of effectiveness.

References

5. NICE (2016) *Headaches in over 12s: diagnosis and management*. Available at: ℘ https://www.nice.org.uk/guidance/cg150/chapter/Recommendations#management-2
6. House of Commons Science and Technology Committee (2010) *Evidence check 2: homeopathy*. Available at: ℘ www.publications.parliament.uk/pa/cm200910/cmselect/cmsctech/45/4502.htm

Further information

Association for Professional Hypnosis and Psychotherapy (*Looking for a therapist?*). Available at: ℘ https://www.aphp.co.uk/
British Acupuncture Council (*Top 10 things to know*). Available at: ℘ www.acupuncture.org.uk
British Chiropractic Association (*Find a chiropractor*). Available at: ℘ www.chiropractic-uk.co.uk
General Osteopathic Council (*Visiting an osteopath*). Available at: ℘ https://www.osteopathy.org.uk/visiting-an-osteopath/

Death confirmation and certification

Around 30% of deaths occur at home in the UK. The GP is often the first to be contacted but a doctor, nurse, or other trained healthcare professional can verify death. The doctor who attended the deceased during their last illness is required to issue a certificate detailing the cause of death. Action to be taken will depend on whether the death is expected or unexpected.

Verification of the fact of death: expected deaths

The nurse has a duty to inform the doctor who has been treating the patient, so that they can certify the death.

Designated nurses may confirm or verify death when: death is expected and occurs in a home, hospice, residential or nursing home, prison, or hospital, and is not accompanied by suspicious circumstance; it has been agreed further intervention would be inappropriate and the appropriate documentation is signed; and death does not require reporting to the coroner. Verification is within 4hrs in a community setting. The nurse can refuse to verify death and request attendance of the responsible doctor or police if there is any unusual situation. The nurse must check specific details of their employer's policy relating to death verification. The policy will usually also state the circumstances in which nurses cannot verify death (e.g. death of a child). Following verification, the family can arrange for removal of the body.

The recognized clinical signs when verifying death are: absence of a carotid pulse (>1min), heart sounds (>1min), and respiratory movements and breath sounds (>1min); fixed, dilated pupils (unresponsive to bright lights); and no response to painful stimuli (e.g. sternal rub).

Parenteral drug administration or any life-prolonging equipment should not be removed prior to verification.

Verification of the fact of death: unexpected deaths

Practitioners visiting in the home finding someone unexpectedly dead should initiate life support (if appropriate) (➲ Adult basic life support and automated external defibrillation p. 792; ➲ Child basic life support p. 800). In unequivocal death (e.g. hypostasis, rigor mortis, massive cranial damage, decomposition), either ☎ 999 or the GP, depending on circumstances and knowledge of the deceased person, and do not move the body. Some organizations have developed protocols for first-contact practitioners, working in out-of-hours services, to verify unexpected deaths at home.

Certification of death

By law, the process of completing the Medical Certificate of Cause of Death must be undertaken by a medical practitioner who attended the deceased person during the last illness. The certificate is usually issued in a sealed envelope, addressed to the registrar, and given to the next of kin to take to register the death.

Medical practitioners report the death to the coroner (procurator fiscal in Scotland) if: a doctor had not seen the patient in the preceding 14 days (28 days in Northern Ireland); within 24hrs of admission to hospital; the death was sudden, violent, unnatural, or suspicious; the cause is unknown or uncertain; the death occurred during surgery or recovery from anaesthetic; the death occurred in prison or policy custody; and the cause was an industrial disease.

The coroner will decide whether a post-mortem and further investigation are required in order to determine the cause of death. Since April 2019, medical examiners have been scrutinizing death certificates, following a reform of the process.

It is good practice for general practices and 1° care nurses to inform other care services (e.g. hospitals, social services involved with the deceased person) of the death, to avoid ongoing appointments, etc. Some general practices keep registers of deaths (➔ General practice p. 18).

Related topics

➔ Coping with bereavement p. 574; ➔ Registration of births, marriages, and deaths p. 842; ➔ Euthanasia, assisted suicide, and assisted dying p. 572; ➔ Sudden infant death syndrome p. 278

Further information

Department of Health and Social Care (*Death certification reforms*). Available at: ℵ https://www.gov.uk/government/consultations/death-certification-reformsdocuments.co.uk/document/cm58/5831/5831.pdf

Royal College of Nursing (*Confirmation or verification of death by registered nurses*). Available at: ℵ https://www.rcn.org.uk/get-help/rcn-advice/confirmation-of-death

Registration of births, marriages, and deaths

It has been a legal requirement since 1837 for UK residents to register births, marriages, and deaths with civil authorities. Registration of stillbirths and adoptions has been required by law since 1927. The registrar of births, marriages, and deaths is an official position in each LA, and they are responsible for the registers for that district. It is a criminal offence not to register births and deaths within specified time periods. Birth, marriage, and death certificates are copies of the entries made in the register for that district. Details of how to find the local registrar are on every council website and in libraries.

Births

All births (including stillbirths) must be registered within 42 days in the district in which the birth occurred, either at the register office or in the hospital before the mother leaves. This can be done by either parent, or both if married. A father not married to the mother can register the birth jointly with her to ensure parental responsibility. ⚠ A father has parental responsibility if he is listed on the birth certificate. If neither the mother nor the father can register the birth, someone present at the birth, or with responsibility for the child, can do so.

Marriages

A man and a woman may marry if both are aged ≥16yrs (those aged 16 and 17yrs need parental consent) and single, widowed, or divorced, or in a civil partnership that has been dissolved, and are not closely related to each other. Same-sex marriage is legal in England, Scotland, and Wales. A transsexual person with a full gender recognition certificate can marry someone of the opposite sex. Details of prohibited marriages of relatives are available through the Citizens Advice Bureau.

Before a marriage ceremony, both parties are required to give notice in their local register office. A marriage can be a civil or religious ceremony, and can take place in any register office or LA-approved premises. The legal requirements for a marriage are that: both parties are free to marry; it is conducted by, or in the presence of, someone authorized to register it; and it is entered into the marriage register in the district where the ceremony takes place.

Civil partnerships

A civil partnership is a legal relationship that is registered by two people of the same or opposite sex who are not related. It can be formed in England, Scotland, Wales, or Northern Ireland, and can only be ended by death or application for dissolution in a court. Civil partnerships can be converted to a marriage in England, Scotland, or Wales.

Deaths

A death must be registered within 5 days in England (8 days in Scotland), but can be delayed for another 9 days if the registrar knows that a medical certificate of death has been issued (➔ Death confirmation and certification p. 840). Deaths reported to coroners cannot be registered until investigations are completed. If the death was at home, the registration is in that district. If the death was in hospital or a care home (➔ Care homes p. 32), then registration is in the district of the institution. Deaths can only be registered by: a relative, present at death or last illness (➔ Carers p. 458), or living in the district where death took place; anyone who was present at the death; the owner/occupier of the public building where the death occurred and who is aware of the death; the person arranging the funeral; and the executor or administrator of the deceased's estate.

The registrar will require the medical certificate of death and, if possible, certificates of birth and marriage and an NHS medical card. Once a death is registered, the registration office issues a certificate to allow the body to be buried or cremated.

Related topics

➔ Postnatal care p. 438; ➔ New birth visits p. 174; ➔ Coping with bereavement p. 574; ➔ Sudden infant death syndrome p. 278; ➔ Euthanasia, assisted suicide, and assisted dying p. 572

Further information

Citizens Advice Bureau (*What to do after a death*). Available at: ℳ https://www.citizensadvice.org. uk/family/death-and-wills/what-to-do-after-a-death/

Citizens Advice Bureau (*Getting married*). Available at: ℳ https://www.citizensadvice.org.uk/family/ living-together-marriage-and-civil-partnership/getting-married/

UK Government (*Register a birth*). Available at: ℳ https://www.gov.uk/register-birth

Index

Note: Tables, figures, and boxes are indicated by t, f, and b following the page number.

A

Abbey Pain Scale 555
abciximab 647
abdominal aortic aneurysm
    screening 388
Abortion Act (1967) 788
abuse
    children 250–1
    vulnerable adults
        454–5, 454b
accident prevention 168–9,
    202–3, 208–9
accountability 83
ACE inhibitors 648
Achilles tendon rupture 735
acne vulgaris 300–1
acral melanoma 682
acromegaly 701
actinic keratosis 683
activities of daily living
    model 111
acupuncture 838
acute cholecystitis 719
acute heart failure 636
acute leukaemia 315
acute low back pain 604
acute otitis media 288
acute pancreatitis 719
Addison's disease 700
ADHD 326–7
adherence 132–3
adhesive capsulitis 734
adolescents 228–9
    anxiety 330
    growth and
        nutrition 234–5
    mental health 246–7
    overweight 302
adoption 255
adrenal disorders 700
adrenal hyperplasia,
    congenital 262
adrenarche 299
adult basic life support 792–
    4, 792f, 793f, 795b
adult learners 54–5
advance care planning 551
advance decisions 471, 551
advanced nurse
    practitioner 40, 41
advance statements 471, 551
adverse drug reactions 130
adverse incidents and
    events 78–9

advocates 123
aerobic fitness 354
ageing, healthy 366–7
    see also older people
Agenda for Change 52
age-related macular
    degeneration 748
Ages and Stages
    Questionnaire 118
airflow obstruction 614
albinism 692
alcohol consumption
    360–1, 423
alcohol hand rubs 98, 98b
alginate dressings 534
allergic rhinitis 695
allergies 694–5, 694t
alopecia 692
alopecia areata 692
alveolitis 752
ambiguous genitalia 262
amblyopia 162
ambulatory oxygen 622
amenorrhoea 779
amiloride 649–50
amlodipine 648
amyotrophic lateral
    sclerosis 672
anaemia 652–4
anal abscess 707
anal cancer 707
anal fissure 706
anaphylaxis 810–13, 812f
anencephaly 274
angina 626–7, 627b
angiotensin-converting en-
    zyme inhibitors 648
angiotensin II antagonists 649
ankle brachial pressure index
    (ABPI) 536, 537t
ankle problems 735
anorexia nervosa
    474–5, 474b
antenatal care and screening
    426–8, 427f
antenatal education 425
anticholinergics 620
anticoagulant therapy 642–4
anti-discriminatory health
    care 81
anti-emetics 559t
anti-inflammatory agents 621
antimalarials 398
antimicrobial
    dressings 534–5

antimicrobial
    stewardship 146
antiplatelets 646–7
antiretroviral therapy 464
anxiety 330, 478–9
    signs and symptoms 478b
aphthous ulcers 696
apocrine glands 229
appendicitis 716
appraisal 52
aprons 100, 101
armed forces veterans 502
aromatherapy 838
arterial leg ulcers 537t
asbestosis 752
Asperger syndrome 323
aspirin 646, 647
assessment tools 118
assisted conception 784
assisted dying/suicide 572–3
assistive technology 834–6
asthma 608–10
    acute (attacks) 612–13
    children 306–7
    drug management 620–1
    inhalers 307, 610
    occupational 752
    primary care services 609
    review and
        monitoring 609
    risk factors for (near-) fatal
        attacks 613
    secondary non-
        pharmacological
        prophylaxis 610
    self-management 609
asylum seekers 10, 444–5
ataxic cerebral palsy 321
atenolol 647
athetoid syndrome 321
athlete's foot 686
atopic eczema 284–5, 684
atorvastatin 649
atrial fibrillation 640, 641
atrophe blanche 540
atrophic vaginitis 786
attention-deficit hyper-
    activity disorder 326–7
audit 70–1, 70f
AUDIT (Alcohol Use
    Disorders Identification
    Test) 360
autistic spectrum
    disorder 322–3
autolytic debridement 529

automated external
    defibrillation 793, 794,
    795*b*, 804
automated peritoneal
    dialysis 755
autonomic dysreflexia 519
autosomal dominant
    inheritance 271
autosomal recessive
    inheritance 272

B

babies
    accident prevention 202–3
    ambiguous genitalia 262
    bathing 194
    birth injuries 258
    bottle feeding 186–7
    breastfeeding 140,
        182–4, 189
    cleft lip and palate 259
    colic 198
    congenital heart
        defects 260–1
    congenital
        impairments 262–3
    cradle cap 194
    crying 198–9
    emotional
        development 210–11
    growth 190
    hair care 194
    hygiene 194–5
    nail care 195
    nappies 195
    neural tube defects 274
    night waking 201
    posseting and
        regurgitation 282
    postnatal care 439
    pre-term 176–7
    projectile vomiting 282
    promoting safe
        development 202–3
    recovery position 796
    registration of birth 842
    sick babies 276–7
    skin cleaning 194
    sleeping 200–1, 200*b*
    soothing 198
    sudden infant death syn-
        drome 177, 278–9
    teething 196
    twins and multiple
        births 180
    weaning 188–9
    weighing and
        measuring 190
    see also newborns
Bacillus cereus 732*t*
backache 432

back pain 264, 604–5
bacterial skin
    infections 680–1
bacterial vaginosis 786
balloon gastrostomies 596
barrier
    contraceptives 416–17
Bartholins gland
    swellings 786
basal cell carcinoma
    374, 682–3
BCG 167, 393, 728
bedwetting 296
bee sting allergy 695
behavioural disorders 326–7
behavioural issues 216–17
behavioural modification 170
Belbin's team roles
    theory 59
benefits 430–1
benign prostatic
    hyperplasia 758
bereavement 574–5
best-interests decisions 470
beta-2 adrenergic
    agonists 620
beta blockers 647–8
biliary colic 719
Billing's method 418
binge eating disorder 475
biomedical model 111
bipolar affective
    disorder 482–4
birth injuries 258
birth marks 178
birth options 434
birth registration 842
bisoprolol 647
bitumen burns 817
blackheads 300
bladder
    overactive 504
    training 506, 506*b*
blame-free culture 78
bleeding
    external 814–15
    palliative care 566–7
blepharitis 746–7
blindness 748–9, 748*b*
blood-borne virus
    exposure 102–3
blood glucose monitoring
    665, 666–7
blood pressure
    measurement 628–9
blue spots 178
body maps 554
body mass index 206, 222–
    3, 342, 346, 347*f*
body odour 229
boil 680, 681

Bolam test 83
bone disorders
    264–6, 738–9
bone fractures 258,
    824, 824*b*
bone tumours 315
bottle feeding 186–7
bowel cancer screening 376
Bowen's disease 683
bow legs 264
brachial plexus palsy 258
Bradshaw's taxonomy of
    needs 111
bradycardia 640
brain tumours 315
Braxton Hicks
    contractions 434
breast awareness 378
breast cancer 378–9, 774–5
breast cysts 772
breastfeeding 140,
    182–4, 189
breast pain 772
breast screening 378–9
breast symptoms 772, 772*b*
breathlessness 560–1
brief interventions 170
Brief Pain Inventory 555
bronchiolitis 288
bronchodilators 620
bulimia nervosa 475
bunion 736
burns 816–17, 816*b*
bursitis 735

C

Caesarean section 436
calcium 343, 704
calcium-channel
    blockers 648
Caldicott guardians and
    principles 89
Calgary-Cambridge consult-
    ation guide 116
Campylobacter jejune 732*t*
cancer
    anal 707
    breast 378–9, 774–5
    cervical 380–5, 381*t*, 776
    childhood 314–15
    colorectal 705
    early signs 372
    lung 751
    ovarian 776
    prevention 372, 374–5
    prostate 759
    skin 374–5, 682–3
    uterine 776
    vaginal 776
    vulval 777
candesartan 649

candida infection 687, 786
capacity 82, 470–1
caps 416–17
captopril 648
caput succedaneum 258
carbohydrate 342
carbohydrate
    counting 664–5
carbuncle 680–1
cardiac glycosides 650
cardiac rehabilitation 634
cardiac rhythms,
    abnormal 640–1
cardiovascular disease, drug
    management 646–50
Care Act (2014) 459
care co-ordination 114
care homes 32–3, 552
care management 114–15
care needs assessment 835
care of next infant 279
care planning 114
Care Quality
    Commission 79
carers 458–60
    assessment 118, 459
    benefits 460
    contribution 459
    impact of caring 458
    support for 460
    young carers 459
Carer's Allowance 460
Carer's Credit 460
Carer's Premium 460
carpal tunnel syndrome 735
carvedilol 647
case closure 115
case finding 114
caseload profiling 64–5
case management 114–15
case managers 22
cataract 748
CD registers 148
cellulitis 548, 681, 681b
central venous
    catheters 582–3
cephalhaematoma 258
cerebral palsy 320–1
cerumen 591
cervical cancer 380–5,
    381t, 776
cervical sample
    taking 384–5
cervical screening
    380–5, 381t
cervical spine injury 796
cervical spondylosis 734
challenging behaviour 457
change, talk of 126
chaperones 84
cheilitis 687

chemical burns 817, 819
chemotherapy 546–7
chest compressions
    adults 794
    children 803b
chickenpox 291t, 293t,
    621, 690–1
child abuse 250–1
child basic life support
    800–4, 801f, 802b,
    803b, 804f
childbirth
    birth options 434
    Caesarean section 436
    episiotomy 436–7
    forceps/ventouse 436
    induced labour 436
    labour 434–5
    postnatal care 438–9
childcare 24
child development
    programme 170
child health promotion pro-
    grammes 152–4, 154t
child protection 248–52
child protection
    conference 252
children
    abuse 250–1
    accident prevention
        168–9, 208–9
    additional communication
        needs 122–3
    ADHD 326–7
    adopted 255
    assessment 156–7, 156f
    asthma 306–7
    autistic spectrum
        disorder 322–3
    behavioural
        disorders 326–7
    behavioural issues 216–17
    bereaved 575
    bone problems 264–6
    cancer 314–15
    cerebral palsy 320–1
    choking 806, 806b, 807f,
        807b, 808b, 808
    communication
        problems 224–5
    complex health
        needs 238–9
    conduct disorder 327
    congenital heart
        defects 260–1
    congenital
        impairments 262–3
    consent 82
    constipation 286–7
    contraception provision
        for 401
    cystic fibrosis 318–19

deafness 268–9
deliberate self-harm 494
dental health 196–7,
    196b, 226
depressive
    behaviours 328–9
developmental progress
    192, 193t, 204, 205t,
    220–1, 220t
development
    screening 118
diabetes 304
diarrhoea 282–3
diet 212, 234
disabled 238–9
eczema 284–5
education 24
emotional
    development 210–11
emotional
    problems 330–1
encopresis 287
endocrine
    problems 304–5
epilepsy 280–1
evidence of harm 250
eye screening 162
febrile convulsions 280
food preferences/
    refusal 213
foods to avoid 213, 235
gastrointestinal
    problems 282–3
genetic problems 270–3
growing pains 265, 735
growth 190–1, 206,
    222–3, 234–5
growth disorders 298–9
Healthy Child Programme
    154, 154t
hearing screening 163
HIV 463
immunization 164–7, 166t
impact of adult health
    problems 159
inborn errors of
    metabolism 305
infections 288–9
infectious diseases 290,
    291t, 293t
infestations 294–5
insect bites and stings 294
as interpreters 122
joint problems 264–6
learning disabilities 456–7
learning problems 224–5
looked-after 254–5
mental health 171, 246–7
in need 24, 158–9
neglect 251
new siblings 217
nocturnal enuresis 296

children (contd)
  nutrition 212–13,
    223, 234–5
  overweight 223, 302
  physical examination 160
  prescribing for 139
  promoting development
    of under-fives 208–9
  protecting/
    safeguarding 248–52
  recovery position 796
  respiratory tract
    infections 288–9
  retention of records 87
  risk of abuse/neglect 250
  screening tests 160–3
  sepsis 827b
  services for 24–5
  sex and relationship
    education 236–7
  sick children 276–7
  sickle cell
    disorders 308–10
  social services 30
  special educational needs
    45, 242–4
  speech and language
    acquisition 218–19
  statistics 152
  temper tantrums 217
  thalassaemia 312
  toilet training 214
  travel vaccination 399
  underweight 223
  urinary tract
    infections 289
  vegan/vegetarian diets
    212, 234
  vision screening 162
  vitamin supplements 189
  vomiting 282–3
  vulnerable 165
  young carers 459
Children Act (1989)
  158, 159
Children Act (2004) 152,
  158, 239
Children and Families Act
  (2014) 238
children's centres 173
chiropractic 839
chlamydia 764
choking 798–9, 799f, 806,
  806b, 807f, 807b,
  808b, 808
cholecystitis 719
cholera vaccination 399
cholesterol 632
chronic heart failure 636
chronic kidney disease
  754–5, 755b
chronic low back pain 604

chronic obstructive pul-
  monary disease 614–15
  drug management 620–1
  exacerbation 618, 619t
  management 616, 617b
  pulmonary
    rehabilitation 616
chronic pancreatitis 719
chronic plaque
  psoriasis 688t
chronic secretory otitis
  media 288
chronic simple
  glaucoma 748
cirrhosis 718
civil partnerships 842
clavicle fracture 258
claw toes 736
cleaning, hygienic 353
cleft lip and palate 259
client-held records 90
clinical audit 70–1, 70f
clinical commissioning
  groups 8
clinical governance 68
clinical medication
  review 142
clinical risk management
  78–9, 78b
clinical supervision 52
clinical waste 106–7, 106t
clitoridectomy 492
clopidogrel 647
closed fracture 824
Clostridium botulinum 732t
Clostridium perfringens 732t
clubfoot 264
coal worker's
  pneumoconiosis 752
cochlear implant 268
coeliac disease 714
cognitive behavioural
  therapy 472
cold burns 817
cold weather 371
colic 198
colorectal cancer 705
colostomy 516–17
Combat Stress 502
combined oral contra-
  ceptive pill 402–4,
  402t, 403b
  missed pill rules 406f
comedones 300
commissioning 12, 13t, 65
common assess-
  ment framework
  156–7, 158–9
common cold 288
communication
  additional communication
    needs 122–3

deaf children 269
dying phase 568
English as a second
  language 122
principles of good
  communication 120–1
problems in
  children 224–5
community dental
  service 20
community development
  335, 338
community-focused health
  promotion 335, 338
Community Health
  Councils 9
community hospitals
  16, 552
community hubs 338
community matron 22, 115
community occupational
  therapists 21
community organization
  theories 334t
community pharmacists 21
community
  physiotherapists 21
community podiatry
  service 21
community practitioner
  nurse prescribers 128
community profiling 64
competency 82
complaints procedures 76
complementary and alter-
  native therapies 838–9
compression-only CPR 794
compression therapy
  542–4, 543t
compromised
  immunity 466
concordance 132
condoms 416
conduct disorder 327
confidentiality 89, 760
  child protection 252
congenital heart
  defects 260–1
congenital
  impairments 262–3
congenital ocular
  opacities 162
CONI 279
conjunctivitis 289,
  293t, 746
connective tissue
  disorders 738–9
consent 55, 82
constipation
  adults 512–13
  children 286–7
  pregnancy 432

consultation models and frameworks 116–17
consumer protection department 27
contact dermatitis 684
contact lens-related red eye 819
continuing professional development 53
continuity of care 598, 598b
continuous ambulatory peritoneal dialysis 755
contraception 400–1
  barrier methods 416–17
  choice of method 400
  combined oral contraceptive pill 402–4, 402t, 403b
  diaphragms and caps 416–17, 416f
  effectiveness of different methods 400t
  emergency 420–1
  female condoms 416
  intrauterine devices 413–14
  intrauterine systems 415
  male condoms 416
  menopause 401
  missed pill rules 406f
  natural family planning 418
  NuvaRing® 402t, 405, 407f
  progestogen injectables 411–12
  progestogen-only pill (mini-pill) 410–11
  progestogen subdermal implants 412
  spermicides 417
  sterilization 418–19
  transdermal patches 402t, 404, 408f
  under 16s 401
contracting 12, 13t, 65
controlled drugs 144–5, 148
Control of Substances Hazardous to Health (2002) 92
cording 775
corneal abrasion 818
corneal ulcer 819
coronary heart disease 624, 625b
corporate caseloads 47
corticosteroids 621
coryza 288
co-sleeping 200
cot death 177, 278–9

counselling 472
Court of Protection 471
cow's milk 187
cradle cap 194
craniosynostosis 299
cri du chat syndrome 271
crime victims 452–3
critical appraisal 72
critical pathway analysis 63
Crohn's disease 712–13, 712b
cross-cutting approaches 14
croup 289
crying 198–9
Cushing's syndrome 700
cyclothymic disorder 483
cystic basal cell carcinoma 683
cystic fibrosis 318–19
cystitis 756
cysts
  breast 772
  ovarian 780
cytomegalovirus 262

D

DAFNE 665
daily living aids 835
damp 26
Data Protection Act (2018) 88
deafness 268–9, 696
death
  certification 840–1
  major causes of 2
  registration 842–3
  verification 840
debridement 528–9, 541
deep vein thrombosis 657–8
defibrillator 793, 794, 795b, 804
delayed puberty 299
deliberate self-harm 494, 495b, 495–6, 823
delinquency 327
dementia 498
  assessment tools 118
  diagnosis 498
  nurse's role 499–500
  Parkinson's disease 674–5
  pharmacological treatment 499
  prognosis 498
  signs and symptoms 498
dental fluorosis 197
dental health 196–7, 196b, 226
dental health promotion programmes 197
dentists 20

Department for Health and Social Services 9
Department of Health 8
Department of Health and Social Care 8
dependence syndrome 476
dependent drinking 361
depression 478, 479–80
  assessment 118
  bipolar affective disorder 482
  palliative care 564
  postnatal 440–1
  signs and symptoms 479b
depressive behaviours 328–9
dermatitis 684–5
dermatophyte infection 686
DESMOND 667
developmental hip dysplasia 264
development of children 192, 193t, 204, 205t, 220–1, 220t
devolution 13t
diabetes insipidus 701
diabetes mellitus 660
  annual review 668
  blood glucose monitoring 665, 666–7
  cardiovascular risk 666, 667
  children 304
  complications 666
  eye problems 666
  foot problems 666
  gestational 661
  hypoglycaemia 665, 667
  hypoglycaemic awareness 665, 667
  insulin therapy 664, 666
  maturity onset diabetes of the young 661
  patient education programmes (DAFNE/ DESMOND) 665, 667
  personalized care plan 667
  prediabetes 661–2
  principles of management 664–8
  renal complications 666
  type 1: 660, 664–6
  type 2: 660–1, 666–7
diabetic ketoacidosis 660, 665, 666
diabetic retinopathy 749
diagnostic model 111
dialysis 755
diaphragms 416–17, 416f
diarrhoea
  children 282–3
  traveller's 397

diet 212, 234, 343, 422
    diabetes 664–5, 666
diffusion of innovation
    theory 334t
digoxin 650
dihydropyridines 648
diltiazem 648
diphtheria 291t
diphtheria vaccination 399
directed enhanced
    services 18–19
disabled children 238–9
discharge from hospital 23
discoid eczema 684
discrimination 81
disease-modifying anti-
    rheumatic drugs 603
dislocated shoulder 734
dispensing medicines 129
dispensing opticians 20
district nursing 32, 50–1
diuretics 649–50
diverticulitis 716
diverticulosis 716
domestic violence 450–1
donor insemination 784
do not attempt car-
    diopulmonary
    resuscitation 551
Down's syndrome 270
dressings 524, 532–5
drugs see medicines
duodenal ulceration 709
duty of care 83
dying 568–9
    services for the dying and
        carers 552
    see also death;
        palliative care
dyscalculia 224
dysfluency 225
dyskinetic syndromes 321
dyslexia 224
dysmenorrhoea 779
dyspareunia 768
dyspepsia 708
dyspraxia 224

E

ear care 590–2
early years services 24
ear wax 591
eating disorders
    474–5, 474b
eccrine glands 229
ECG 584–5, 584f
E. coli 732t
eczema 284–5, 684–5
eczema herpeticum 690
Edinburgh Postnatal
    Depression Scale 440–1

education
    advanced nurse
        practitioners 41
    antenatal 425
    children and young
        people 24
    district nurses 51
    health visitors 47
    practice nurses 41
    school nurses 43
    see also schools
Edward's syndrome 270
elbow problems 735
elderly
    healthy ageing 366–7
    physical activity 355
    prescribing for
        138–9, 138b
electrical burns 817
electrocardiogram
    584–5, 584f
electronic records 87b
EllaOne® 420–1
embryo donation 784
emergencies see first aid
    and emergencies
emergency
    accommodation 447
emergency
    contraception 420–1
emotional abuse 251
emotional
    development 210–11
emotional
    problems 330–1
enalapril 648
encephalocoele 274
encopresis 287
endocrine problems 304–5
end-of-life 550, 572–3
endometriosis 780
end-stage renal
    disease 754–5
enduring power of
    attorney 471
energy requirements 342
engagement, patient 340
England
    commissioning 12, 13t
    NHS 8
English as a second
    language 122
enteral tube feeding 594–6
Enterobius vermicularis
    293t, 295
environmental health
    services 27
epidemiological-focused
    health promotion
    approaches 335
epilepsy 280–1, 740–2
episiotomy 436–7
Equality Act (2010) 81, 836

equality impact
    assessment 81
equity 14
Erb's palsy 258
erectile dysfunction 769
erythema infectiosum 291t
erythrodermic
    psoriasis 688t
Escherichia coli 732t
estimated average require-
    ments for energy 342
estimated delivery date 424
ethics 56–7
euthanasia 572–3, 572b
evidence-based clinical
    practice 72
evidence-based healthcare
    72–3, 72b
Evra® 408f
excision (female genital
    mutilation) 492
exercise 354–5
    diabetes 665, 666
expert patients 340
expressing milk 183
express verbal consent 82
express written
    consent 82
externalizing
    disorders 326–7
extrinsic allergic
    alveolitis 752
exudate 522, 531, 541
eye problems 289, 746–9
    diabetes 666
    new babies 179
    screening children 162
    trauma 818–19, 818b
eye protection 101

F

face masks 100, 101
facial palsy 258
facial psoriasis 688t
faecal incontinence 514–15
faith healing 838
falls prevention 368–9
faltering weight gain 191
families
    assessment 156–7, 156f
    services for 24–5
    social services 30
    support for parents 172
family information
    services 24
fasting glucose 661–2
FAST test 830, 830b
fatigue 562
fats 342
fear 330
febrile convulsions 280

female genital mutilation (FGM) 492, 493t
fertility awareness 423
fertility problems 784
fetal alcohol syndrome 423
fibre 342
fibro-adenoma 772
fibroids 780
5th disease 291t
film dressings 533
first aid and emergencies
  adult basic life support 792–4, 792f, 793f, 795b
  anaphylaxis 810–13, 812f
  bleeding 814–15
  burns and scalds 816–17, 816b
  child basic life support 800–4, 801f, 802b, 803b, 804f
  choking 798–9, 799f, 806, 806b, 807f, 807b, 808b, 808
  consent 82
  eye trauma 818–19, 818b
  fractures 824, 824b
  hypothermia 819, 819b
  palliative care 566–7
  poisoning and overdoses 822–3
  recovery position 794, 796
  sepsis 826, 827b, 828b, 828
  sprains and strains 824, 824b
  tracheostomy 589
first parenting programmes 173
Five Year Forward View 112
flat feet 264, 736
flexibility 354
flexural psoriasis 688t
floaters 747
flu
  exclusion time 293t
  immunization 392
  pandemic 726–7, 726b
  seasonal 720
fluoride supplements 197
fluoride varnish 197
foam dressings 533
focal epilepsy 740
folate deficiency 653–4
folliculitis 680
food allergies and intolerances 189, 284, 695
food hygiene and safety 27b, 352–3

food poisoning 27b, 422–3, 730–1, 732t
food preferences/refusal 213
foods to avoid in children 213, 235
foot
  diabetes 666
  musculoskeletal problems 735–6
forced expiratory volume in 1s (FEV₁) 606, 606t
forced vital capacity (FVC) 606, 606t
forceps delivery 436
foreign bodies
  airway 798–9, 806–8
  eye 819
formula milk 186
foundation trusts 8
Foyers 447
fractures 258, 824, 824b
fragile X syndrome 272–3
frailty 678
Fraser Guidelines 401
Freedom of Information Act (2000) 88
free prescription entitlement 134
frozen shoulder 734
full medication review 142
fungal infections 686–7
fungating wounds 530–1
furosemide 649, 650
furuncle 680, 681

G

galactosaemia 305
gallstones 719
GANTT chart 63, 63f
gastric ulceration 709
gastritis 708
gastroenteritis 293t
gastro-oesophageal reflux disease 708
gastrostomy tubes 594–5
gender
  cause of death 2
  life expectancy 2
generalized anxiety disorder 330
General Medical Service contract 18–19
general palliative care 550, 552
general practice 18–19
  dispensing practices 19
  list closures 19
  new patient health check 387
  out of hours 19

practice nurses 40–1
registration with 19
removal from practice list 19
retention of records 87
storage of medicines 148
generic long-term conditions model 6
genetic counselling 422
genetic problems 270–3
genetic screening 422
genital herpes 764
genitals
  ambiguous 262
  new babies 179
genital warts 764
genu varum 264
gestational diabetes mellitus 661
gingivitis 696
glandular fever 293t, 721
glaucoma 748
glomerulonephritis 754
gloves 100, 101
glucose (fasting) 661–2
glue ear 288
glyceryl trinitrate 627, 646
glycogen storage diseases 272
glycoprotein IIb/IIIa inhibitors 647
glycosylated haemoglobin (HbA1C) 665, 666–7
GMS contract 18–19
goggles 100
goitre 702
Gold Standard Framework 551
golfer's elbow 735
gonorrhoea 765
GORD 708
governance 57
GPIIa/IIIa inhibitors 647
GPs 18
GP specialties 18
grand mal epilepsy 740
Graves' disease 305, 702
gravitational eczema 684
grief 574–5
Groshong line 592
group health promotion 335, 336–7
growing pains 265, 735
growth 190–1, 206, 222–3, 234–5
growth charts 190–1, 191f, 206
growth disorders 298–9
GTN 627, 646
guidelines 72
gum inflammation 696
guttate psoriasis 688t
gypsies 448–9

H

haemodialysis 755
Haemophilus influenzae 291t
haemorrhage see bleeding
haemorrhoids 432, 706
hair
  baby hair care 194
  excess hairiness 692
  loss 692
  new babies 178
hair follicle infections 680–1
hallux valgus 736
hammer toes 736
hand hygiene 98–9, 98b
handling aids 96–7
handling patients 96–7, 97b
hand problems 735
harlequin colour
  change 178
hay fever 695
HbA1C 665, 666–7
HDL cholesterol 632
head
  growth abnormalities 299
  newborns 178
head lice 293t, 294–5
health and safety at
  work 92–3
Health and Safety at Work
  Act (1974) 27b, 92
Health and Safety
  Executive 79
Health and Social Care Act
  (2012) 12, 42
Health and Social Care
  Board 8
Health and Social Care
  Trusts 8
Health and Well-being
  Boards 15
health belief model 334t
healthcare rights 80
healthcare waste
  106–7, 106t
health impact
  assessment 14
health inequalities 2
health needs assessment
  15, 110–12
health promotion
  ageing 366–7
  child programmes
    152–4, 154t
  dental health 197
  group work 335, 336–7
  models and approaches
    334–5, 334t
  in schools 230–1
  sexual health 761
  travel 396–7
health visitors 14, 46–7

Health Watch 8, 12
healthy ageing 366–7
Healthy Child Programme
  154, 154t
healthy eating 342–3, 344b
Healthy Start 431
hearing aids 268
hearing problems
  268–9, 696
hearing screening 163
heart defects 260–1
heart failure 636–8, 637b
heart rhythms,
  abnormal 640–1
heat exhaustion 370
heat rash 178
heatstroke 370
heel prick blood
  samples 160
Helicobacter pylori 708
'hello my name is …'
  campaign 118
hepatitis A 293t, 724
hepatitis A vaccination
  393, 399
hepatitis B 102, 293t,
  724–5, 724b
hepatitis B vaccination
  393, 399
hepatitis C 102, 293t, 725
hepatitis E 725
herbal medicine 838
hernias 716–17
  hiatus 709
  incisional 717
  umbilical 178, 717
herpes simplex 293t,
  690, 721
herpes varicella zoster see
  chickenpox
herpes zoster 691, 721
hiatus hernia 709
Hickman line 592
hierarchy of evidence 72b
high-density lipoprotein 632
highly active antiretroviral
  therapy (HAART) 464
hip disorders of
  childhood 264
hirsutism 692
HIV 293t, 462–4
  exposure 102, 103b
  prevention 462
  progression 462, 463t
  testing 763
Hodgkin's lymphoma 315
homelessness 26, 446–7
homeopathy 165, 838
homes
  adaptations 834, 835
  assistive
    technology 834–6

chemotherapy in 546–7
housing issues 26, 446–7
hygiene 352–3
palliative care in 550–1
storing medicines 148–9
visiting 94–5, 172
Home-Start 173
home tutoring 24
honey dressings 535
hormone replacement
  therapy 365
horseshoe kidney 263
hospices 552
hospital at home 23
hospital discharge 23
hostels 447
hot flushes 365
hot weather 370–1, 370b
housing 26, 446–7
housing associations 26
Human Fertilization/
  Embryology Act
  (1990) 788
human immunodeficiency
  virus (HIV) 293t, 462–4
  exposure 102, 103b
  prevention 462
  progression 462, 463t
  testing 763
human papilloma virus
  testing 382
Human Rights Act
  (1998) 80, 81
humerus fracture 258
hydrocolloid dressings 533
hydrofibre dressings 534
hydrogel dressings 533
hygiene
  babies 194–5
  food 27b, 352–3
  hands 98–9, 98b
  in the home 352–3
hypercalcaemia 704
  palliative care 566
hypercholesterolaemia 632–3
hyperglycaemic
  hyperosmolar state 667
hyperlipidaemia 632
hypersensitivity
  pneumonitis 752
hypertension 628–30
hyperthyroidism 305, 702
hypertrichosis 692
hypnotherapy 838–9
hypocalcaemia 704
hypoglycaemia 304,
  665, 667
hypopituitarism 701
hypospadias 262
hypothermia 819, 819b
hypothyroidism 304, 702–3
hysterectomy 782–3

I

ICSI 784
ileal conduit 517
ileostomy 516–17
immunizations
  administration 390–1
  children 164–7, 166*t*
  targeted adult 392–3
  travellers 399
immunodeficiency 466
impaired fasting glucose/
  glucose tolerance 661–2
impetigo 293*t*, 680
implied consent 82
inborn errors of
  metabolism 305
incisional hernia 717
incontinence
  faecal 514–15
  urinary *see* urinary
    incontinence
independent mental cap-
  acity advocates 471
independent nurse
  prescribers 128
indigestion 432
individual health needs
  assessment 110–12
individual health
  promotion 335
induced labour 436
indwelling catheters 508–10
inequalities in health 2
infants
  basic life support 800–4,
    801*f*, 802*b*, 803*b*, 804*f*
  growth 190
  mortality 2
  prescribing for 139
  see also babies; children
infection
  bacterial skin 680–1
  childhood 288–9
  congenital 262
  fungal 686–7
  upper respiratory
    tract 288
  urinary tract 289,
    510, 756
  viral 690–1, 720–1
  wounds 526–7
infectious disease 27*b*, 290,
  291*t*, 293*t*, 467
  notifications 104–5, 104*b*
infectious
  mononucleosis 293*t*
infectious waste 106
infertility 784
infestations 294–5
infibulation (female genital
  mutilation) 492

inflammatory bowel disease
  712–13, 712*b*
influenza
  exclusion time 293*t*
  immunization 392
  pandemic 726–7, 726*b*
  seasonal 720
information provision 121
ingrowing toe nail 736
inhalers 307, 610
injection techniques 576–8
inner consultation 116
innovation 62–3
INR testing 643
insect bites and stings
  294, 695
instrumental delivery 436
insulin therapy 664, 666
integrated assessment 112,
  158–9, 238
integrated care
  pathways 73
integrated care systems 13*t*
Integrated Research
  Application System
  (IRAS) 57
international normalized
  ratio (INR) testing 643
interpreters 122
intersectoral work 14
intertrigo 687
intestinal obstruction 717
intimate examinations 84
intracytoplasmic sperm
  injection 784
intramuscular
  injections 576–7
intrauterine devices
  413–14, 421
intrauterine
  insemination 784
intrauterine systems 415
in vitro fertilization 784
iodine dressings 534
iron 343
iron deficiency anaemia 652
irritable bowel syndrome 710
irritable hip 264
isosorbide dinitrate/
  mononitrate 646
IVF 784

J

Japanese B encephalitis
  vaccination 399
jewellery 98
joint disorders 264–6
Joint Health and Well-being
  Strategies 15
Joint Strategic Needs
  Assessments 15

junior staff, duty of care 83
juvenile idiopathic (chronic)
  arthritis 265

K

Keele STarT Back Screening
  Tool 604
kerion 686
Klinefelter's syndrome 271
Klumpke's palsy 258
knock knees 264

L

labour 434–5
  induction 436
language
  acquisition 218–19
lanugo 178
large for gestational
  age 190
larval therapy 529
laryngectomy 586, 589
laryngitis 698–9
lasting power of attorney
  470, 471
latex gloves 100
laundry 353
laxatives 513
LDL cholesterol 632
leadership 60–1
learning disabilities 456–7
  sexual health 770–1
learning problems 224–5
leg cramps 735
leg ulcers
  arterial 537*t*
  assessment 536–8
  compression therapy
    542–4, 543*t*
  venous 537*t*, 540–4
leisure activities 25
lentigo maligna
  melanoma 682
leukaemia 315
leukotriene receptor
  antagonists 621
Levonelle® 420
levonorgestrel 420
libido 769
life expectancy 2
lipodermatosclerosis 540
lisinopril 648
Listeria monocytogenes 732*t*
liver disease
  cirrhosis 718
  prescribing 140
local authority housing 26
local commissioning
  groups 8
local health boards 9

locally enhanced services 18
loneliness 28
lone working 94–5
long-acting beta-2 agonists 620
long-acting muscarinic antagonists 620
long-term conditions 6, 114
long-term oxygen therapy 622
looked-after children 254–5
losartan 649
loss 574–5
low back pain 604–5
low birthweight 190
low-density lipoprotein 632
low income benefits 791
lung disease
  cancer 751
  occupational 752
lung function 606–7
lymphoedema 548–9, 775
lymphogranuloma venereum 765
lymphoma 315

M

macrocephaly 299
macular degeneration 748
malaria 398
malignant fungating wounds 530–1
malignant melanoma 374, 375, 682
malnutrition 350–1
Malnutrition Universal Screening Tool 350, 351t
mammography screening 378–9
mania 482, 482t
manual handling 96–7, 97b
manual lymphatic drainage 549
marble bone disease 266
Marfan's disease 266
marriage 842
Maslow's hierarchy of needs 111
mastalgia 772
maternal health 438
maternity allowance 431
maternity benefits 430–1
Maternity Exemption Certificate 134
maternity leave 430
maternity records 87
maternity rights 430
maturity onset diabetes of the young 661

McGill Pain Questionnaire 555
measles 291t, 293t
mechanical debridement 529
meconium 179
Medical and Healthcare Products Regulatory Agency 79
Medical Exemption Certificate 134
medicines
  adherence 132–3
  administration 129, 145
  adverse drug reactions 130
  concordance 132
  controlled drugs 144–5, 148
  dispensing 129
  disposal 149
  errors in dispensing or administration 129
  feeding tubes 595–6
  help with costs 134–5
  management teams 21
  optimization 128–30
  out-of-date/ unwanted 149
  reviewing 142–3
  in schools 44–5
  storage 148–9
  transportation 149
  see also prescribing
medicines use review 142
meningitis vaccination 392, 399
meningococcal disease 293t
meningocoele 274
menopause 364–5, 401
menorrhagia 778–9
menstrual problems 778–9
mental capacity 82, 470–1
Mental Capacity Act (MCA, 2005) 470
mental health
  armed forces veterans 502
  assessment tools 118
  children and adolescents 171, 246–7
Mental Health Act (1983, amended 2007) 487
mental illness 87
mesothelioma 752
metastatic spinal cord compression 566
metformin 666
methicillin-resistant Staphylococcus aureus 722–3
metoprolol 647

microcephaly 299
midwives 14
migraine 744
milia 178
minerals 343
Mini-Mental State Examination 118
mini-pill 410–11
miscarriage 784
mixed incontinence 504
MMR 164
molluscum contagiosum 690
mood 229
morphoeic basal cell carcinoma 683
motivational interviewing 126
motor fitness 354
motor neurone disease 672–3
mouth-to-nose ventilation 794
mouth ulcers 698
moving patients 96–7, 97b
MRC dyspnoea scale 614t
MRSA 722–3
multidisciplinary specialist teams 16
multiple births 180
multiple sclerosis 670–1
mumps 291t, 293t
muscular endurance 354
muscular strength 354
musculoskeletal problems 734–5
myelomeningocoele 274
myoclonic epilepsy 740
myxoedema 702–3

N

nail psoriasis 688t
nappies 195
nasogastric tubes 594
National Health Service see NHS
National Institute for Health Research 56
National Reporting and Learning System 79
natural family planning 418
nausea 432, 558, 559t
nebulizers 623
neck problems 734
neglect 251
negligence 83
neighbour (inner consultation) 116
neonatal hypothyroidism 304
nephroblastoma 315

nephrotic syndrome 754
neural tube
  defects 274–5
neuroblastoma 315
neurogenic bladder 518
neurogenic bowel 518–19
new birth visits 174–5
newborns
  appearance 178–9
  birth injuries 258
  blood spot
    screening 160–1
  first nappies 179
  hearing screening 163
  new birth visits 174–5
  pre-term 176–7
new patient health
  check 387
new roles, duty of care 83
Nexplanon® 412
NHS 8–9
  Bowel Cancer Screening
    Programme 376
  Breast Screening
    Programme 378–9
  care home fees 32
  commissioning 12, 13t
  entitlements 10
  Friends and Family
    Test 75
  Healthcare Leadership
    Model 60
  Health Check 387
  health, safety and
    welfare 93
  Knowledge and Skills
    Framework 52
  Overall Patient
    Experience Survey 75
  public health 14
  Research Ethics
    Committees 56
  trusts 8
nicotine replacement
  therapy 357
nifedipine 648
night shelters 447
Nightstop 447
night sweats 365
nitrates spray 627, 646
NMC
  Code 80
  continuing professional
    development 53
nocturnal enuresis 296
nodular basal cell
  carcinoma 683
nodular melanoma 682
nodular squamous cell
  carcinoma 683
noise problems 27b
nondihydropyridines 648

non-gonococcal
  urethritis 765
non-Hodgkin's
  lymphoma 315
non-melanoma skin cancer
  374, 375, 682–3
non-vitamin K oral anti-
  coagulants 642, 644
norovirus 732t
Northern Ireland, NHS 8
notifiable diseases
  104–5, 104b
nummular eczema 684
nurse independent
  prescribers 128
nurse practitioner 40, 41
nurse prescribing 128
nursery schools 24
nurses, public health
  role 14
Nursing and Midwifery
  Council (NMC)
  Code 80
  continuing professional
    development 53
nutrition 212–13, 223,
  234–5, 342–3, 344b
nutritional supplements 351
NuvaRing® 402t, 405, 407f

O

obesity 348–9
  prevention 234–5
occupational
  exposure 102–3
occupational health and
  safety 27b
occupational lung
  disease 752
occupational therapists 21
Office of the Public
  Guardian 471
older people
  healthy ageing 366–7
  physical activity 355
  prescribing for
    138–9, 138b
oncology records 87
oocyte donation 784
open fracture 824
opticians 20
organizational change
  theory 334t
orthodontics 226
osteoarthritis 600–1
osteogenesis
  imperfecta 265
osteomalacia 738
osteomyelitis 265, 738
osteopathy 839
osteopetrosis 266

osteosarcoma 315
otitis media 288
out of hours 19
ovarian cancer 776
ovarian cysts 780
overactive bladder 504
overdoses 822–3
overflow incontinence 504
overseas visitors, en-
  titlement to NHS
  treatment 10
overweight 223,
  302, 348–9
ovulation estimation 418
oxygen therapy 622

P

Paget's disease of bone 738
pain
  assessment and man-
    agement 554–5,
    555f, 556t
  in labour 434
  palliative care 554–5
palliative care
  breathlessness 560–1
  children 314–15
  depression 564
  dying phase 568–9
  emergencies 566–7
  fatigue 562
  at home 550–1
  nausea and vomiting
    558, 559t
  pain management 554–5
  spiritual care 564
  syringe drivers 570
palpitations 640
pancreatitis 719
pandemic influenza
  726–7, 726b
paratyphoid 293t
parent advisory models 170
parents
  antenatal education 425
  childcare options 24
  child mental health 171
  good enough
    parenting 172
  support for 172–3
  working with 170–1
Parkinson's disease 674–5
paronychia 687
partial sight 748–9, 748b
participatory learning 336
partnership approaches to
  health promotion 338
partnership intersectoral
  work 14
passive smoking 356
paste bandaging 285

Patau's syndrome 270
paternity leave and pay 431
Patient and Client Council 8
patient and public
  involvement 8, 9
patient engagement 340
patient experience 75
patient group
  directions 129
patient-held records 90
patient records see records
patient-reported outcome
  measures 75
patient's home see homes
patient-specific
  direction 129
payment exemption
  certificates 134
peak expiratory flow
  rate 606–7
Pediculus capitis 293t, 294–5
peer support 172
PEG 594
pelvic floor exercises
  506, 506b
pelvic organ prolapse 781
Pendleton consultation
  model 116
Pension Credit 460
peptic ulceration 709
percutaneous endoscopic
  gastrostomy 594
peri-menopause 364
perindopril 648
peripherally inserted central catheter 582–3
permissions 57
pernicious anaemia 654
personal development
  plan 53
Personal Medical Service
  contract 18
personal protective
  equipment 100–1
pertussis 291t, 293t
pes planum 264, 736
pest control 27b
petit mal epilepsy 740
pharmacists 20–1
phenylketonuria 305
phlebotomy 580–1
phobias 330–1
photokeratitis 819
phototherapy 689
physical abuse 251
physical activity 354–5
  diabetes 665, 666
physiotherapists 21
phytonutrients 343
pigmentation 692
piles see haemorrhoids
pilonidal sinus 707

pituitary disorders 701
pituitary tumours 701
pityriasis versicolor 687
planning tools 63
plantar fasciitis 735
plastic aprons 100, 101
play 24
PMS contract 18
pneumococcal
  immunization 392
pneumoconiosis 752
pneumonia 289, 750
pneumonitis 752
podiatrists 20
poisoning 822–3
poliomyelitis 291t
poliomyelitis
  vaccination 399
pollution control 27b
polycystic ovary
  syndrome 780
polygenic inheritance 273
pompholyx 684
Portacath 592
portal hypertension 718
port wine stain 178
posseting 282
post-exposure prophylaxis
  103b, 103
postnatal care 438–9
postnatal depression 440–1
  assessment 118
post-operative wound
  care 524–5
post-partum psychosis 486
post-partum sepsis 829b
post-traumatic stress
  disorder (PTSD)
  490–1, 490t
postural hypotension 629b
posture 264
pravastatin 649
precocious puberty 299
preconceptual care 422–3
prediabetes 661–2
preferred priorities for
  care 551
pregnancy 424
  antenatal care and
    screening 426–8, 427f
  antenatal education 425
  backache 432
  birth options 434
  constipation 432
  diabetes 661, 665, 667
  estimated delivery
    date 424
  gestational diabetes 661
  haemorrhoids 432
  indigestion 432
  maternity benefits 430–1
  maternity leave 430

maternity rights 430
micturition 433
nausea and vomiting 432
prescribing 139
previous problems 423
sepsis 829b
termination 788–9
trimesters 424
twin and multiple 180
varicosities 432
premature ejaculation 769
premature menopause 364
premenstrual
  syndrome 778
pre-payment
  certificates 135
prescribing
  advisors 21
  breastfeeding 140
  controlled drugs 144
  infants and children 139
  liver disease 140
  non-medical 128
  nurse prescribing 128
  older people 138–9, 138b
  pregnancy 139
  renal disease 140
  ten-step model 136
prescription
  intervention 142
prescription review 142
prescriptions
  controlled drugs 144
  forms (FP10) 128
  free prescription
    entitlement 134
  payment exemption
    certificates 134
  pre-payment
    certificates 135
  security issues 137
  writing 137
pressure ulcers 519
  prevention 520–1
  risk assessment 118
pre-term infants 176–7
primary care
  asthma services 609
  care homes 32
  clinical audit 70–1, 70f
  co-commissioning 13t
  core elements 16
  definition 4
  overview of services 16
  range of services and
    professionals 20–1
  termination of
    pregnancy 788
  WHO vision 4b
primary care nursing 35–66
  appraisal 52
  clinical supervision 52

continuing professional
  development 53
district nursing 50–1
general practice
  nursing 50–1
health visiting 46–7
innovation 62–3
leadership 60–1
learning to work in pri-
  mary care 38
project planning 62–3
research in 56–7, 56f
school nursing 42–5
stakeholder
  management 62
teaching 54–5
teamwork 58–9
using information for
  practice 64–6
work roles 36–7
primary care
  pharmacists 21
private sector housing
  26, 27b
professional
  accountability 83
professional conduct 80
profiling 64–6
progestogen
  injectables 411–12
progestogen-only
  contraceptive pill
  (mini-pill) 410–11
progestogen subdermal
  implants 412
progressive bulbar
  palsy 672
progressive muscular
  atrophy 672
Prohibition of Female
  Genital Mutilation
  (Scotland) Act
  (2005) 492
projectile vomiting 282
project planning 62–3
proper officer 27b
propranolol 647
prostate cancer 759
prostate specific
  antigen 759
prostatitis 758
protein 342
protocols 72
pruritus 787
PSA test 759
PSHE 230–1
psoriasis 688–9, 688t
psychoanalytical
  therapy 472
psychodynamic therapy 472
psychosis 486–7
  Parkinson's disease 675

symptoms 487t
puberty 221, 228–9
  delayed 299
  precocious 299
pubic lice 765
public experience 75
public health
  definition 4
  in NHS 14
public interest 89
Public Interest Disclosure
  Act (1998) 85
puerperal psychosis 486
pulled elbow 735
pulmonary
  rehabilitation 616
pupil referral units 24, 45
pustular psoriasis 688t
pyelonephritis 756

Q

Quality and Outcomes
  Framework 74
quality governance 68

R

rabies 396
rabies vaccination 399
radical hysterectomy 782
radiologically inserted
  gastrostomy 594
ramipril 648
rape 761
rapid-response
  schemes 23
Raynaud's syndrome 739
reablement schemes 23
records 86–8
  access to 88
  electronic 87b
  leg ulcers 538
  patient-held 90
  retention 87
  storage 86, 87b
  urinary catheters 510
  what to include 86
  wound assessment 523
recovery position 794, 796
red eye 747b
  contact lens-related 819
reflexology 839
refugees 10, 444–5
regurgitation 282
relaxation techniques 359
remote consultation 124–5
renal problems 140, 754–5
renal stones 754
rented accommodation
  26, 27b
repetitive strain injury 735

Reporting of Injuries,
  Diseases and
  Dangerous Occurrences
  Regulations 92
rescue breaths 794,
  802b, 803b
research in primary care
  56–7, 56f
respiratory tract
  infections 288–9
retinal detachment 749
retinoblastoma 315
rhabdomyosarcoma 315
rheumatoid arthritis 602–3
RICE 824
rickets 738
RIDDOR 92
RIG 594
rings 98
ringworm 293t, 686
risk management 62,
  78–9, 78b
rodent ulcer 682–3
roseola infantum 291t
rubella 262, 291t, 293t, 422

S

safety representatives 92
Salmonella infection 732t
Sarcoptes scabie 293t, 295
scabies 293t, 295
scalds 816–17, 816b
scalp
  psoriasis 688t
  ringworm 686
scarlet fever 291t, 293t
schizophrenia 486, 487t, 487
schools
  food in 223, 235
  health promotion in
    (PSHE) 230–1
  medicines in 44–5
  notifiable diseases 105
  nursing in 42–5
  sex and relationship
    education 236–7
  special schools 45
sciatica 604
scoliosis 265
Scotland, NHS 9
Scottish Health Council 9
screening
  abdominal aortic
    aneurysm 388
  antenatal 426–8, 427f
  bowel cancer 376
  cervical 380–5, 381t
  children 160–3
  mammography 378–9
  preconceptual 422
  programmes 362

seasonal influenza 720
  immunization 392
seborrhoeic dermatitis 684
seizures 740–2
self-care model 111
self-harm 494, 495b, 495–6, 823
Self-Management UK 340
separation anxiety 330
separation anxiety disorder 330
sepsis 826, 827b, 828b, 828
  palliative care 566
septic arthritis 265
service user experience 75
sex and relationship education 236–7
sex chromosome abnormalities 271
sex differences see gender
sex-linked disorders 272–3
sexual abuse 251
sexual assault 761
sexual health 760
  adults with learning disability 770–1
  confidentiality 760
  consultations 762–3
  health promotion 761
  partner notification 760
  physical examination 762
  referral to GUM clinics 763
  sexual history 762
  sexual problems 768–9
  STI testing 762
sexually transmitted infections 764–6
  testing for 762
sharp debridement 528
sharps injuries 108
sheltered housing 26
shingles 293t, 691, 721
shingles vaccination 393
short-acting beta-2 agonists 620
short-acting muscarinic antagonists 620
short stature 298
shoulder problems 734
sickle cell disorders 308–10
silicosis 752
silver dressings 534
simvastatin 649
single assessment processes 112
sinusitis 699
skin
  adolescent spots 229
  bacterial infections 680–1
  cancer 374–5, 682–3
  dermatitis 684–5

eczema 284–5, 684–5
fungal infections 686–7
new babies 178
pigmentation 692
psoriasis 688–9, 688t
viral infections 690–1
skin tunnelled long-term catheter 582–3
skull asymmetry 299
sleep
  adolescents 229
  babies 200–1, 200b
slipped capital femoral epiphysis 264
small for gestational age 190
SMART objectives 62
smoking cessation 356–7, 423
soap and water 99
social care
  assessment of need for 112
  night sitters 552
social change 335
social cohesion 338
social learning theory 334t
social prescribing 338
social services 30–1, 249
social support 24, 28
social work teams 31
sodium cromoglycate 621
solar UV index 375
solution-focused therapy 473
sore throat 288, 698–9
soya-based formula 186
spastic cerebral palsy 320
special educational needs 45, 242–4
specialist nurses 16
specialist palliative care 550, 552
special schools 45
specific learning difficulties 224
specific phobias 330–1
speech and language acquisition 218–19
speech and language therapists 21
spermicides 417
spider naevi 178
spina bifida 274–5
spina bifida occulta 274
spinal cord injury 518–19, 518t, 796
spinal problems 264–5
spiritual care 564
spirometry 606, 606t
spironolactone 649
sports 25, 226, 734

spots 229
sprains and strains 824, 824b
squamous cell carcinoma 374, 683
stages of change model 334t
stakeholder management 62
stammering 225
standardized assessment tools 118
Staphylococcus aureus 722, 732t
  methicillin-resistant (MRSA) 722–3
staple removal 524–5
stasis eczema 684
statement of special educational needs 45
statins 649
status epilepticus 740
statutory maternity pay 430
Stemmer's sign 548
step-down schemes 23
sterilization surgery 418–19
sticky eyes 179
stoma care 516–17, 588, 596
stork marks 178
strawberry marks 178
stress incontinence 504
stress management 358–9
stroke 830, 830b
students, duty of care 83
subconjunctival haemorrhage 747
subcutaneous injections 577–8
substance use 476, 477t
subtotal hysterectomy 782
suctioning 587
sudden infant death syndrome 177, 278–9
suicide 494–6
  assisted 572–3
  risk 487
sunbeds 374
sunlamps 374
sunscreen 374–5
superficial spreading basal cell carcinoma 683
superficial spreading malignant melanoma 682
superior vena cava obstruction 566
supplementary prescribers 128
supported housing 26
suprapubic catheters 508–9

Sure Start maternity grants 431
surgical debridement 528
sustainability and transformation partnerships 13t
sweat glands 229
sympathomimetic agents 620
syphilis 765–6
syringe drivers 570
systemic lupus erythematosus 739

T

tachycardia 640
talipes 264
talking therapies 472–3
tall stature 298
tamoxifen 774
tar burns 817
teaching in primary care 54–5
team formulation theory 58–9
team roles theory 59
teamwork 58–9
teenagers 232–3
  see also adolescents
teething 196
telehealth and telecare 832
telephone consultations and triage 124–5
temper tantrums 217
temporal lobe epilepsy 740
tennis elbow 735
terminal care 550
termination of pregnancy 788–9
testes
  self-examination 386
  undescended 262
testicular cancer 386
tetanus vaccination 399
thalassaemia 312
thelarche 299
thiomersal 164
threadworm 293t, 295
throat soreness 288, 698–9
thrombophlebitis 656–7
thrush 687, 786
thyroid disorders 702–3
thyroxine 702
ticagrelor 647
tick-borne encephalitis vaccination 399
tinea 293t, 686
tinea capitis 686
tinea corporis 686
tinea cruris 686
tinea manium 686

tinea pedis 686
tinea unguium 686
tinnitus 696
toe nail, ingrowing 736
toilet training 214
tonsillitis 288, 698–9
tooth care 196–7, 196b, 226
torticollis 265, 734
total cholesterol 632
total hysterectomy (with salpingo-oophorectomy) 782
total incontinence 504
totally implanted venous access device 582
toxic nodular goitre 702
toxic shock syndrome 778
toxoplasmosis 262, 423
tracheostomy 586–9
training
  advanced nurse practitioners 41
  district nurses 51
  health visitors 47
  practice nurses 41
  school nurses 43
transient ischaemic attack 830
transition of young people to adult services 468
travel, safety issues 95
travel health 394
  health insurance 397
  health promotion 396–7
  vaccinations 399
travellers 448–9
traveller's diarrhoea 397
triage 124
trichomonas vaginalis 766
triglyceride 632
triiodothyronine 702
tuberculosis 293t, 728–9
Tuckman's team formulation theory 58–9
tunnelled long-term catheter 582–3
Turner's syndrome 271
twin and multiple births 180
type 1 diabetes 660, 664–6
type 2 diabetes 660–1, 666–7
typhoid 293t
typhoid vaccination 399

U

UK Clinical Research Network 56
UK health profile 2
ulcerated squamous cell carcinoma 683

ulcerative colitis 712–13, 712b
ulipristal acetate 420–1
umbilical hernia 178, 717
umbilicus 178
UN Convention on the Rights of the Child (1989) 24
underweight 223
undescended testes 262
Universal Plus 47
unplanned hospital admission 22
upper respiratory tract infections 288
urge incontinence 504
urinary catheters 508–10
urinary incontinence 504–7
  bladder training 506, 506b
  mixed incontinence 504
  overflow incontinence 504
  pelvic floor exercises 506, 506b
  stress incontinence 504
  total incontinence 504
  urge incontinence 504
urinary tract infection 289, 756
  catheter-associated 510
urostomy 517
urticaria 178
uterine cancer 776
uterine prolapse 781

V

vaginal cancer 776
vaginal diaphragms and caps 416–17, 416f
vaginal discharge 786
vaginal dryness 365
vaginal ring pessaries 781
vaginismus 768
varicella zoster see chickenpox
varicose eczema 684
varicose veins 656
varicosities 432
vegan/vegetarian diets 212, 234, 343
venepuncture 580–1
venous eczema 684
venous hypertension 540
venous leg ulcer 537t, 540–4
ventouse 436
verapamil 648
verbal consent 82
vernix 178
verrucae 293t, 690
very low birthweight 190

veterans 502
Vibrio cholera 732*t*
Vibrio parahaemolyticus 732*t*
vicarious liability 83
victim support 452–3
viral hepatitis see hepatitis A; hepatitis B; hepatitis C; hepatitis E
viral infections 690–1, 720–1
virtual wards 23
vision screening 162
visual acuity 162
visual analogue scales 554
vitamin B12 deficiency 652–3
vitamins 343
vitamin supplements 189
vitiligo 692
vomiting
  children 282–3
  palliative care 558, 559*t*
  pregnancy 432
vulnerable adolescents 229, 233
vulnerable adults
  abuse 454–5, 454*b*
  social services 30–1
vulnerable children 165
vulval cancer 777
vulval dystrophy 787
vulval intraepithelial neoplasia 787
vulval itching 787
vulval skin changes 787
vulval swelling 787
vulvodynia 768

W

waist circumference 342
Wales, NHS 9

walk-in centres 16
warfarin 642–3
War Pension Exemption Certificate 134
warts 293*t*, 690
  genital 764
washing hands 99
wasp sting allergy 695
waste management 106–7, 106*t*
Waterlow Score Card 118
weaning 188–9
weather extremes 370–1, 370*b*
weight
  management 348–51
welfare benefits 430–1
wet combing 294
wet wrapping 285
wheelchairs 835
whiplash 734
whistleblowing 85
WHO
  pain relief ladder 555*f*
  primary care vision 4*b*
Whooley Questions for Depression 118
whooping cough 291*t*, 293*t*
Wilms' tumour 315
working parents 24
Working Together to Safeguard Children–England 248
workload profiling 65–6
wounds
  assessment 522–3
  cleansing 524
  closure 524
  debridement 528–9, 541
  dressings 524, 532–5
  healing phases 532

healing by primary intention 524
healing by secondary intention 524
infected 526–7
malignant
  fungating 530–1
post-operative care 524–5
staple removal 524–5
wrist problems 735
written consent 82
written information 121
written prescriptions 137
wry neck 265

X

xanthines 620

Y

yeast infections 686, 687
yellow fever vaccination 399
young carers 459
young people
  assessment 156–7, 156*f*
  deliberate self-harm 194
  learning disabilities 456–7
  in need 158–9
  retention of records 87
  sepsis 828*b*
  services for 24–5
  social services 30
  transition to adult services 468
  see also adolescents; children
youth offending team 25